Anatomy

An Essential Textbook

Second Edition

Anne M. Gilroy, MA
Associate Professor
Department of Radiology
University of Massachusetts Medical School
Worcester, Massachusetts

Illustrations by
Markus Voll
Karl Wesker

650 illustrations

Thieme
New York • Stuttgart • Delhi • Rio de Janeiro

Thieme Medical Publishers, Inc.
333 Seventh Ave.
New York, NY 10001

Vice President and Editorial Director,
    Educational Products: Anne M. Sydor
Development Editor: Julie Montalbano
Production Editor: Barbara Chernow
Director, Editorial Services: Mary Jo Casey
International Production Director: Andreas Schabert
International Marketing Director: Fiona Henderson
International Sales Director: Louisa Turrell
Director of Sales, North America: Mike Roseman
Senior Vice President and Chief Operating Officer:
    Sarah Vanderbilt
President: Brian D. Scanlan
Compositor: Carol Pierson, Chernow Editorial Services, Inc.
Printer: Replika Press Ltd.
Illustrations: Markus Voll and Karl Wesker

Library of Congress Cataloging-in-Publication Data

Names: Gilroy, Anne M., author. | Voll, Markus M., illustrator. |
    Wesker, Karl, illustrator.
Title: Anatomy : an essential textbook / Anne M. Gilroy ;
    illustrations by Markus Voll, Karl Wesker.
Description: Second edition. | New York : Thieme, [2017] |
    Includes index.
Identifiers: LCCN 2017006504 (print) | LCCN 2017008004
    (ebook) | ISBN 9781626234390 (alk. paper) | ISBN
    9781626234406
Subjects: | MESH: Anatomy | Examination Questions | Atlases
Classification: LCC QM23.2 (print) | LCC QM23.2 (ebook) | NLM
    QS 18.2 | DDC 612.0076—dc23
LC record available at https://lccn.loc.gov/2017006504

Important note: Medicine is an ever-changing science undergoing continual development. Research and clinical experience are continually expanding our knowledge, in particular our knowledge of proper treatment and drug therapy. Insofar as this book mentions any dosage or application, readers may rest assured that the authors, editors, and publishers have made every effort to ensure that such references are in accordance with **the state of knowledge at the time of production of the book.**

Nevertheless, this does not involve, imply, or express any guarantee or responsibility on the part of the publishers in respect to any dosage instructions and forms of applications stated in the book. **Every user is requested to examine carefully** the manufacturers' leaflets accompanying each drug and to check, if necessary in consultation with a physician or specialist, whether the dosage schedules mentioned therein or the contraindications stated by the manufacturers differ from the statements made in the present book. Such examination is particularly important with drugs that are either rarely used or have been newly released on the market. Every dosage schedule or every form of application used is entirely at the user's own risk and responsibility. The authors and publishers request every user to report to the publishers any discrepancies or inaccuracies noticed. If errors in this work are found after publication, errata will be posted at www.thieme.com on the product description page.

Some of the product names, patents, and registered designs referred to in this book are in fact registered trademarks or proprietary names even though specific reference to this fact is not always made in the text. Therefore, the appearance of a name without designation as proprietary is not to be construed as a representation by the publisher that it is in the public domain.

To my mother, Mary Gilroy, a woman of courage and love;
To Colin and Bryan, my strength and sanity;
And once more, to my Dad.

Contents

Acknowledgements

Special thanks to authors Michael Schuenke, Erik Schulte, and Udo Schumacher of the award-winning three-volume *Thieme Atlas of Anatomy* and illustrators Markus Voll and Karl Wesker for their work over the course of many years

For their careful and thoughtful review of the manuscript, thanks to

Brian R. MacPherson, PhD
Department of Anatomy and Neurobiology
University of Kentucky School of Medicine
Lexington, Kentucky

Carmen E. Rexach, PhD
Department of Biological Sciences
Mount San Antonio College
Walnut, California

For their contributions to the problems sets, thanks to

Frank J. Daly, PhD
Department of Biomedical Sciences
University of New England
School of Osteopathic Medicine
Biddeford, Maine

Geoffrey Guttman, PhD
Department of Cell Biology and Anatomy
University of North Texas Health Science Center
Texas College of Osteopathic Medicine
Fort Worth, Texas

Contributor: Clinical Imaging Basics
Joseph Makris, MD
Department of Radiology
University of Massachusetts Medical School
Worcester, Massachusetts
Children's Diagnostic Imaging of Atlanta
Atlanta, Georgia

Krista S. Johansen, MD
Department of Biomedical Sciences
Edward Via Virginia College of Osteopathic Medicine
Blacksburg, Virginia

Center for Human Anatomy Education
Monash University
Melbourne, Victoria, Australia

Preface to the Second Edition

In the four years since the release of the 1st edition of *Anatomy – An Essential Textbook,* I have been both relieved and encouraged by the enthusiastic response from students. In that first volume, we offered a somewhat unique and untested format that combined systemic and regional approaches that were presented via prioritized bulleted explanations. We integrated this with summary tables, clinical correlations, and stunning Thieme illustrations to create a learning tool that students from a wide diversity of anatomy programs have embraced.

The challenge of undertaking a 2nd edition was equally humbling and exciting. I was eager for the opportunity to respond to student feedback and did so by enhancing some sections through additional images and clinical applications, and revising or expanding text and adding summary tables in sections that needed clarity. I also wanted to push the boundaries of innovation just a little further by including more clinical images and updating concepts, correlations and perspectives in ways we hadn't considered in the first edition. Finally, it was important to address the myriad of errors and omissions that linger, here and in every publication, despite the efforts of a meticulous editorial team. One hopes, then, that the content of a 2nd edition is a more complete, current, and accurate depiction of what anatomy educators believe to be essential. For students, a new edition should offer a user-friendly organization and presentation, one that's formulated with insight into modern learning practices. Hopefully, this newest effort will be an even more useful guide for them as they negotiate the complex and often overwhelming universe of anatomic study.

Despite many additions, this new text follows the general scheme of the 1st edition. The introductory chapter covers basic concepts and a summary of anatomical systems. Regional units begin with an overview of systems followed by chapters that focus on organ and functional anatomy. Readers will notice increased content in the first chapter with more detailed explanations, particularly relating to the vascular and nervous systems. There's also some minor reorganization of later chapters that attempt to better represent the flow of content in most anatomy curricula (e.g., the pharynx has been moved out of the neck section and into the chapter on the deep regions of the head). All sections are generously populated with an additional 25 tables (totaling 120) and an expanded library of 650 images.

One of the most interesting changes for this edition is the introduction of illustrated clinical correlations. Now, many of the 175 clinical and developmental correlates are coordinated with new pathological or procedural images and schematics. New "Note" boxes that provide detailed information on singular topics (e.g., functional aspects of the circulatory system) also appear throughout the text.

The most dramatic addition to this 2nd edition is the inclusion of radiographic material. At Thieme, we recognize that radiology has infiltrated every aspect of medicine from diagnosis to treatment. Physicians who lack the ability to utilize this resource are severely disadvantaged in today's clinical world. As medical educators, few of us are qualified to teach clinical radiology, but as anatomists it is our responsibility to expose our students to the radiographic representation of anatomic structure. Therefore, we have made an effort in this edition to add radiographs wherever appropriate. We also created a new section in each unit called *Clinical Imaging Basics.* Included in these is a discussion of the usefulness of different imaging modalities in that particular anatomic region, sample images that demonstrate important structures and relationships, and tips on examining and interpreting those images.

Many dedicated hands have touched this manuscript over the last year and I owe thanks to the entire Thieme team for their support and expertise. My sincere thanks goes to Julie Montalbano, my Developmental Editor, who has been a key asset in this project. Her dogged sense of organization saved me from the chaos that usually accompanies such endeavors. I appreciated her open response to new ideas and relied on her encouragement more than she knows. Thank you also to Torsten Scheihagen, Managing Editor, who interpreted and transcribed the long list of additions, deletions, and revisions that belong to this new edition. Finally, thank you to Barbara Chernow, Production Editor, and her excellent team. I recognize that this was a challenging volume to format and I appreciate their diligence and persistence in attending to every detail.

My colleague Dr. Joseph Makris, a radiologist and medical educator, was largely responsible for the new *Clinical Imaging Basics* sections. It's been a delight and privilege to work with him and I look forward to more collaborations. As in the 1st edition, I've drawn extensively from the most recent edition of the *Atlas of Anatomy* (Gilroy, MacPherson 2016, 3rd ed.) and I'm particularly grateful to my coauthor, Dr. Brian MacPherson. Many of the expanded explanations and imagery for the head and neck unit were based on his outstanding work in the atlas. The *Thieme Atlas of Anatomy* 3-volume set was an essential source for that atlas, as well as for this text, and I'm deeply indebted to authors Michael Schuenke, Erik Schulte, and Udo Schumacher and the illustrators Markus Voll and Karl Wesker. Their innovative perspectives and outstanding talent continue to inspire me and greatly influence my work as an educator and an author. Finally, thanks to all of colleagues and students who provided the feedback that initiated the revisions contained here. My humble hope is that this new edition meets, and perhaps exceeds, their expectations.

Anne M. Gilroy
Worcester, Massachusetts

Unit I Introduction to Anatomic Systems and Terminology

1 Introduction to Anatomic Systems and Terminology

Anatomy of the human body can be studied by inspection of all the systems that occupy a specific region or by considering the global aspects of a particular system throughout the entire body. The first approach tends to focus on anatomic relationships while the second is better suited to studying physiologic influences. Most systems, however, are conveniently confined to one or two regions, and in this text are discussed in the units devoted to those regions. Some systems, however, (those included in this chapter) are more pervasive throughout the body, and a fundamental understanding of their basic organization is important before undertaking the study of the systems they support.

1.1 Structural Design of the Human Body

The most preliminary inspection of the human body reveals that it is structurally divided into a head and neck region, a trunk, and paired upper and lower extremities (limbs). Each is further divided into smaller regions (**Fig. 1.1; Table 1.1**). These house the

structures that make up the functional organ systems that perform the basic bodily functions (**Table 1.2**). Although the primary organ of a system is often confined to a single anatomic region (e.g., the brains resides in the head), systems extend beyond regional borders, both anatomically and physiologically, to integrate their influences on normal function and growth.

Table 1.1 **Regional Subdivisions of the Body**

Head
Neck
Trunk
• Thorax (chest)
• Abdomen
• Pelvis
Upper limb
• Shoulder girdle
• Free upper limb
Lower limb
• Pelvic girdle
• Free lower limb

Table 1.2 **Functional Subdivisions by Organ Systems**

Locomotor system (musculoskeletal system)
• Skeleton and skeletal connections (passive part)
• Striated skeletal musculature (active part)
Viscera
• Cardiovascular system
• Hemolymphatic system
• Endocrine system
• Respiratory system
• Digestive system
• Urinary system
• Male and female reproductive system
Nervous system
• Central and peripheral nervous system
• Sensory organs
The skin and its appendages

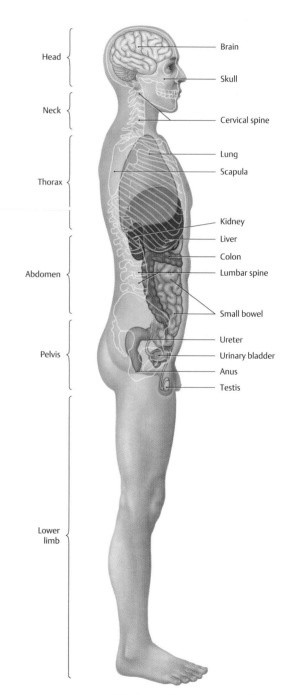

Fig. 1.1 **Structural design of the human body: location of the internal organs.**

Head — Brain
— Skull
Neck — Cervical spine
Thorax — Lung
— Scapula
Abdomen — Kidney
— Liver
— Colon
— Lumbar spine
— Small bowel
Pelvis — Ureter
— Urinary bladder
— Anus
— Testis
Lower limb

1.2 Terms of Location and Direction, Cardinal Planes, and Axes

— All locational and directional terms used in anatomy, and in medical practice, refer to the human body in the **anatomic position,** in which the body is upright, arms at the side, with the eyes, palms of the hands, and feet directed forward (**Fig. 1.2, Table 1.3**).

— Three perpendicular cardinal planes and three axes based on the three spatial coordinates can be drawn through the body (**Fig. 1.3**).

- The **sagittal plane** passes through the body from front to back, dividing it into right and left sides.
- The **coronal plane** passes through the body from side to side, dividing it into front (anterior) and back (posterior) parts.

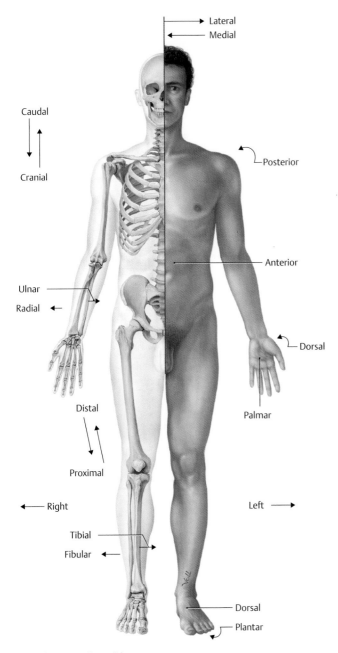

Fig. 1.2 Anatomic position
Anterior view.

Table 1.3 **General Terms of Location and Direction**

Term	Explanation
Upper Body (Head, Neck, and Trunk)	
Cranial	Pertaining to, or located toward, the head
Caudal	Pertaining to, or located toward, the tail
Anterior	Pertaining to, or located toward, the front; synonym: ventral (used for all animals)
Posterior	Pertaining to, or located toward, the back; synonym: dorsal (used for all animals)
Superior	Upper or above
Inferior	Lower or below
Axial	Pertaining to the axis of a structure
Transverse	Situated at right angles to the long axis of a structure
Longitudinal	Parallel to the long axis of a structure
Horizontal	Parallel to the plane of the horizon
Vertical	Perpendicular to the plane of the horizon
Medial	Toward the median plane
Lateral	Away from the median plane (toward the side)
Median	Situated in the median plane or midline
Peripheral	Situated away from the center
Superficial	Situated near the surface
Deep	Situated deep beneath the surface
External	Outer or lateral
Internal	Inner or medial
Apical	Pertaining to the top or apex
Basal	Pertaining to the bottom or base
Sagittal	Situated parallel to the sagittal suture
Coronal	Situated parallel to the coronal suture (pertaining to the crown of the head)
Limbs	
Proximal	Close to, or toward, the trunk, or toward the point of origin
Distal	Away from the trunk (toward the end of the limb), or away from the point of origin
Radial	Pertaining to the radius or the lateral side of the forearm
Ulnar	Pertaining to the ulna or the medial side of the forearm
Tibial	Pertaining to the tibia or the medial side of the leg
Fibular	Pertaining to the fibula or the lateral side of the leg
Palmar (volar)	Pertaining to the palm of the hand
Plantar	Pertaining to the sole of the foot
Dorsal	Pertaining to the back of the hand or top of the foot

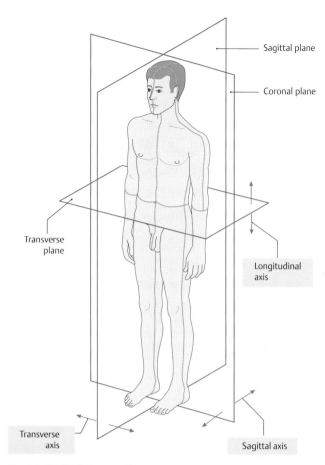

Fig. 1.3 Cardinal planes and axes
Neutral position, left anterolateral view.

1.3 Landmarks and Reference Lines

— In surface anatomy, palpable structures or visible markings on the surface of the body are used to identify the location of underlying structures. **Reference lines** are vertical or transverse planes that connect palpable structures or markings (**Tables 1.4, 1.5,** and **1.6;** see also **Fig. 1.5**).

A Anterior view.

B Right lateral view.

Table 1.4 **Anterior and Lateral Reference Lines on Trunk**

Anterior midline	Passes through the center of the sternum
Sternal line	Passes along the lateral border of the sternum
Midclavicular line	Passes through the midpoint of the clavicle
Parasternal line	Passes through a point midway between the sternal and midclavicular lines
Anterior axillary line	Marks the anterior axillary fold formed by the pectoralis major muscle
Posterior axillary line	Marks the posterior axillary fold formed by the teres major muscle
Midaxillary line	Marks the midpoint between the anterior and posterior axillary lines

- The **transverse** (axial, horizontal, cross-sectional) **plane** divides the body into upper and lower parts. A particular transverse section is often given the designation of the corresponding vertebral level, such as *T4,* which passes through the fourth thoracic vertebra.
- The **longitudinal axis** passes along the height of the body in a craniocaudal direction.
- The **sagittal axis** passes from the front to the back (or the back to the front) of the body in an anteroposterior direction.
- The **transverse** (horizontal) **axis** passes through the body from side to side.

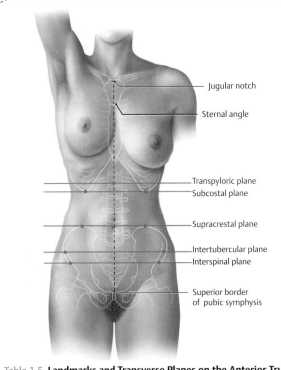

Table 1.5 **Landmarks and Transverse Planes on the Anterior Trunk**

Jugular notch	Marks the superior border of the manubrium
Sternal angle	Marks the junction of manubrium and body of the sternum
Transpyloric plane	Passes through the midpoint between the jugular notch and pubic symphysis
Subcostal plane	Marks the lowest level of the thoracic cage, the tenth costal cartilage
Supracrestal plane	Connects the top of the iliac crests
Intertubercular plane	Passes through the iliac tubercles
Interspinal plane	Connects the anterior superior iliac crests

Table 1.6 **Vertebral Spinous Processes and Posterior Landmarks**

C7	The vertebra prominens
T3	Level of the medial edge of spines of the scapulae
T7	Level of the inferior angles of the scapulae
T12	Level of the lower limit of the thoracic cavity
L4	Level of the iliac crests
S2	Level of the posterior superior iliac spine

1.4 The Integumentary System

The skin (integument), the largest organ of the body, protects underlying tissue from biologic, mechanical, and chemical injury; regulates body temperature; and participates in metabolic processes, such as the synthesis of vitamin D.

— The skin is composed of
- an outer waterproof avascular layer, the **epidermis,** which has a superficial layer of keratinized cells that shed continuously and a deep basal layer of regenerating cells, and
- an inner richly vascularized and innervated layer, the **dermis,** which supports the epidermis and contains hair follicles.

1.5 Fascia

Fascia is a sheet of connective tissue that lies between the skin and underlying muscles and bone (**Fig. 1.4**).

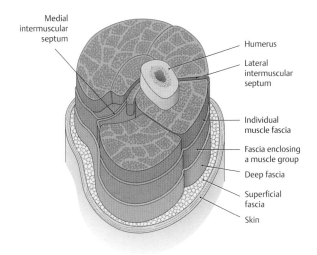

Fig. 1.4 **Fascia**
Cross section through the right arm, proximal view.

- **Superficial fascia,** a layer of varying thickness that lies deep to the skin, is composed of loose connective tissue and fat. Superficial nerves and vessels traverse this layer.
- **Deep fascia,** a dense connective tissue layer, lies under (deep to) the superficial fascia and is devoid of fat. It forms an investing layer, which envelops neurovascular structures and muscles of the limbs, trunk wall, head, and neck. Invaginations of the deep fascia of the limbs form **intermuscular septa** that separate limb musculature into functional groups (compartments).

1.6   The Skeletal System

The bones and cartilages of the body, which make up the skeletal system, provide leverage for muscles and protect the internal organs. Bone is also the site for calcium storage and blood cell production.

- There are two anatomic divisions of the skeleton (**Fig. 1.5**):
  - The **axial skeleton,** which consists of the skull, vertebrae, sacrum, coccyx, ribs, and sternum
  - The **appendicular skeleton,** which includes the clavicle and scapula of the pectoral girdle, the coxal bones of

Fig. 1.5 Human skeleton
Left forearm is pronated, and both feet are in plantarflexion.

the pelvic girdle, and the bones of the upper and lower limbs
— **Periosteum** is a thin layer of fibrous connective tissue that coats the outer surface of each bone **(Fig. 1.6)**. **Perichondrium** forms a similar layer around cartilaginous structures. These tissues nourish and assist in the healing of the underlying bone.
— All bones have a superficial layer of dense **compact** (cortical) **bone** that surrounds a less dense **cancellous** (spongy) **bone.** In some areas of the bone, a **medullary cavity** contains yellow (fatty) or red (blood cell or platelet-forming) **bone marrow.**

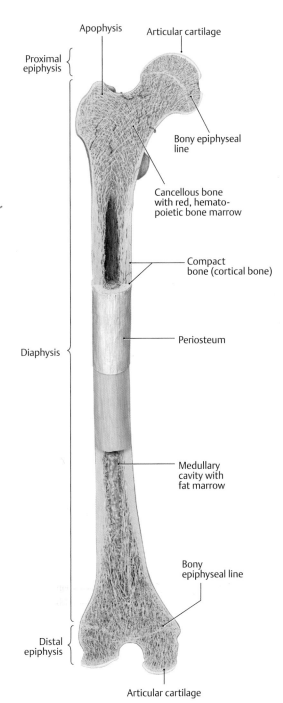

Fig. 1.6 Structure of a typical long bone
Illustrated for the femur. Coronal cuts through the proximal and distal parts of an adult femur.

— Bones develop from **mesenchyme** (embryonic connective tissue) through two processes of ossification (bone formation).
  • The clavicle and some bones of the skull develop by **membranous ossification,** in which the bones form through direct ossification of mesenchymal templates that are set down during the embryonic period.
  • Most bones, including the long bones of the limbs, develop by **endochondral ossification,** in which a cartilaginous template, formed from mesenchyme, is laid down during the fetal period. Over the first and second decades of life, bone replaces most of the cartilage.
    ○ Within each bone undergoing endochondral ossification, bone formation occurs first at a **primary ossification center,** which is in the **diaphysis** (shaft) of the long bones. **Secondary ossification centers** appear later at the **epiphyses** (growing ends) of the bones.
— Long bones of the skeleton increase in length through growth of the epiphyses and diaphysis on either side of the **epiphyseal plate,** an intervening cartilaginous area. During childhood and adolescence the epiphyseal plates gradually shorten as they are replaced by bone. In the adult these areas are completely ossified, and only thin **epiphyseal lines** remain.
— **Apophyses,** bony outgrowths that lack their own growth center, serve as attachment sites for ligaments or tendons. Specific apophyses are referred to as condyles, tubercles, spines, crests, trochanters, or processes.
— **Ligaments** are connective tissue bands that connect bones to each other or to cartilage. (Within the body cavities, the term *ligament* refers to folds or condensations of a serous or fibrous membrane that support visceral structures.)
— Joints are classified according to the type of tissue that connects the bones.
  • **Syndesmoses** (fibrous joints), such as those found in the sutures of the skull and interosseous membrane of the forearm, are united by fibrous tissue and allow minimal movement **(Fig. 1.7).**
  • **Synchondroses** (cartilaginous joints) are united either by fibrocartilaginous segments, such as the costal cartilages of the ribs, intervertebral disks, and pubic symphysis **(Fig. 1.8A,B)**, or by articular cartilage, often found in temporary

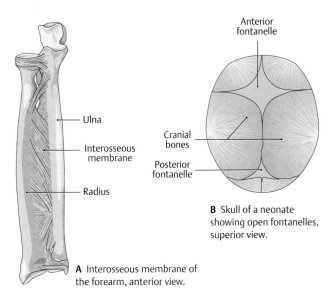

A Interosseous membrane of the forearm, anterior view.

B Skull of a neonate showing open fontanelles, superior view.

Fig. 1.7 Syndesmoses

A Costal cartilages.

B Pubic symphysis and intervertebral disks.

C Hip bone before closure of the growth plates.

Fig. 1.8 Synchondroses

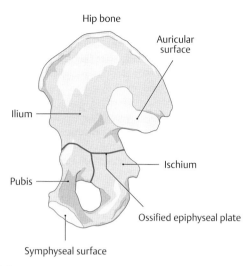

Fig. 1.9 Synostoses
Hip bone (fusion of the ischium, ilium, and pubis).

joints, such as those that join the ilium, ischium, and pubis of the hip bone (**Fig. 1.8C**). Subsequent fusion of these temporary joints creates **synostoses** (sites of bony fusion) (**Fig. 1.9**).

• **Synovial joints,** the most common type of joint, allow free movement (**Fig. 1.10**) and typically have
  ◦ a **joint cavity** that is enclosed by a fibrous **joint capsule** and lined by a **synovial membrane,** which secretes a thin film of lubricating **synovial fluid;**
  ◦ articulating ends of the bones that are covered by articular (hyaline) cartilage; and
  ◦ extrinsic ligaments on the outer surface, which reinforce the joints.
  ◦ Some synovial joints also contain intrinsic ligaments and intra-articular fibrocartilaginous structures.
— **Bursae** are closed sacs that contain a thin film of fluid and are lined with a synovial membrane. Commonly found around joints of the limbs, bursae cushion prominent bony processes from external pressure and prevent friction where tendons cross bony surfaces.

EXTRA-ARTICULAR AND INTRA-ARTICULAR STRUCTURES OF SYNO-VIAL JOINTS (SEE FIG. 1.10) The joint capsule of a synovial joint is composed of an outer fibrous membrane and an inner synovial membrane. The intima (innermost lining) of the synovial membrane produces the synovial fluid, which lubricates and nourishes intra-articular structures.

— Ligaments of synovial joints act as primary joint stabilizers. They may be:
  • Extra-capsular (e.g., fibular collateral ligament of the knee), which lie outside the fibrous capsule.
  • Intra-capsular, which run either with the fibrous membrane (e.g., medial collateral ligament of the knee) or between the fibrous and synovial membranes (e.g., cruciate ligaments).
— Menisci, articular disks, and articular labra are intra-articular structures composed of connective tissue and fibrocartilage:
  • Menisci are crescent-shaped structures found in the knee joint. They act as shock absorbers and modify the incongruity of the articulating surfaces.
  • Articular disks divide joints into separate chambers and are found in the sternoclavicular and proximal wrist joints.
  • Articular labra are wedge-shaped structures that line the glenoid of the scapula and acetabulum of the coxal (hip) bone, thus enlarging the articular surfaces of the shoulder and hip joints.

A Schematic.

B Intracapsular structures of the knee joint.

Fig. 1.10 **Structure of a synovial joint**

1.7   The Muscular System

The muscular system is composed of muscles and their tendons, which produce movement through contraction of muscle cells.

— **Muscle cells** are the structural units of the muscular system. Connective tissue binds muscle cells (fibers) together to form bundles, which in turn are bound together to form muscles (**Fig. 1.11**).

— A **motor unit** is the functional unit of muscles and describes the group of muscle fibers innervated by a single motor neuron. Motor units are relatively small in muscles that perform fine movements but larger in muscles that are responsible for maintaining posture or performing gross movements.

— Muscles function through tensing and contraction of the muscle fibers, which provide movement and stability

  • **Phasic contractions** can change the length of the muscle through shortening (**concentric contractions**), or lengthening (**eccentric contractions**), or simply increasing the muscle tension (**isometric contractions**).

  • **Tonic contractions** contribute to stability of joints and position but do not provide any movements.

  • **Reflexive contractions** are involuntary and are responsive to muscle stretch.

— Muscle tissue is classified by location (somatic or visceral), appearance (striated or nonstriated), and innervation (voluntary or involuntary).

— **Somatic**, or **skeletal muscles**, the most prevalent type, are found in the neck, trunk wall, and limbs, where they move and support the skeleton (**Fig. 1.12**). They are multinucleated, striated, and voluntary.

  • Somatic muscle fibers are interwoven with three sheaths of connective tissue including the **endomysium**, the innermost sheath, which surrounds and condenses muscle fibers into primary bundles; the **perimysium,** which surrounds and condenses primary bundles into secondary bundles; and the **epimysium**, a loose connective tissue layer that surrounds the muscle and lies deep to the muscle fascia.

  • **Muscle fascia** is the tough connective tissue sheath that encloses the muscle, maintains its shape, and allows frictionless movement between muscles and muscle groups.

  • **Tendons**, dense fibrous bands, connect muscles to their bony attachments. **Aponeuroses** are tendons that form flat

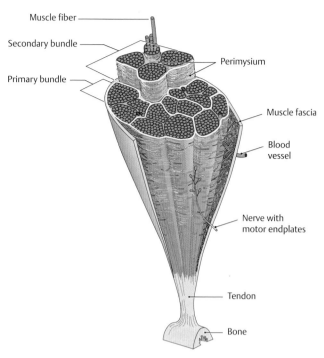

Fig. 1.11 Structure of a skeletal muscle
Cross section through a skeletal muscle.

Muscle fiber

Secondary bundle

Primary bundle

Perimysium

Muscle fascia

Blood vessel

Nerve with motor endplates

Tendon

Bone

sheets, which attach the muscle to the skeleton, other muscles, or organs.

  • Muscles shapes are described according to the arrangement of the muscle fibers as pennate (uni-, bi-, multi-), fusiform, circular, convergent, or parallel.

  • **Tendon (synovial) sheaths**, such as those found in the wrist and ankle, facilitate the movement of tendons over bone. Similar to a synovial joint capsule, they are composed of an outer fibrous membrane lined with a two-layered synovial membrane. The space between the synovial layers is filled with synovial fluid.

— **Visceral muscles,** considered involuntary**,** alter the shape of internal structures, such as the heart and gastrointestinal tract. There are two types:

  • **Cardiac muscle**, which makes up the thick muscular layer (myocardium) of the heart, is striated.

  • **Smooth muscle,** which found in the walls of blood vessels and hollow internal organs, is nonstriated.

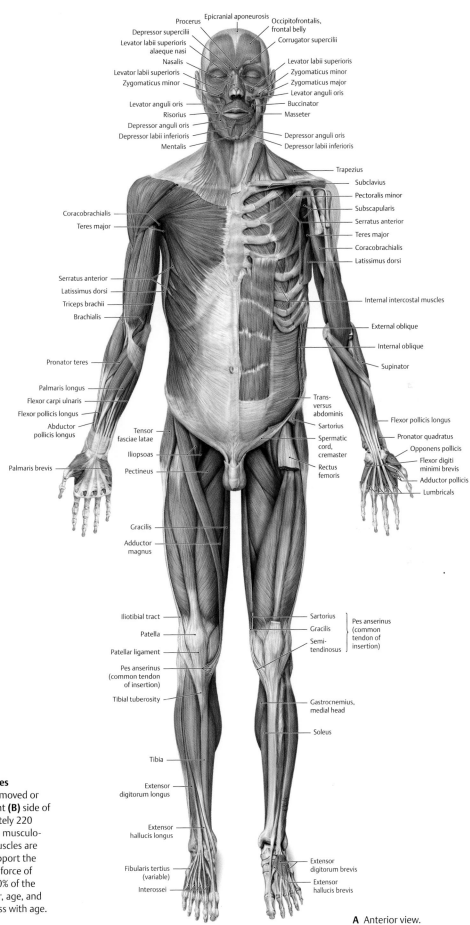

Fig. 1.12 Overview of skeletal muscles
Some superficial muscles have been removed or windowed on both the left **(A)** and right **(B)** side of the body. Skeletal muscles (approximately 220 individual muscles) make up the active musculoskeletal system. Two thirds of these muscles are found in the lower limb where they support the upright stance of the body against the force of gravity. They make up an average of 40% of the total body weight (varying with gender, age, and physical condition) but decrease in mass with age. (*continued on page 12*)

A Anterior view.

Sternocleidomastoid

Thoracolumbar fascia
(= deep layer of
nuchal fascia)

Scapular spine

Teres major

Thoracolumbar fascia,
superficial layer

Aponeurosis of origin of
latissimus dorsi

Brachioradialis

Extensor carpi radialis brevis

Anconeus

Extensor carpi ulnaris

Flexor carpi ulnaris

Abductor pollicis longus

Extensor pollicis brevis

Second dorsal
interosseus

Third dorsal
interosseus

Iliac
crest

Extensor
digiti minimi

Tensor
fasciae latae

Abductor digiti
minimi

Fourth dorsal
interosseus

Adductor
magnus

Gracilis

Semimembranosus

Popliteal fossa

Plantaris

Semispinalis capitis

Splenius cervicis

Rhomboid minor

Clavicle

Acromion

Scapula, medial border

Serratus anterior

Latissimus dorsi

Extensor carpi radialis longus

Extensor carpi radialis brevis

Supinator

Flexor digitorum profundus

Brachioradialis

Extensor pollicis brevis

Abductor
digiti minimi

Dorsal
interossei

Tensor
fasciae latae

Gemellus
superior

Gemellus
inferior

Obturator
internus

Quadratus
femoris

Adductor
magnus

Semitendinosus

Biceps femoris,
long head

Plantaris

Gastrocnemius

Fibularis
brevis

Fibularis
longus

B Posterior view.

Fig. 1.12 (*continued*) **Overview of skeletal muscles**

1.8 The Circulatory System

The heart and blood vessels, which make up the circulatory system (**Figs. 1.13** and **1.14**), transport blood to tissues of the body for the exchange of gases, waste products, and nutrients.

- The muscular heart provides the pumping action that maintains the flow of blood through the vessels.
- The blood vessels of the circulatory system (**Fig. 1.15**) are classified as follows:
  - **Arteries,** which transport blood away from the heart and branch into many smaller **arterioles**
  - **Veins,** which carry blood toward the heart and are formed by the convergence of many small **venules**

- ○ Many veins, particularly in the limbs, have multiple valves along their length to prevent backward flow due to gravity.
- ○ The veins are divided into **superficial veins,** which travel in the superficial fascia, and **deep veins,** which accompany the arteries. **Perforator veins** connect the superficial and deep venous circulations.
- ○ Veins are more numerous and more variable than arteries and often form venous plexuses (networks), which are named for the structure they surround (e.g., uterine venous plexus).
  - **Capillaries,** which form networks that intervene between the arteries and veins at the **terminal vascular beds,** where gas, nutrient, and waste exchange occurs

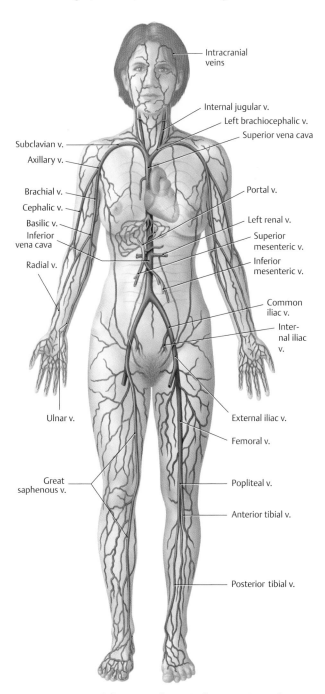

Fig. 1.13 Overview of the principal arteries in the systemic circulation
Anterior view.

Fig. 1.14 Overview of the principal veins in the systemic circulation
Anterior view. The portal circulation of the liver is shown in purple.

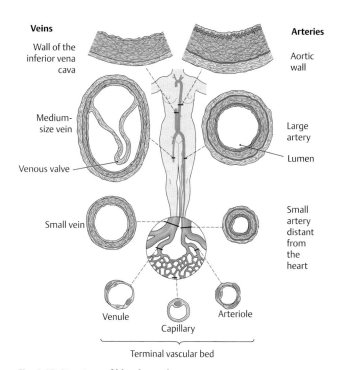

Fig. 1.15 **Structure of blood vessels**
Blood vessels in different regions of the systemic circulation, shown in cross section.

- **Sinusoids,** which are wide, thin-walled vessels that replace capillaries in some organs, such as the liver

NOTE

FUNCTIONAL ASPECTS OF THE CIRCULATORY SYSTEM Blood is transported through the circulatory system along a pressure gradient that is influenced by the size, number, and structure of the vessels through which it flows **(Fig. 1.16)**. Relatively high pressure is maintained in the arterial system. Large elastic type arteries can accommodate the intermittent volume ejected from the heart while more distal muscular arteries, through vasodilation (expansion) and vasoconstriction (contraction), can control vascular resistance and regulate local blood flow.

The venous system maintains a much lower pressure, and veins have comparatively thinner walls and larger diameters. They can accommodate up to 80% of the total blood volume and therefore serve an important reservoir function. Return of venous blood to the heart is aided by factors such as (a) venous valves that prevent backflow, (b) arteriovenous coupling that transmits the arterial pulse to accompanying veins, and (c) the pumping action of surrounding muscles **(Fig. 1.17)**.

Terminal vascular beds, formed by the extensive branching of capillaries, connect the arterial and venous circulations. These vascular networks are characterized by a large increase in cross-sectional area and a corresponding decrease in the flow velocity, which is necessary for the exchange process between the blood and interstitial fluid. Flow through these vascular beds can be regulated locally by contraction and relaxation of precapillary sphincters. Only one fourth to one third of capillary networks are perfused under normal resting conditions.

Fig. 1.16 **Pressure gradients in the circulatory system**
(*Note:* No distinction is made between the systemic and pulmonary systems in the diagram; Klinke R, Sibernagel S. Lehbuch der Phyiologic. 3rd ed. Stuttgart: Thieme; 2001.)

— The circulatory system has two circuits **(Fig. 1.18)**:
  1. The **pulmonary circulation** transports oxygen-poor blood from the right side of the heart to the lungs through **pulmonary arteries.** Oxygen-rich blood from the lungs flows back to the left side of the heart through **pulmonary veins.**
  2. The **systemic circulation** distributes oxygen-rich blood from the left side of the heart to body tissues through the systemic arteries (the **aorta** and its branches). Oxygen-poor blood returns to the heart through the systemic veins (the **superior** and **inferior venae cavae** and their tributaries—sometimes referred to as the **caval system—** and the coronary sinus).

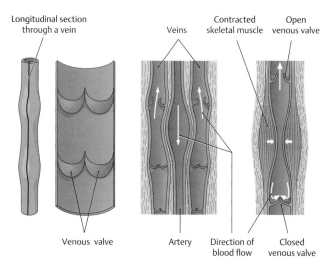

Fig. 1.17 **Venous return to the heart**

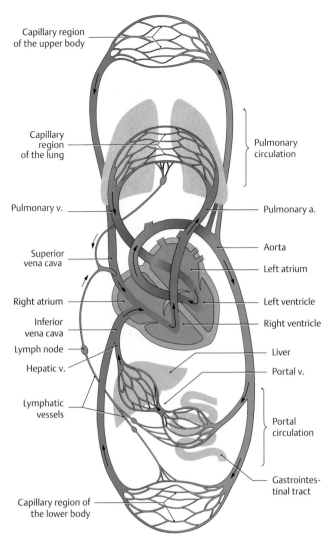

Fig. 1.18 Circulation
Schematic showing the pulmonary and systemic circulations. The portal circulation through the liver is part of the systemic circulation. Arteries are shown in red, veins in blue, and lymphatic vessels in green.

— A **portal circulation** is a route within the systemic circulation that diverts blood to a second capillary network before returning it to the systemic veins. The largest of these, the **portal system** in the liver, diverts blood from the gastrointestinal tract to the capillaries (sinusoids) in the liver before returning it to the systemic veins. A similar portal system is found in the pituitary gland.

— An **anastomosis,** a communication between blood vessels, allows blood to bypass its normal route and flow through an alternate, or collateral, route. Although blood volume through the anastomosis is usually minimal, it increases when the lumen of vessels along the normal route is obstructed.

— **End arteries** are vessels that lack anastomoses. Gradual narrowing of end arteries stimulates the formation of new vessels, but an abrupt obstruction of an end artery can cause necrosis (death) of the target tissue.

1.9 The Lymphatic System

The lymphatic system, which runs parallel to the circulatory system, consists of lymph, lymphatic vessels, and lymphoid organs.
— The lymphatic system performs the following functions:
  • Drains excess extracellular fluid from body tissues and returns it to veins of the systemic circulation
  • Mounts an immune response in the body
  • Transports fat and large protein molecules that cannot be taken up by venous capillaries
— Lymphoid organs and tissues that are part of the body's immune system include the thymus, bone marrow, spleen, lymph nodes, and tonsils. They also include bronchus-associated lymphatic tissue (BALT) in the airway and gut-associated lymphatic tissue (GALT), such as Peyer's patches and the vermiform appendix, within the gastrointestinal tract **(Fig. 1.19)**.
— **Lymph,** extracellular fluid that is extracted by lymph capillaries and transported by lymphatic vessels, is a clear, watery substance similar to blood plasma.
— The conducting vessels of the lymphatic system include
  • blind-ended **lymphatic capillaries** that begin in the tissues and drain to lymphatic vessels;
  • **lymphatic vessels,** which are interposed with lymph nodes along their length and drain to lymphatic trunks; and

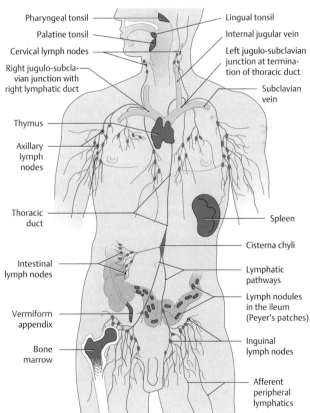

Fig. 1.19 Lymphatic system
The lymphatic system parallels the veins of the circulatory system and includes lymph nodes, lymphatic vessels, and lymphatic organs.

- • two major **lymphatic trunks,** the thoracic duct (left lymphatic trunk) and right lymphatic trunk, which drain into large veins of the neck.
- — The **thoracic duct** (left lymphatic duct), which arises from the **cisterna chyli** (chyle cistern), a dilated lymphatic vessel in the abdomen, is the larger of the two major lymphatic trunks. It drains lymph from the right and left lower quadrants and left upper quadrant of the body. The smaller **right lymphatic duct** drains only the right upper quadrant of the body **(Fig. 1.20)**.
- — Lymph carried by the thoracic duct and right lymphatic duct returns to the systemic venous circulation at the **left** and **right venous angles** (junction of the internal jugular and subclavian veins), also known as the jugulosubclavian junction, in the neck **(Fig. 1.21)**.

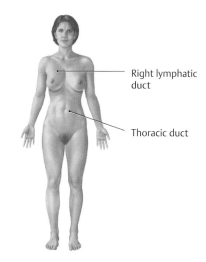

Fig. 1.20 Lymphatic drainage by body quadrants

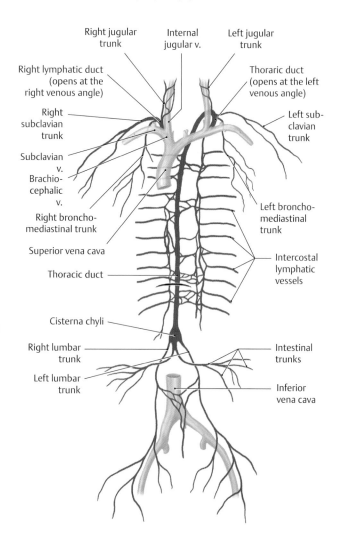

Fig. 1.21 Lymphatic pathways

Anterior view. The right lymphatic duct (~ 1 cm long) collects lymph from the right upper quadrant of the body and empties into the right venous angle at the junction of the right internal jugular vein with the right subclavian vein. Its major tributaries are

- — the right jugular trunk (right half of the head and neck),
- — the right subclavian trunk (right upper limb, right side of the chest and back wall), and
- — the right bronchomediastinal trunk (organs of the right thoracic cavity).

The thoracic duct is approximately 40 cm long and transports lymph from the entire lower half of the body and left upper quadrant. It empties into the left venous angle between the left internal jugular vein and left subclavian vein. Its main tributaries are

- — the left jugular trunk (left half of the head and neck),
- — the left subclavian trunk (left upper limb, left side of the chest and back wall),
- — the intestinal trunks (abdominal organs), and
- — the right and left lumbar trunks (right and left lower limb; pelvic viscera; right and left pelvic, abdominal, and back wall).

The intercostal lymphatic vessels transport lymph from the left and right intercostal spaces to the lymphatic duct.

1.10 The Nervous System

The nervous system receives, transmits, and integrates information throughout the body through the conduction of nerve impulses. This complex system can be classified according to many different criteria. Although these classifications are somewhat artificial, they are useful for understanding the numerous interconnections within the nervous systems **(Fig. 1.22)**.

— The nervous system has two major structural, or anatomic, divisions **(Fig. 1.23)**:
  - A **central nervous system** (CNS), which consists of the brain and spinal cord, where information about the body's internal and external environment is processed
  - A **peripheral nervous system** (PNS), which consists of 12 pairs of cranial nerves, 31 pairs of spinal nerves, and autonomic (visceral) nerves; peripheral nerves transmit information between the CNS and "target" organs and tissues in the rest of the body.

— The nervous system can also be divided into functional divisions **(Fig. 1.24)**. Both the CNS and PNS contain components of each functional division.
  - The **somatic nervous system** controls voluntary functions such as contraction of skeletal muscles.
  - The **autonomic** (visceral) **nervous system** controls involuntary functions such as gland secretion.

— **Nerve cells** or **neurons,** the functional unit of the nervous system found in the CNS and PNS, are specialized for conducting nerve impulses. They generate electrical signals, the action potential, and pass them on to other nerve or muscle cells. A variety of neurons can be described based on their appearance but the basic structure remains similar. The typical **neuron (Fig. 1.25A)** has
  - a **cell body** (soma). An aggregate of cell bodies in the CNS is a **nucleus;** an aggregate of cell bodies in the PNS is a **ganglion.**

- multiple short branching **dendrites**, which receive information from other neurons and transmit impulses toward the cell body.
- a single long **axon** or nerve fiber, which transmits impulses away from the cell body. Bundles of axons in the CNS form **tracts;** bundles of axons in the PNS form **nerves.**

— Neurons transmit electrical signals from cell to cell across junctions called **synapses**. At the synapse the electrical impulse of the **presynaptic** nerve fiber initiates the release of a chemical signal, or transmitter, which generates an electrical impulse in the receptor, or **postsynaptic** nerve cell **(Fig 1.25B)**.

— Neurons are classified by function as
  - **sensory** (afferent) **nerves**, which carry information regarding pain, temperature, and pressure to the central nervous system (CNS) from peripheral structures.
  - **motor** (efferent) **nerves**, which transmit impulses from the CNS that elicit responses from peripheral target organs.

— **Neuroglia**, or **glial** cells, the non-neuronal cellular components of the nervous system, act as supporting cells and perform a variety of metabolic functions. Glial cells are responsible for producing the **myelin sheath**, a lipid-rich layer that surrounds axons and increases the speed of impulse conduction **(Fig. 1.26)**. The myelin-producing cells in the PNS are called **Schwann cells** and in the CNS are called **oligodendrocytes**.

Fig. 1.23 **Topography of the nervous system**
Posterior view.

Labels: Brain, Spinal cord, Brachial plexus, Intervertebral foramina, Spinal ganglia, Spinal nerves, Lumbosacral plexus

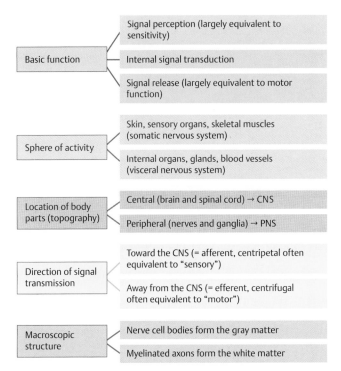

Basic function	Signal perception (largely equivalent to sensitivity)
	Internal signal transduction
	Signal release (largely equivalent to motor function)

| Sphere of activity | Skin, sensory organs, skeletal muscles (somatic nervous system) |
| | Internal organs, glands, blood vessels (visceral nervous system) |

| Location of body parts (topography) | Central (brain and spinal cord) → CNS |
| | Peripheral (nerves and ganglia) → PNS |

| Direction of signal transmission | Toward the CNS (= afferent, centripetal often equivalent to "sensory") |
| | Away from the CNS (= efferent, centrifugal often equivalent to "motor") |

| Macroscopic structure | Nerve cell bodies form the gray matter |
| | Myelinated axons form the white matter |

Fig 1.22 **Classification of the nervous system—overview**

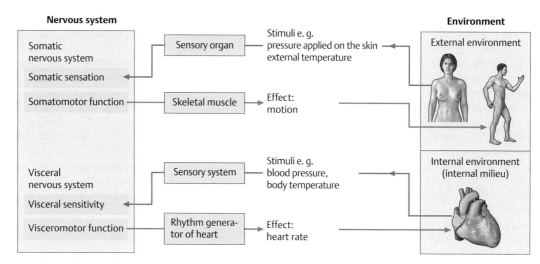

Fig. 1.24 **Functional classification of the nervous system**

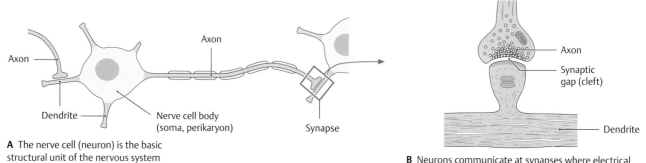

A The nerve cell (neuron) is the basic structural unit of the nervous system

Fig. 1.25 **Nerve cell and synapse**

B Neurons communicate at synapses where electrical signals initiate the release of neurotransmitters (chemical transmitters), which create an excitatory or inhibitory response at the target (postsynaptic) neuron.

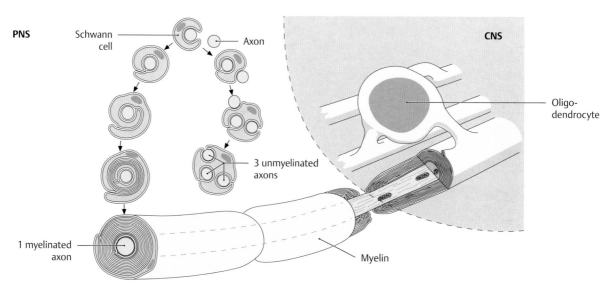

Fig. 1.26 **Glial cells in the CNS and PNS**
Glial cells form myelin sheaths around axons. This increases the speed with which impulses travel in the nervous system. In myelinated axons, multiple layers of glial membrane surround a single axon forming a distinct myelin sheath. In unmyelinated axons, a glial cell surrounds and supports multiple axons without forming a myelin sheath.

The Central Nervous System

The detailed anatomy of the central nervous system is most appropriately described in texts on neuroanatomy, and therefore is not included in this text. However, because an appreciation of its structure is essential to understanding the functioning of peripheral structures, a brief overview is included here, with further discussions to follow in Section 2.2 (spinal cord) and Section 18.2 (brain).

— The brain and spinal cord of the central nervous system (**Fig. 1.27**) consist of
  - **gray matter,** which contains the cell bodies, dendrites, and unmyelinated axons of neurons;
  - **white matter,** which contains the myelinated axons of neurons; and
  - neuroglial cells, which are abundant in both white and gray matter.

— The brain resides in the cranial cavity of the skull. Gray matter forms the cortex (outer layer) of the brain and surrounds the inner areas of white matter. Axonal tracts of the white matter link regions of the brain with each other and with the spinal cord.

— The brain (**Fig. 1.28**) is subdivided into
  - **cerebral hemispheres**
  - **diencephalon**
  - **cerebellum**
  - **brainstem**

— The bony vertebral column encloses the spinal cord. Gray matter in the spinal cord is located centrally and is surrounded by white matter tracts. The gray matter forms an H-shaped area that consists of bilateral
  - **anterior horns,** which contain motor neurons;
  - **posterior horns,** which contain sensory neurons;
  - **lateral horns** in the thoracic and upper lumbar region, which contain visceromotor neurons.

A Coronal section through the brain.

B Transverse section through the spinal cord.

Fig. 1.27 Gray and white matter in the central nervous system
Nerve cell bodies appear gray in gross inspection, whereas nerve cell processes (axons) and their insulating myelin sheaths appear white.

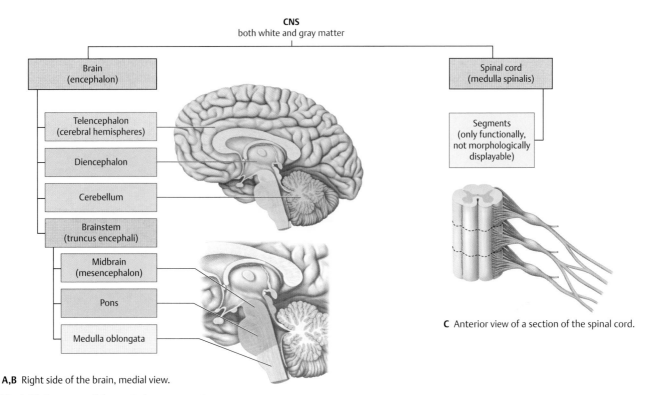

A,B Right side of the brain, medial view.

Fig. 1.28 Structure of the central nervous system

The Peripheral Nervous System

— The peripheral nervous system includes the peripheral parts of the autonomic and somatic divisions. Components of each system **(Fig. 1.29)** are found in

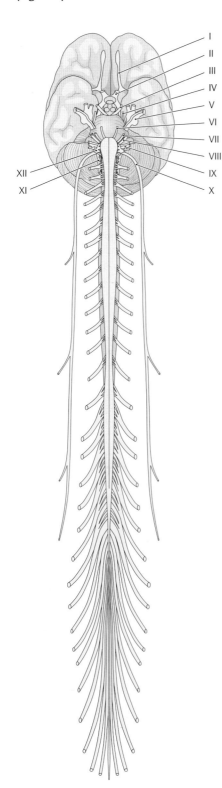

Fig. 1.29 Spinal nerves and cranial nerves
Anterior view. Thirty-one pairs of spinal nerves arise from the spinal cord in the peripheral nervous system, compared with 12 pairs of cranial nerves that arise from the brain. The cranial nerve pairs are traditionally designated by Roman numerals.

- 12 pairs of **cranial nerves** (traditionally designated, in order from cranial to caudal, by Roman numeral) that arise from the brain and primarily innervate structures of the head and neck. The **vagus nerve** (cranial nerve X) also innervates viscera of the thorax and abdomen.
- 31 pairs of **spinal nerves** that arise from the spinal cord and exit the vertebral column through **intervertebral foramina** (openings between vertebrae). Spinal nerves are named for the section of the spinal cord from which they arise (e.g., T4 is the fourth segment of the thoracic part of the spinal cord).

— Most nerves of the peripheral nervous system are **mixed nerves** that contain motor and sensory fibers **(Fig. 1.30)**.
- The combination of fiber types that are found in the somatic nervous system are:
  ○ **somatic sensory fibers,** which transmit the information from skin and skeletal muscles
  ○ **somatic motor fibers,** which innervate skeletal muscles
- Fiber types found in the autonomic nervous system are:
  ○ **visceral sensory fibers,** which transmit information from smooth muscle, cardiac muscle, and internal organs
  ○ **visceral motor fibers,** which innervate smooth muscle, cardiac muscle, and glands
- In addition to those named above, cranial nerves may also contain special fiber types that are associated with structures in the head:
  ○ **Special somatic sensory fibers,** which conduct information from the retina of the eye, and auditory and vestibular apparatus of the ear
  ○ **Special visceral sensory fibers,** which transmit information from the taste buds of the tongue and olfactory mucosa
  ○ **Special visceral motor,** which innervate skeletal muscles that originate from the branchial arches

— The somatic component of the nervous system transmits the motor output to, and sensory input from, structures over which we have voluntary and conscious control. (Consider a simple activity like walking, in which we have control over the movement of our legs and are aware of the pain elicited by an arthritic knee joint or a splinter in the sole of the foot.)

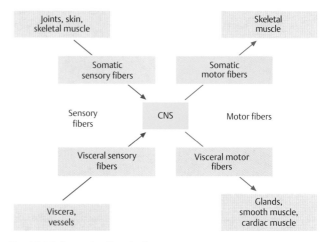

Fig. 1.30 Information flow in the nervous system
Fibers that carry information to the central nervous system (CNS) are called sensory or afferent fibers; fibers that carry signals away from the CNS are called motor or efferent fibers.

Table 1.7 **Effects of the Sympathetic and Parasympathetic Nervous Systems**

Organ	Sympathetic Nervous System	Parasympathetic Nervous System
Eye	Pupillary dilation	Pupillary constriction and increased curvature of the lens
Salivary glands	Decreased salivation (scant, viscous)	Increased salivation (copious, watery)
Heart	Elevation of the heart rate	Slowing of the heart rate
Lungs	Decreased bronchial secretions; bronchial dilation	Increased bronchial secretions; bronchial constriction
Gastrointestinal tract	Decreased secretions and motor activity	Increased secretions and motor activity
Pancreas	Decreased secretion from the endocrine part of the gland	Increased secretion
Male sex organs	Ejaculation	Erection
Skin	Vasoconstriction, sweat, secretion, piloerection	No parasympathetic innervation

— The autonomic component transmits the motor output to, and sensory input from, structures that function without conscious control. Its two divisions work to excite **(sympathetic)** or relax **(parasympathetic)** visceral responses based on internal and external stimuli **(Table 1.7)**. Together they work to maintain a stable (homeostatic) internal environment. (Consider the increase in heart rate when you have won the lottery and the crucial corresponding slowing of the heart rate when you need to sleep.)

— The somatic and autonomic nervous systems each have their own network of nerves that transmit information between the CNS and PNS. Although somatic and autonomic nerves may travel together, the nerve fibers remain anatomically and functionally distinct.

— Most cranial nerves and all spinal nerves carry somatic nerve fibers, although some also carry autonomic fibers including
  • cranial nerves III, VII, IX, and X (parasympathetic), and
  • spinal nerves T1–L2 (sympathetic) and S2–S4 (parasympathetic).

— Nerves from each system typically form nerve plexuses (i.e., somatic nerve plexus, autonomic nerve plexus). Each contains nerves arising from multiple levels of the spinal cord.
  • Somatic plexuses are made up of large, distinct, easily identifiable nerve roots and give rise to nerves that are given descriptive names (median n., femoral n.).
  • Autonomic plexuses appear as dense mats of thin hair-like nerves that frequently extend peripherally along major arteries.

— Both somatic and autonomic nerves carry motor information from the CNS to a peripheral structure, but the type of target organ they innervate and the response they elicit is very different.
  • Somatic nerves initiate voluntary responses (such as contraction of the biceps).
  • Autonomic nerves initiate visceral responses (such as secretion of pancreatic juices).

— Both somatic and autonomic nerves carry sensory information from target organs to the CNS.
  • Sensations carried by visceral (autonomic) sensory fibers are vague and poorly localized (such as nausea).
  • Sensations carried by somatic sensory fibers are sharp and localized (such as a paper cut).

  • In all cases, the cell bodies of peripheral sensory neurons lie in sensory (spinal/dorsal root) ganglia that lie outside the CNS.

— **Splanchnic nerves** are nerves of the autonomic nervous system. They innervate visceral structures (splanchnic refers to internal organs or viscera). They may carry either sympathetic or parasympathetic fibers (never both) and contain no somatic fibers. All splanchnic nerves contain visceral sensory and visceral motor fibers.

1.11 Body Cavities and Internal Organ Systems

The large organs of the endocrine, respiratory, digestive, urinary, and reproductive systems are housed in the thoracic, abdominal, and pelvic cavities. These large spaces are divided into serous cavities and connective tissue spaces.

— A serous cavity is a fully enclosed potential space that is lined by a serous (fluid secreting) membrane. The outer, or **parietal,** layer of this membrane lines the inner wall of the cavity. It is continuous with the inner, or **visceral,** layer that reflects from the wall to cover or enclose the viscera within the cavity. The large serous cavities include:
  • In the thorax
    ○ paired **pleural cavities**, which contain the lungs
    ○ a **pericardial cavity,** which contains the heart
  • In the abdomen and pelvis
    ○ a **peritoneal cavity**, which contains the gastrointestinal tract and its accessory structures

— Connective tissue spaces are potential spaces that lie outside the serous cavities. They are often defined by adjacent layers of fascia or may lie between opposing serous cavities. Major examples include:
  • The **deep cervical space** between fascial layers of the neck
  • The **mediastinum**, which lies between the pleural cavities in the thorax
  • The **retroperitoneal space**, which lies posterior to the peritoneal cavity in the abdomen, and its continuation into the pelvis below the peritoneum, where it is known as the **subperitoneal space**. Urinary and reproductive organs, as well as the major vascular structures, reside within these extraperitoneal spaces.

Unit I   Clinical Imaging Basics Introduction

Imaging is the primary diagnostic method used by physicians in nearly all medical specialties. All physicians should have a basic understanding of radiology concepts and how imaging can be optimally utilized in the care of their patients. The clinical imaging basics covered in this text are meant to be a brief introduction to the extraordinary diagnostic and therapeutic capabilities of radiology.

The four most commonly used imaging modalities are

1. Radiographs (X-rays)
2. CT (computed tomography)
3. MRI (magnetic resonance imaging)
4. Ultrasound

X-Rays

— X-rays are a form of electromagnetic energy and are ionizing radiation. An X-ray tube generates energy in the form of photons, which are directed toward the patient. An electronic detector is positioned behind the patient, which detects the photons (X-ray energy) that pass through the patient to produce an image (**Fig. 1.31**). The degree to which that energy is able to pass through different tissues of the body produces the light, dark, and intermediate grays that are seen on the image. Tissues are rendered as
  • white when the energy is blocked (metal)
  • black when the energy is not blocked (air)
  • gray when the energy is partially blocked (soft tissues)
— The amount of X-ray energy passing through the body depends on the type of tissue encountered by the X-ray beam and the thickness of the tissues. Based on these principles, five densities can be identified on a radiograph (**Table 1.8**).
— Additional descriptive terms are "opacity," "density," and "shadow," which indicate a whiter area on the x-ray; "lucency" indicates a blacker area.
— The image created is a summation of shadows based on the type and thickness of tissues the X-ray photons encounter (**Fig. 1.32**). This summation of shadows creates a two-dimensional representation of the three-dimensional structure of the body. Because it is frequently difficult to determine the depth of a structure in a two-dimensional image, an additional orthogonal (right angle) projection

Table 1.8   **Radiographic Densities**

Tissue	Radiographic Density
Air	Dark black
Fat	Light black
Water and soft tissue	Shades of gray
Bone (calcium)	White
Metal	Bright white

may be required to "construct" a three-dimensional visualization (**Fig. 1.33**).
— The position of the patient and direction of the x-ray beam are manipulated to optimize image quality, obtain positional information accurately, and produce different physical and physiologic effects (such as fluid moving to the most dependent part of the patient). The resulting image is described in terms of both patient position and x-ray beam direction, for example, upright posteroanterior (PA) view (**Fig. 1.34**) or supine lateral view.
Standard patient positions include
  • Upright (standing or sitting up)
  • Supine (lying on back)

Fig. 1.31 **Example of a simplified schematic of X-ray machine.** (From Gunderman R. Essential Radiology, 3rd ed. New York: Thieme; 2014.)

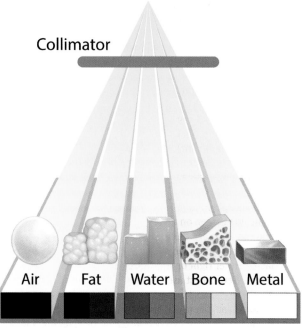

Fig. 1.32 **The effects of density (tissue type) and thickness of tissue on the exposure of an X-ray image using the five basic X-ray densities.** Note that air virtually blocks none of the beam (all energy passes through), whereas metal virtually blocks all of the X-ray energy.

Fig. 1.33 Abdominal radiograph in a patient who swallowed multiple foreign objects. The objects are two forks, one plastic hairbrush with partially metallic bristles, and one plastic pen with a metallic tip. As the image is a summation of the shadows produced by the objects and the tissue, it is impossible to know based on this single X-ray if the objects are in front of or behind the patient, or if they are indeed inside the abdomen. Given the patient's history of swallowing foreign objects, however, we deduce that they are inside the gastrointestinal tract. A lateral view (orthogonal to the frontal view) could confirm this. Using the frontal and lateral view can help triangulate the position of the objects and visualize the abdomen in three dimensions. (From Gunderman R. Essential Radiology, 3rd ed. New York: Thieme; 2014.)

- Prone
- Decubitus (lying on the side)
- Oblique

Standard direction of X-ray beams include

- PA (posteroanterior)
- AP (anteroposterior)
- Lateral

— Radiographs are oriented in a standard fashion.

- Frontal images are viewed with the patient in the anatomic position (facing the observer). The patient's right side is seen on the observer's left and vice versa, and each side is labeled as R or L.
- The lateral projection can be viewed with the patient facing either right or left, but should be consistent. The lateral view is best used in conjunction with the frontal view; the two orthogonal projections can be used to "triangulate" the precise location of specific pathologic findings. The lateral view is also helpful in seeing "hidden" areas on the frontal view such as behind the sternum and heart.

— When evaluating radiographs, a systematic approach is important and should include a checklist of major anatomic structures, which are discussed in the appropriate units.

A Standing (upright) posteroanterior (PA) radiograph being produced in an X-ray room.

B Resultant normal upright PA chest radiograph.

Fig. 1.34 Positioning of patient and direction of X-ray beam.

CT (Computed Tomography)

— CT scans are created by rotating an X-ray beam around the patient. The computer reconstructs these data into image sets of consecutive sections or "slices" (**Fig. 1.35;** see also **Fig. 1.37**). The exquisite anatomic detail on each slice lacks the "shadow summation" of overlapping structures that can make viewing regular X-rays difficult. Because the CT scan is made up of a large number of individual X-rays, the radiation dose is considerably higher. For this reason CT scanning is used judiciously.

— The images produced are based on the computer calculation of the absorption coefficient for each image voxel and expressed in Hounsfield units (Hounsfield was one of the discoverers of CT). Water is arbitrarily set to 0 Hounsfield

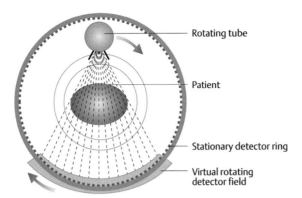

Fig. 1.35 How computed tomography (CT) scanners work.
The X-ray tube rotates continuously around the patient, as the patient, lying on the table, slides through the machine. The curved X-ray detector is opposite to the X-ray tube and registers the amount of X-ray energy that passes through the body. Taking into account the tube position and patient position at each time point of measurement, the computer constructs a data matrix and ultimately a set of images. (From Eastman G, et al. Getting Started in Radiology. Stuttgart: Thieme; 2005.)

Fig. 1.36 Example of single axial slice from a normal abdominal CT.
This image is shown in soft tissue windows to highlight the solid organs and blood vessels.

units; more dense structures are lighter (bone), and less dense structures are darker (air).

— Individual CT slices are oriented in the transverse (axial) plane and, by convention, are viewed from the inferior perspective (looking from the feet toward the head) **(Fig. 1.36)**. However, CT scanners can also generate a volume of data that can be viewed in any plane, including three dimensions (3D reconstruction). Additionally, individual images can be "windowed," which involves changing the brightness or the contrast, to optimize the appearance of structures with specific densities, such as a bone or soft tissue "window."

MRI (Magnetic Resonance Imaging)

— A magnetic resonance image is produced by the interactions of a strong magnetic field on the protons within cells and a radiofrequency energy pulse that disturbs the protons. These spinning protons produce a "signal" that is picked up by a receiver and converted via computerized mathematical manipulation into images.

— MRIs are especially useful because they lack ionizing radiation, produce superb soft tissue contrast, and can be oriented in any plane **(Fig. 1.37)**. Disadvantages include the

A Axial slice of CT scan of the brain in a young woman with blurry vision. This scan is normal.

B Axial slice from an MRI at the same location in the same patient, showing bright spots in the white matter, indicating multiple sclerosis. (Courtesy of Joseph Makris, MD, UMass Medical Health Care Center.)

Fig. 1.37 Example of the improved soft tissue contrast and sensitivity of magnetic resonance imaging (MRI).

high cost, long study acquisition time, and small confined space that patients must tolerate. MRI machines look similar to CT machines, but the tube that the patient slides into is smaller in diameter and longer.

— MRI images are traditionally viewed in the axial, sagittal, and coronal planes, but these can be skewed to optimize "out of plane" structures such as the heart. As in CT, axial images are viewed as if the patient is supine and the observer is looking superiorly from the feet (i.e., inferior view).

— An MRI exam consists of multiple sequences with each sequence highlighting different types of tissue. The same tissues can look different on different sequences. The two basic MRI sequences are T1 and T2 (T represents time constant).
  • T1 sequence: fluid appears dark (black).
  • T2 sequence: fluid appears bright (white).
  • Cortical bone usually appears black on all sequences.

Ultrasound

— Ultrasound images are created by using a transducer, which emits high-frequency sound waves that penetrate the body. It then "listens" for the return echo, similar to the way sonar operates in a submarine (**Fig. 1.38**). Because tissues of different densities attenuate the sound wave to different degrees, the returning echo produces an image of varying shades of gray (**Fig. 1.39**).

— Ultrasound travels most easily through water, which appears black on the image, but it travels poorly through air and bone, which block the sound energy and appear white on the image. Common terms used to describe ultrasound images include *hypoechoic*, meaning blacker, and *hyperechoic* or *echogenic*, meaning gray or white.

— Ultrasound is relatively inexpensive and is radiation free, so it is used whenever possible and is the primary imaging modality in pediatrics, obstetrics, and when imaging both male and female gonads.

— Ultrasound can also make use of the Doppler effect to identify and characterize motion. In medical imaging, Doppler is

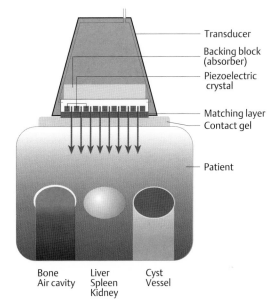

Transducer
Backing block (absorber)
Piezoelectric crystal
Matching layer
Contact gel
Patient

Bone   Liver   Cyst
Air cavity   Spleen   Vessel
              Kidney

Fig. 1.38 Schematic of ultrasound probe held against patient's skin. Gel is used to acoustically couple the probe to the patient. Sound waves travel into the patient and are absorbed, reflected, or scattered based on type of tissue and tissue interfaces. The probe listens for the return echoes and the computer reconstructs the echoes into a two-dimensional image slice. (From Eastman G, et al. Getting Started in Radiology. Stuttgart: Thieme; 2005.)

primarily used to characterize flow in blood vessels and to assess heart physiology. Color Doppler encodes direction and velocity into colors. By convention, blood flowing toward the ultrasound transducer is red and blood flowing away from the transducer is blue (regardless of vessel type). Spectral Doppler gives a graphical representation of the speed of flow with respect to time and thus can demonstrate characteristics of arterial vs. venous flow and identify abnormal flow patterns.

Abdominal wall

Cranial

Caudal

Fig. 1.39 Example ultrasound image of a normal left kidney. The probe was positioned on the abdomen such that the kidney could be seen oriented longitudinally. The image is through the mid-kidney. Ultrasound differentiates the renal pyramids, which are blacker because of higher relative water content. The renal sinus fat is shown to be whiter. Note the liver tissue anterior and superior to the kidney. (From Gunderman R. Essential Radiology, 3rd ed. New York: Thieme; 2014.)

Unit I Review Questions: Introduction

1. Which of the following is associated with membranous bone formation?
   - A. Primary ossification center
   - B. Epiphyses
   - C. Direct ossification of mesenchymal templates
   - D. Long bones of the limbs
   - E. Diaphysis

2. A portal system is associated with
   - A. venous shunts that divert blood toward the heart
   - B. the pulmonary circulation
   - C. arterial-venous anastomoses
   - D. capillary beds in the liver
   - E. lymphatic capillaries

3. In the anatomic position the
   - A. eyes are directed forward
   - B. palms are directed forward
   - C. body is erect with arms at the sides
   - D. feet are directed forward
   - E. All of the above

4. Which of the following is true of splanchnic nerves?
   - A. They synapse in ganglia near their target organ.
   - B. They innervate viscera of the abdomen.
   - C. They may carry sympathetic fibers.
   - D. They may carry parasympathetic fibers.
   - E. All of the above

5. A 43-year-old high school teacher complained to her physician of abdominal bloating and pelvic pain. Radiographic studies showed a large tumor involving her right ovary. Although the patient was scheduled for surgery to remove the tumor, the physician was concerned about the spread of the cancer along lymphatic channels. What is the lymphatic drainage pattern of pelvic viscera?
   - A. Ipsilateral drainage to the right and left lymphatic ducts
   - B. Contralateral drainage to the right and left lymphatic ducts
   - C. Bilateral drainage to the right and left lymphatic ducts
   - D. All pelvic viscera drain to the right lymphatic duct.
   - E. All pelvic viscera drain to the left lymphatic duct.

Answers and Explanations

1. **C.** In the process of membranous ossification, embryonic mesenchymal templates are replaced by bone (Section 1.5).
   A. A primary ossification center, usually in the shaft of the long bones, is the site at which endochondral ossification begins.
   B. Epiphyses, located on either end of the long bones, are the secondary ossification centers for endochondral ossification.
   D. Long bones of the limbs undergo endochondral bone formation, in which a cartilaginous template forms from the embryonic mesenchyme before being replaced by bone.

   E. A diaphysis is the shaft of a long bone, which undergoes endochondral ossification.

2. **D.** The body's largest portal system diverts blood from capillary beds in the gastrointestinal tract to secondary capillary beds in the liver before returning it to systemic veins (Section 1.7).
   A. A portal system diverts venous blood from one capillary network to another, instead of allowing it to flow directly into systemic veins toward the heart.
   B. A portal system is a venous system within the systemic (general body) circulation, but not within the pulmonary (lung) circulation.
   C. A portal system diverts blood from one capillary network to another, unlike arterial-venous anastomoses, which divert blood away from capillary beds.
   E. Lymphatic capillaries are restricted to the lymphatic system and are not involved with portal venous systems.

3. **E.** The anatomic position is the standard position of the body used in medical references. The body is upright, facing the observer, with arms at the side and the head, eyes, palms, and feet directed forward (Section 1.1).
   A. Eyes are directed forward, and other positions are correct as well (E).
   B. Palms are directed forward, and other positions are correct as well (E).
   C. Body is erect with arms at side, and other positions are correct as well (E).
   D. Feet are directed forward, and other positions are correct as well (E).

4. **E.** All of the above (Section 1.9).
   A. Splanchnic nerves synapse near their target organ either in prevertebral ganglia or in small ganglia on the viscera. B through D are correct also (E).
   B. Splanchnic nerves are autonomic nerves that innervate viscera in the thorax, abdomen, and pelvis. A, C, and D are correct also (E).
   C. Sympathetic fibers arise from the T1–L2 spinal cord to form thoracic, lumbar, and sacral splanchnic nerves. A, B, and D are correct also (E).
   D. Parasympathetic fibers arise from the S2–S4 spinal cord and form pelvic splanchnic nerves. A through C are correct also (E).

5. **E.** The left lymphatic duct receives lymph from the entire body below the diaphragm, as well as from the left side of the thorax, head, and neck and the left upper limb (Section 1.8). The right lymphatic duct receives lymph only from the right side of the thorax, head, and neck and the right upper limb.
   A. Viscera from the right and left sides of the pelvis drain to the left lymphatic duct.
   B. All pelvic viscera drain to the left lymphatic duct.
   C. All pelvic viscera drain to the left lymphatic duct.
   D. Only the right upper quadrant of the body drains to the right lymphatic duct.

Unit II   Back

2   Back

2 Back

2.1 The Vertebral Column

The back includes the vertebral column, the spinal cord and spinal nerves, and the overlying muscles and skin.

General Features

— The vertebral column
  • encloses and protects the spinal cord,
  • supports the head and trunk,
  • provides an attachment for the limbs, and
  • transfers the weight of the body to the lower limbs.
— The vertebral column, which extends from the skull to the coccyx, comprises 33 vertebrae and the intervening intervertebral disks, which are divided among five regions **(Fig. 2.1)**:
  • 7 cervical vertebrae
  • 12 thoracic vertebrae
  • 5 lumbar vertebrae
  • 5 fused sacral vertebrae
  • 4 (3–5) fused coccygeal vertebrae

CLINICAL CORRELATION

OSTEOPOROSIS The spine is the primary target for degenerative diseases of the skeleton, such as osteoporosis, in which the rate of reabsorption by osteoclasts exceeds that of bone formation by osteoblasts. The resulting loss of bone mass predisposes the individual to compression fractures of the spine.

— Within each region, individual vertebrae are identified by number, a designation often referred to as a **vertebral level** (such as T8 vertebral level).
— Vertebrae increase in size from the cervical to the lumbar regions and decrease in size from the top of the sacrum to the coccyx.
— The **kyphotic curvatures** of the thoracic and sacral regions of the vertebral column, known as primary curvatures, are curved posteriorly and are present in the fetus. The **lordotic curvatures** of the cervical and lumbar regions, curved anteriorly, are secondary curvatures that develop postnatally **(Fig. 2.2)**.

CLINICAL CORRELATION

ABNORMAL CURVATURES OF THE VERTEBRAL COLUMN: KYPHOSIS, LORDOSIS, AND SCOLIOSIS Kyphosis ("hunchback"), an excessive anterior curvature of the thoracic spine, is often seen in elderly women. Although it may be congenital or posture related, it is usually secondary to degenerative changes (collapse) of the vertebral bodies. Lordosis ("swayback"), an excessive posterior curvature of the lumbar spine, frequently develops as a temporary side effect during pregnancy, but in nonpregnant individuals it may have pathologic or even weight-related causes. Scoliosis is a lateral curvature of the spine and may be congenital or neuromuscular, caused by diseases such as cerebral palsy and muscular dystrophy.

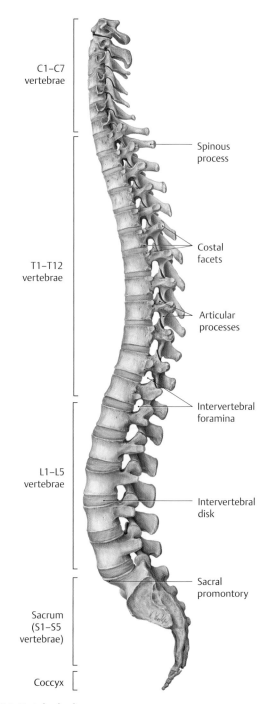

C1–C7 vertebrae

Spinous process

Costal facets

T1–T12 vertebrae

Articular processes

Intervertebral foramina

L1–L5 vertebrae

Intervertebral disk

Sacral promontory

Sacrum (S1–S5 vertebrae)

Coccyx

Fig. 2.1 Vertebral column
Left lateral view.

— **A vertebral canal** passes through the center of the vertebral column and encloses the spinal cord, the spinal meninges (membranes surrounding the spinal cord), and the roots of the spinal nerves, and associated vasculature (see Section 2.2).

II BACK

Fig. 2.2 MRI of the spine

Labels (top to bottom, left side):
- Cervical vertebrae C1–C7
- Thoracic vertebrae T1–T12
- Lumbar vertebrae L1–L5
- Sacrum (sacral vertebrae) S1–S5
- Coccyx (coccygeal vertebrae) Co1-Co3 or Co4

Labels (top to bottom, right side):
- Nuchal lig.
- Dens of axis (C2)
- Vertebra prominens (C7)
- Body of thoracic vertebra T1
- Vertebral canal
- Spinal cord (thoracic part)
- Intervertebral disk
- Supraspinous lig.
- Interspinous ligs.
- Body of lumbar vertebra L1
- Conus medullaris
- Cauda equina
- Spinous process
- Dural sac
- Sacrum (S1)
- Sacral promontory
- Coccyx

— **Intervertebral foramina,** openings between vertebrae, allow the passage of spinal nerves.
— **Spinal cord segments** emit paired spinal nerves, and both the segment and the spinal nerve pair are identified by region and number (such as L4). Spinal cord segments do not necessarily lie adjacent to vertebra of the same number.

Regional Characteristics of Vertebrae

Most vertebrae share a typical form (**Fig. 2.3**), although specific features vary by region.

— Most vertebrae have the following:
  • An anterior vertebral body

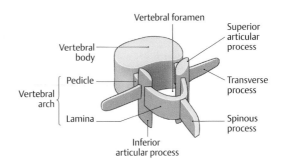

Fig. 2.3 Structural elements of a vertebra
Left posterosuperior view. With the exception of the atlas (C1) and axis (C2), all vertebrae consist of the same structural elements.

Labels:
- Vertebral foramen
- Superior articular process
- Vertebral body
- Pedicle
- Transverse process
- Vertebral arch
- Lamina
- Spinous process
- Inferior articular process

Fig. 2.4 Cervical spine
Bones of the cervical spine, left lateral view.

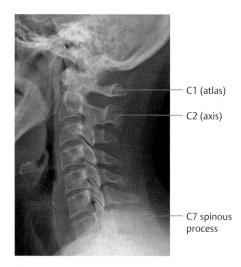

Fig. 2.5 Radiograph of the cervical spine
Left lateral view.

- • A posterior vertebral arch formed by paired pedicles and paired laminae (the pedicles attach to the vertebral body, and the paired laminae join to form a spinous process)
- • Paired transverse processes that project laterally from the vertebral arch
- • Superior and inferior articular processes that articulate with the vertebrae above and below
- • A vertebral foramen encircled by the vertebral body and vertebral arch (the combined vertebral foramina of all vertebrae form the vertebral canal)
- — Cervical vertebrae, the smallest of all of the vertebrae, support the head and form the posterior skeleton of the neck (**Figs. 2.4** and **2.5**). The seven cervical vertebrae are characterized as typical or atypical.
  - • Typical cervical vertebrae (**Fig. 2.6A**)
    - ◦ C3–C6 have a small body, a large vertebral foramen, and often bifid (two-pronged) spinous processes.
  - • Atypical cervical vertebrae
    - ◦ C1, the **atlas,** lacks a vertebral body and spinous process (**Fig. 2.6B**). It has anterior and posterior vertebral arches that are connected on each side by **lateral masses.** C1 articulates with the occipital bone of the skull and C2.
    - ◦ C2, the axis, has a peglike **dens** projecting superiorly from its body that articulates with the anterior arch of C1 (**Fig. 2.6C**).

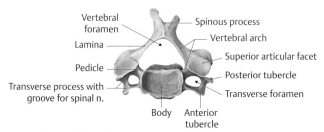

A Typical cervical vertebra (C4), superior view.

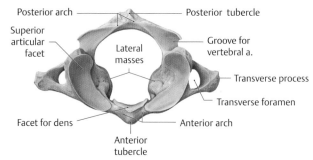

B Atlas (C1), superior view.

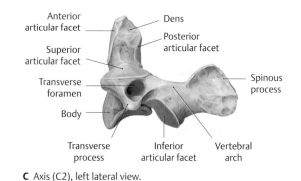

C Axis (C2), left lateral view.

Fig. 2.6 Cervical vertebrae

- ○ C7, the **vertebra prominens,** has a long, palpable spinous process.
- • All cervical vertebrae have paired **transverse foramina,** openings formed by the anterior and posterior tubercles of each transverse process.
— Paired **vertebral arteries** ascend in the neck through the transverse foramina of C1–C6, pass through a groove on the posterior arch of C1, and enter the skull through a large opening, the **foramen magnum.**
— Thoracic vertebrae (**Fig. 2.7**) have
- • long spinous processes that project inferiorly,
- • heart-shaped vertebral bodies,
- • **superior** and **inferior articular facets** that are oriented in the coronal plane, and
- • **costal facets** that articulate with the ribs.
— Lumbar vertebrae (**Figs. 2.8** and **2.9**), the largest vertebrae, have
- • large bodies;
- • short, broad spinous processes; and
- • an **interarticular part** (pars interarticularis), part of the lamina between the superior and inferior articular facets, that forms the neck of the "Scottie dog" seen on oblique views of lumbar spine radiographs. It is a common site of vertebral fractures.
— The five sacral vertebrae are fused into a single bone, the **sacrum** (**Figs. 2.10** and **2.11**), which forms the posterosuperior wall of the pelvis and articulates laterally with the hip bones. The sacrum contains
- • the **sacral canal,** a continuation of the vertebral canal, which is open inferiorly at the **sacral hiatus;**
- • the **median sacral crest,** the fused spinous processes of the sacral vertebrae;
- • paired **medial sacral crests** that end inferiorly as the **sacral cornua** on either side of the sacral hiatus;
- • four pairs of **anterior** and **posterior sacral foramina** for the passage of spinal nerve branches; and
- • the **promontory,** formed by the anterior lip of the S1 vertebral body.
— The small coccygeal vertebrae, usually four (but this can vary from three to five), fuse into a single triangularly shaped bone, the **coccyx,** which articulates with the sacrum at the **sacrococcygeal joint.**

DEVELOPMENT CORRELATION

SPINA BIFIDA Spina bifida is a congenital defect associated with the incomplete fusion of the vertebral arches (usually L5 and S1). In the mild form, spina bifida occulta, the defect is small and asymptomatic and is often marked only by a patch of hair, birthmark, or dimple over the affected vertebrae. Severe forms such as spina bifida cystica are caused by incomplete closure of the embryonic neural tube, resulting in incomplete development of the spinal cord, meninges, and overlying vertebrae. Severe cases are associated with neurologic deficits and herniation of the spinal cord and meninges through the vertebral arch defect.

A Bones of the thoracic spine, left lateral view.

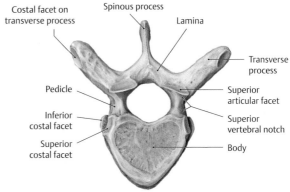

B Typical thoracic vertebra (T6), superior view.

Fig. 2.7 Thoracic spine

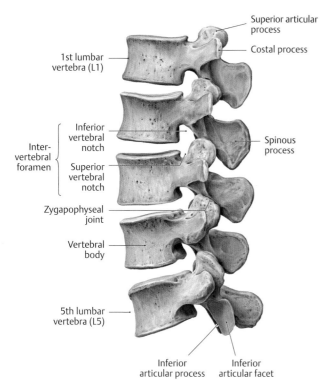

Superior articular process

Costal process

1st lumbar vertebra (L1)

Inferior vertebral notch

Inter-vertebral foramen

Superior vertebral notch

Spinous process

Zygapophyseal joint

Vertebral body

5th lumbar vertebra (L5)

Inferior articular process

Inferior articular facet

A Bones of the lumbar spine, left lateral view.

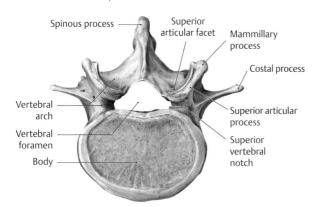

Spinous process

Superior articular facet

Mammillary process

Costal process

Vertebral arch

Vertebral foramen

Body

Superior articular process

Superior vertebral notch

B Typical lumbar vertebra (L4), superior view.

Fig. 2.8 Lumbar spine

CLINICAL CORRELATION

SPONDYLOLYSIS AND SPONDYLOLISTHESIS Spondylolysis is a fracture across the interarticular part of the lamina, usually at L5, and appears as a collar on the "Scottie dog" seen on lumbar radiographs. When the defect is bilateral, the vertebral body may separate from its vertebral arch and shift anteriorly relative to the vertebra below it, a condition known as spondylolisthesis. Mild cases can be asymptomatic, but more severe cases compress the spinal nerves and cause pain in the lower limbs and back.

Fig. 2.9 Radiograph of the lumbar spine.
Left lateral view.

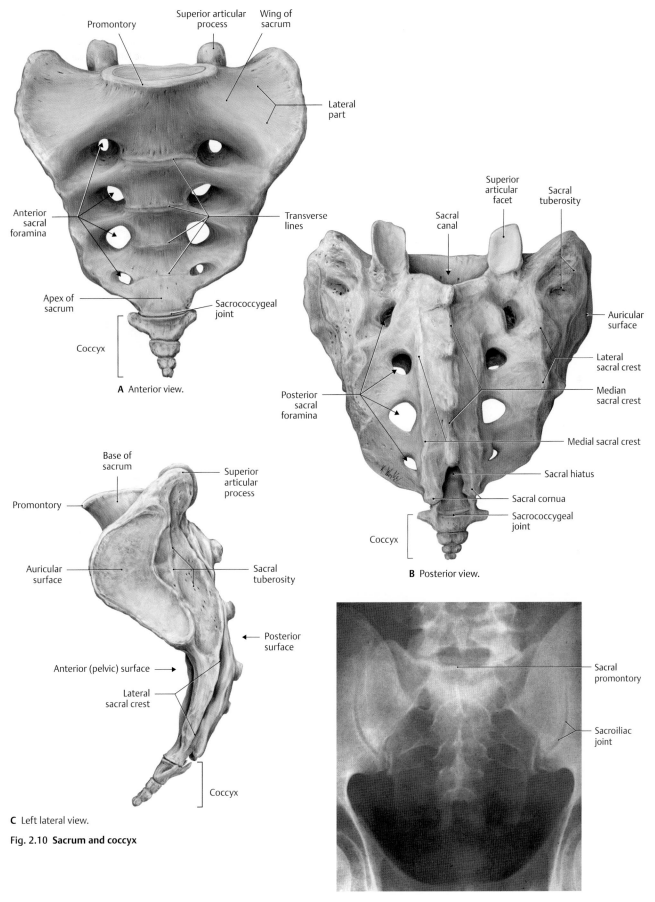

A Anterior view.

Promontory

Superior articular process

Wing of sacrum

Lateral part

Anterior sacral foramina

Transverse lines

Apex of sacrum

Sacrococcygeal joint

Coccyx

B Posterior view.

Sacral canal

Superior articular facet

Sacral tuberosity

Auricular surface

Lateral sacral crest

Median sacral crest

Posterior sacral foramina

Medial sacral crest

Sacral hiatus

Sacral cornua

Sacrococcygeal joint

Coccyx

C Left lateral view.

Base of sacrum

Superior articular process

Promontory

Auricular surface

Sacral tuberosity

Posterior surface

Anterior (pelvic) surface

Lateral sacral crest

Coccyx

Fig. 2.10 Sacrum and coccyx

Sacral promontory

Sacroiliac joint

Fig. 2.11 Radiograph of the sacrum.
Anteroposterior view.

Joints of the Vertebral Column

Joints of the vertebral column include articulations between adjacent vertebral bodies and articulations between adjacent vertebral arches. Joints also form between the vertebral column and the skull (**Table 2.1**). Individual vertebral joints allow small local movements, but the combination of these movements over multiple vertebral levels accounts for the considerable flexibility of the vertebral column.

— **Craniovertebral joints (Fig. 2.12)** are synovial joints between the skull and C1, and between C1 and C2:

  • Paired **atlanto-occipital joints** between the occipital bone of the skull and the atlas (C1) allow flexion and extension of the head (as when nodding "yes").

  • **Atlantoaxial joints,** which include one median and two lateral articulations between the atlas and axis (C1 and C2), allow rotation of the head (as when saying "no").

CLINICAL CORRELATION

INJURIES OF THE CERVICAL SPINE The laxity of the cervical spine makes it prone to hyperextension injuries, such as "whiplash," the excessive and often violent backward movement of the head, resulting in fractures of the dens of the axis and traumatic spondylolisthesis (see box Spondylolysis and Spondylolisthesis, on page 32). Patient prognosis is largely dependent on the spinal level of the injuries.

— **Uncovertebral joints** form between the **uncinate processes** (lateral lips on the superior edges of the vertebral bodies) of C3–C7 vertebrae and the vertebral bodies immediately superior to them.

  • These joints, which are not present at birth, form during childhood, probably as a result of a fissure in the cartilage of the intervertebral disk that then assumes a joint-like character.

— **Intervertebral joints** form between **intervertebral (IV) disks** and the articular surfaces of vertebral bodies. There are no IV disks between C1 and C2.

  • The IV disks act as shock absorbers and are composed of an outer fibrous ring, the **anulus fibrosus,** and a gelatinous core, the **nucleus pulposus (Fig. 2.13).**

Table 2.1 **Joints of the Vertebral Column**

Craniovertebral joints		
①	Atlanto-occipital joints	Occiput-CI
②	Atlantoaxial joints	C1–C2
Joints of the vertebral bodies		
③	Uncovertebral joints	C3–C7
④	Intervertebral joints	C2–S1
Joints of the vertebral arch		
⑤	Zygapophyseal joints	C1–S1

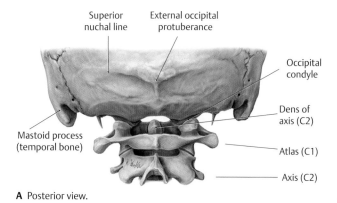

A Posterior view.

Fig. 2.12 Craniovertebral joints

Superior nuchal line
External occipital protuberance
Occipital condyle
Dens of axis (C2)
Mastoid process (temporal bone)
Atlas (C1)
Axis (C2)

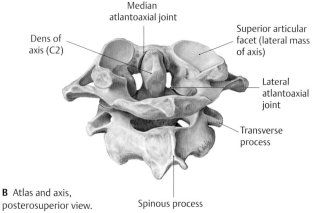

B Atlas and axis, posterosuperior view.

Median atlantoaxial joint
Superior articular facet (lateral mass of axis)
Dens of axis (C2)
Lateral atlantoaxial joint
Transverse process
Spinous process

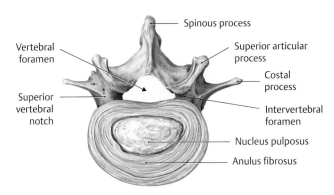

Fig. 2.13 Intervertebral disk
Fourth lumbar vertebra, superior view.

- The height of the IV disk relative to the height of the vertebral body determines the degree of mobility of the joint; mobility is greatest in the cervical and lumbar regions.
- The differences between anterior and posterior heights of the cervical and lumbar disks contribute to the lordotic curvatures.

— **Zygapophyseal joints,** also known as **facet joints,** are synovial joints that join the superior and inferior articular facets of adjacent vertebrae. The orientation of these joints differs between regions and influences the degree and direction of movement of the vertebral column.
  • In the cervical region, the joints are mostly in the horizontal plane and allow movement in most directions.

CLINICAL CORRELATION

HERNIATION OF INTERVERTEBRAL DISKS As elasticity of the anulus fibrosus declines with age, compressive forces can cause the nucleus pulposus to protrude through weakened areas. If the fibrous ring of the anulus ruptures posteriorly, the herniated material may compress the contents of the dural sac, but posterolateral herniations that compress spinal nerves are most common, particularly at the L4–L5 or L5–S1 level. In the lumbar region, where spinal nerves exit the vertebral canal above the IV disk, the hernia is likely to compress the spinal nerve inferior to that level (e.g., a herniation of the L4–L5 disk will impact the L5 spinal nerve), and pain is felt along the corresponding dermatome **(Fig. 2.14)**.

A Superior view.

B Midsagittal T2-weighted MRI.

Posterior herniation **(A,B)**. In the MRI a conspicuously herniated disk at the level of L3-L4 protrudes posteriorly. The dural sac is deeply indented at that level. CSF, cerebrospinal fluid.

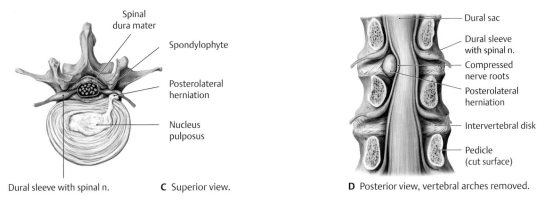

C Superior view.

D Posterior view, vertebral arches removed.

Posterolateral herniation **(C,D)**. A posterolateral herniation may compress the spinal nerve as it passes through the intervertebral foramen. If more medially positioned, the herniation may spare the nerve at that level but impact nerves at inferior levels.

Fig. 2.14 Disk herniation in the lumbar spine

- In the thorax, the joints largely lie in the coronal plane, limiting movement to lateral flexion.
- In the lumbar region, the joints are in the sagittal plane, facilitating flexion and extension.

AGE-RELATED CHANGES IN VERTEBRAE With advancing age, a decrease in bone density and aging of the IV disks can lead to an increase in compressive forces on the vertebral joints. Subsequent degenerative changes can include the depletion of articular cartilage and the formation of osteophytes (bony spurs). Osteophyte formation at the periphery of the vertebral bodies where they join the IV disks is known as spondylosis. Similar degenerative changes of the zygapophyseal joints indicate osteoarthritis, common in the cervical and lumbar spine but also manifested in the joints of the hand, hip, and knee.

Vertebral Ligaments

Vertebral ligaments support the joints of the vertebral column.
— Ligaments that support the cranial vertebral joints (**Fig. 2.15**) include
  - the **atlanto-occipital membranes,** which connect the occipital bone of the skull to the anterior and posterior arches of the atlas (C1);
  - the **alar ligaments,** which secure the dens of C2 to the skull; and
  - the **cruciform ligament,** formed by longitudinal fascicles (fibers) and a transverse ligament, which secures the dens against the anterior arch of the atlas.

A Posterior longitudinal ligament. *Removed:* Spinal cord; vertebral canal windowed.

B Cruciform ligament of atlas (*). *Removed:* Tectorial membrane.

Fig. 2.15 Dissection of the craniovertebral joint ligaments
Posterior view.

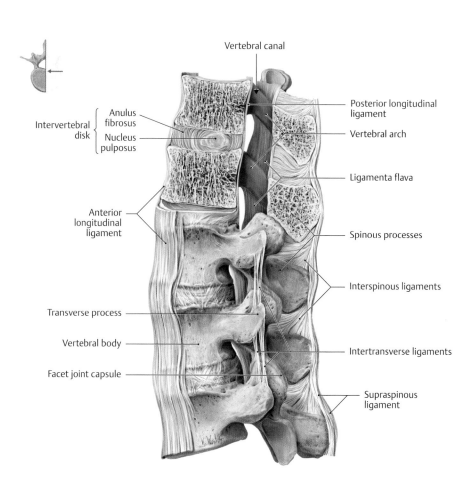

Fig. 2.16 Ligaments of the vertebral column: thoracolumbar junction
Left lateral view of T11–L3, with T11–T12 sectioned in the midsagittal plane.

— Two longitudinal ligaments (**Figs. 2.16** and **2.17**) join all of the vertebral bodies:

1. The **anterior longitudinal ligament,** a broad fibrous band extending from the occipital bone of the skull to the sacrum, attaches to the anterior and lateral surfaces of the vertebral bodies and IV disks and prevents hyperextension.

2. The **posterior longitudinal ligament,** a thin fibrous band extending from C2 to the sacrum along the anterior aspect of the vertebral canal, attaches primarily to the IV disks and offers weak resistance to hyperflexion. Superiorly, this ligament extends into the skull as the **tectorial membrane** (see **Fig. 2.15A**).

— Ligaments that join the vertebral arches (**Fig. 2.18**) include the following:

- the paired **ligamenta flava,** which join the laminae of adjacent vertebrae on the posterior wall of the vertebral canal. They limit flexion and provide postural support of the vertebral column (see also **Fig. 2.16**).

- the **supraspinous ligament,** which connects the posterior ridge of the spinous processes

- the **nuchal ligament,** a finlike expansion of the supraspinous ligament in the neck that extends from the occipital bone to the spinous process of C7

— Additional vertebral ligaments connect elements of the vertebral arches and spinous processes (see **Fig. 2.16**).

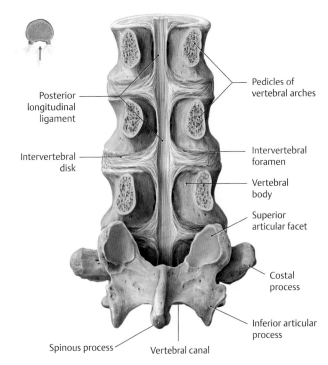

Fig. 2.17 Posterior longitudinal ligament
Posterior view of opened vertebral canal at level of L2–L5. *Removed:* L2–L4 vertebral arches at pedicular level.

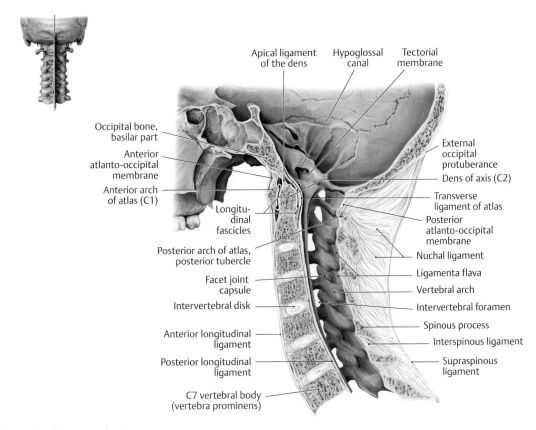

Fig. 2.18 Ligaments of the cervical spine
Midsagittal section, left lateral view. The nuchal ligament is the broadened, sagittally oriented part of the supraspinous ligament that extends from the vertebra prominens (C7) to the external occipital protuberance.

Neurovasculature of the Vertebral Column

— The following arteries **(Fig. 2.19)** supply the vertebrae, vertebral ligaments, meninges, and spinal cord:
  • The segmental arteries, paired branches of the descending aorta such as the **posterior intercostal** and **lumbar arteries,** that arise in the thoracic and lumbar regions
  • Branches of the **subclavian artery** in the neck, including the vertebral and **ascending cervical arteries**
  • The **iliolumbar, medial,** and **lateral sacral arteries** in the pelvis

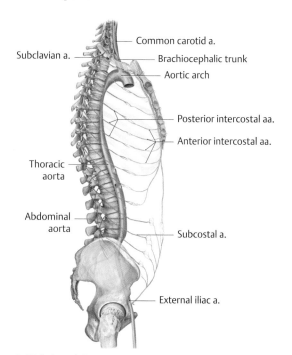

A Right lateral view.

— The **vertebral venous** (Batson) **plexus** surrounds the vertebral bodies and drains the spinal cord, meninges, and vertebrae **(Fig. 2.20)**.
  • **Anterior** and **posterior external plexuses** surround the vertebrae, and **anterior** and **posterior internal plexuses** lie within the epidural space in the vertebral canal.
  • Both the internal and external plexuses drain into **intervertebral veins,** which in turn drain to **vertebral veins** of the neck (see **Fig. 2.25A;** see also **Fig. 17.29**) and segmental veins (paired tributaries of the inferior vena cava and azygos system) in the thoracic, lumbar, and sacral regions.
  • The veins of the vertebral venous plexus have few valves; thus, there is free venous communication between the skull, neck, thorax, abdomen, and pelvis.
— Lymphatic drainage from the vertebrae and vertebral ligaments generally follows the arteries that supply each region and end in cervical, thoracic, lumbar, and sacral lymph nodes.
— Posterior rami and meningeal branches of anterior rami of spinal nerves innervate the vertebrae, vertebral ligaments, and spinal meninges.
— Posterior rami of spinal nerves innervate the skin and intrinsic muscles of the back (see **Fig 2.28**).

CLINICAL CORRELATION

METASTASIS AND THE VERTEBRAL VENOUS PLEXUS The vertebral venous plexus links the venous drainages of viscera in the thorax, abdomen, and pelvis and the venous sinuses of the brain. These communications have been identified as a likely route of metastases of carcinoma of the prostate (commonly), breast, and lung (less commonly) to the central nervous system and bone.

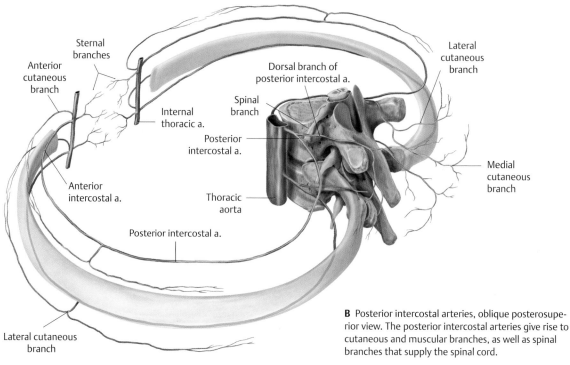

B Posterior intercostal arteries, oblique posterosuperior view. The posterior intercostal arteries give rise to cutaneous and muscular branches, as well as spinal branches that supply the spinal cord.

Fig. 2.19 Arteries of the trunk

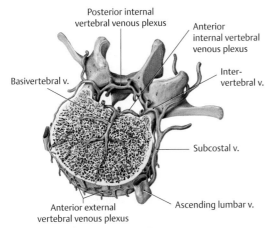

A Vertebral venous plexuses, superior view.

2.2   The Spinal Cord

The spinal cord is the part of the central nervous system that relays information between the brain and the body. The spinal cord, along with its spinal nerves, surrounding membranes (the **meninges**), and associated vasculature, is enclosed within the vertebral canal.

Structure of the Spinal Cord

— The spinal cord, continuous with the **medulla oblongata** of the brain (see **Fig. 18.11A**) superiorly, exits the skull base through the **foramen magnum** of the occipital bone. It descends within the vertebral canal and terminates as the **conus medullaris** adjacent to the L1 vertebra (**Fig. 2.21;** see also **Fig. 17.8**).

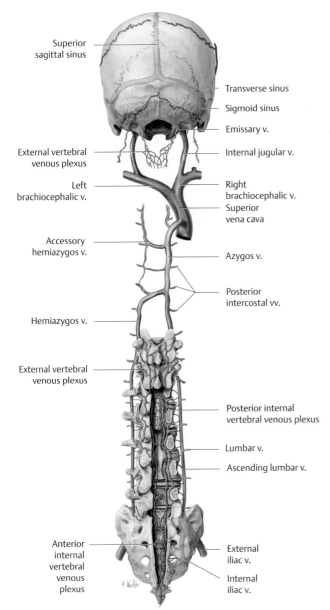

B Vertebral venous plexus, posterior view with vertebral canal windowed in the lumbar and sacral spine.

Fig. 2.20 Vertebral venous plexus
The intervertebral and basivertebral veins connect the internal and external venous plexuses, which drain into the azygos system.

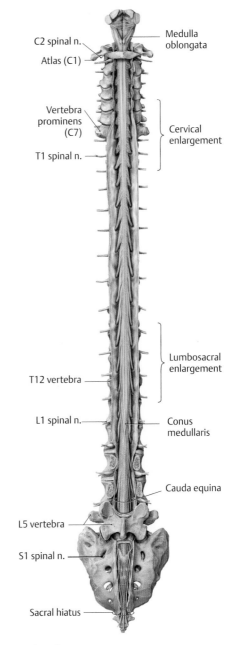

Fig. 2.21 Spinal cord in situ
Posterior view with vertebral canal windowed.

— During development, the longitudinal growth of the vertebral column exceeds that of the spinal cord. At birth the conus medullaris is at the level of the L3 vertebra, but in the adult it lies adjacent to the L1/L2 intervertebral disk.

— Because the adult spinal cord is considerably shorter than the vertebral column, occupying only the superior two thirds of the vertebral canal, most spinal cord segments do not lie adjacent to the vertebral level of the same number (**Fig. 2.22**).

— The spinal cord consists of 31 segments, each of which innervates a specific area of the trunk or limbs. Each spinal cord segment has paired **spinal nerves** that contain both sensory and motor neurons.

— Two swellings occur in the regions of the spinal cord that innervate the limbs:

   • The **cervical enlargement** at C4–T1 is related to the brachial plexus, a plexus of nerves that innervate the upper limb.

   • The **lumbosacral enlargement** at T11–S1 is related to the lumbar and sacral plexuses, nerve plexuses that innervate the abdominal wall and lower limb.

Meninges of the Spinal Cord

The spinal **meninges** are membranes that surround the spinal cord and nerve roots and that contain the **cerebrospinal fluid** (a fluid that cushions and nourishes the brain and spinal cord) (**Figs. 2.23** and **2.24**); see also Section 18.2).

— The three layers of spinal meninges are continuous with the meninges that surround the brain:

   1. **Dura mater,** a tough outer layer that forms the **dural sac** enclosing the spinal cord and extending along the nerve roots to the intervertebral foramina. The dural sac begins

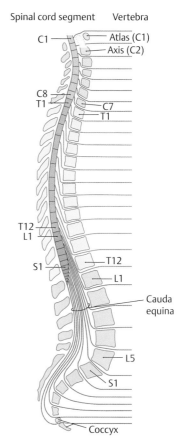

Spinal cord segment　　Vertebra

Fig. 2.22 Spinal cord segments and vertebral levels
The spinal cord is divided into four major regions: cervical, thoracic, lumbar, and sacral. Spinal cord segments are numbered by the exit points of their associated spinal nerves.

Fig. 2.23 Spinal cord and its meningeal layers
Posterior view. The dura mater is opened, and the arachnoid mater is sectioned.

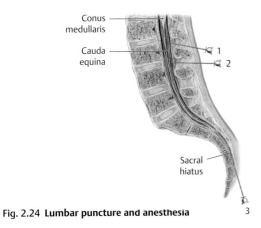

Conus
medullaris

Cauda
equina

1

2

Sacral
hiatus

3

Fig. 2.24 Lumbar puncture and anesthesia

at the foramen magnum of the skull and ends at the level
of S2.
2. **Arachnoid mater,** a delicate middle layer that is connected
   to the underlying membrane by **arachnoid trabeculae**
   (strands of connective tissue).
3. **Pia mater,** a thin layer that adheres to the surface of the
   spinal cord. **Denticulate ligaments,** transverse extensions
   of the pia mater, attach to the dura mater and suspend the
   spinal cord within the dural sac.

— The **filum terminale,** a thin cord of pia mater, extends from
  the conus medullaris to the apex of the dural sac. There it is
  surrounded by spinal dura mater and extends to the end of
  the vertebral canal, where it anchors both membranes to the
  coccyx.
— Three spaces separate the layers of meninges **(Fig. 2.25):**
  • The **epidural space** lies between the bony wall of the
    vertebral canal and the dura mater. It contains fat and the
    vertebral venous plexus.

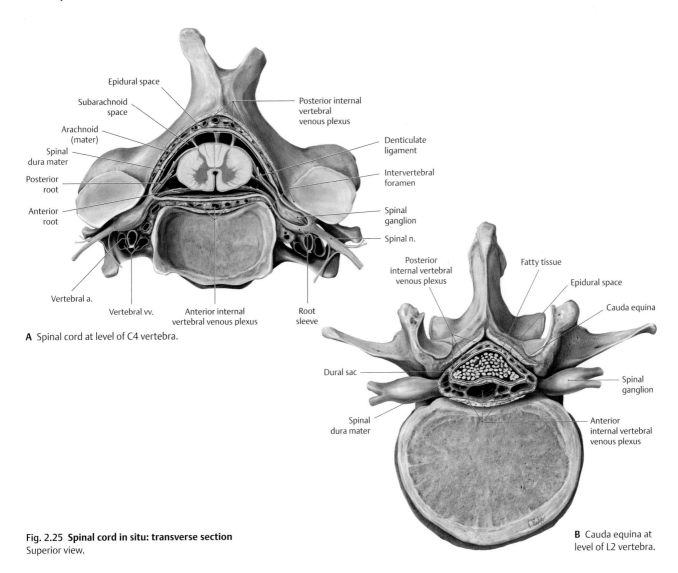

Epidural space

Subarachnoid
space

Arachnoid
(mater)

Spinal
dura mater

Posterior
root

Anterior
root

Vertebral a.

Vertebral vv.

Anterior internal
vertebral venous plexus

Root
sleeve

Posterior internal
vertebral
venous plexus

Denticulate
ligament

Intervertebral
foramen

Spinal
ganglion

Spinal n.

A Spinal cord at level of C4 vertebra.

Posterior
internal vertebral
venous plexus

Fatty tissue

Epidural space

Cauda equina

Dural sac

Spinal
dura mater

Spinal
ganglion

Anterior
internal vertebral
venous plexus

Fig. 2.25 Spinal cord in situ: transverse section
Superior view.

B Cauda equina at
level of L2 vertebra.

- The **subdural space,** a potential space between the dura and arachnoid layers, contains a thin film of lubricating fluid.
- The **subarachnoid space** lies deep to the arachnoid layer and contains the cerebrospinal fluid. The **lumbar cistern** is an enlargement of the subarachnoid space within the dural sac inferior to the conus medullaris.

Blood Supply to the Spinal Cord (Fig. 2.26)

— Longitudinal spinal arteries supply the superior part of the spinal cord.
  - A single **anterior spinal artery** arises from the two vertebral arteries (branches of the subclavian arteries) and supplies the anterior two thirds of the spinal cord.
  - Paired **posterior spinal arteries** arise from the vertebral arteries (or one of their branches, the posterior cerebellar artery) and supply the posterior third of the spinal cord.
— **Anterior** and **posterior segmental medullary arteries** are large, irregularly spaced vessels that communicate with the spinal arteries.
  - They arise from branches of the subclavian artery and segmental arteries in the thoracic and lumbar region.
  - The medullary arteries enter the vertebral canal through the intervertebral foramina and are found mainly at the cervical and lumbar enlargements.
— The **great anterior segmental medullary artery** (of Adamkiewicz), a single large, usually left-sided vessel, can provide an important contribution to the circulation of the lower two thirds of the spinal cord.
  - It arises as a branch of a lower thoracic or lumbar segmental artery.
  - It enters the vertebral canal through an intervertebral foramen in the lower thorax or upper lumbar region.
— The **anterior** and **posterior radicular arteries** are small arteries that supply the roots of the spinal nerves and the superficial **gray matter** of the spinal cord. They do not communicate with the spinal arteries.
— Veins of the spinal cord, which are more numerous than the arteries, have the same distribution, anastomose freely with one another, and drain into the internal vertebral plexus **(Fig. 2.27)**.

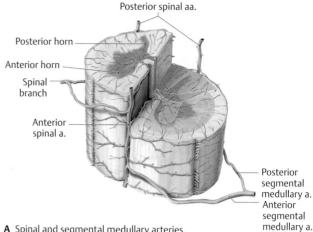

A Spinal and segmental medullary arteries.

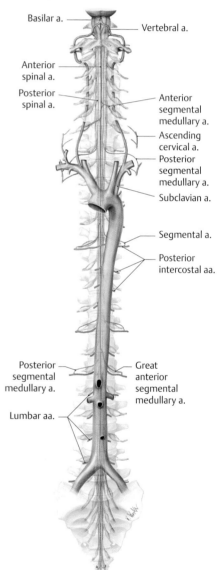

B Arterial supply system.

Fig. 2.26 Arteries of the spinal cord
The unpaired anterior and paired posterior spinal arteries typically arise from the vertebral arteries. As they descend within the vertebral canal, the spinal arteries are reinforced by anterior and posterior segmental medullary arteries. Depending on the spinal level, these reinforcing branches may arise from the vertebral, ascending or deep cervical, posterior intercostal, lumbar, or lateral sacral arteries.

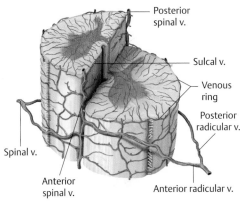

Posterior
spinal v.

Sulcal v.

Venous
ring

Posterior
radicular v.

Spinal v.

Anterior
spinal v.

Anterior radicular v.

A Spinal and radicular veins.

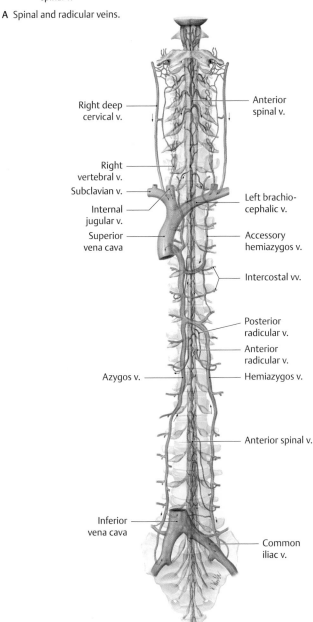

Right deep
cervical v.

Anterior
spinal v.

Right
vertebral v.

Subclavian v.

Internal
jugular v.

Left brachio-
cephalic v.

Superior
vena cava

Accessory
hemiazygos v.

Intercostal vv.

Posterior
radicular v.

Anterior
radicular v.

Azygos v.

Hemiazygos v.

Anterior spinal v.

Inferior
vena cava

Common
iliac v.

B Venous drainage system.

Fig. 2.27 Veins of the spinal cord
The interior of the spinal cord drains via venous plexuses into an anterior
and a posterior spinal vein. The radicular and spinal veins connect the
veins of the spinal cord with the internal vertebral venous plexus. The
intervertebral and basivertebral veins connect the internal and external
vertebral venous plexuses, which drain into the azygos system.

2.3 Spinal Nerves

Spinal nerves transmit information between peripheral body tissues and the spinal cord. A single pair of spinal nerves arises from
each spinal cord segment.
— There are 31 pairs of spinal nerves: 8 cervical, 12 thoracic,
   5 lumbar, 5 sacral, and 1 coccygeal.
— Spinal nerves arise bilaterally from each spinal cord segment
   (**Fig. 2.28**). They are formed by the merging of
   • an **anterior root** carrying motor (efferent) fibers whose
      cell bodies are located in the anterior horn of the spinal
      cord, and
   • a **posterior root** carrying sensory (afferent) fibers whose
      cell bodies are located in a spinal ganglion located outside
      the spinal cord.
— Spinal nerves from each spinal cord segment pass through
   the intervertebral foramina at the corresponding vertebral
   level.
   • Cervical nerves C1–C7 exit the vertebral canal superior
      to the vertebra of the same number (e.g., C4 spinal nerve
      exits between C3 and C4 vertebrae).
   • C8 spinal nerve exits below the C7 vertebra (between the
      C7 and T1 vertebrae).
   • Spinal nerves T1–Co1 exit the canal inferior to the
      corresponding vertebra.
— Because the spinal cord is shorter than the vertebral column,
   nerve roots from the lower spinal cord (L2–Co1) must
   descend below the conus medullaris within the lumbar
   cistern of the dural sac before exiting through the respective
   intervertebral foramina. This loose group of nerve roots
   within the dural sac is called the **cauda equina** (see **Figs. 2.22**
   and **2.25B**).

Peripheral Nerve Pathways of the Somatic Nervous system

The somatic nervous system innervates structures under conscious
control including the skin and skeletal muscles.
— As spinal nerves emerge from the intervertebral foramen,
   they split to form rami (branches) that contain both sensory

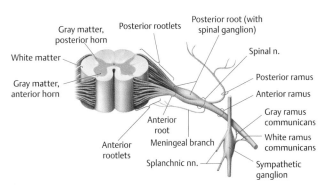

Gray matter,
posterior horn

Posterior rootlets

Posterior root (with
spinal ganglion)

White matter

Spinal n.

Gray matter,
anterior horn

Posterior ramus

Anterior ramus

Gray ramus
communicans

White ramus
communicans

Anterior
root

Meningeal branch

Anterior
rootlets

Splanchnic nn.

Sympathetic
ganglion

Fig. 2.28 Structure of a spinal cord segment
Anterior view. The spinal cord consists of 31 segments, each of which
gives rise to a pair of spinal nerves that innervate a specific area in the
trunk or limbs, Afferent (sensory) posterior rootlets and efferent (motor)
anterior rootlets form the posterior and anterior roots, respectively. The
two roots fuse within the intervertebral foramen to form a mixed spinal
nerve. Subsequent branches of the spinal nerve contain both motor and
sensory fibers (except the meningeal branch, which is only sensory).

and motor fibers (except C1, which contains only motor fibers) (see **Fig 2.28**).

- **Posterior rami** innervate skin and muscles of the back and scalp.
- **Anterior rami** form peripheral nerves and plexuses that innervate the rest of the body.

— Posterior rami do not form plexuses, and most are referred to by the spinal cord segment from which they originate (e.g., T4 posterior ramus). The suboccipital n. (C1), greater occipital n. (C2), and 3rd occipital n. (C3) that innervate the scalp are the only individually named posterior rami (**Fig. 2.29A**).

— Anterior rami have a larger distribution than posterior rami, and most have a more complex course (**Fig. 2.29**).

- Anterior rami of thoracic spinal nerves do not form plexuses but become **intercostal nerves,** which run in the spaces between ribs to innervate the thoracic and anterolateral abdominal walls.

- Anterior rami of the cervical, lumbar, and sacral regions form plexuses that give rise to multi-segmental nerves that may carry only sensory or only motor fibers, or they may be mixed nerves, carrying both sensory and motor fibers. These nerves are usually given specific names (e.g., radial n., femoral n.). These somatic plexuses include:
  - ◦ Cervical plexus (C1–C4) innervates muscles of the neck and skin over the neck and scalp.
  - ◦ Brachial plexus (C5–T1) innervates the pectoral girdle and upper limb.
  - ◦ Lumbar plexus (L1–L4) innervates the lower anterior abdominal wall and anterior thigh.
  - ◦ Sacral plexus (L4–S3) innervates the gluteal region, posterior thigh, and leg.

— In somatic nerve plexuses, sensory nerve fibers associated with a single spinal cord segment are distributed among several peripheral nerves. Traveling from the periphery toward the

Spinal Cord Segment	Anterior Branches (anterior rami)	Posterior Branches (posterior rami)
C1		Suboccipital nerve
C2	Cervical plexus	Greater occipital nerve
C3		Third occipital nerve
C4		
C5	Branchial plexus	
C6		
C7		
C8		
T1		
T2		
T3		
T4		
T5		
T6	Intercostal nerves	
T7		
T8		Posterior rami
T9		
T10		
T11		
T12		
L1		
L2		
L3	Lumbar plexus	
L4		
L5		
S1		
S2	Sacral plexus	
S3		
S4		
S5	Coccygeal plexus	
Co1		
Co2		

A Anterior and posterior branches of the spinal nerves.

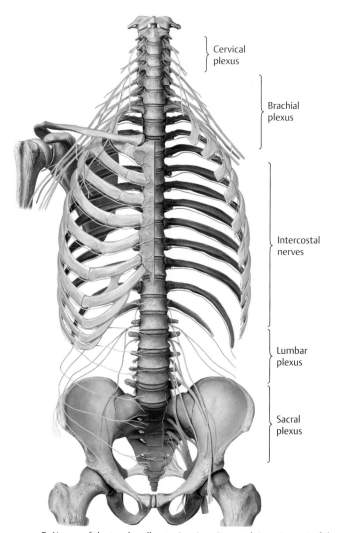

B Nerves of the trunk wall, anterior view. *Removed:* Anterior part of the left half of the thoracic cage.

Fig. 2.29 **Nerves of the trunk wall**

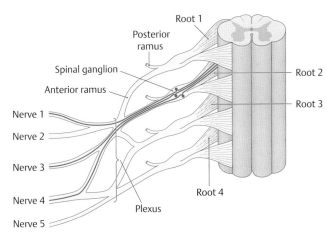

Fig. 2.30 Principles of plexus formation: sensory nerves
The axons, which form the afferents from a dermatome, extend from that dermatome to a single root in the spinal cord.

spinal cord, the sensory fibers converge to enter the spinal cord via the posterior root. There they synapse with sensory neurons in the posterior horn of the spinal cord (**Fig. 2.30**).

— Sensory roots from each spinal cord segment correspond to the sensory (cutaneous) innervation of a particular area of skin, known as a **dermatome (Fig. 2.31)**. Because sensory fibers from each segment are distributed among multiple peripheral nerves, there is a large area of overlap between adjacent dermatomes. Thus, the lesion of a single sensory nerve root (such as by the impingement of a herniated disk) would have a minimal effect.

— Typically peripheral sensory nerves carry fibers from several spinal cord levels. Lesions of a sensory nerve, therefore, would affect a larger cutaneous territory covering multiple dermatomes (**Fig. 2.32**).

— Cutaneous sensations transmitted by somatic sensory nerves include those of pain, pressure (touch), and temperature. Sensory nerves also transmit a sense of position, or **proprioception,** that provides information about the spatial position of the limbs.

— Similar to the distribution of sensory fibers in a plexus, motor fibers from multiple spinal cord levels may combine in a peripheral nerve to innervate a single skeletal muscle. In other cases, muscles may be innervated by a single spinal cord segment. Muscles are divided into two groups based on their innervation patterns (**Fig. 2.33**):

  • **Monosegmentally** innervated muscles are innervated by motor neurons from a single spinal cord segment.

  • **Polysegmentally** innervated muscles are innervated by neurons whose nuclei extend over several spinal cord segments.

— M**yotomes** represent the muscle mass that is innervated by a single spinal cord segment. For example, although the femoral n. and the obturator n. both contain anterior rami of L2–L4, they innervate different muscles. The L2 myotome would comprise all of the muscle fibers innervated by the L2 spinal segment, whether carried in the femoral n. or obturator n.

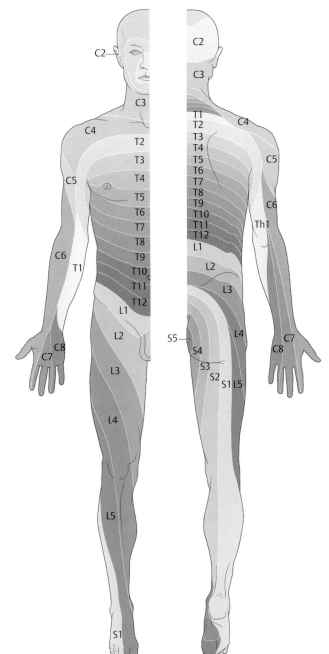

Fig. 2.31 Dermatomes of the head, trunk, and limbs
Each spinal cord segment innervates a particular skin area (dermatome). Dermatomes are band-like areas of skin innervated by a pair of spinal nerves arising from a single spinal cord segment. Since spinal nerve C1 carries only motor fibers, there is no corresponding dermatome.

— Muscles that are innervated by a single segment of the spinal cord (monosegmental) can be evaluated clinically by testing a corresponding **reflex**. Reflexes, such as the patellar tendon reflex, are mediated by motor (efferent limb) and sensory (afferent limb) neurons that are located within a single segment of the spinal cord.

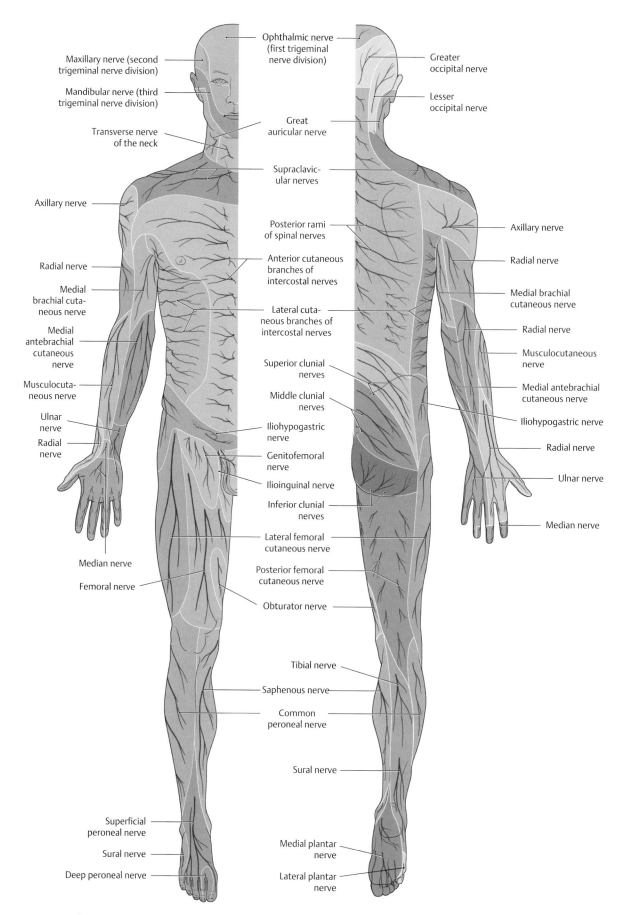

Fig. 2.32 Pattern of peripheral sensory cutaneous sensation
Sensory loss patterns that are associated with a peripheral nerve lesion overlap multiple dermatomes.

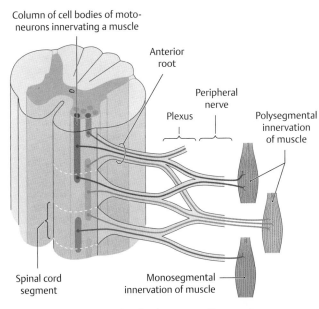

Fig. 2.33 **Monosegmental and polysegmental innervation**

Peripheral Nerve Pathways of the Autonomic Nervous System

The autonomic nervous system, the visceral part of the peripheral nervous system, innervates blood vessels, glands, smooth muscle, and cardiac muscle.

— The autonomic nervous system consists of two divisions that often have antagonistic effects on the same organ (**Fig. 2.34;** see **Table 1.7**):
  • The **sympathetic division** allows the body to respond to stress ("fight or flight").
  • The **parasympathetic division** allows the body to maintain, or return to, a state of homeostasis ("rest and digest").

— Nerve pathways of both the sympathetic and parasympathetic systems consist of a two-neuron chain between the central nervous system (CNS) and the target organ: a proximal **preganglionic** (presynaptic) **neuron** and distal **postganglionic** (postsynaptic) **neuron** that synapse with each other in an intervening ganglion (**Fig. 2.35**).

— The sympathetic division is known as the **thoracolumbar** component because its nerves arise from the lateral horn of

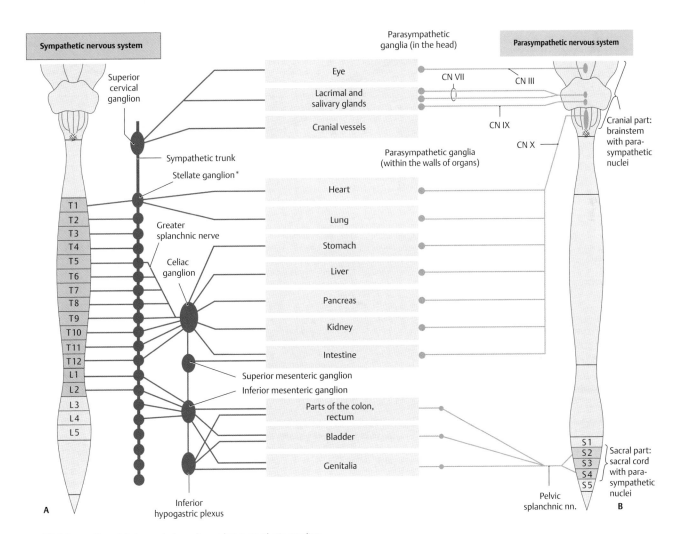

*Stellate ganglion = inferior cervical ganglion and T1 sympathetic ganglion

Fig. 2.34 **Autonomic nervous system**
The autonomic nervous system is subdivided into **(A)** sympathetic (thoracolumbar) and **(B)** parasympathetic (craniosacral) divisions. Each utilizes a two-neuron pathway in which preganglionic neurons synapse with postganglionic neurons in peripheral autonomic ganglia.

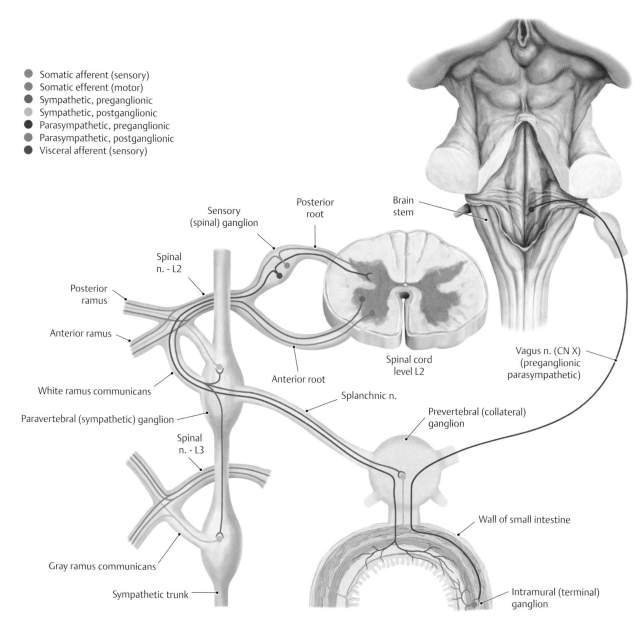

- Somatic afferent (sensory)
- Somatic efferent (motor)
- Sympathetic, preganglionic
- Sympathetic, postganglionic
- Parasympathetic, preganglionic
- Parasympathetic, postganglionic
- Visceral afferent (sensory)

Sensory (spinal) ganglion

Posterior root

Brain stem

Spinal n. - L2

Posterior ramus

Anterior ramus

Spinal cord level L2

Vagus n. (CN X) (preganglionic parasympathetic)

White ramus communicans

Anterior root

Splanchnic n.

Paravertebral (sympathetic) ganglion

Prevertebral (collateral) ganglion

Spinal n. - L3

Wall of small intestine

Gray ramus communicans

Sympathetic trunk

Intramural (terminal) ganglion

Fig. 2.35 **Circuitry of the autonomic nervous system**

the spinal cord in the thoracic and lumbar regions (T1–L2). They exit through the intervertebral foramina with the motor fibers of the corresponding spinal nerves.

— In addition to sympathetic nerves, the sympathetic system includes paired **sympathetic trunks**, chains of **paravertebral ganglia** that contain the cell bodies of postganglionic sympathetic nerves**.** The trunks run along each side of the vertebral bodies from C1 to S5. The paravertebral ganglia are connected to spinal nerves via

- **gray rami communicans,** which connect paravertebral ganglia at all levels (C1–S5) to the corresponding spinal nerve; and
- **white rami communicans**, which connect only paravertebral ganglia between T1 and L2 to the corresponding spinal nerve.

— Shortly after emerging from the vertebral column, the preganglionic sympathetic fibers leave the spinal nerve via white rami communicans to enter the paravertebral ganglion.

From this point the sympathetic fibers can take three different routes:

- They can synapse with the postganglionic neuron in the paravertebral ganglia at that level and return to the spinal nerve via the gray rami communicans. As part of the spinal nerve, these fibers will follow the sensory and motor fibers of the anterior and posterior rami to innervate structures in the dermatome.
- They can course up or down within the trunk to synapse with ganglia at other levels. The postganglionic fibers then join the spinal nerves at those levels. This route allows sympathetic fibers to be distributed to spinal nerves along the entire length of the spinal cord, and thus to all regions of the body, even though they originate only from the thoracolumbar segment.
- They can pass through the paravertebral ganglia without synapsing to form **thoracic, lumbar,** or **sacral splanchnic nerves**. These synapse in **prevertebral ganglia**, such as the

celiac ganglion (see Section 8.2). Postganglionic fibers contribute to autonomic plexuses in the thorax, abdomen, and pelvis that travel along periarterial routes to innervate viscera in those regions.

— The parasympathetic division is known as the **craniosacral** component because its nerves arise from the brain and the S2–S4 segments of the sacral spinal cord.

  • Preganglionic parasympathetic fibers that arise from the brain travel with cranial nerves III, VII, IX, and X and synapse in parasympathetic ganglia of the head or, in the case of the vagus nerve, ganglia near the target organ. The neural pathways involved are discussed in detail in Section 18.3.

    ○ The vagus nerve is the only cranial nerve that extends inferior to the neck. Its parasympathetic fibers reach as far as the transverse colon in the abdomen. Thus, it provides parasympathetic innervation to all thoracic viscera and most of the abdominal viscera.

  • Similar to sympathetic fibers in the thoracolumbar region, sacral parasympathetic nerves leave the spinal cord with the motor nerves of the corresponding somatic spinal nerves (S2–S4). These preganglionic parasympathetic fibers are known as **pelvic splanchnic nerves.** They contribute to autonomic plexuses in the pelvis and abdomen and synapse in small ganglia located close to, or within, their target organ.

— Smooth muscle in the skin and body wall (important for vasoconstriction, piloerection, gland secretion) does not receive any parasympathetic innervation. Sympathetic innervation is responsible for constriction of blood vessels; vasodilation results when sympathetic stimulation ceases.

— The autonomic nervous system also contains visceral sensory fibers that convey sensations from physiologic processes, such as distension of the bladder. Nociceptive (pain) fibers have been shown to accompany both sympathetic and parasympathetic nerves.

  • Nociceptive fibers from viscera travel in the splanchnic nerves to sympathetic ganglia and reach the spinal nerve by way of the white rami communicans. Like somatic sensory neurons, their cell bodies are located in spinal ganglia. They enter the posterior horn of the spinal cord through the posterior roots.

  • Nociceptive fibers traveling with cranial parasympathetic fibers have their cell bodies in the inferior or superior ganglia of the vagus nerve (cranial nerve X). Those traveling with sacral parasympathetic nerves have their cell bodies in the sacral spinal ganglia of S2–S4.

CLINICAL CORRELATION

REFERRED PAIN Referred pain is a sensation that originates from viscera but is perceived as if coming from an overlying or nearby somatic structure. It occurs because the somatic and visceral sensory fibers converge onto the same spinal cord segment. Diaphragmatic irritation from a splenic abscess, for example, is typically referred to the shoulder because both the diaphragm and the skin over the shoulder convey sensory information to C3–C5 segments of the spinal cord **(Fig. 2.36).**

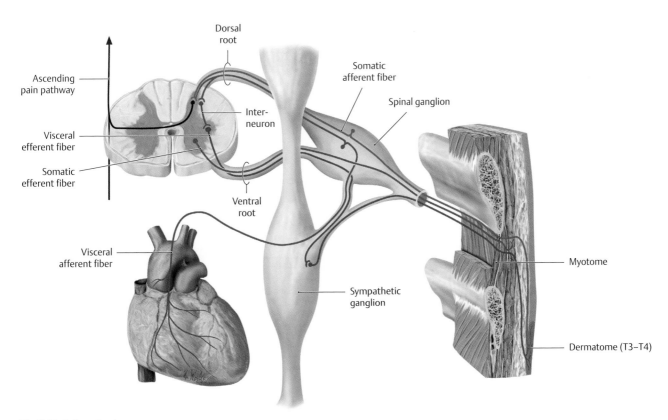

Fig. 2.36 Referred pain
It is believed that nociceptive sensory fibers from dermatomes (somatic pain) and internal organs (visceral pain) terminate on the same relay neurons in the spinal cord. The convergence of somatic and visceral sensory fibers confuses the relationship between the perceived and actual sites of pain, a phenomenon known as referred pain. The pain is typically perceived at the somatic site given that somatic pain is well localized while visceral pain is not.

2.4 Muscles of the Back and Suboccipital Region

- **Extrinsic muscles,** the most superficial muscles that overlie the back, stabilize and move the upper limb. (See Chapter 14 for a discussion of the muscles of the upper limb.)
  - Extrinsic muscles include the trapezius, latissimus dorsi, levator scapulae, and rhomboid major and minor.
- **Intrinsic muscles,** which attach to vertebrae or ribs, move and support the vertebral column **(Table 2.2)**.
  - They are arranged in superficial, intermediate, and deep layers **(Figs. 2.37** and **2.38)**.
  - The superficial layer includes the **splenius** muscle group that covers the deeper neck muscles laterally and posteriorly. These muscles extend and rotate the head and neck. They extend superolaterally from the spinous processes of cervical and upper thoracic vertebrae to the occipital bone and transverse processes of C1 and C2.
  - The intermediate layer includes the **erector spinae** muscle group that extends from the midline of the back to the angle of the ribs laterally. These large muscles are the

main extensors and stabilizers of the thoracic and lumbar vertebral column. They include:
  - the **iliocostalis,** the most lateral column that arises from the **thoracolumbar fascia,** the sacrum, iliac crest, and ribs and extends superolaterally to the ribs and to cervical and lumbar vertebrae.
  - the **longissimus,** the middle column that arises from the sacrum, iliac crest, spinous processes of lumbar vertebrae, and transverse processes of thoracic and cervical vertebrae. It inserts superiorly on the temporal bone of the skull, to cervical, thoracic and lumbar vertebrae and to the ribs.
  - the **spinalis,** the most medial column that extends between the spinous processes of cervical and thoracic vertebrae.

Table 2.2 **Muscles of the Back and Suboccipital Region**

Muscle Group	Innervation	Action
Intrinsic muscles of the back		
Superficial layer Splenius capitis Splenius cervicis	Posterior rami of cervical spinal nerves	Extend, rotate, and laterally flex the head and cervical spine
Intermediate layer (erector spinae) Spinalis Longissimus Iliocostalis	Posterior rami of spinal nerves	Extend and laterally flex the spine
Deep layer Transversospinalis group Rotatores (brevis and longus) Multifidus Semispinalis Deep segmental group Interspinals Intertransversarii Levatores costarum	Posterior rami of spinal nerves	Extend, rotate, and laterally flex the head and spine
Muscles of the suboccipital region		
Rectus capitis posterior major Rectus capitis posterior minor Obliquus capitis superior Obliquus capitis inferior	Suboccipital n. (C1)	Extend and rotate the head

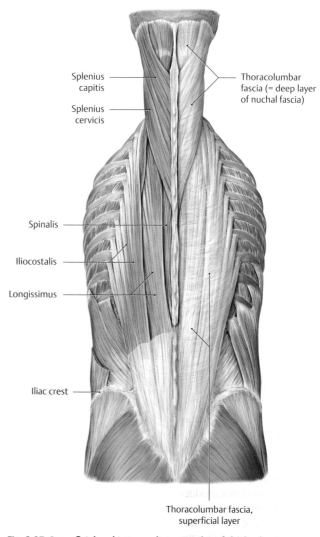

Fig. 2.37 Superficial and intermediate muscles of the back
Posterior view. *Removed:* Thoracolumbar fascia *(left)*.

Labels on figure:
Splenius capitis
Splenius cervicis
Thoracolumbar fascia (= deep layer of nuchal fascia)
Spinalis
Iliocostalis
Longissimus
Iliac crest
Thoracolumbar fascia, superficial layer

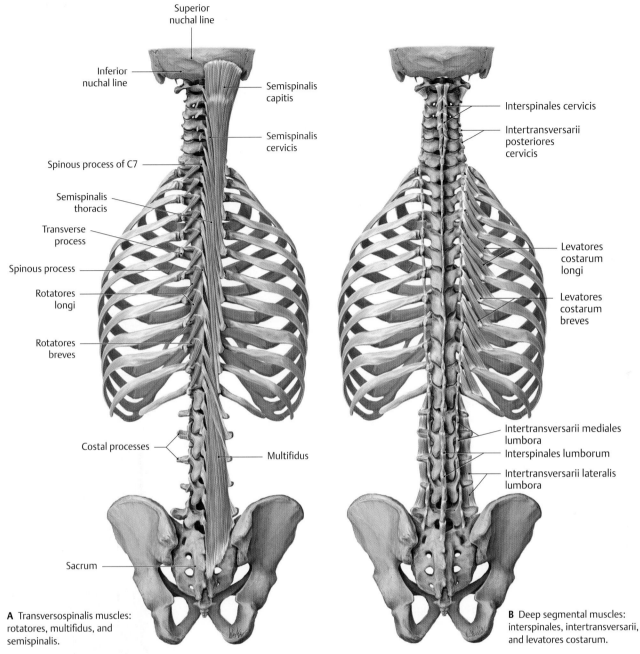

A Transversospinalis muscles: rotatores, multifidus, and semispinalis.

B Deep segmental muscles: interspinales, intertransversarii, and levatores costarum.

Fig. 2.38   Deep intrinsic back muscles
Posterior view.

- The deep layer includes short muscles at multiple vertebral levels that produce small movements along the entire vertebral column. They are divided into a **transversospinalis** muscle group and a **deep segmental** muscle group. The transversospinalis muscles extend between the transverse and spinous processes of the vertebrae. They include:

  ○ the **semispinalis** muscles, the most superficial group
  ○ the **multifidus,** most prominent in the lumbar region
  ○ the **rotatores,** the deepest muscles of the transversospinalis group, best developed in the thoracic region
- The deep segmental muscles are minor muscles of the back. They include the **interspinales** and **intertransversarii**

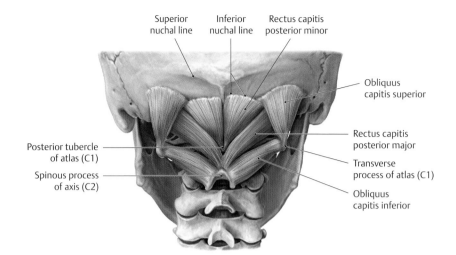

Fig. 2.39 Short nuchal and craniovertebral joint muscles
Suboccipital muscles, posterior view.

that connect adjacent vertebrae, and the **levatores costarum** that connect vertebrae to ribs.

- A deep fascia that encloses the intrinsic muscles runs laterally from the posterior midline to the cervical and lumbar transverse processes and to the ribs. This **thoracolumbar fascia** continues into the neck as the deep layer of the **nuchal fascia,** the posterior extension of the **cervical fascia** (see Section 21.2).

— Muscles of the posterior neck occupy the small **suboccipital compartment (Fig. 2.39)** that is inferior to the base of the skull and deep to the trapezius and intrinsic back muscles that extend into the neck. The suboccipital muscles arise from C1 or C2 and extend upward to insert on the occipital bone or transverse process of C1. All assist in the positioning of the head and are innervated by the suboccipital nerve, the posterior ramus of C1. They include the **rectus capitis posterior major, rectus capitis posterior minor, obliquus capitis inferior,** and **obliquus capitis superior.**

— Posterior intercostal and lumbar arteries (branches of the descending aorta and subclavian artery) supply the skin and muscles of the back. The veins of the back accompany the arteries and are tributaries of the azygos system.

— Posterior intercostal and lumbar veins accompany the corresponding arteries to drain muscles of the back. These veins are tributaries of the azygos system, which communicates with both the vertebral venous plexus and the vena cavae.

— Posterior rami of intercostal and lumbar nerves supply the skin and intrinsic muscles of the back (**Figs. 2.40** and **2.41**).

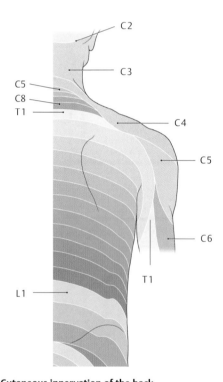

Fig. 2.40 Cutaneous innervation of the back
Dermatomes: segmental (radicular) cutaneous innervation of the back.
Note: The posterior ramus of C1 is purely motor; there is consequently no C1 dermatome.

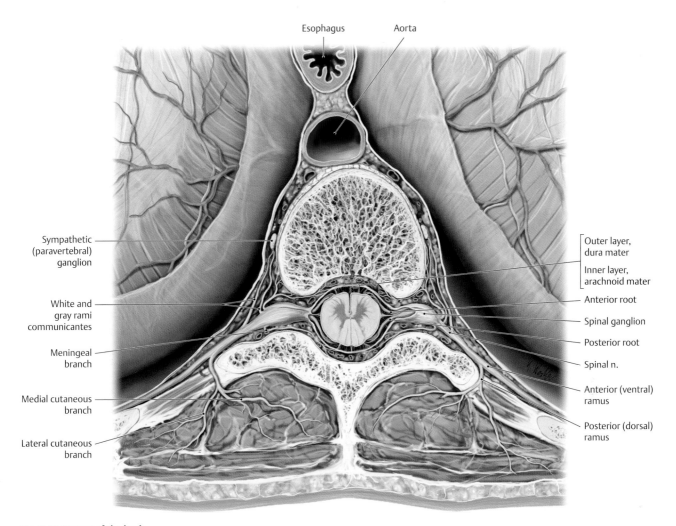

Esophagus

Aorta

Sympathetic
(paravertebral)
ganglion

White and
gray rami
communicantes

Meningeal
branch

Medial cutaneous
branch

Lateral cutaneous
branch

Outer layer,
dura mater

Inner layer,
arachnoid mater

Anterior root

Spinal ganglion

Posterior root

Spinal n.

Anterior (ventral)
ramus

Posterior (dorsal)
ramus

Fig. 2.41 Nerves of the back
Cross section through the vertebral column and spinal cord with surrounding musculature, superior view.

Unit II   Clinical Imaging Basics of the Spine

Radiographs provide a fast initial assessment of overall alignment of the spine and are often the first imaging study obtained in trauma patients. However, nondisplaced fractures may be invisible on X-ray and only detected with the high resolution and detail of computed tomography (CT). Because X-ray and CT do not show soft tissues well, magnetic resonance imaging (MRI) is used for optimal evaluation of the spinal cord, nerve roots, ligaments, and intervertebral disks. The fully developed adult spine is not suitable for ultrasound analysis as the bones of the vertebrae block the sound waves. In infants, the posterior aspect of the vertebral bodies are not yet ossified, allowing for sound transmission into the spinal canal from the infants back. This anatomic consideration, the infant's small size, and the lack of radiation make ultrasound ideal for evaluation of the spinal cord and spinal canal in infants (**Table 2.3**).

Radiographic examination of the spine should include both frontal and lateral views. This is especially important for assessing alignment. Note that in both views the vertebral bodies appear as rectangles, the result of the "summation shadow" (**Figs. 2.42** and **2.43**). The spinous processes and the pedicles of each vertebra, superimposed on the vertebral bodies, are easily seen on the frontal radiographs because of the brightness of the cortical edges. The facet joints are best assessed on the lateral view. CT provides superior details of the vertebral column and has the additional advantage of being able to be reconstructed into three-dimensional (3D) images that allow the radiologist to optimize the evaluation of pathologic conditions (**Fig. 2.44**). This can be compared to the soft tissue detail that is best evaluated in an MRI (**Fig. 2.45**).

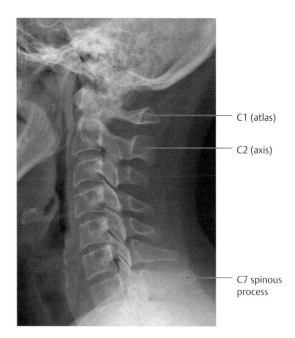

C1 (atlas)

C2 (axis)

C7 spinous process

Fig. 2.42 Radiograph of the cervical spine
Left lateral view.
In a normal radiograph of the spine, the vertebral bodies appear roughly rectangular in shape and the corners of each vertebral body line up with the corners of the vertebral body above and below it. The intervertebral disk spaces are uniform from level to level and the spinous process of each vertebra is easily identified.

Table 2.3 **Suitability of Imaging Modalities for the Back and Spine**

Modality	Clinical Notes
Radiographs (X-rays)	Excellent for first-line evaluation of alignment of the vertebral column and assessment for fractures in trauma patients; vertebral anatomy is well depicted
CT (computed tomography)	Although important soft structures are not well seen, other anatomic relationships are seen with exceptional detail; more sensitive than radiographs for the evaluation of fractures (especially nondisplaced fractures) and injuries to the posterior structures
MRI (magnetic resonance imaging)	Best for evaluation of the disks, nerve roots, spinal cord, ligaments, and other soft tissues
Ultrasound	Used only in young infants whose spinal column is not fully ossified, allowing for excellent imaging of the infant spinal cord

Body of vertebra

Spinous process

Transverse process

Pedicle

Intervertebral disk

Fig. 2.43 Anteroposterior (AP) radiograph of the lower thoracic spine
Anterior view.
As in the cervical spine, vertebral bodies are rectangular and the intervertebral disk spaces are uniform. Alignment is assessed by lining up the corners of each vertebral body with the adjacent vertebra. The spinous processes and the pedicles of each vertebra are well defined on the frontal radiographs, but are superimposed on the vertebral bodies.

Fig. 2.44 CT reconstruction of the spine
Midsagittal section.
This midsagittal section represents a single slice of a digitally reconstructed CT scan. This image is a single slice of the midline that was digitally "reconstructed" in the sagittal plane from the original CT images. The spine is easier to evaluate in this plane because the relationships between vertebrae are better depicted. This image is presented in the "bone window," which is best for evaluating the osseous structures. The multiple densities (whiter spots) throughout many of the vertebral bodies are metastatic lesions from prostate cancer, referred to as sclerotic or blastic lesions because there is increased bone at the metastatic focus. Although these may be visible on an X-ray of the spine, they are more obvious with CT. As with radiographs, the edges of each vertebral body should line up with the edges of the vertebral body above and below.

Thoracic vertebral body T12 — Mamillary process
— Erector spinae
Lumbar vertebral body L2 —
Inferior vena cava — Spinal ganglion L2
— Lamina
Intervertebral disk L3/L4 (nucleus pulposus) — Intervertebral foramen
— Inferior articular process
Superior articular process — Zygapophyseal joint
Common iliac a. — Multifudus
Promontory of sacrum —
Sacrum (S1) — Gluteus maximus

Fig. 2.45 MRI of the lumbar spine
Parasagittal section through the lateral edges of the vertebral bodies and the intervertebral foramina. Left lateral view.
(*Fat = white, muscles = black, nerve roots = light gray, bone = dark gray.*)
This image demonstrates MRI's superior ability to show soft tissues, an advantage over radiographs and CT. The intervertebral foramina are clearly visualized with the dark nerve roots surrounded by fat within the intervertebral foramina. If this patient had a disk herniation, the disk tissue would be clearly visible intruding into the spinal canal. Note the white nucleus pulposus in the middle of the intervertebral disks.

Unit II Review Questions: Back

1. During the surgical repair of an aortic aneurysm in a 62-year-old patient, the left T10 intercostal artery that supplied the great anterior segmental artery (of Adamkiewicz) was inadvertently ligated. A likely consequence of this would be a disruption of the blood supply to
    A. the cervical enlargement of the spinal cord
    B. the lumbosacral enlargement of the spinal cord
    C. the lower thoracic vertebrae
    D. the deep intrinsic muscles of the back
    E. the posterior one third of the spinal cord

2. A 57-year-old woman who runs a 4-mile route three times a week complained to her primary care physician of low back pain and an irritating paresthesia (tingling) along the inner aspect of her right leg. Electromyographic studies identified a lesion of her L4 spinal nerve on the right side. The L4 spinal nerve
    A. carries only sensory fibers
    B. contributes to both the lumbar and sacral nerve plexuses
    C. contains sympathetic nerve fibers that innervate pelvic viscera
    D. exits the intervertebral foramen between the L3 and L4 vertebrae
    E. innervates intrinsic muscles and skin of the back via its anterior ramus

3. The filum terminale is best described as
    A. an extension of the arachnoid mater that connects to the pia mater
    B. a transverse ligament that suspends the spinal cord within the dural sac
    C. an extension of the pia mater that descends within the lumbar cistern
    D. a ligament that connects the spinous processes of the vertebrae
    E. an extension of the pia mater that anchors the conus medullaris to the L2 vertebra

4. The nerves that descend within the lumbar cistern of the dural sac are called
    A. lumbar plexus
    B. sacral plexus
    C. cauda equina
    D. posterior rami
    E. sacral spinal nerves

5. An 87-year-old man sees his primary care physician with a complaint of mental confusion and back pain. Although the physician considers that these symptoms may be a normal consequence of the patient's age, examination reveals that the patient has advanced prostate cancer that has spread to his brain and vertebral column. The probable route of metastasis is identified as the vertebral venous plexus, which
    A. drains the vertebrae and intervertebral disks but does not drain the spinal cord
    B. lies within the subarachnoid space

    C. consists of veins with multiple valves along their length
    D. consists of paired longitudinal veins within the vertebral canal
    E. is a valveless system of veins

6. A 47-year-old construction worker presented to his physician with debilitating pain in his lower back and lower limb. Radiographic studies showed a herniated intervertebral disk at the L4–L5 vertebral level. Which of the following is true?
    A. The herniated disk most likely signals a weakness of the anterior longitudinal ligament.
    B. A posterior herniation of this disk could result in compression of the adjacent spinal cord.
    C. Pain from this hernia would most likely be felt along the L4 dermatome.
    D. The herniation is the result of a loss of elasticity of the anulus fibrosus, which allowed protrusion of the nucleus pulposus.
    E. None of the above

7. The splenius muscle group
    A. lies deep to the trapezius
    B. is enclosed by the thoracolumbar fascia
    C. extends the cervical spine and head
    D. is innervated by posterior rami of cervical spinal nerves
    E. All of the above

8. A 92-year-old woman remains mentally alert and physically active but has lost several inches in height, and her posture is stooped forward. Her geriatrician explains that this exaggerated curvature is due to degeneration of the bodies of two of her thoracic vertebrae that often occurs in older women as a result of decreased bone density. The curvature exhibited by this patient is known as
    A. scoliosis
    B. spondylolysis
    C. lordosis
    D. kyphosis
    E. spondylosis

9. The spinal cord terminates caudally as the
    A. denticulate ligament
    B. filum terminale
    C. conus medullaris
    D. lumbar cistern
    E. sacral hiatus

10. Which of the following ligaments would prevent hyperextension of the vertebral column?
    A. Anterior longitudinal ligament
    B. Posterior longitudinal ligament
    C. Ligamentum flavum
    D. Alar ligament
    E. Cruciform ligament

11. Which of the following vertebral characteristics is paired with the correct vertebral region?
  - **A.** Promontory—sacral
  - **B.** Vertebral prominens—thoracic
  - **C.** Dens—thoracic
  - **D.** Transverse foramen—lumbar
  - **E.** Costal facet—cervical

Answers and Explanations

1. B. The great anterior segmental artery (of Adamkiewicz) supplies the inferior two thirds of the spinal cord, which includes the region of the lumbosacral enlargement (T11–S1) (Section 2.2).

    A. The great anterior segmental artery (of Adamkiewicz) supplies the inferior two thirds of the spinal cord, which does not include the region of the cervical enlargement (C4–T1).

    C. Vertebrae are supplied by segmental arteries of the descending aorta, as well as by branches of the subclavian arteries and arteries of the pelvis.

    D. Intrinsic muscles of the back get their blood supply from posterior branches of the intercostal and lumbar arteries.

    E. The posterior spinal arteries that usually arise from the vertebral arteries in the neck supply the posterior third of the spinal cord.

2. B. The lumbar plexus includes anterior rami of spinal nerves L1–L4, and the sacral plexus includes anterior rami of spinal nerves L4–S4 (Section 2.3).

    A. All spinal nerves carry both sensory and motor fibers

    C. Sympathetic fibers are carried only in spinal nerves between T1 and L2.

    D. Except for nerves in the cervical region, spinal nerves exit below the vertebra of the corresponding number; thus, L4 exits between the L4 and L5 vertebrae.

    E. Intrinsic muscles and skin of the back are innervated by posterior rami of spinal nerves.

3. C. The filum terminale is a filament of pia mater that runs within the lumbar cistern with the cauda equina, from the conus medullaris to the end of the dural sac. Inferior to the dural sac, it is surrounded by spinal dura mater and extends to the coccyx (Section 2.2).

    A. The arachnoid trabeculae connect the arachnoid mater to the pia mater.

    B. Denticulate ligaments suspend the spinal cord within the dural sac.

    D. The supraspinous ligament connects the spinous processes of all thoracic, lumbar, and sacral vertebrae. In the cervical region it expands as the nuchal ligament, a finlike ligament that attaches superiorly to the occipital bone.

    E. The end of the spinal cord, the conus medullaris, lies adjacent to the L2 vertebra but is not attached to it.

4. C. Because the spinal cord is shorter than the vertebral column, spinal nerves L2–Co1 descend as a group (cauda equina) within the dural sac before exiting at the appropriate intervertebral foramen (Section 2.3).

    A. The lumbar plexus forms outside the vertebral canal on the posterior abdominal wall and contains only anterior rami of lumbar spinal nerves (L1–L4).

    B. The sacral plexus forms outside the vertebral canal on the posterior wall of the pelvis and contains only anterior rami of L4–S4 spinal nerves.

    D. The nerves of the cauda equina are spinal nerves, which contain both anterior and posterior rami.

    E. The cauda equina contains both lumbar and sacral spinal nerves.

5. E. The vertebral venous plexus is a valveless system that allows communication between the caval and azygos systems, which drain the trunk, and the venous sinuses of the brain (Section 2.1).

    A. The vertebral venous plexus drains the vertebrae, meninges, and spinal cord.

    B. The internal vertebral venous plexus lies in the epidural space. The external plexus surrounds the outside of the vertebral column.

    C. The vertebral venous plexus is a valveless system that allows communication between the caval and azygos systems, which drain the trunk, and the venous sinuses of the brain.

    D. The venous plexus consists of interconnecting veins that form an internal plexus within the vertebral canal and an external plexus that surrounds the vertebrae.

6. D. Loss in elasticity of the fibrous ring, which may occur with aging, allows herniation of the nucleus pulposus (Section 2.1).

    A. The anterior longitudinal ligament supports the vertebral bodies and disks anteriorly. The posterior longitudinal ligament supports the disks posteriorly where herniation normally occurs.

    B. The spinal cord ends at L2 and is not present in this part of the vertebral canal.

    C. The L4 spinal nerve exits the intervertebral foramen superior to the intervertebral disk and is usually unaffected by the herniation. The hernia would compress the next inferior spinal nerve, L5, and pain would be felt along that dermatome.

    E. Not applicable

7. E. All of the above (Section 2.4)

    A. The splenius muscles are superficial intrinsic back muscles that lie deep to the trapezius, an extrinsic muscle of the upper back. B through D are also correct (E).

    B. All intrinsic back muscles, including the splenius group, are enclosed by the deep fascia of the back, the thoracolumbar fascia. A, C, and D are also correct (E).

    C. Splenius muscles extend the cervical spine and head when working bilaterally. Unilaterally, they flex and rotate the head to the same side. A, B, and D are also correct (E).

    D. The splenius muscles are innervated by the posterior rami of C1–C6 spinal nerves. A through C are also correct (E).

8. D. Kyphosis is an abnormal posterior curvature of the thoracic spine often seen in older women (Section 2.1).

    A. Scoliosis is a lateral curvature of the spine.

    B. Spondylolysis refers to a fracture or defect across the interarticular part of the lamina of the lumbar vertebrae.

    C. Lordosis is an exaggerated anterior curvature of the lumbar spine often seen in pregnant women.

    E. Spondylosis is a degeneration of the intervertebral disk and corresponding vertebral body that results in osteophyte formation.

9. **C.** The spinal cord terminates caudally as the conus medullaris. This usually corresponds to the L1–L2 vertebral level in an adult (Section 2.2).

    A. Denticulate ligaments are transverse extensions of the pia mater that attach to dura mater and suspend the spinal cord within the dural sac.

    B. Pia mater terminates caudally as the filum terminale.

    D. The lumbar cistern is part of the subarachnoid space that lies between the conus medullaris and the inferior end of the dural sac.

    E. The sacral hiatus is the inferior opening of the sacral canal, which is a continuation of the vertebral canal.

10. **A.** The anterior longitudinal ligament attaches the anterior and lateral surfaces of the vertebral bodies and intervertebral disks and prevents hyperextension (Section 2.1).

    B. The posterior longitudinal ligament attaches primarily to the intervertebral disks and produces weak resistance to hyperflexion.

    C. The ligamenta flava join the laminae of adjacent vertebrae. They limit flexion and provide postural support of the vertebral column.

    D. The alar ligaments secure the dens of C2 to the skull.

    E. The cruciform ligament, formed by longitudinal fibers and a transverse ligament, secure the dens against the anterior arch of the atlas.

11. **A.** The anterior lip of S1 forms the promontory of the sacrum (Section 2.1).

    B. The vertebral prominens is the C7 vertebra, named for its long palpable spinous process.

    C. Only the C2 vertebra has a dens, the peg-like process that articulates with C1.

    D. Only cervical vertebrae have transverse foramina.

    E. Only thoracic vertebrae have costal facets where they articulate with the ribs.

Unit III   Thorax

3 Overview of the Thorax

The thorax is the region of the trunk between the neck and abdomen. The thoracic cavity, surrounded by a bony cage that protects the thoracic contents, is open to the neck but separated from the abdomen by a muscular diaphragm. The viscera of the thorax include the primary organs of the respiratory and cardiovascular systems, as well as components of the gastrointestinal, endocrine, and lymphatic systems.

3.1 General Features

— The thorax is divided into two lateral compartments, the **pulmonary cavities,** which contain the lungs and pleural sacs, and a central compartment, the **mediastinum,** which contains the heart, pericardial sac, trachea and bronchi, esophagus, thymus, and neurovasculature **(Fig. 3.1; Table 3.1)**.
— **A pericardial sac** surrounds the heart, and a **pleural sac** surrounds each lung. These closed membranous sacs contain a thin layer of serous fluid that ensures frictionless movement, which is crucial to the function of these organs.
— The lungs are the organs of respiration. They communicate with the **tracheobronchial tree** (the passages for air between the lungs and outside environment) and the heart through the **hilum,** an indentation on the medial surface of each lung.
— The heart is a four-chambered muscular organ that functions as a dual pump that propels blood through the body. Each pump is made up of two chambers: a thin-walled **atrium** and a thick-walled **ventricle.**

— During a cardiac cycle, the right pump receives deoxygenated blood from the **systemic circulation** (circulation of blood through all regions of the body except the lungs) and directs it to the **pulmonary circulation** in the lungs. The left pump receives oxygenated blood from the pulmonary circulation and returns it to the systemic circulation for the distribution of oxygen and nutrients **(Fig. 3.2)**.
— Coordinated contraction of atria and ventricles, known as the **cardiac cycle,** is self-moderated by specialized tissue within the cardiac muscle that makes up the heart's **conduction system.**

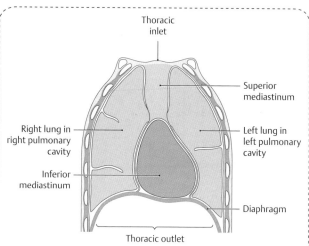

Table 3.1 **Major Structures of the Thoracic Cavity**

Mediastinum	Superior mediastinum		Thymus, great vessels, trachea, esophagus, and thoracic duct
	Inferior mediastinum	Anterior	Thymus
		Middle	Heart, pericardium, and roots of great vessels
		Posterior	Thoracic aorta, thoracic duct, esophagus, and azygos venous system
Pulmonary cavities	Right pulmonary cavity		Right lung, pleura
	Left pulmonary cavity		Left lung, pleura

Fig. 3.1 Radiograph of the thorax
Anteroposterior chest radiograph, anterior view.

3.2   Neurovasculature of the Thorax

The "great vessels," which include the pulmonary arteries and veins, the aorta, the superior vena cava, and the inferior vena cava, direct blood into and out of the heart and lungs. Their branches and further details of their anatomy, along with more detailed descriptions of lymphatic drainage and nerves of the thorax, are discussed in Chapters 5 and 6 on the mediastinum and pulmonary cavities.

Arteries of the Thorax

— The **pulmonary trunk** directs deoxygenated blood from the right side of the heart into the pulmonary circulation. It arises from the right ventricle on the anterior surface of the heart, passes superiorly and posteriorly, and, under the arch of the aorta, divides into **right** and **left pulmonary arteries (Fig. 3.3)**.
— One pulmonary artery enters each lung, where it branches into generations of smaller vessels that accompany the respiratory passages. The pulmonary arteries transport deoxygenated blood to the small respiratory units in the lungs.
— The **thoracic aorta** arises from the left side of the heart and carries oxygenated blood that is distributed to the systemic circulation. It is divided into three sections:
  • The **ascending aorta** arises from the left ventricle of the heart and ascends to the level of the fourth thoracic vertebra. The right and left coronary arteries are its only branches.
  • The **aortic arch** (radiographically, the "aortic knob") ascends anterior to the right pulmonary artery and the

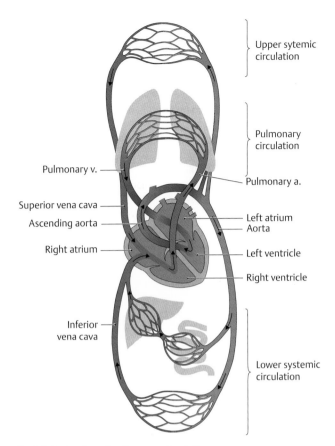

Fig. 3.2   Systemic and pulmonary circulation
Red, oxygenated blood; *blue*, deoxygenated blood.

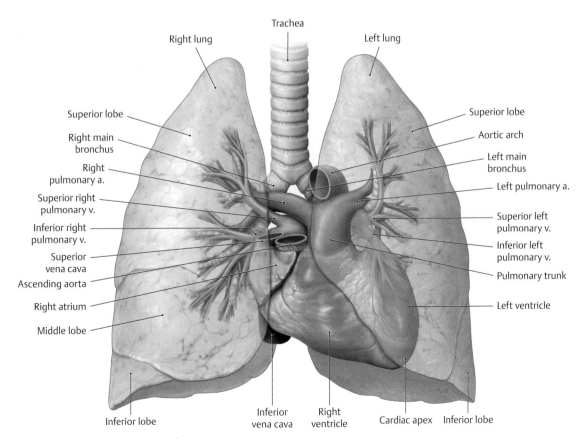

Fig. 3.3   Pulmonary arteries and veins
Distribution of the pulmonary arteries and veins, anterior view.

bifurcation of the trachea (where the trachea splits into right and left bronchi). It courses posteriorly and to the left, arching over the structures entering the left lung, and then turns inferiorly to descend to the left of the trachea and esophagus. It terminates on the left side of the T4 vertebral body. Three large branches arise from the arch (**Fig. 3.4**):

- ○ The **brachiocephalic trunk,** which ascends posterior to the right sternoclavicular joint, where it bifurcates into the **right common carotid** and **right subclavian arteries**

- ○ The **left common carotid artery,** which enters the neck posterior to the left sternoclavicular joint
- ○ The **left subclavian artery,** which arises from the distal segment of the arch and enters the neck posterior to the left sternoclavicular joint
- • The **descending aorta,** a continuation of the aortic arch, descends within the posterior mediastinum, where it passes posterior to the root of the left lung and anterior and to the left of the thoracic vertebral bodies. It passes into the abdomen through the diaphragm at T12. Its thoracic branches (**Fig.3.5**) are

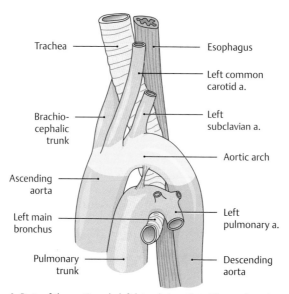

A Parts of the aortic arch, left lateral view. *Note:* The aortic arch begins and ends at the level of the sternal angle (T4-T5).

B Aortic arch angiogram.

Fig. 3.4 **Thoracic aorta**

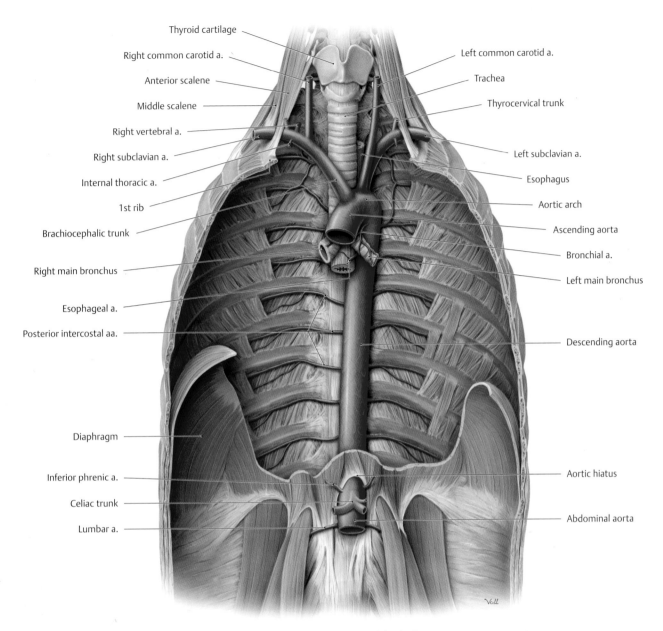

Thyroid cartilage
Right common carotid a.
Anterior scalene
Middle scalene
Right vertebral a.
Right subclavian a.
Internal thoracic a.
1st rib
Brachiocephalic trunk
Right main bronchus
Esophageal a.
Posterior intercostal aa.
Diaphragm
Inferior phrenic a.
Celiac trunk
Lumbar a.

Left common carotid a.
Trachea
Thyrocervical trunk
Left subclavian a.
Esophagus
Aortic arch
Ascending aorta
Bronchial a.
Left main bronchus
Descending aorta
Aortic hiatus
Abdominal aorta

Fig. 3.5 Thoracic aorta in situ, anterior view. *Removed:* Heart, lungs, and portions of the diaphragm.

- o the **posterior intercostal arteries,** which run anteriorly within the 3rd through the 11th intercostal spaces (between the ribs), where they anastomose with the anterior intercostal arteries; and
  - o the visceral branches to the esophagus, trachea, bronchi, and pericardium.
- — The **internal thoracic arteries** arise from the subclavian arteries in the neck and descend deep to the ribs on either side of the sternum. Their branches supply the thoracic and abdominal walls **(Fig. 3.6):**

- The **anterior intercostal arteries,** which run within the intercostal spaces
- The **musculophrenic arteries,** terminal branches of the internal thoracic arteries, which arise at the level of the sixth costal cartilage and follow the lower margin of the ribcage laterally
- The **superior epigastric arteries,** terminal branches of the internal thoracic arteries, which run inferiorly to supply muscles of the anterior abdominal wall

Fig. 3.6 Arteries of the thoracic wall
Anterior view.

Labels (clockwise from top):
Right common carotid a.
Right subclavian a.
Left common carotid a.
Superior thoracic a.
Thyrocervical trunk
Vertebral a.
Thoracoacromial a.
Brachiocephalic trunk
Left subclavian a.
Axillary a.
Internal thoracic a.
2nd intercostal a.
Sternoclavicular joint
Thoracic aorta
Posterior intercostal a.
Thoraco-dorsal a.
Dorsal ramus
Lateral thoracic a.
Internal thoracic a.
Anterior intercostal aa.
Anterior intercostal a.
Abdominal aorta
Superior epigastric a.
Musculophrenic a.
Aortic bifurcation

Veins of the Thorax (Fig. 3.7)

— **Internal thoracic veins,** which receive the anterior intercostal veins, accompany the internal thoracic arteries and drain into the brachiocephalic veins of the superior mediastinum.
— The **right** and **left brachiocephalic veins,** which drain the head, neck, and upper limb, form behind the clavicle by the convergence of the internal jugular and subclavian veins. The left brachiocephalic vein, which is longer than the right, crosses the midline just anterior to the branches of the aortic arch and converges with the right brachiocephalic vein to form the superior vena cava.
— The **superior vena cava,** which returns deoxygenated blood from the upper body to the heart, forms on the right side, posterior to the costal cartilage of the first rib by the junction of the brachiocephalic veins. It descends behind and to the right side of the aorta and drains into the superior pole of the right atrium.
— The **inferior vena cava,** which returns deoxygenated blood to the heart from the abdomen, pelvis, and lower limbs, enters the right atrium after passing through the diaphragm from the abdomen. Only a small portion, therefore, is located within the thorax.
— The **pulmonary veins,** two on each side (often three on the left side), carry oxygenated blood from the lungs to the left side of the heart (see **Fig. 3.3**).

— The **azygos system** drains veins of the thoracic and antero-lateral abdominal walls (**Fig. 3.8**; see also **Fig. 3.7**).
  • The **azygos vein** ascends along the right side of the thoracic vertebral bodies as it drains the **posterior intercostal veins** of the thoracic wall on that side. It arches over the root of the right lung to empty into the superior vena cava.
  • The **accessory hemiazygos** and **hemiazygos veins** run along the left side of the thoracic vertebrae and drain the thoracic wall on the left side. They cross the midline independently (or they may join to form a single vessel) to drain into the azygos vein on the right side.
  • The azygos and hemiazygos veins are the continuations of the **ascending lumbar veins** in the abdomen, which

CLINICAL CORRELATION

SUPERIOR VENA CAVA SYNDROME The superior vena cava syndrome is an obstruction of the superior vena cava (SVC), which in the majority of cases is caused by mediastinal tumors such as metastatic lung carcinoma (the upper lobe of the right lung lies next to the SVC), lymphoma, breast cancer, or thyroid cancer. Noncancerous causes include thromboses (blood clots) that obstruct the lumen and infections that produce scarring. The onset of symptoms is usually gradual and includes dyspnea (shortness of breath) and swelling of the face, neck, and arms.

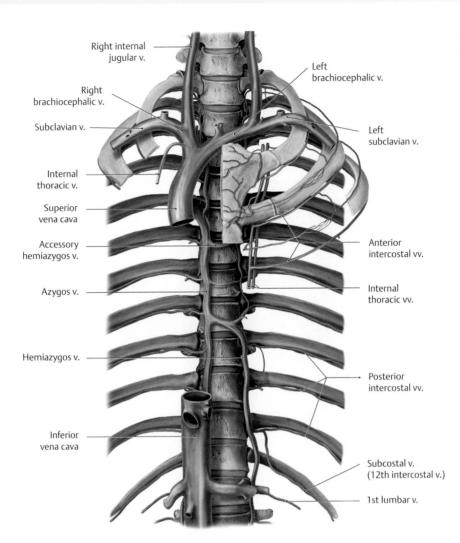

Fig. 3.7 Veins of the thoracic wall
Anterior view with rib cage opened. *Removed:* Clavicle.

Right internal jugular v.

Right brachiocephalic v.

Subclavian v.

Internal thoracic v.

Superior vena cava

Accessory hemiazygos v.

Azygos v.

Hemiazygos v.

Inferior vena cava

Left brachiocephalic v.

Left subclavian v.

Anterior intercostal vv.

Internal thoracic vv.

Posterior intercostal vv.

Subcostal v. (12th intercostal v.)

1st lumbar v.

Fig. 3.7 Veins of the thoracic wall
Anterior view with rib cage opened. *Removed:* Clavicle.

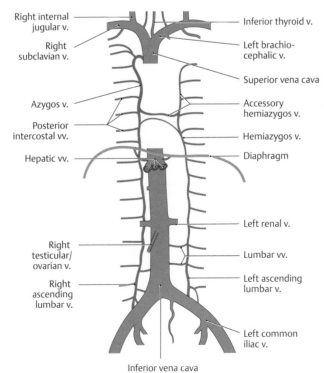

Right internal jugular v.

Right subclavian v.

Azygos v.

Posterior intercostal vv.

Hepatic vv.

Right testicular/ ovarian v.

Right ascending lumbar v.

Inferior thyroid v.

Left brachio-cephalic v.

Superior vena cava

Accessory hemiazygos v.

Hemiazygos v.

Diaphragm

Left renal v.

Lumbar vv.

Left ascending lumbar v.

Left common iliac v.

Inferior vena cava

Fig. 3.8 Azygos system
Anterior view.

communicate with the inferior vena cava. Thus the azygos system links the drainages of the superior and inferior vena cavae and provides a collateral (alternate) pathway for blood back to the heart.

- **Mediastinal, esophageal,** and **bronchial veins** in the thorax, and the vertebral venous plexus (see Section 2.2) are also tributaries of the azygos system.

Lymphatics of the Thorax (see Fig. 1.20)

— The **thoracic duct,** the main lymphatic vessel of the body,
  - drains the abdomen, pelvis, and lower limbs, and the left side of the thorax, head, neck, and left upper limb;
  - enters the thorax from its origin in the abdomen and passes superiorly in the midline of the posterior mediastinum; and
  - terminates at the junction of the left subclavian and left internal jugular veins (jugulosubclavian junction or "venous angle") in the neck.
— The **right lymphatic duct,** which has a variable form,
  - drains lymph from the right side of the thorax, head, and neck, and the right upper limb; and
  - usually terminates at the junction of the right subclavian and right internal jugular veins (the jugulosubclavian junction).
— Lymph from most thoracic structures drains through chains of lymph nodes that empty into **bronchomediastinal trunks** in the mediastinum (**Figs. 3.9** and **3.10**). This includes

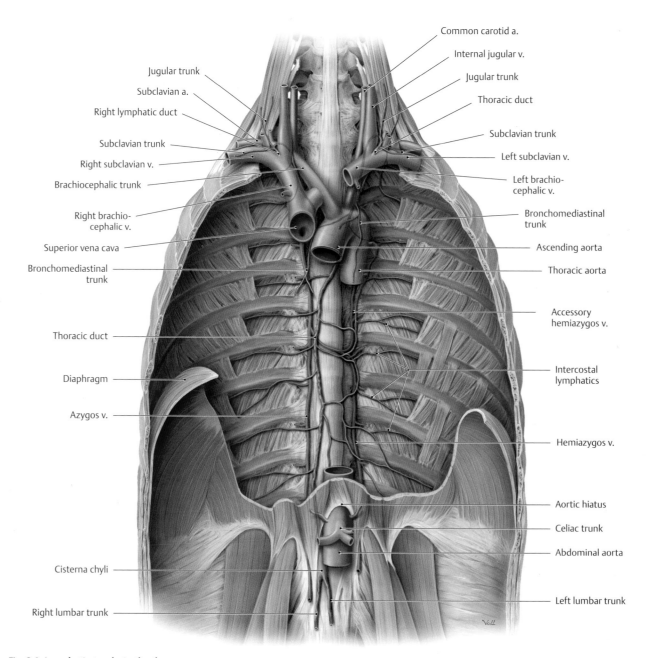

Common carotid a.

Internal jugular v.

Jugular trunk

Thoracic duct

Subclavian trunk

Left subclavian v.

Left brachio-
cephalic v.

Bronchomediastinal
trunk

Ascending aorta

Thoracic aorta

Accessory
hemiazygos v.

Intercostal
lymphatics

Hemiazygos v.

Aortic hiatus

Celiac trunk

Abdominal aorta

Left lumbar trunk

Jugular trunk

Subclavian a.

Right lymphatic duct

Subclavian trunk

Right subclavian v.

Brachiocephalic trunk

Right brachio-
cephalic v.

Superior vena cava

Bronchomediastinal
trunk

Thoracic duct

Diaphragm

Azygos v.

Cisterna chyli

Right lumbar trunk

Fig. 3.9 Lymphatic trunks in the thorax
Anterior view of opened thorax.

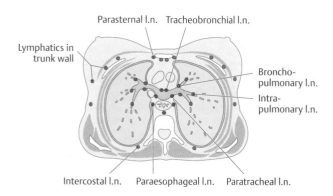

Parasternal l.n.   Tracheobronchial l.n.

Lymphatics in
trunk wall

Broncho-
pulmonary l.n.

Intra-
pulmonary l.n.

Intercostal l.n.   Paraesophageal l.n.   Paratracheal l.n.

Fig. 3.10 Thoracic lymph nodes
Transverse section at the level of the tracheal bifurcation (at approximately T4), viewed from below. Topographically, the thoracic lymph
nodes can be divided into three broad groups:
— Lymph nodes in the thoracic wall (pink)
— Lymph nodes in the lung and at the divisions of the bronchial tree
  (blue)
— Lymph nodes associated with the trachea, esophagus, and pericardium
  (green)

- parasternal and intercostal lymph nodes of the thoracic wall and superior surface of the diaphragm;
- bronchopulmonary and intrapulmonary lymph nodes of the lungs and bronchi; and
- tracheobronchial, paratracheal, and paraesophageal lymph nodes of the heart, pericardium, trachea, and esophagus.
— The bronchomediastinal trunks may empty into the thoracic and right lymphatic ducts, but, more commonly, they empty directly into the subclavian veins in the neck.

Nerves of the Thorax (Figs. 3.11, 3.12, 3.13)

— Pairs of **posterior intercostal nerves** arise from the anterior rami of T1–T11 and pass along the inferior edge of the ribs on their deep surface.
  - The nerves innervate the muscles between the ribs, overlying muscles and skin of the thoracic wall and the breast.
— **Phrenic nerves** arise in the neck from anterior rami of C3, C4, and C5 ("to keep the diaphragm alive") and descend into the thorax.
  - On the right, the nerve runs along the superior vena cava; on the left, it crosses lateral to the aortic arch.
  - Both nerves pass anterior to the hila of the lungs as they descend to the diaphragm between the pericardial and pleural sacs.

- The phrenic nerves innervate the pericardium, the medial part of the pleura, and the diaphragm.
— The **thoracic sympathetic trunks** run along either side of the thoracic vertebral column.
  - Sympathetic (paravertebral) ganglia at each spinal level communicate with spinal nerves through white and gray rami communicans.
  - The T1 ganglion may combine with the ganglion at C8 to form a large stellate (star-shaped) ganglion.
  - Splanchnic nerves, derived from the sympathetic trunk, pass medially to contribute to the autonomic plexuses of the thorax, which innervate thoracic viscera.
— Nerves derived from the thoracic sympathetic trunk, called the **greater** (T5 to T9 or T10), **lesser** (T10–T11), and **least splanchnic nerves** course inferomedially along the thoracic vertebral bodies into the abdomen. They contain preganglionic fibers that synapse in prevertebral ganglia of abdominal autonomic nerve plexuses **(Table 3.2)**.
— The **vagus nerves** (cranial nerve X) descend from the neck into the thorax.
  - The right vagus courses behind the superior vena cava, medial to the arch of the azygos vein; the left vagus runs lateral to the aortic arch.
  - Both vagus nerves pass posterior to the hilum of the lung before merging on the wall of the esophagus.

Trachea

Right subclavian a.

Right recurrent laryngeal n.

Right vagus n.

Intercostal n.

Right main bronchus

Esophagus, thoracic part

Sympathetic trunk

Anterior vagal trunk with esophageal plexus

Greater splanchnic n.

Left common carotid a.

Left vagus n.

Left recurrent laryngeal n.

Aortic arch

Left main bronchus

Thoracic aorta

Sympathetic trunk

Diaphragm

Anterior gastric plexus

Stomach

Fig. 3.11 Nerves of the posterior mediastinum
Anterior view.

Fig. 3.12 Nerves of the thorax
Anterior view of opened thorax.

- The vagus nerves contribute parasympathetic fibers to the cardiac, pulmonary, and esophageal plexuses (**Table 3.3**).
- The **left recurrent laryngeal nerve,** a branch of the left vagus nerve, passes under the aortic arch, posterior to the **ligamentum arteriosum** (see Section 5.6), and turns superiorly to ascend in the neck in the groove between the trachea and esophagus.
  - The right recurrent laryngeal nerve, a branch of the right vagus, recurs around the subclavian artery in the neck and is not a thoracic structure.
- The **esophageal plexus** surrounds the lower esophagus.
  - It is composed of preganglionic parasympathetic fibers from the right and left vagus nerves and postganglionic fibers from the thoracic sympathetic trunk.

- **Anterior** and **posterior vagal trunks** arise from the plexus and pass into the abdomen, anterior and posterior to the esophagus.
- The **cardiac plexus (Figs. 3.12** and **3.13)**, which is located above the heart in the concavity of the arch of the aorta, continues along the coronary arteries. It innervates the conducting system of the heart and contains
  - preganglionic sympathetic fibers from T1 to T5 and postganglionic sympathetic fibers from cardiopulmonary branches of the cervical and thoracic sympathetic trunk;
  - preganglionic parasympathetic fibers from cardiac branches of the vagus nerve that arise in the cervical region and contributions from the recurrent laryngeal nerves; and

Table 3.2 **Peripheral sympathetic nervous system**

Origin of Preganglionic Fibers*	Ganglion Cells	Course of Postganglionic Fibers	Target
Spinal cord	Sympathetic trunk	Follow intercostal nn.	Blood vessels and glands in chest wall
		Accompany intrathoracic aa.	Visceral targets
		Gather in greater and lesser splanchnic nn.	Abdomen

*The axons of preganglionic neurons exit the spinal cord via the anterior roots and synapse with postganglionic neurons in the sympathetic ganglia.

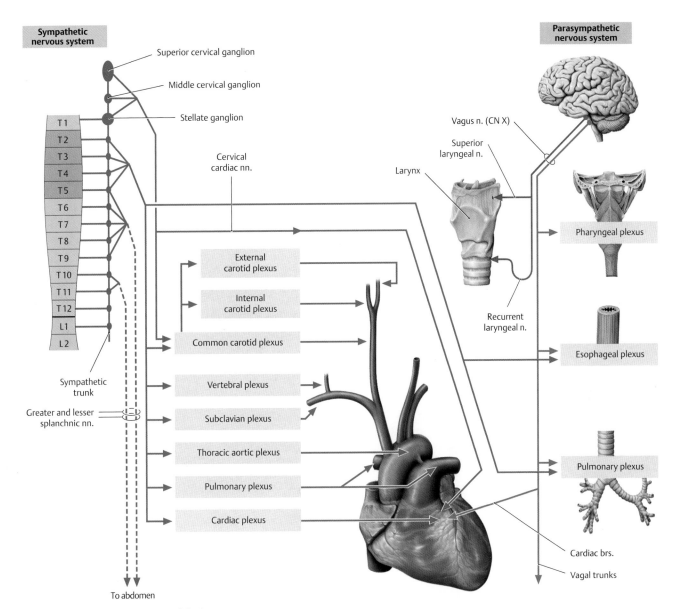

Fig. 3.13 Autonomic innervation of the heart
Schematic.

- visceral sensory fibers that travel with sympathetic and parasympathetic nerves.
- The **pulmonary plexus** is a continuation of the cardiac plexus onto the bifurcation of the trachea and the bronchi that penetrate the hilum of each lung.

- It regulates the constriction and dilation of the pulmonary vessels and respiratory passages.
- It transmits sensation from the lung and visceral, or inner, layer of the pleural sac that is adherent to the surface of the lung.

Table 3.3 **Peripheral Parasympathetic Nervous System**

Origin of Preganglionic Fibers	Course of Postganglionic Motor Axons		Target
Brainstem	Vagus n. (CN X)	Cardiac brs.	Cardiac plexus
		Esophageal brs.	Esophageal plexus
		Tracheal brs.	Trachea
		Bronchial brs.	Pulmonary plexus (bronchi, pulmonary vessels)

*The ganglion cells of the parasympathetic nervous system are scattered in microscopic groups in their target organs. The vagus n. thus carries the preganglionic motor axons to these targets.
CN, cranial n.

4 Thoracic Wall

A bony and muscular cage, which communicates superiorly with the neck and inferiorly with the abdomen, encloses and protects the thoracic contents. A superficial layer of extrinsic muscles overlies the thoracic cage, although these muscles act primarily on the upper limb. The breast, a derivative of the epidermis (outermost layer of skin), is a prominent superficial structure of the thoracic wall.

4.1 The Breast

General Features

The breast is made up of the **mammary gland,** a modified sweat gland, and its supporting fat and fibrous tissue (**Figs. 4.1, 4.2, 4.3**). Breasts remain rudimentary in males but are prominent structures of the female pectoral region.

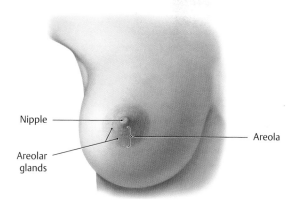

Fig. 4.1 Surface anatomy of the breast
Right breast, anterior view.

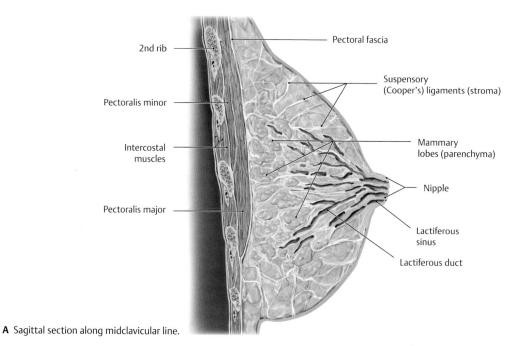

A Sagittal section along midclavicular line.

B Duct system and portions of a mammary lobe. In the nonlactating breast (shown here), the lobules contain clusters of rudimentary acini.

Fig. 4.2 Structure of the breast

C Structure of a mammary lobe.

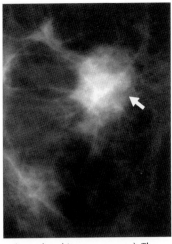

Nipple —

A Normal mammogram.

B Mammograms of invasive duct carcinoma (irregular white areas, *arrows*). The large lesion has changed the architecture of the neighboring breast tissue.

Fig. 4.3 Mammogram of the breast

— Female breasts extend from the lateral border of the sternum to the midaxillary line and overlie the 2nd through 6th ribs.
— The breast is embedded in the subcutaneous layer of the skin overlying the deep fascia of the pectoralis major and serratus anterior muscles.
— The **retromammary space** is a plane of loose connective tissue that separates the breast from underlying fascia of the pectoralis major muscle and allows movement of the breasts on the thoracic wall.
— The highest prominence of the breast, the **nipple,** is located at the center of the areola. Circularly arranged smooth muscle fibers cause erection of the nipple in response to cold or tactile stimulation. In men and young women, the nipple is at the T4 vertebral level, but in older women this location varies considerably.
— The **areola,** the pigmented skin surrounding the nipple, contains sebaceous glands whose oily secretions lubricate the area during nursing.
— An **axillary tail,** or small finger of glandular tissue, may extend into the axilla (armpit) along the lower edge of the pectoralis muscle.
— The volume of fat, not the volume of glandular tissue, largely determines the differences in breast size among women.

Mammary Gland

The mammary gland has two components:
— The **parenchyma,** or milk-producing part of the gland (see **Fig. 4.2A**)
  • The parenchyma consists of lobes divided into 15 to 20 lobules, which contain grapelike clusters of **alveoli,** hollow balls lined by secretory cells.
  • **Lactiferous ducts** in the parenchyma drain each lobule and open at the nipple. Deep to the areola, each duct has a small, dilated portion called the **lactiferous sinus** where, in lactating females, a small amount of milk is stored.
— The **stroma,** or fibrous framework, of the gland that separates the lobules and supports the lobes
  • Stroma is attached to the overlying dermis of the skin by **suspensory (Cooper) ligaments,** which are particularly strong on the superior surface of the breast.

Neurovasculature of the Breast

— Anterior intercostal branches and medial mammary branches (from perforating branches) of the internal thoracic artery, **lateral thoracic** and **thoracoacromial branches** of the axillary artery, and the 2nd, 3rd, and 4th posterior intercostal arteries supply the breast (see **Fig. 3.5**).
— Venous blood drains primarily to the axillary vein but also to the internal thoracic vein.
— Most lymph (> 75%) from the breast drains (particularly from the lateral quadrant) to axillary lymph nodes (**Fig. 4.4**); from there it travels to nodes around the clavicle and the ipsilateral lymphatic duct.
  • Some lymph may drain to deep pectoral nodes, where it joins the bronchomediastinal drainage in the mediastinum.
  • Medial portions of the breast may drain to parasternal nodes and to the contralateral breast; inferior segments may drain to abdominal nodes.

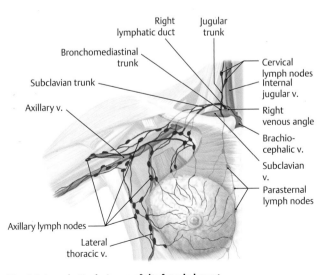

Fig. 4.4 Lymphatic drainage of the female breast
Axillary, parasternal, and cervical lymph nodes. Right thoracic and axillary region with the arm abducted, anterior view.

Fig. 4.5 **Origin of malignant breast tumors by quadrant**

— The anterior and lateral cutaneous branches of the 4th, 5th, and 6th intercostal nerves innervate the breast.

CLINICAL CORRELATION

CARCINOMA OF THE BREAST The most common type of breast cancer, invasive ductal carcinoma, arises from the lining of the lactiferous ducts. Typically, it metastasizes through lymphatic channels, most abundantly to axillary nodes from the supralateral quadrant **(Fig. 4.5)**, but it may also travel to supraclavicular nodes, the contralateral breast, and the abdomen. Obstruction of the lymphatic drainage causes edema, and fibrosis (shortening) of the suspensory ligaments can cause a pitted appearance of the skin. Through venous communication with the azygos system and vertebral venous plexus, breast cancer can metastasize to the vertebrae, cranium, and brain. Elevation of the breast with contraction of the pectoralis major muscle suggests invasion of the pectoralis fascia and retromammary space.

4.2   The Thoracic Skeleton

The thoracic skeleton protects the thoracic viscera and provides attachment for the upper limb. The thoracic cage includes the sternum, 12 pairs of ribs, and the 12 thoracic vertebrae **(Fig. 4.6;** see also Section 2.1).

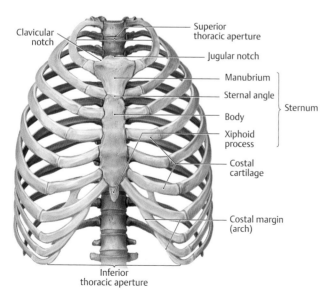

Fig. 4.6 **Thoracic skeleton**
Anterior view.

The Sternum

The **sternum** is a flat, elongated bone that has three parts:

1. The **manubrium,** which articulates laterally with the costal cartilages (cartilage that attaches the ribs to the sternum) of the 1st and 2nd ribs. A deep **jugular notch** separates the right and left sternoclavicular joints, where the manubrium articulates with the clavicles.
2. The **body,** which is fused superiorly with the manubrium at the **manubriosternal joint.** Laterally, the body articulates with costal cartilages of the 2nd to 7th ribs.
3. The **xiphoid process,** the lowest part of the sternum, which joins superiorly with the body of the sternum at the xiphisternal joint.
   • The **sternal angle** is an important surface landmark on the anterior thoracic wall that provides orientation to the internal anatomy of the thorax. It is a palpable ridge that marks the fusion of the manubrium and body of the sternum. A horizontal plane through the sternal angle intersects
   ◦ the articulation between the sternum and the costal cartilages of the 2nd ribs,
   ◦ the division of the mediastinum into superior and inferior regions,
   ◦ the origin and termination of the aortic arch,
   ◦ the bifurcation of the trachea, and
   ◦ the T4–T5 intervertebral disk.

The Ribs

— The ribs are numbered 1 to 12 from superior to inferior, and each rib articulates with a thoracic vertebra of the same number.
— The ribs hang obliquely downward from their articulation with the vertebral column. Their anterior ends may be two to five vertebral levels lower than their posterior attachment **(Fig. 4.7)**.
— Ribs 1 to 10 articulate anteriorly with a cartilaginous segment called the **costal cartilage.**
— The ribs are classified according to their articulation with the sternum (see **Fig. 4.7**):
   • **True ribs** (1 to 7) articulate directly with the sternum via individual costal cartilages.
   • **False ribs** (8 to 10) articulate indirectly with the sternum through costal cartilages that are connected to the cartilage superior to it.

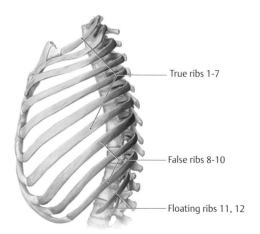

Fig. 4.7 **Types of ribs**
Left lateral view.

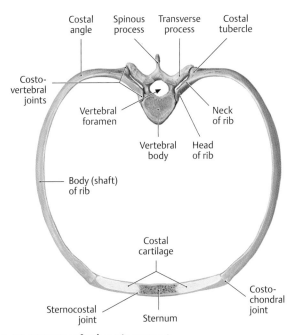

Fig. 4.8 **Structure of a thoracic segment**
Superior view of 6th rib pair.

- **Floating ribs** (11 and 12) have no connection to the sternum.
— Most ribs articulate at three joints (**Fig. 4.8**):
  1. **Costochondral joints** between the bony segments of ribs 1 to 10 and their respective **costal cartilages**
  2. **Sternocostal joints** between the sternum and costal cartilages of ribs 1 to 7 on each side
  3. **Costovertebral joints** between the ribs and vertebrae. These joints may contain multiple articulations.
     - The **costal tubercle** of each rib articulates with the costal facet on its accompanying vertebra (see **Fig. 2.7A**).

- The **heads** of ribs 2 to 10 articulate with the vertebra of the same number and with the vertebra superior to them. Ribs 1, 11, and 12 articulate only with their own vertebra.

Thoracic Apertures

— The thoracic cage has superior and inferior openings (see **Fig. 4.6**):
  - The **superior thoracic aperture (thoracic inlet)**, which is bounded by the T1 vertebra, the 1st ribs, and the manubrium of the sternum. The thorax communicates with the neck through this opening.
  - The **inferior thoracic aperture (thoracic outlet)**, which is bounded by the T12 vertebra, the 11th and 12th ribs, the **costal margin** (lower border of the thoracic cage), and the xiphoid process. A muscular diaphragm closes this aperture, separating the thoracic cavity from the abdominal cavity (see Section 4.3).

4.3 Muscles of the Thorax

Muscles of the Thoracic Wall (Fig. 4.9; Table 4.1)

— Extrinsic muscles of the upper limb, including the **pectoralis major, pectoralis minor,** and **serratus anterior,** cover the

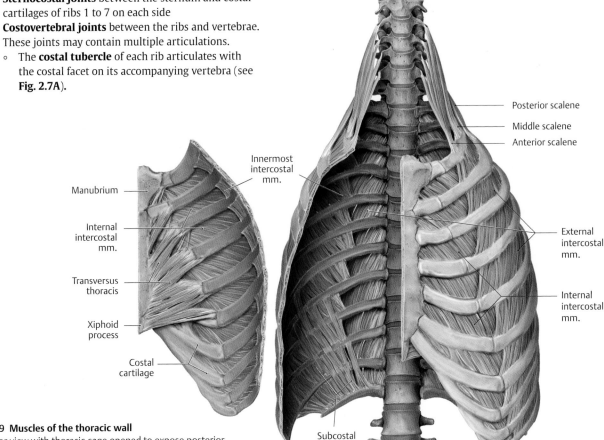

Fig. 4.9 **Muscles of the thoracic wall**
Anterior view with thoracic cage opened to expose posterior surface of anterior wall.

Table 4.1 **Muscles of the Thoracic Wall**

Muscle		Origin	Insertion	Innervation	Action
Scalene mm.	Anterior scalene	C3–C6 (transverse processes, anterior tubercles)	1st rib (anterior scalene tubercles)	C3–C6	Raise the upper ribs during inspiration
	Middle scalene	C3–C7 (transverse processes, posterior tubercles)	1st rib (posterior to groove for subclavian a.)		
	Posterior scalene	C5–C7 (transverse processes, posterior tubercles)	2nd rib (outer surface)		
Intercostal mm.	External intercostal mm.	Lower margin of rib to upper margin of next lower rib (courses obliquely forward and downward from costal tubercle to chondro-osseous junction)		1st to 11th intercostal nn.	Raise the ribs during inspiration
	Internal intercostal mm.	Lower margin of rib to upper margin of next lower rib (courses obliquely forward and upward from costal angle to sternum)			Lower the ribs during expiration
	Innermost intercostal mm.				
Subcostal mm.		Lower margin of lower ribs to inner surface of ribs two to three ribs below		Adjacent lower intercostal nn.	Lower the ribs during expiration
Transversus thoracis		Sternum and xiphoid process (inner surface)	2nd to 6th ribs (costal cartilage, inner surface)	2nd to 6th intercostal nn.	Weakly lower the ribs during expiration

thorax. Although they mainly move or stabilize the upper limb, these muscles also assist in movements of the ribs during deep inspiration. (See Chapter 13, Overview of the Upper Limb.)

— The **anterior scalene, middle scalene,** and **posterior scalene muscles** originate on the transverse processes of the cervical vertebrae and insert onto the 1st and 2nd ribs. They assist the intrinsic thoracic muscles during inspiration and are considered extrinsic muscles of respiration.

— Intrinsic muscles of the thoracic wall are the chief muscles that move the ribs during respiration.

- The **intercostal muscles** occupy the intercostal spaces between the ribs. They extend from the inferior border of one rib to the superior border of the next inferior rib. The intercostal muscles move the ribs primarily during forced respiration. During quiet respiration, they stabilize the thoracic wall. They include
  - the **external intercostal muscles,** with fibers directed inferoanteriorly, which make up the most superficial layer
  - the **internal intercostal** and **innermost intercostal muscles,** which occupy the middle and deepest layers of the thoracic wall, respectively, with their fibers directed inferoposteriorly

- The **subcostal muscles** are most prominent along the lower thoracic wall, where they cross the inner surface of one or two intercostal spaces.
- The **transversus thoracic muscles** consist of four of five thin slips that extend superiorly and laterally from the posterior surface of the sternum to the ribs.

The Thoracic Diaphragm

The **thoracic diaphragm** (or simply, the **diaphragm**), a musculo-tendinous sheet that separates the thorax from the abdomen, is the principal muscle of respiration. The diaphragm forms the floor of the thorax, the roof of the abdomen, and a portion of the posterior abdominal wall (**Fig. 4.10**).

— The skeletal muscle fibers of the diaphragm originate along the costal margin, the vertebral bodies of L1–L3, the **medial** and **lateral arcuate ligaments,** and the xiphoid process. They insert on the diaphragm's **central tendon.**

— **Right** and **left crura,** extensions of the posterior diaphragm, attach to the bodies of the lumbar vertebrae, with the right crus extending slightly lower than the left crus.

— The domes on the right and left sides of the diaphragm are asymmetric; the right hemidiaphragm is generally higher than the left.

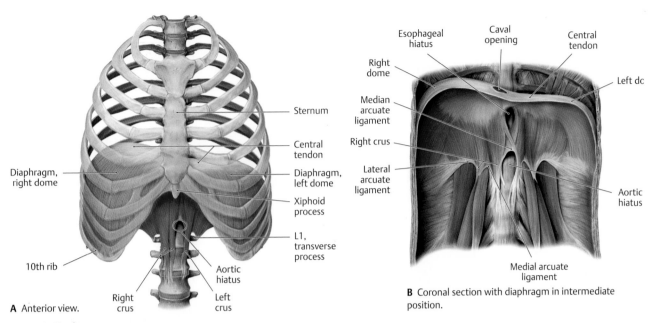

A Anterior view.

B Coronal section with diaphragm in intermediate position.

Fig. 4.10 Diaphragm
The diaphragm, which separates the thorax from the abdomen, has two asymmetric domes and three apertures (for the aorta, vena cava, and esophagus).

— During full expiration the diaphragm is 4 to 6 cm higher than during full inspiration. During expiration it ascends to the level of the 4th or 5th rib on the right and slightly lower on the left, although this varies with respiration, posture, and body type.

— The diaphragm has three openings to allow the passage of structures between the thorax and abdomen (**Fig. 4.11**):
  1. The **caval aperture** (hiatus), which is a passage for the inferior vena cava through the central tendon at the T8 vertebral level.
  2. The **esophageal aperture** (hiatus), which is an opening at the T10 vertebral level for the esophagus, the anterior and posterior vagal trunks, and left gastric artery and vein.It is usually formed by the right crus of the diaphragm (occasionally by the right and left crura) that, when contracted, forms a sphincter around the esophagus.
  3. The **aortic aperture (hiatus)**, which is a passageway for the aorta between the right and left crura as it passes behind the diaphragm at T12. The thoracic duct, and often the azygos and hemiazygos veins, also passes through this aperture.

— The inferior phrenic arteries, branches of the abdominal aorta (or celiac trunk), are the primary blood supply to the diaphragm. The superior phrenic, pericardiacophrenic, and musculophrenic arteries make additional contributions (**Fig. 4.12**).

— Venous blood drains to the azygos system through posterior intercostal and superior phrenic veins.

— The phrenic nerve (C3–C5) provides all of the motor and most of the sensory innervation to the diaphragm. The subcostal and lower intercostal nerves supply sensory innervation to the periphery of the diaphragm (**Fig. 4.13**).

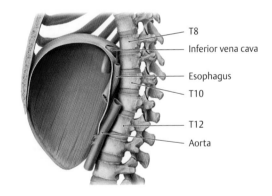

Fig. 4.11 Diaphragmatic apertures
Left lateral view.

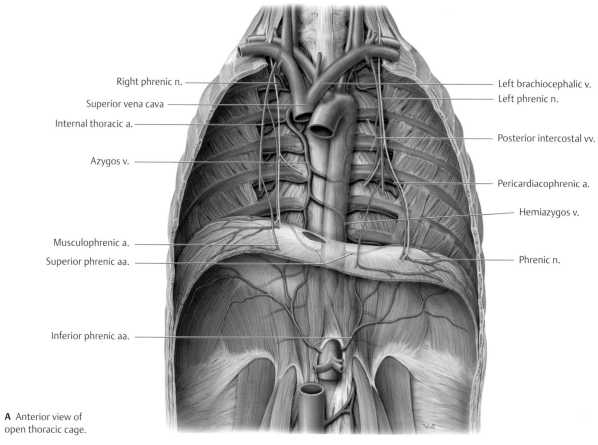

Right phrenic n.

Superior vena cava

Internal thoracic a.

Azygos v.

Musculophrenic a.

Superior phrenic aa.

Inferior phrenic aa.

Left brachiocephalic v.

Left phrenic n.

Posterior intercostal vv.

Pericardiacophrenic a.

Hemiazygos v.

Phrenic n.

A Anterior view of open thoracic cage.

Spinal cord

Sympathetic trunk   Thoracic aorta   Hemiazygos v.

Intercostal n.

Azygos v.

Right superior phrenic a.

Inferior vena cava

Parietal pleura, costal part

Musculophrenic a. (from internal thoracic a.)

Parietal pleura, costal part

Parietal pleura, diaphragmatic part

Left superior phrenic a. (from thoracic aorta)

Parietal pleura, mediastinal part

Esophagus

Phrenic n., pericardiacophrenic a. and v.

Pericardium

Internal thoracic a. and vv.

Sternum

B Superior view of diaphragm.

Fig. 4.12 Neurovasculature of the diaphragm

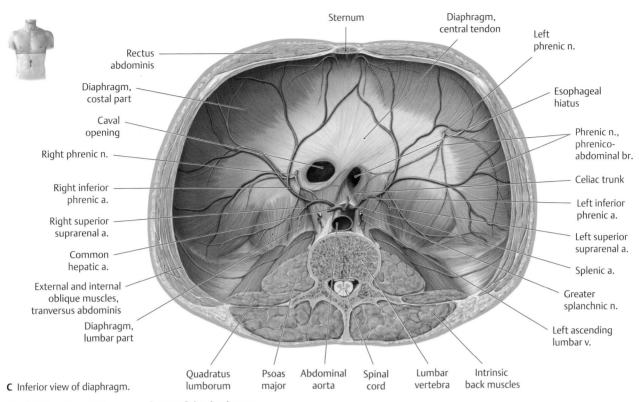

Sternum

Diaphragm, central tendon

Left phrenic n.

Rectus abdominis

Diaphragm, costal part

Esophageal hiatus

Caval opening

Phrenic n., phrenico-abdominal br.

Right phrenic n.

Celiac trunk

Right inferior phrenic a.

Left inferior phrenic a.

Right superior suprarenal a.

Left superior suprarenal a.

Common hepatic a.

Splenic a.

External and internal oblique muscles, tranversus abdominis

Greater splanchnic n.

Diaphragm, lumbar part

Left ascending lumbar v.

Quadratus lumborum

Psoas major

Abdominal aorta

Spinal cord

Lumbar vertebra

Intrinsic back muscles

C Inferior view of diaphragm.

Fig. 4.12 (*continued*) **Neurovasculature of the diaphragm**

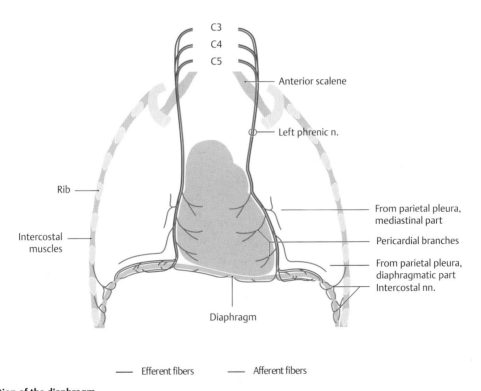

C3

C4

C5

Anterior scalene

Left phrenic n.

Rib

Intercostal muscles

From parietal pleura, mediastinal part

Pericardial branches

From parietal pleura, diaphragmatic part

Intercostal nn.

Diaphragm

—— Efferent fibers   —— Afferent fibers

Fig. 4.13 Innervation of the diaphragm
Anterior view. The phrenic nerve lies on the lateral surface of the fibrous pericardium together with the pericardiacophrenic arteries and veins. *Note:* The phrenic nerve also innervates the pericardium.

4.4　Neurovasculature of the Thoracic Wall

— Intercostal neurovascular bundles course along the inferior surface of the ribs within the costal groove **(Fig 4.14)**.
  • Anterior intercostal arteries (branches of the internal thoracic arteries) and posterior intercostal arteries (branches of the thoracic aorta and axillary arteries) supply the muscles and skin of the thoracic wall (see **Fig. 3.6**).
  • Intercostal veins drain primarily to the azygos system but also into the brachiocephalic and internal thoracic veins, which join the superior vena cava (see **Fig. 3.7**).

— The **thoracoepigastric vein** is a superficial vein that drains the subcutaneous tissue of the anterolateral thoracic and abdominal walls. It drains superiorly to the axillary vein of the upper limb and inferiorly to the superficial epigastric vein **(Fig. 4.15)**.
— The thoracic wall is drained by three major groups of lymph nodes:
  • The **parasternal nodes,** which are scattered along the internal thoracic artery. They receive lymph from the breast, anterior thoracic wall, liver, and upper deep surface of the anterior abdominal wall.
  • The **intercostal nodes,** which are located in the intercostal spaces near the heads and necks of the ribs. They

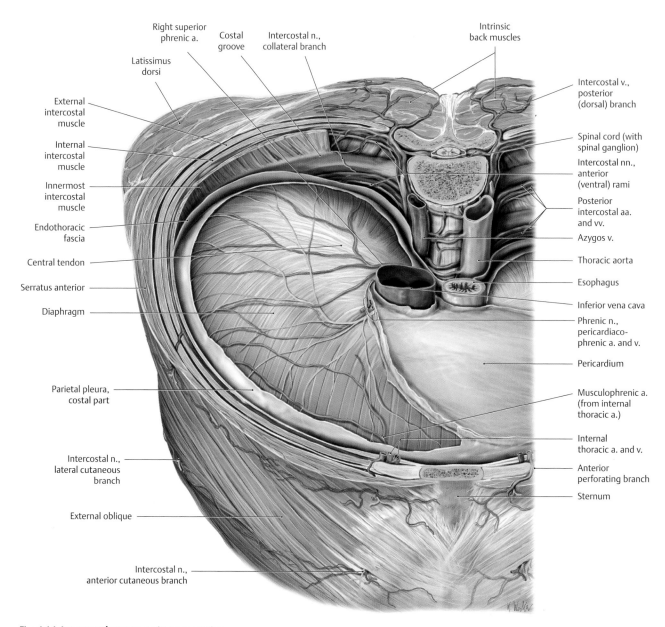

Fig. 4.14 Intercostal structures in cross section
Transverse section, anterosuperior view.

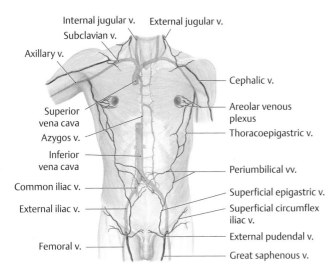

Fig. 4.15 **Superficial veins**
Anterior view. The thoracoepigastric veins are a potential superficial collateral venous drainage route in the event of superior or inferior vena cava obstruction.

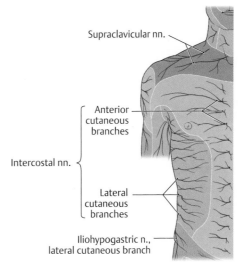

A Sensory nerves of the anterior thoracic wall.

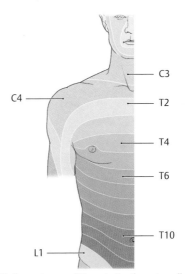

B Dermatomes of the anterior thoracic wall.
Landmarks: T4 generally includes the nipple; T6 innervates the skin over the xiphoid.

Fig. 4.16 **Cutaneous innervation of the thoracic wall**
Anterior view.

drain the posterolateral part of the chest and mammary glands.
- The **diaphragmatic nodes,** which are located on the superior surface of the diaphragm. They drain the central tendon of the diaphragm, the fibrous pericardium, and the superior surface of the liver.
— Intercostal nerves T1–T11 innervate the muscles of the thoracic wall. In the midaxillary line these nerves give off a lateral cutaneous branch that supplies the superficial muscles and skin of the thorax (**Fig. 4.16**).
— Intercostal nerves and vessels are protected within the **costal groove** on the deep inferior edge of the ribs (see **Fig. 4.14**). Within this bundle of neurovascular structures, the nerve runs inferior to its accompanying vessels.
— The 7th through 11th intercostal nerves continue anteriorly from the intercostal space to innervate the anterior abdominal wall.
— Landmark dermatomes on the thoracic wall include T4 at the nipple and T6 over the xiphoid process.

5 Mediastinum

The **mediastinum** is the region within the thorax between the right and left pulmonary cavities (**Fig 5.1**; see **Table 3.1**). The sternum and the costal cartilages of ribs 1 through 7 form its anterior boundary, and the thoracic vertebrae form its posterior boundary.

The mediastinum contains the heart, great vessels, and pericardium, as well as the esophagus, trachea, thymus, and associated neurovasculature (**Fig. 5.2**).

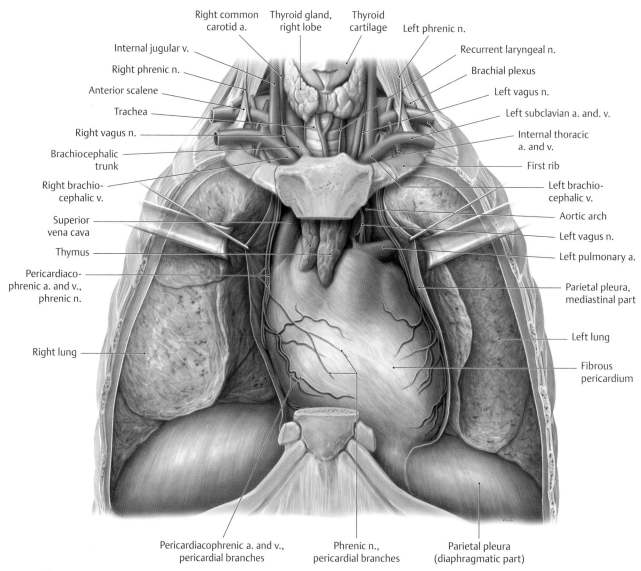

Fig. 5.1 Thoracic cavity
Opened thoracic cavity. *Removed:* Thoracic wall; connective tissue of anterior mediastinum.

5.1   Regions of the Mediastinum (Table 5.1)

— A horizontal plane passing through the sternal angle (at the T4-T5 intervertebral disk) divides the region into a **superior mediastinum,** bounded above by the superior thoracic aperture, and an **inferior mediastinum** limited inferiorly by the thoracic diaphragm.

— The inferior mediastinum is further divided into
  - the **anterior mediastinum,** a narrow space posterior to the sternum and anterior to the pericardium;
  - the **middle mediastinum,** the largest section of the inferior mediastinum, which contains the pericardium, heart, and major vessels; and
  - the **posterior mediastinum,** a small area posterior to the pericardium and anterior to the 5th through 12th thoracic vertebrae.

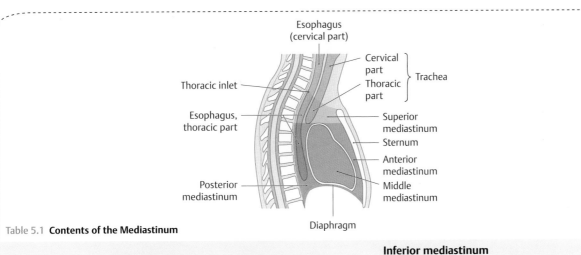

Table 5.1 Contents of the Mediastinum

| | Superior mediastinum ○ | Inferior mediastinum | | |
		Anterior ○	Middle ○	Posterior ○
Organs	• Thymus • Trachea • Esophagus	• Thymus, inferior aspects (especially in children)	• Heart • Pericardium	• Esophagus
Arteries	• Aortic arch • Brachiocephalic trunk • Left common carotid a. • Left subclavian a.	• Smaller vessels	• Ascending aorta • Pulmonary trunk and branches • Pericardiaco-phrenic aa.	• Thoracic aorta and branches
Veins and lymph vessels	• Superior vena cava • Brachiocephalic vv. • Thoracic duct and right lymphatic duct	• Smaller vessels, lymphatics, and lymph nodes	• Superior vena cava • Azygos v. • Pulmonary vv. • Pericardiaco-phrenic vv.	• Azygos v. • Accessory hemiazygous and hemiazygous vv. • Thoracic duct
Nerves	• Vagus nn. • Left recurrent laryngeal n. • Cardiac nn. • Phrenic nn.	• None	• Phrenic nn.	• Vagus nn.

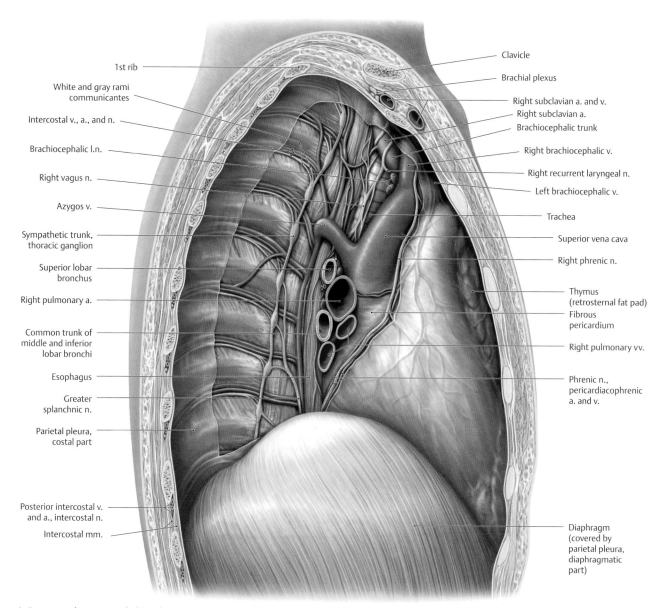

1st rib

White and gray rami communicantes

Intercostal v., a., and n.

Brachiocephalic l.n.

Right vagus n.

Azygos v.

Sympathetic trunk, thoracic ganglion

Superior lobar bronchus

Right pulmonary a.

Common trunk of middle and inferior lobar bronchi

Esophagus

Greater splanchnic n.

Parietal pleura, costal part

Posterior intercostal v. and a., intercostal n.

Intercostal mm.

Clavicle

Brachial plexus

Right subclavian a. and v.

Right subclavian a.

Brachiocephalic trunk

Right brachiocephalic v.

Right recurrent laryngeal n.

Left brachiocephalic v.

Trachea

Superior vena cava

Right phrenic n.

Thymus (retrosternal fat pad)

Fibrous pericardium

Right pulmonary vv.

Phrenic n., pericardiacophrenic a. and v.

Diaphragm (covered by parietal pleura, diaphragmatic part)

A Parasagittal section, right lateral view. Note the many structures passing between the superior and inferior (middle and posterior) mediastinum.

Fig. 5.2 Mediastinum
Divisions of the mediastinum.

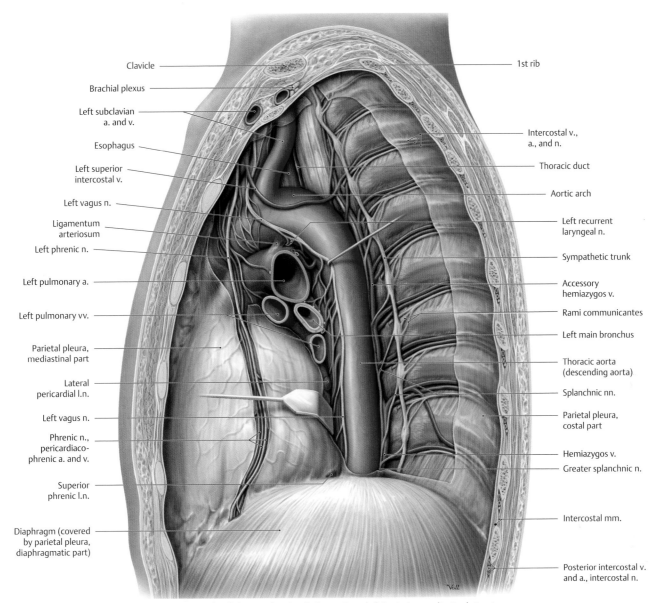

Clavicle

Brachial plexus

Left subclavian a. and v.

Esophagus

Left superior intercostal v.

Left vagus n.

Ligamentum arteriosum

Left phrenic n.

Left pulmonary a.

Left pulmonary vv.

Parietal pleura, mediastinal part

Lateral pericardial l.n.

Left vagus n.

Phrenic n., pericardiaco-phrenic a. and v.

Superior phrenic l.n.

Diaphragm (covered by parietal pleura, diaphragmatic part)

1st rib

Intercostal v., a., and n.

Thoracic duct

Aortic arch

Left recurrent laryngeal n.

Sympathetic trunk

Accessory hemiazygos v.

Rami communicantes

Left main bronchus

Thoracic aorta (descending aorta)

Splanchnic nn.

Parietal pleura, costal part

Hemiazygos v.

Greater splanchnic n.

Intercostal mm.

Posterior intercostal v. and a., intercostal n.

B Parasagittal section, left lateral view. *Removed:* Left lung and parietal pleura. *Revealed:* Posterior mediastinal structures.

Fig. 5.2 (*continued*) **Mediastinum**

5.2   Anterior Mediastinum

Thymus

The thymus is a gland of the immune system, responsible for maturation of T-lymphocytes (see **Fig. 5.1**).

— In childhood, the thymus presents as a large bilobed organ that overlies the heart and great vessels in the superior and anterior mediastinum (**Fig. 5.3**).
— At puberty, high levels of circulating sex hormones cause the gland to atrophy.

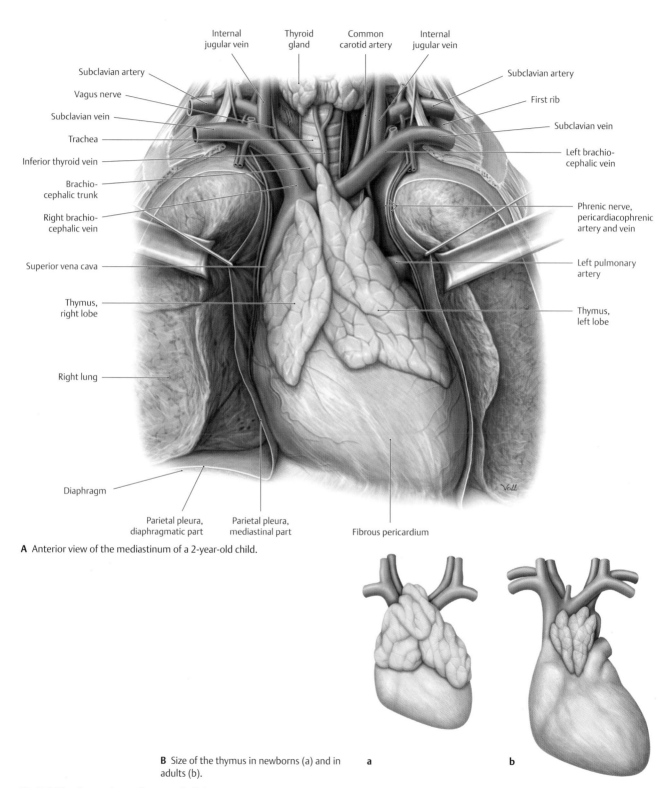

A Anterior view of the mediastinum of a 2-year-old child.

B Size of the thymus in newborns (a) and in adults (b).

a   **b**

Fig. 5.3   The thymus in newborns and adults
The thymus of newborns is much larger than those of adults and extends inferiorly into the anterior part of the inferior mediastinum. Because it atrophies during puberty, the thymus in adults is small and extends only into the superior mediastinum.

5.3 Middle Mediastinum: Pericardium and Pericardial Cavity

Pericardium

The **pericardium,** a double-layered fibroserous membrane, forms the **pericardial sac** that surrounds the heart and the origins of the great vessels (**Figs. 5.4, 5.5, 5.6, 5.7**).

— The pericardium is composed of two layers: an outer fibrous layer and an inner serous layer.

1. The outer **fibrous pericardium** is composed of tough inelastic connective tissue. It is attached inferiorly to the diaphragm and is continuous superiorly with the tunica adventitia (outer layer) of the great vessels.

2. The thin **serous pericardium** consists of parietal and visceral layers.

   ○ The **parietal layer of serous pericardium** lines the inner surface of the parietal pericardium.

   ○ The **visceral layer of serous pericardium** firmly adheres to the outer surface of the heart as the **epicardium.** This layer is continuous with the parietal layer of the serous pericardium at the root of the great vessels.

— **Pericardiacophrenic arteries,** branches of the internal thoracic arteries, provide the main blood supply to the pericardium. Veins that accompany the arteries drain into the superior vena cava.

— The vagus (cranial nerve X) and phrenic nerves (C3–C5) and branches from the sympathetic trunks innervate the pericardium.

— Pericardial pain is often referred via the phrenic nerve to the skin of the ipsilateral supraclavicular region (dermatomes C3–C5).

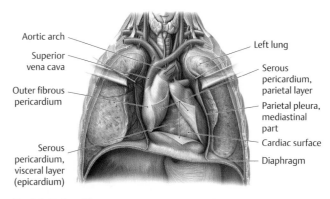

Fig. 5.4 Pericardium
Anterior view of opened thorax. *Removed:* Thymus. *Reflected:* Flaps of the fibrous pericardium.

CLINICAL CORRELATION

PERICARDITIS Pericarditis is an inflammation of the pericardium, which causes sharp, retrosternal or epigastric pain and a characteristic pericardial friction rub (a sound like the rustle of silk) that is heard on auscultation. This is caused by friction from the roughened layers of the inflamed pericardium rubbing together. Pericarditis can lead to pericardial effusion (fluid in the pericardial cavity) or cardiac tamponade (abnormal accumulation of fluid in the pericardial cavity that prevents venous return to the heart) and may be accompanied by dyspnea (shortness of breath) and peripheral edema (swelling).

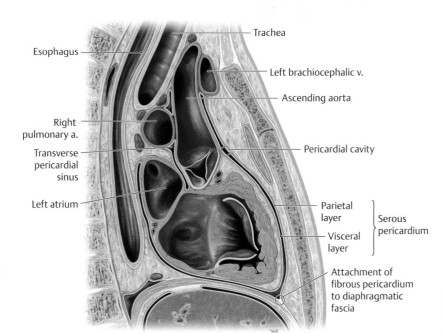

Fig. 5.5 Serous pericardial reflections
Sagittal section through the mediastinum. Note the continuity of the parietal serous and visceral serous pericardia.

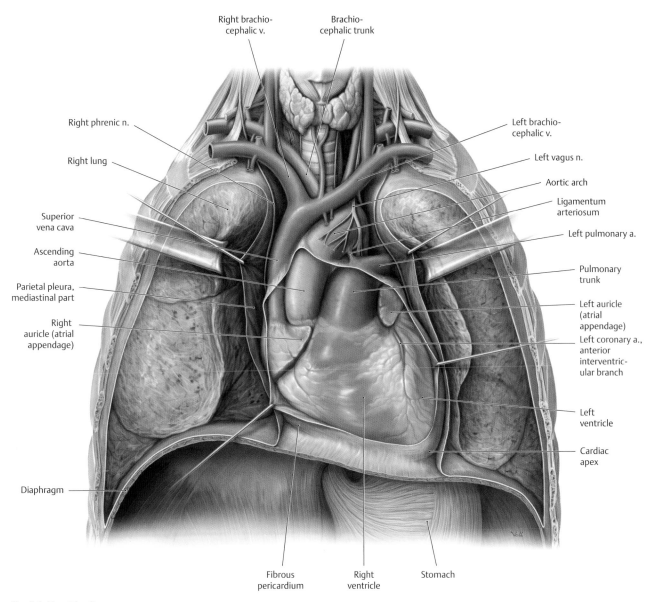

Fig. 5.6 Heart in situ
Anterior view of the opened thorax. *Removed:* Thymus and anterior pericardium. *Revealed:* Heart.

Superior vena cava

Ascending aorta

Left auricle (atrial appendage)

Heart, diaphragmatic surface

Coronary sinus

Left vagus n.

Pericardiacophrenic a. and v., left phrenic n.

Pulmonary trunk

Left pulmonary vv.

Oblique pericardial sinus

Right pulmonary v.

Inferior vena cava

Fig. 5.7 Posterior pericardial cavity
Anterior view. The heart has been elevated to partially visualize the posterior pericardial cavity and the oblique pericardial sinus.

The Pericardial Cavity

The **pericardial cavity** is the space within the pericardial sac between the parietal and visceral layers of the serous pericardium (see **Fig. 5.5**).

— The pericardial cavity is filled with a thin layer of serous fluid that allows for frictionless movement of the heart.

— Two pericardial recesses form where the serous pericardium reflects around the roots of the great vessels (**Figs. 5.5, 5.7 and 5.8**):

1. The **transverse pericardial sinus** is a passage between the inflow channels (superior vena cava and pulmonary veins)

CLINICAL CORRELATION

CARDIAC TAMPONADE Cardiac tamponade is a life-threatening condition in which fluid collects in the pericardial space. The increased intrapericardial pressure restricts the filling of the heart during diastole and reduces cardiac output but increases the heart rate. Inhibition of venous return to the heart causes peripheral edema, hepatomegaly (enlarged liver), and increased venous pressure (often noted by distension of the internal jugular vein). Pericardiocentesis, aspiration of the fluid from the pericardial space, can relieve the tamponade.

Left recurrent laryngeal n.

Ligamentum arteriosum

Ascending aorta

Transverse pericardial sinus

Superior vena cava

Right pulmonary vv.

Inferior vena cava

Sternum

Left vagus n.

Pulmonary trunk

Left phrenic n.

Left pulmonary vv.

Parietal pleura, mediastinal part

Oblique pericardial sinus

Serous pericardium, parietal layer

Fibrous pericardium

Attachment of fibrous pericardium to central tendon of diaphragm

Fig. 5.8 Pericardial recesses
Posterior pericardium, anterior view. *Removed:* Anterior pericardium and heart. *Revealed:* The posterior pericardium and the oblique pericardial sinus. The *double-headed arrow* indicates the course of the transverse pericardial sinus, the passage between the reflections of the serous layer of the pericardium around the arterial and venous great vessels of the heart.

and the outflow channels (aorta and pulmonary trunk) of the heart.

2. The **oblique pericardial sinus** is a recess of the pericardial cavity posterior to the heart between the right and left pulmonary veins.

5.4   Middle Mediastinum: The Heart

General Features

— The heart is a hollow muscular organ located in the middle mediastinum within the pericardial sac. It rests on the central tendon of the diaphragm and is flanked on either side by the right and left pulmonary cavities.

— The heart has a conical shape. The **base,** anchored by the great vessels, is on its superior and posterior surfaces. The **apex,** located approximately at the 5th intercostal space, projects anteriorly, inferiorly, and to the left and moves freely within the pericardial sac.

— Internally, the heart is divided into four chambers: the right and left atria and the right and left ventricles.

  • The right and left atria, separated by an **interatrial septum,** are the inflow chambers of the heart, receiving blood from the systemic circulation on the right and pulmonary circulation on the left.

  • The right and left ventricles, separated by an **interventricular septum,** are the outflow chambers of the heart. Blood flows from the right ventricle into the pulmonary circulation and from the left ventricle into the systemic circulation.

— Two small appendages, the **right** and **left auricles,** are extensions of the atria and are visible externally.

— The surfaces of the heart **(Fig. 5.9)** are

  • the **sternocostal surface** on the anterior side of the heart, formed mostly by the right ventricle with portions of the right atrium and left ventricle;

  • the base on the posterior and superior sides of the heart, formed by the left atrium and a portion of the right atrium; and

  • the **diaphragmatic surface** on the inferior side of the heart, formed by the left and right ventricles.

— The borders of the heart define the cardiac shadow that is seen on radiographic images **(Table 5.2; Fig. 5.10).**

— Three grooves on the external surface of the heart can be used to determine the position of the chambers:

  1. The **coronary sulcus** encircles the heart between the atria and ventricles. Because the heart has an oblique orientation, the sulcus is nearly vertical.

  2. The **anterior interventricular sulcus** is a longitudinal groove on the anterior surface of the heart that marks the position of the interventricular septum.

  3. The **posterior interventricular sulcus** is a longitudinal groove on the diaphragmatic surface of the heart that marks the position of the interventricular septum.

— The **crux** of the heart is a point on the posterior surface of the heart where the coronary (atrioventricular) and interventricular sulci meet. It marks the junction of the four chambers of the heart.

— The wall of the heart consists of three layers:

  1. The **epicardium,** the thin outermost layer, formed by the visceral layer of the serous pericardium

  2. The **myocardium,** the thick layer of cardiac muscle, thickest in the walls of the ventricles

  3. The **endocardium,** the thin internal layer, which lines the chambers and valves of the heart

— A **cardiac skeleton** of dense fibrous connective tissue forms four **fibrous anuli** (rings) and intervening **trigones** that separate the chambers of the heart, provide anchoring points for cardiac muscle fibers and cardiac valves, and insulate electrical impulses of the heart's conduction system **(Fig. 5.11).**

Left subclavian a.
Left common carotid a.
Aortic arch
Brachio-cephalic trunk
Ligamentum arteriosum
Right pulmonary a.
Left pulmonary a.
Superior vena cava
Left pulmonary vv.
Ascending aorta
Pulmonary trunk
Right auricle
Left auricle
Right atrium
Fibrous pericardium (cut edge)
Coronary (right atrioventricular) sulcus
Anterior interventricular sulcus
Right ventricle
Left ventricle
Inferior vena cava
Cardiac apex

A Anterior (sternocostal) surface.

Fig. 5.9 Surfaces of the heart
The heart has three surfaces: anterior (sternocostal), posterior (base), and inferior (diaphragmatic).

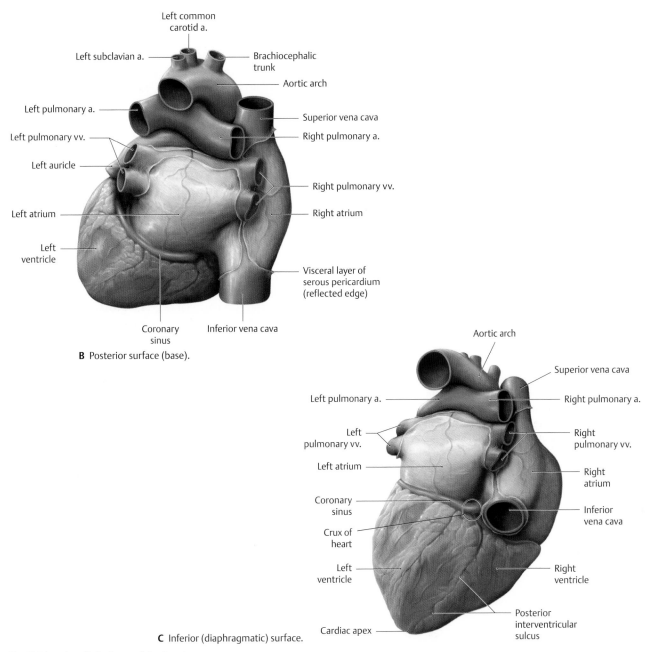

B Posterior surface (base).

C Inferior (diaphragmatic) surface.

Fig. 5.9 (continued) Surfaces of the heart

Table 5.2 Borders of the Heart

Border	Defining Structures
Right cardiac border	Right atrium
	Superior vena cava
Apex	Left ventricle
Left cardiac border	Aortic arch ("aortic knob")
	Pulmonary trunk
	Left atrium
	Left ventricle
Inferior cardiac border	Left ventricle
	Right ventricle

Fig. 5.10 Radiographic appearance of the heart

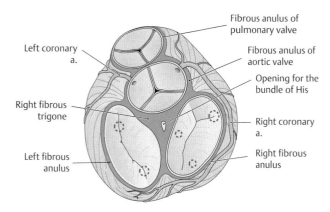

Fig. 5.11 Cardiac skeleton
Superior view. *Red dotted circles* indicate attachment sites of papillary muscles on valves.

The Atria (Figs. 5.12 and 5.13)

The **atria** are the thin-walled inflow chambers of the heart.

— The right atrium receives the superior and inferior venae cavae from the systemic circulation and the cardiac veins from the heart. The left atrium receives the pulmonary veins from the lungs.

— Each atrium is associated with an auricle, a small pouch that expands the capacity of the atrium and whose roughened walls contain pectinate muscles.

— A depression on the right ride of the interatrial septum, the **oval fossa** (fossa ovalis), is a remnant of the **oval foramen** (foramen ovale), an opening through which blood was shunted from the right to left atria in the prenatal circulation.

— The right atrium is divided into two parts by a muscular ridge, the **terminal crest** (crista terminalis). The ridge is evident on the outside of the heart as the **terminal sulcus.** The two parts of the right atrium are

1. the **venous sinus** (sinus venarum), a smooth-walled region on the posterior wall that contains the openings of

the superior vena cava, inferior vena cava, coronary sinus, and anterior cardiac veins; and

2. the **atrium proper,** the anterior muscular portion that, like the right auricle, contains pectinate muscles.

— The left atrium is smaller but thicker walled than the right atrium and receives the four to five pulmonary veins from the lungs. The atrial walls are smooth, with the pectinate muscles confined to the left auricle.

The Ventricles

The ventricles are thick-walled chambers that connect to the outflow channels of the heart: the right ventricle to the pulmonary artery and the left ventricle to the aorta (see **Figs. 5.12** and **5.13**).

— The walls of the ventricles are marked with a meshwork of thick muscular ridges known as **trabeculae carneae.**

— Most of the interventricular septum is muscular, but there is a small membranous part at the superior end that is a common site of septal defects.

— The right ventricle is the smaller and thinner walled of the two ventricles. A muscular ridge, the **supraventricular crest,** separates it into two parts:

1. The **right ventricle proper,** the inflow portion of the ventricle that receives blood from the right atrium

   ○ An **anterior** and a **posterior papillary muscle** arise from its floor, and a **septal papillary muscle** arises from the interventricular septum.

   ○ A muscular **septomarginal trabecula** (moderator band) extends from the septum to the base of the anterior papillary muscle and carries a part of the electrical conduction system (the right branch of the atrioventricular bundle) that facilitates the coordinated contraction of the papillary muscle.

2. The **conus arteriosus** (infundibulum), the smooth-walled outflow channel through which blood flows into the pulmonary trunk

— The left ventricle, which includes the apex of the heart, is the thickest-walled chamber of the heart. Similar to the

A Right ventricle, anterior view.

Fig. 5.12 Chambers of the heart

Superior vena cava

Right pulmonary a.

Left atrium

Right pulmonary vv.

Interatrial septum

Oval fossa

Inferior vena cava

Ascending aorta

Pulmonary trunk

Right auricle

Terminal crest

Pectinate muscles

Right ventricle

Right atrioventricular orifice with atrioventricular valve

Eustachian valve at orifice of inferior vena cava

Thebesian valve at orifice of coronary sinus

B Right atrium, right lateral view.

Left pulmonary a.

Pulmonary trunk

Pectinate muscles

Anterior papillary muscle

Trabeculae carneae of interventricular septum

Tendinous cords

Cardiac apex

Aortic arch

Right pulmonary a.

Left auricle

Left superior pulmonary v.

Valve of oval fossa

Left atrium

Interatrial septum

Inferior vena cava

Posterior papillary muscle

Left atrioventricular valve

C Left atrium and ventricle, left lateral view. Note the irregular trabeculae carneae characteristic of the ventricular wall.

Fig. 5.12 (*continued*) **Chambers of the heart**

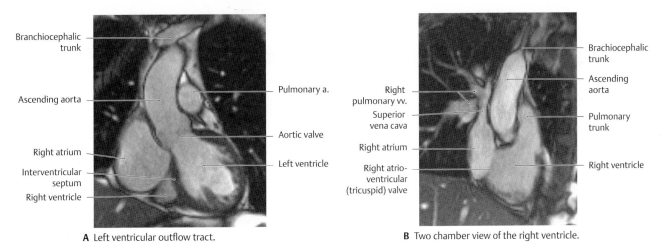

Branchiocephalic trunk

Ascending aorta

Right atrium

Interventricular septum

Right ventricle

Pulmonary a.

Aortic valve

Left ventricle

A Left ventricular outflow tract.

Right pulmonary vv.

Superior vena cava

Right atrium

Right atrioventricular (tricuspid) valve

Branchiocephalic trunk

Ascending aorta

Pulmonary trunk

Right ventricle

B Two chamber view of the right ventricle.

Fig. 5.13 MRI of the Heart

right ventricle, the left is divided into inflow and outflow portions:

1. The **left ventricle proper,** which receives blood from the left atrium. A large anterior and small posterior papillary muscle arise from its floor
2. The **aortic vestibule,** the smooth-walled outflow channel through which blood flows into the aorta

---

DEVELOPMENTAL CORRELATION

TETRALOGY OF FALLOT Tetralogy of Fallot is a rare combination of four congenital cardiac defects: pulmonary stenosis, overriding aorta, ventricular septal defect (VSD), and right ventricular hypertrophy. Symptoms include cyanosis, dyspnea (shortness of breath), fainting, finger clubbing, fatigue, and prolonged crying in infants.

Valves of the Heart

There are two types of cardiac valves: atrioventricular and semilunar (**5.14**).

1. **Atrioventricular valves** separate the atria from the ventricles and prevent regurgitation of blood into the atria during contraction of the ventricles (see **Fig. 5.12**).
   - The atrioventricular valves are made up of cusps, thin leaflets with free inner margins and outer margins that are attached to the fibrous rings of the cardiac skeleton.
   - Slender threads called **tendinous cords** (chordae tendineae) attach the free edges of the valve leaflets to the papillary muscles in the ventricles. These cords maintain closure of the valves and prevent regurgitation of blood during ventricular contraction. Each cusp attaches to tendinous cords from more than one papillary muscle.

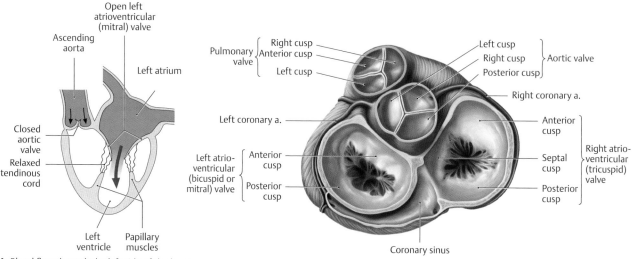

A Blood flow through the left side of the heart during ventricular diastole (relaxation of the ventricles), anterior view. *Closed:* Semilunar valves. *Opened:* Atrioventricular valves.

B Superior view of cardiac valves during ventricular diastole. *Closed:* Semilunar valves. *Opened:* Atrioventricular valves. *Removed:* Atria and great arteries.

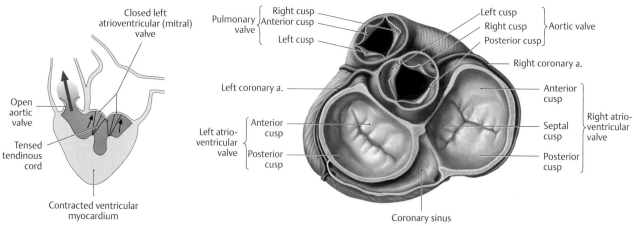

C Blood flow through the left side of the heart during ventricular systole (contraction of the ventricles). *Closed:* Atrioventricular valves. *Opened:* Semilunar valves.

D Superior view of cardiac valves during ventricular systole. *Closed:* Atrioventricular valves. *Opened:* Semilunar valves. *Removed:* Atria and great arteries.

Fig. 5.14 Cardiac valves

- The atrioventricular valves include
  - the **tricuspid valve,** which separates the right atrium from the right ventricle and is composed of anterior, posterior, and septal cusps; and
  - the **bicuspid** (or **mitral**) **valve,** which separates the left atrium from the left ventricle and is composed of anterior and posterior cusps. The anterior cusp is immediately adjacent to, and continuous with, the wall of the aorta.

CLINICAL CORRELATION

MITRAL VALVE PROLAPSE Mitral valve prolapse is a condition in which one or both leaflets of the mitral valve prolapse (evert) into the left atrium, allowing regurgitation of blood through the mitral valve during systole. This condition is usually asymptomatic but is noted by a midsystolic click (valve prolapsing) and murmur (regurgitation).

2. **Semilunar valves** prevent outflow from the ventricles as the chambers fill and backflow of blood into the ventricles after it has been expelled.
   - Each valve is composed of three semilunar cusps with free inner margins and attached outer margins. A **sinus,** or pocket, is created between each cusp and the vessel wall. The thickened free margin of the cusp, the **lunule,** is the point of contact of the cusps. A **nodule** marks the center of the lunule.
   - The semilunar valves include the following:
     - The **pulmonary semilunar valve (pulmonary valve),** is located in the pulmonary trunk at the top of the conus arteriosus, where it moderates blood flow through the right ventricular outflow channel. Its cusps are in the anterior, right, and left positions.
     - The **aortic semilunar valve (aortic valve)** is located within the aorta immediately adjacent to the mitral valve, where it moderates blood flow through the left ventricular outflow channel. Its cusps are in the posterior, right, and left positions. The coronary arteries arise from the sinuses above the right and left cusps.

CLINICAL CORRELATION

AORTIC VALVE STENOSIS Stenosis of the aortic valve is the most common valve abnormality. Calcifications of the valve leaflets narrow the outflow tract and lead to overload of the left ventricle, resulting in left ventricular hypertrophy.

Heart Sounds and Auscultation Sites

When the heart valves close, they produce characteristic sounds described as "lub dub."
- Closure of the tricuspid and mitral valves during contraction of the ventricles produces the first sound ("lub").
- Closure of the pulmonary and aortic valves as the ventricles relax produces the second sound ("dub").
- The sounds, carried by the blood as it flows into the next vessel or chamber, are best distinguished at **auscultation sites** downstream from the valves (**Table 5.3**).

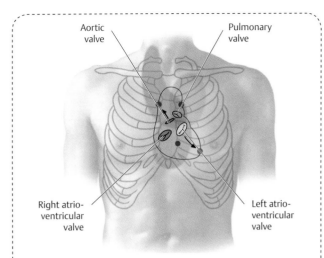

Table 5.3 **Position and Auscultation Sites of Cardiac Valves**

Valve	Anatomical Projection	Auscultation Site
Aortic valve	Left sternal border (at level of 3rd rib)	Right 2nd intercostal space (at sternal margin)
Pulmonary valve	Left sternal border (at level of 3rd costal cartilage)	Left 2nd intercostal space (at sternal margin)
Left atrioventricular valve	Left 4th/5th costal cartilage	Left 5th intercostal space (at midclavicular line) or cardiac apex
Right atrioventricular valve	Sternum (at level of 3rd costal cartilage)	Left 5th intercostal space (at sternal margin)

Note: Auscultation sites of the cardiac valves, indicated by *colored dots*. Valvular heart disease causes turbulent blood flow through a valve; this produces a murmur that may be detected in the *colored region* around the valve.

Conduction System of the Heart (Fig. 5.15)

The conduction system of the heart generates and transmits impulses that modulate the contraction of the cardiac muscle. It consists of nodes, which initiate the impulses, and conducting fibers, which distribute the impulses to cardiac muscle to effect a coordinated contraction of the heart chambers.
- The **sinoatrial (SA) node,** the pacemaker of the heart, initiates and coordinates the timing of the contraction of the heart chambers.
  - At a frequency of 60 to 70 beats per minute, the SA node transmits impulses to both atria and to the atrioventricular node.
  - It is subepicardial, located on the external surface of the heart, just within the myocardium of the right atrium at the junction with the superior vena cava.
  - A branch of the right coronary artery usually supplies the SA node.
- The **atrioventricular (AV) node** is stimulated by the SA node and transmits impulses to the AV bundle.

A **Anterior view.** *Opened:* All four chambers.

B **Right lateral view.** *Opened:* Right atrium and ventricle.

C **Left lateral view.** *Opened:* Left atrium and ventricle.

Fig. 5.15 Cardiac conduction system

- It is subendocardial, located at the base of the interatrial septum above the septal cusp of the tricuspid valve.
- The AV nodal artery, usually a branch of the right coronary artery, arises near the origin of the posterior interventricular artery at the crux of the heart.
— The **atrioventricular (AV) bundle** (of His) arises from cells of the AV node and transmits impulses to the walls of the ventricles.
  - It runs first along the membranous part of the interventricular septum and then divides into **right** and **left bundle branches** that descend to the apex on either side of the muscular part of the septum.
  - The bundle branches end as **Purkinje fibers,** modified cardiac fibers, which ascend within the muscular walls of the ventricles.

CLINICAL CORRELATION

ATRIOVENTRICULAR HEART BLOCK AV heart block is a partial or complete blockage of the conduction of electrical impulses between the atria and ventricles. This causes bradycardia (slow heartbeat) and arrhythmias (irregular heartbeat) and ultimately prevents the heart from effectively contracting and delivering blood to the body. Although heart block may be congenital, it is frequently the result of damage to the heart muscle after myocardial infarction (MI).

The Cardiac Cycle

The heart's conduction system moderates the cardiac cycle, the coordinated **systole** (contraction) and **diastole** (relaxation) of the

A,B Ventricular diastole.

C,D Ventricular systole.

Fig. 5.16 The cardiac cycle

atria and ventricles. **Fig. 5.16** summarizes the sequence of events of the cycle.

1. In the initial phase of diastole, the atria and ventricles are relaxed, and the AV and semilunar valves are closed.

2. In late diastole, the atria fill, the AV valves open, and blood flows passively into the ventricles.
3. Stimulation from the SA node initiates the contraction of the atria, forcing the remaining atrial blood volume into the ventricles.
4. As pressure in the ventricles rises above that in the atria, the AV valves close.
5. Stimulation from the AV node and the AV bundles initiates contraction of the ventricles (ventricular systole).
6. Rising intraventricular pressure forces the semilunar valves to open. Blood is ejected from the right ventricle into the pulmonary trunk and from the left ventricle into the aorta.
7. Relaxation of the ventricles (ventricular diastole) causes backward flow in the pulmonary trunk and aorta and closure of the pulmonary and aortic valves.

5.5 Middle Mediastinum: Neurovasculature of the Heart

Coronary Arteries (Figs. 5.17, 5.18, 5.19; Table 5.4)

The **right** and **left coronary arteries** arise from the ascending aorta just superior to the right and left cusps of the aortic valve. In the initial phase of ventricular diastole, the local surge in aortic pressure caused by the backflow closes the aortic valve and drives blood into the coronary arteries. Blood flow in the arteries is greatest during diastole because of the compression of arteries within the myocardium during systole.

— The right and left coronary arteries supply the myocardium and epicardium of the heart.

• The **right coronary artery** descends within the coronary sulcus around the right side of the heart. Its major branches and their distribution are

  ○ the **SA nodal artery,** which supplies the right atrium and the SA node;

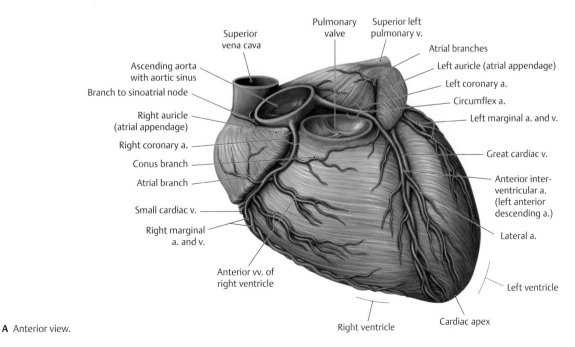

A Anterior view.

Fig. 5.17 Coronary arteries and cardiac veins (continued on page 96)

B Posteroinferior view. *Note:* The right and left coronary arteries typically anastomose posteriorly at the left atrium and ventricle.

Fig. 5.17 (*continued*) **Coronary arteries and cardiac veins**

- - the **right marginal branch,** which supplies the apex and part of the right ventricle;
  - the **posterior interventricular branch,** which supplies the right and left ventricles and posterior third of the interventricular septum and anastomoses with the interventricular branch of the left coronary artery near the apex on the diaphragmatic surface; and
  - the **AV nodal artery,** which supplies the AV node.
- The **left coronary artery,** typically larger than the right coronary artery, arises from the aorta posterior to the

pulmonary trunk. After a short but variable course, it divides into two large branches, the **anterior interventricular** (left anterior descending, LAD) **artery,** which descends in the anterior interventricular sulcus, and the **circumflex artery,** which runs around the left side of the heart in the coronary sulcus. Their branches and distributions include
- the anterior interventricular artery, which supplies the anterior aspects of the right and left ventricles and the anterior two thirds of the interventricular septum, including the AV bundle of the conducting system; and

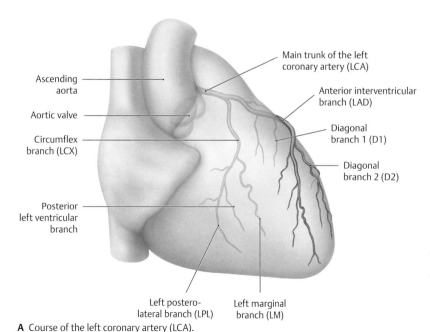

A Course of the left coronary artery (LCA).

B Selective coronary angiography of the LCA. (From Thelen M, et al. Bildgebende Kardiodiagnostik/ Cardiac Imaging. Stuttgart: Thieme; 2007.)

Fig. 5.18 Selective coronary angiography of the left coronary artery in right anterior oblique (RAO) projection
Note: In RAO projections, the spinal column is always projected on the left side.

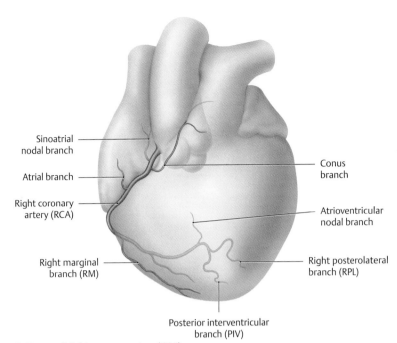

Sinoatrial nodal branch

Atrial branch

Right coronary artery (RCA)

Right marginal branch (RM)

Conus branch

Atrioventricular nodal branch

Right posterolateral branch (RPL)

Posterior interventricular branch (PIV)

A Course of right coronary artery (RCA).

B Selective coronary angiography of the RCA. (From Thelen M. et al. Bildgebende Kardiodiagnostik/Cardiac Imaging. Stuttgart: Thieme; 2007.)

Fig. 5.19 Selective coronary angiography of the right coronary artery in LAO projection
Note: In left anterior oblique (LAO) projections, the spinal column is always projected on the right side.

○ the circumflex artery, which supplies the left atrium and, via its **left marginal branch,** the left ventricle. In ~ 40% of the population, an **SA nodal branch** arises to supply the SA node.

— Variation in the coronary circulation is common but the descriptive language is misleading. The word *dominant* refers not to the artery that supplies the greater volume of cardiac tissue (that is almost always the left coronary artery), but to the artery that gives rise to the posterior interventricular branch.

• A right dominant circulation occurs in about two thirds of the population. The posterior interventricular branch arises from the right coronary artery and supplies the posterior third of the interventricular septum.

• Approximately 15% of people exhibit left dominance in which the posterior interventricular artery is a branch of

the circumflex artery. In these cases, the entire interventricular septum and the AV node are supplied by the left coronary artery.

• Approximately 15% of people have a shared dominance in which branches from both coronary arteries run in the interventricular groove and jointly supply the interventricular septum.

CLINICAL CORRELATION

ANGINA Angina (angina pectoris), a sudden, crushing substernal pain, is a result of myocardial ischemia (insufficient blood supply) caused by a narrowing of the coronary arteries. Exercise following a heavy meal, stress, or even cold weather can trigger an episode. Although angina pain may be severe, it is relieved by a short rest and does not result in infarction of cardiac muscle.

Fig. 5.20 Severe stenosis *(arrow)* of the left circumflex artery
(From Claussen CD, et al. Pareto Reihe Radiologie. Herz/Pareto Series Radiology. Heart. Stuttgart: Thieme; 2007.)

CLINICAL CORRELATION

CORONARY ARTERY DISEASE Coronary artery disease results in ischemia of the myocardium and is a leading cause of death in the United States. In atherosclerosis of the coronary arteries, lipid deposits build up on the inner wall of the vessel and gradually narrow the lumen **(Fig. 5.20)**. In acute disease a fragment of plaque breaks off and completely obstructs the vessel. This creates a necrotic (dead) area of myocardium known as a myocardial infarction. Chronic disease is characterized by a gradual narrowing of the vessels. Overtime a collateral circulation develops that circumvents the narrowed segment and may prevent, or limit, damage from other ischemic events.

Table 5.4 **Branches of the Coronary Arteries**

Left coronary artery circumflex a.	Right coronary artery branch to sinoatrial node
• Atrial branch • Left marginal a. • Posterior left ventricular a.	
	Conus branch
	Atrial branch
	Right marginal a.
Anterior interventricular a. (left anterior descending a.)	Posterior interventricular (descending) a.
• Conus branch • Lateral branch • Interventricular septal branches	• Interventricular septal branches
	Branch to atrioventricular node
	Right posterolateral a.

CLINICAL CORRELATION

CORONARY ARTERY BYPASS GRAFT Coronary artery bypass graft (CABG) is a surgical procedure performed to bypass atherosclerotic narrowings of the coronary arteries that are the cause of anginal pain. If left untreated, these narrowings can eventually occlude the vessel and lead to myocardial infarction (MI). The internal thoracic artery and the great saphenous vein are most commonly used as the bypass vessel.

Coronary Veins (see Fig. 5.17)

— The **coronary sinus,** which receives most of the venous return from the heart, runs in the posterior coronary sulcus between the left atrium and ventricle. The **thebesian valve** guards the orifice of the coronary sinus where it drains into the right atrium near the opening of the inferior vena cava (see **Fig. 5.12B**).

— The large veins of the heart are tributaries of the coronary sinus.

  • The **great cardiac vein** travels with the anterior interventricular artery and drains the left atrium and both ventricles.

  • The **posterior left ventricular** vein drains the diaphragmatic surface of the left ventricle.

  • The **posterior interventricular (middle cardiac) vein** runs in the posterior interventricular groove with the posterior interventricular artery and drains the posterior part of the interventricular septum.

  • The **small cardiac vein,** which drains the posterior right atrium and the right ventricle, accompanies the right coronary artery in the atrioventricular groove.

— **Anterior cardiac veins** drain the anterior surface of the right ventricle and open directly into the right atrium.

Lymphatic Drainage of the Heart

— Lymphatic vessels of the heart have a crossed drainage pattern. Lymph from the left atrium and ventricle drains via a left coronary trunk to inferior tracheobronchial nodes. Efferents from these nodes usually drain to the right venous junction via the bronchomediastinal trunk. Lymph from the right ventricle and atrium drains via a right coronary trunk that runs along the ascending aorta to brachiocephalic nodes near the left venous junction (**Fig. 5.21**).

— The pericardium usually drains to the right and left venous junctions via superior phrenic nodes and bronchomediastinal

A Lymphatic drainage of the left chambers, anterior view.

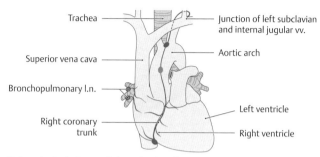

B Lymphatic drainage of the right chambers, anterior view.

Fig. 5.21 Lymphatic drainage of the heart
A unique "crossed" drainage pattern exists in the heart: lymph from the left atrium and ventricle drains to the right venous junction, whereas lymph from the right atrium and ventricle drains to the left venous junction.

trunks, but it may also drain superiorly to the brachiocephalic nodes.

Innervation of the Heart

The autonomic nerves of the cardiac plexus innervate the conduction system of the heart (**Fig. 5.22**, also see **Fig. 3.13**); they therefore regulate the heart rate but do not initiate the heartbeat.

— Sympathetic innervation increases the rate and force of contractions by increasing the response of the SA and AV nodes. It also allows dilation of the coronary arteries.

— Parasympathetic innervation decreases the rate of contractions and causes vasoconstriction of the coronary arteries.

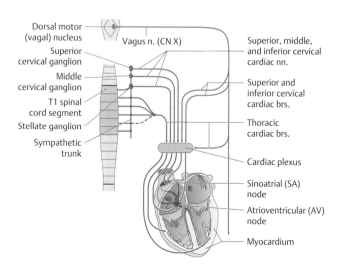

Fig. 5.22 Autonomic innervation of the heart
Schematic.

— Visceral sensory fibers innervating the baroreceptors (receptors that measure blood pressure) and chemoreceptors (receptors that measure blood CO_2) in the heart and aortic arch travel with the parasympathetic fibers of the vagus nerve.

— Visceral sensory fibers carrying pain sensation travel with sympathetic fibers to the T1–T5 spinal cord.

5.6 Prenatal and Neonatal Circulation

Prenatal Circulation

Fetal shunts that direct the flow of blood through the liver, heart, and lungs create a prenatal circulation that differs from that of the adult. The numbered steps in **Fig. 5.23** illustrate the blood flow in the fetal circulation:

1. Fetal blood supplied with oxygen and nutrients in the placenta courses through the umbilical vein toward the liver of the fetus.

2. Although a portion of the blood is distributed to the liver, over half bypasses the liver and is redirected through a shunt, the **ductus venosus,** which empties directly into the inferior vena cava. This blood mixes with smaller amounts from the liver and lower parts of the body before entering the right atrium of the heart.

3. The **eustachian valve** (see **Fig. 5.12B**) at the orifice of the inferior vena cava directs this well-oxygenated mixture across the right atrium into the left atrium through the oval foramen on the interatrial septum. The higher systolic pressure in the right atrium relative to that in the left creates this right-to-left shunt.

From the left atrium, the flow continues into the left ventricle, the aorta, and the systemic circulation of the head and neck. Thus the most highly oxygenated and nutrient-rich blood from the placenta is directed into the coronary, carotid, and subclavian arteries to supply the upper body, especially the heart and developing brain.

4. Oxygen-depleted blood entering the right atrium from the superior vena cava is directed downward through the tricuspid valve into the right ventricle and out through the pulmonary trunk.

Because the high vascular resistance in the lungs prevents much blood from entering the pulmonary arteries, most is

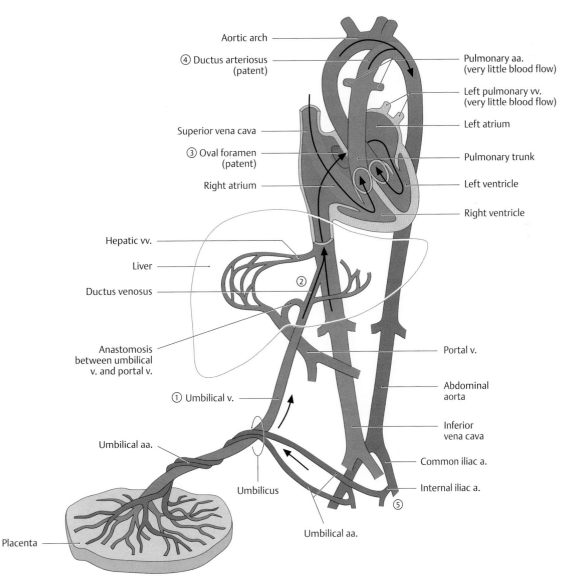

Fig. 5.23 Prenatal circulation
After Fritsch H, Kuhnel W. Taschenatlas der Anatomie. Bd.2.7. Aufl. Stuttgart: Thieme; 2001.

diverted to the descending aorta through the **ductus arteriosus,** a connection between the pulmonary trunk and the aortic arch.

5. The blood entering the aorta from the ductus arteriosus mixes with some blood from the aortic arch. This partially oxygenated blood flows into the descending aorta and is distributed to the lower body, or back to the placenta by way of the paired umbilical arteries.

Cardiovascular Changes at Birth

At birth, a series of changes occurs in the cardiovascular system (**Figs. 5.24** and **5.25A; Table 5.5**).

1. Pressure in the right atrium decreases as a result of
   a. ligation of the umbilical vein, which cuts off blood flow from the placenta; and
   b. the onset of pulmonary respiration, which dramatically decreases the pulmonary blood pressure and increases blood flow to the lungs.

2. As a result of increased flow through the lungs, there is a decreased blood flow through the ductus arteriosus, which constricts within 10 to 15 hours of birth. In the adult, the remnant of this structure is the **ligamentum arteriosum.**

3. Blood returning to the heart through the pulmonary veins increases pressure in the left atrium.

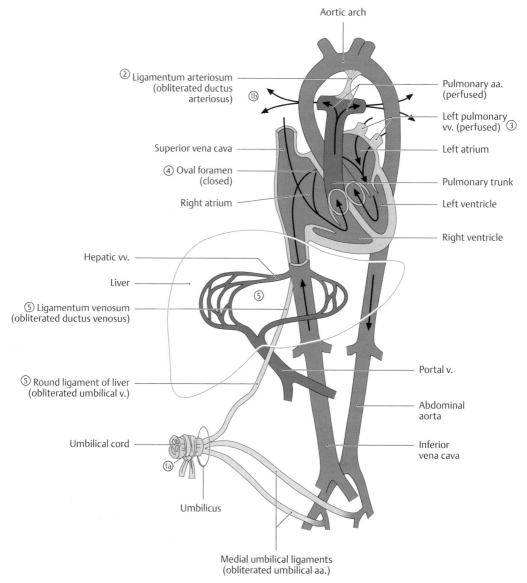

Fig. 5.24 Postnatal circulation
After Fritsch H, Kuhnel W. Taschenatlas der Anatomie. Bd.2.7. Aufl. Stuttgart: Thieme; 2001.

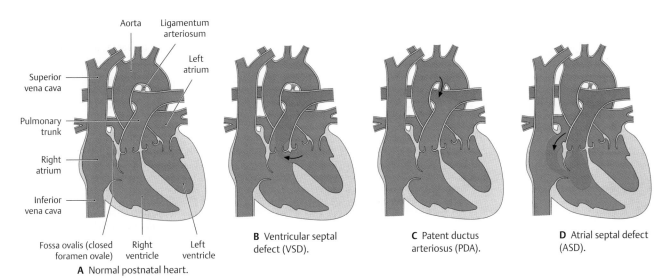

B Ventricular septal defect (VSD).

C Patent ductus arteriosus (PDA).

D Atrial septal defect (ASD).

A Normal postnatal heart.

Fig. 5.25 **Congenital heart defects**.

4. Increased pressure in the left atrium, coupled with a corresponding decrease in pressure in the right atrium, causes a functional closure of the oval foramen (foramen ovale) within

DEVLEOPMENT CORRELATION

PATENT DUCTUS ARTERIOSUS The opening of the pulmonary circulation at birth causes the ductus arteriosus to constrict, probably in response to an increase in local oxygen tension. If the ductus remains open, as a patent ductus arteriosus (PDA), deoxygenated blood continues to enter the descending aorta **(Fig. 5.25C)**. There may be no symptoms if the defect is small, but larger defects may cause failure to thrive, dyspnea (shortness of breath), fatigue, tachycardia (increased heart rate), and cyanosis. Because prostaglandins maintain patency of the ductus during fetal life, premature infants whose ductus does not constrict spontaneously at birth may be treated with prostaglandin inhibitors.

DEVELOPMENT CORRELATION

ATRIAL SEPTAL DEFECT Atrial septal defects (ASDs) **(Fig. 5.25D)** are among the most common congenital cardiac anomalies and are particularly associated with Down syndrome. Most ASDs result from a failure of the oval foramen to close at birth, but they may also result from incomplete development of the septal components. ASDs result in left-to-right shunting and an increase in blood volume through the pulmonary circulation. Small ASDs are often asymptomatic, but larger ASDs will cause hypertrophy of the right atrium, right ventricle, and pulmonary arteries due to the fluid overload.

hours of birth. Complete closure of the oval foramen usually occurs after several months, forming the **oval fossa** (fossa ovalis) in the adult heart.

5. Functional closure of the umbilical arteries, umbilical vein, and ductus venosus occurs within minutes of birth, although the obliteration of the lumen in each vessel may take several months. The remnants of these vessels in the adult are ligamentous structures.

DEVELOPMENT CORRELATION

COARCTATION OF THE AORTA Coarctation, or stenosis, of the aorta usually occurs in proximity to the ligamentum arteriosum, where it limits (or obstructs) the normal blood flow from the aortic arch through the descending aorta. When the narrowing is distal to the ligamentum (postductal stenosis), an effective collateral circulation links the proximal and distal aortic segments via the internal thoracic arteries and their intercostal branches **(Fig. 5.26)**. The intercostal arteries may become large and tortuous enough to form notches along the lower margins of the ribs.

Fig. 5.26 **Coarctation: postductal stenosis**.
Magnetic resonance angiography of an aortic isthmus stenosis in an adult with severe stenosis and pronounced collateral vessels.

Table 5.5 **Derivatives of Fetal Circulatory Structures**

Fetal Structure	Adult Remnant
Ductus arteriosus	Ligamentum arteriosum
Oval foramen	Oval fossa
Ductus venosus	Ligamentum venosum
Umbilical v.	Round ligament of the liver (ligamentum teres)
Umbilical a.	Medial umbilical ligament

5.7   Superior and Posterior Mediastinum

Many of the large arteries and veins of the thorax—superior vena cava (SVC), inferior vena cava (IVC), aorta, common carotid and subclavian arteries—pass through the superior and posterior mediastinum en route to the neck or the abdomen or both. They are accompanied by the vagus, phrenic, and cardiac nerves. These structures are listed in **Table 5.1** and described in detail in Section 3.2. Only viscera of the superior and posterior mediastinum will be discussed in this section.

Esophagus

The esophagus, the thoracic segment of the gastrointestinal tract, is a narrow, but highly distensible, muscular tube. It connects the pharynx in the neck to the stomach in the abdomen (**Fig. 5.27**).

— The esophagus descends anterior to the thoracic vertebral bodies in the posterior mediastinum. Superiorly, it lies posterior to the trachea; inferiorly, it lies posterior to the left atrium of the heart.

— In the upper thorax, the esophagus descends on the right side of the aorta. Before passing through the esophageal aperture of the diaphragm, the esophagus passes first anterior to, and then to the left of, the aorta.

— The upper esophagus is composed mostly of striated muscle arranged in inner circular and outer longitudinal layers. Striated muscle is gradually replaced by smooth muscle fibers inferiorly.

— Three constrictions narrow the lumen of the esophagus (**Fig. 5.28**):

1. The **upper esophageal sphincter,** created by the cricopharyngeus muscle (part of the inferior constrictor muscle of the pharynx), which surrounds the upper esophageal opening in the neck
2. The **middle esophageal constriction,** created by the aortic arch and left main bronchus
3. The **lower esophageal constriction,** or **cardiac sphincter,** created by circular muscles of the distal esophagus, folds in the mucosa formed by a submucosal venous plexus, and the muscular esophageal aperture of the diaphragm

— The blood supply to the upper, middle, and lower esophagus arises from vessels in the neck (inferior thyroid), thorax (esophageal branches of the descending aorta), and abdomen (left gastric and left inferior phrenic), respectively.

— The veins of upper and middle esophageal segments drain into the azygos system. Veins of the lower esophageal segment drain inferiorly along inferior phrenic veins into the

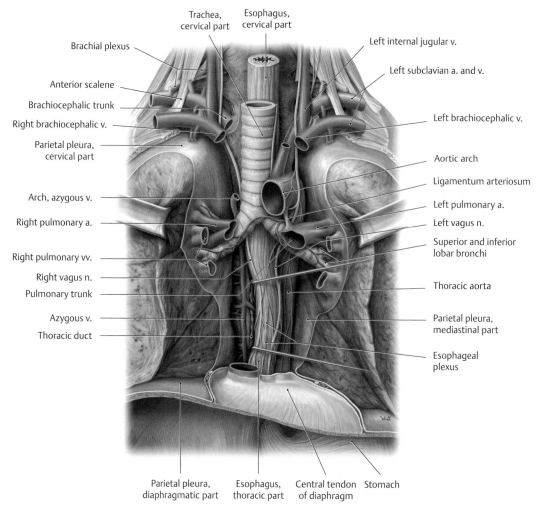

Fig. 5.27 Esophagus in situ
Anterior view.

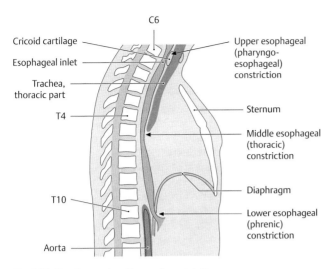

Fig. 5.28 Esophagus: location and constrictions
Esophageal constrictions, right lateral view.

hepatic portal system (the venous drainage for organs of the abdominal gastrointestinal tract).

— The **esophageal plexus,** formed by the right and left vagus nerves with contributions from the greater splanchnic nerves, innervates the esophagus.

CLINICAL CORRELATION

ACHALASIA Achalasia is a deficiency of inhibitory neurons in the lower part of the esophagus. These neurons are responsible for overriding the normal resting tonic contraction of the smooth muscle cells in the lower esophageal sphincter. Their deficiency results in failure of the sphincter to relax during swallowing. As food accumulates above the sphincter, there is an increased risk of aspiration pneumonia.

Trachea and Bronchi

The trachea, located in the superior mediastinum, is the proximal part of the **tracheobronchial tree,** a passageway for air between the lungs and the external environment. The distal part of this passageway, the **bronchial tree,** extends into the lungs and is discussed with the pulmonary cavities in Chapter 6.

— As the trachea descends through the superior mediastinum, slightly to the right of the midline, it lies anterior to the esophagus and posterior to the great vessels.

— C-shaped cartilaginous rings form the skeleton of the trachea and prevent collapse of the lumen. A muscular membrane connects the ends of the rings posteriorly (**Fig. 5.29**).

— The **carina,** a wedge-shaped cartilage, marks the bifurcation of the trachea into a **right** and **left bronchus** at the T4-T5 vertebral level.

— Of the two main bronchi, the right is shorter, wider, and more vertical than the left, and therefore is more prone to obstruction by foreign objects.

— Descending branches of the inferior thyroid artery in the neck (see **Fig. 21.17C**), as well as bronchial arteries that arise from the descending aorta (see **Fig. 3.5**), supply the trachea. Venous blood drains to the inferior thyroid veins.

— Thoracic splanchnic nerves and parasympathetic fibers from the vagus (cranial nerve X) nerve innervate the trachea via the pulmonary plexus.

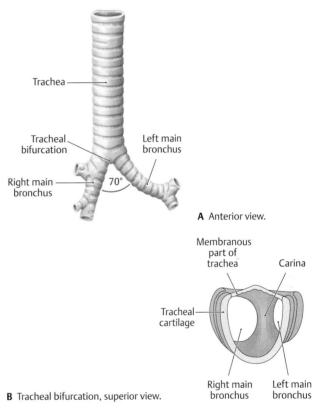

B Tracheal bifurcation, superior view.

Fig. 5.29 Trachea

6 Pulmonary Cavities

The right and left pulmonary cavities, which flank the mediastinum laterally and anteriorly, extend superiorly above the costal cartilages of the first rib and inferiorly to the thoracic diaphragm (see **Table 3.1**). Each pulmonary cavity contains a lung and bronchial tree and a pleural sac.

6.1 The Pleura and Pleural Cavity

The Pleura

The **pleura** is a fibroserous membrane that surrounds each lung and lines the pulmonary cavities (**Fig. 6.1**).

— The pleura is composed of two layers:

- The **parietal pleura,** which is a continuous layer that lines the inner wall of the thoracic cavity, the superior surface of the diaphragm, and the mediastinum. Its parts are named according to location: cervical, costal, diaphragmatic, and mediastinal (**Fig. 6.2**).
- The **visceral pleura,** which covers the surface of the lung and extends into its fissures.

— The visceral and parietal layers are continuous with one another at the hilum of the lung (see Section 6.2). Together they form the inner and outer walls of a closed pleural sac that contains a **pleural cavity** (**Fig. 6.3**).

— The **pulmonary ligament** is a double-layered fold of visceral and parietal pleura that extends vertically from the hilum to the diaphragm along the mediastinal border of each lung (see **Fig. 6.5B,D**).

— The blood supply and innervation of the pleura are derived from nerves and vessels that supply adjacent structures.

- Visceral pleura shares the neurovasculature of the lungs and bronchi.
- Parietal pleura shares the neurovasculature of the thoracic wall, pericardium, and diaphragm.

CLINICAL CORRELATION

PLEURITIS Inflammation of the pleura, or pleuritis, creates friction between the visceral and parietal layers that produces a sharp, stabbing pain as the layers glide over one another during respiration. The inflammation may also produce adhesions between the two layers.

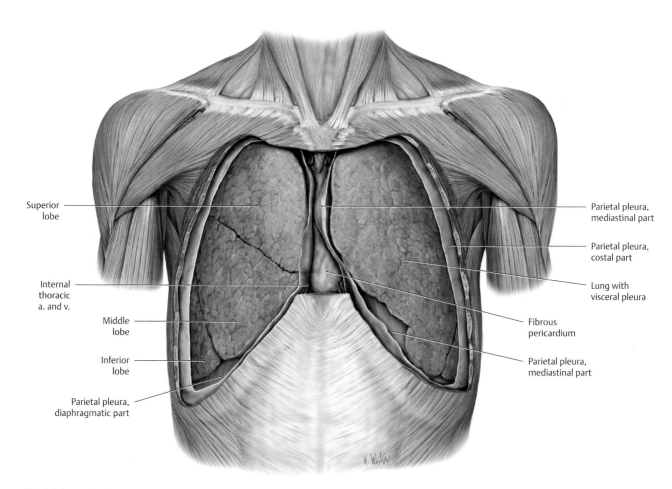

Superior lobe — Parietal pleura, mediastinal part — Parietal pleura, costal part — Lung with visceral pleura — Internal thoracic a. and v. — Middle lobe — Fibrous pericardium — Inferior lobe — Parietal pleura, mediastinal part — Parietal pleura, diaphragmatic part

Fig. 6.1 Lungs in situ
Anterior view. *Removed*: Anterior thoracic wall and costal part of the parietal pleura.

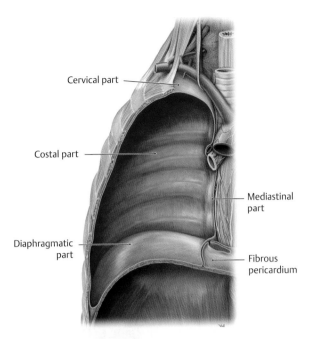

Fig. 6.2 Parts of the parietal pleura
Anterior view. *Opened:* Right pleural cavity.

The Pleural Cavity

The **pleural cavity,** the cavity within the pleural sac, is the potential space between the visceral and parietal layers of pleura (see **Fig. 6.3**).

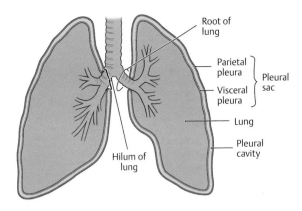

Fig. 6.3 Pleura and pleural cavity
Schematic.

— The pleural cavity contains a thin layer of serous fluid, which lubricates the adjacent pleural surfaces, facilitates the movement of the lung, and maintains surface tension that is crucial to respiration.

— On most surfaces, the two pleural layers approximate one another, but the lung and its visceral pleura are somewhat smaller than the outer wall of the pleural cavity and its lining of parietal pleura. Two recesses that form as a result of this discrepancy accommodate the expansion of the lungs during inspiration (**Fig. 6.4**):

• The **costodiaphragmatic recess** forms where the diaphragmatic pleura reflects from the perimeter of the diaphragm to meet the costal pleura on the thoracic wall.

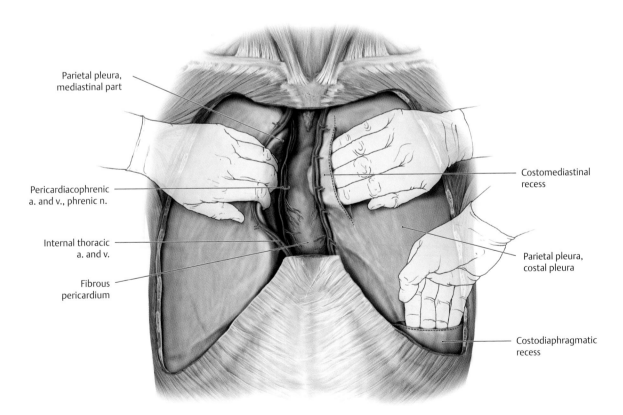

Fig. 6.4 Costomediastinal and costodiaphragmatic recesses
On the left side of the thorax, the examiner's fingertips are placed in the costomediastinal and costodiaphragmatic recesses. These recesses are formed by the acute reflection of the costal part of the parietal pleura onto the fibrous pericardium (costomediastinal) or diaphragm (costodiaphragmatic).

- The **costomediastinal recess** forms between the pericardial sac and the sternum, where the mediastinal pleura reflects to meet the costal pleura.

CLINICAL CORRELATION

PNEUMOTHORAX Pneumothorax is a condition in which air enters the pleural space. It may result from a tear in the chest wall and parietal pleura (such as from a stab wound) or a tear of the visceral pleura (such as from a rupture of a pulmonary lesion). Air in the pleural space decreases the negative pressure that normally keeps the lungs inflated and leads to a partial or complete lung collapse.

CLINICAL CORRELATION

TENSION PNEUMOTHORAX Tension pneumothorax is a life-threatening condition in which air accumulates in the pleural space and becomes trapped because the injured tissue acts as a one-way valve. This causes complete collapse of the lung on the affected side and a shifting of the heart to the opposite side, thus compromising venous return and cardiac output. This mediastinal shift also compresses the opposite lung and impairs its ventilatory capacity.

CLINICAL CORRELATION

PLEURAL EFFUSION Pleural effusion is a condition in which there is excess fluid in the pleural space. Effusions are designated by their protein concentration into transudates (low protein) and exudates (high protein). Transudates are usually caused by congestive heart failure or fluid overload (causing increased venous pressure). Less commonly they are caused by liver failure or renal disease. Exudates may leak from the pleural capillaries in inflammatory states, pneumonia, tuberculosis (TB), and lung cancer. Symptoms include dyspnea (shortness of breath), cough, and dull chest pain. Pleural effusions are treated by draining the fluid through a procedure known as thoracentesis (see Thoracentesis box, below).

CLINICAL BLUE BOX>

CHYLOTHORAX Chylothorax is a type of pleural effusion (fluid in the pleural space) in which chyle leaks from the thoracic duct or one of the main lymphatic vessels and accumulates in the pleural space.

CLINICAL CORRELATION

THORACENTESIS Thoracentesis (chest drain) is a procedure in which a needle is inserted into the pleural cavity to drain fluid, blood, or pus. In an upright patient the fluid accumulates in the costodiaphragmatic recesses. In order to access these recesses without damaging the inferior border of the lung, the diaphragm, the liver, or the spleen, the needle is usually inserted at the posterior axillary line in the 7th intercostal space or in the mid-axillary line at the 7th or 8th intercostal space. The needle is inserted above the rib to avoid the intercostal neurovascular bundle that runs in the costal groove along the lower margin of the rib.

6.2 The Lungs

General Features (Fig. 6.5; Table 6.1)

— Each lung has costal, mediastinal, and diaphragmatic surfaces.
— The **apex** of each lung projects into the neck above the first costal cartilage; the **base** of each lung rests on the diaphragm.
— The **root** of the lung, which connects the lung to the mediastinum, contains the pulmonary vessels, nerves, and bronchi. The root enters the lung at the **hilum,** an indentation on the mediastinal surface (**Fig. 6.6;** see **Fig. 6.3**).
— Fissures, lined by visceral pleura, divide each lung into lobes: three lobes on the right and two lobes on the left.
— Thin connective tissue septa (intersegmental septa) that are continuous with the visceral pleura subdivide lobes of the lungs into discrete pyramidal-shaped units called **bronchopulmonary segments (Fig. 6.7)**.

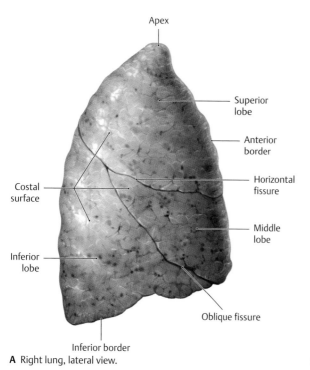

A Right lung, lateral view.

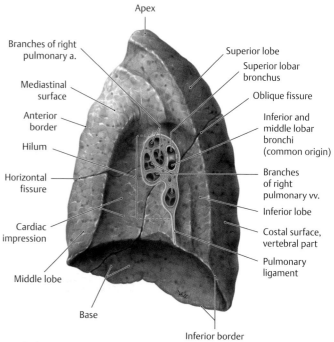

B Right lung, medial view.

Fig. 6.5 Gross anatomy of the lungs

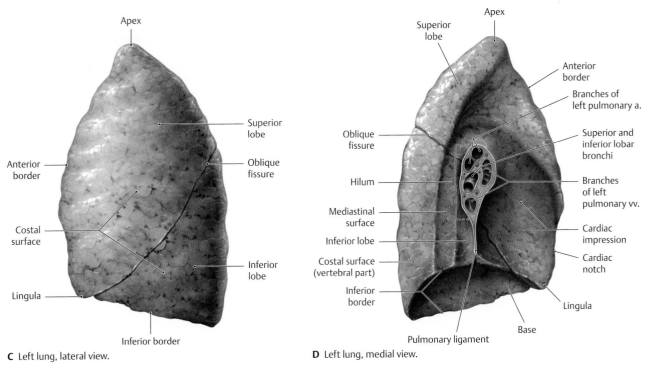

Apex

Superior
lobe

Oblique
fissure

Anterior
border

Costal
surface

Lingula

Inferior
lobe

Inferior border

C Left lung, lateral view.

Apex

Superior
lobe

Anterior
border

Branches of
left pulmonary a.

Oblique
fissure

Superior and
inferior lobar
bronchi

Hilum

Branches
of left
pulmonary vv.

Mediastinal
surface

Inferior lobe

Cardiac
impression

Costal surface
(vertebral part)

Cardiac
notch

Inferior
border

Lingula

Pulmonary ligament

Base

D Left lung, medial view.

Fig. 6.5 (*continued*) **Gross anatomy of the lungs**

Ascending aorta

Superior vena cava

Right pulmonary a.

Right inferior
lobar bronchus

Pulmonary trunk

Left pulmonary v.

Left atrium

Left inferior lobar bronchus

Esophagus

Azygous v.

Descending aorta

W: 477
L: 43
360

A Axial section at the
level of the right
pulmonary artery.

Right auricle

Superior vena cava

Left atrium

Esophagus

Conus arteriosus

Ascending aorta

Left ventricle

Left pulmonary v.

Descending aorta

W: 477
L: 43
60

B Axial section at the
level of the left
pulmonary artery.

Fig. 6.6 CT of the thorax at the level of the hila of the lungs

Table 6.1 **Structure of the Lungs**

	Right Lung	**Left Lung**
Lobes	Superior, middle, inferior	Superior, inferior
Fissures	Oblique, horizontal	Oblique
Bronchopulmonary Segments	10	8–10
Unique Features	Larger and heavier than the left, but shorter and wider due to higher right hemidiaphragm	Superior lobe characterized by the lingula and a deep cardiac notch

CLINICAL CORRELATION

CARCINOMA OF THE LUNG Carcinoma of the lung accounts for ~ 20% of all cancers and is mainly caused by cigarette smoking. It arises first in the lining of the bronchi and metastasizes quickly to bronchopulmonary lymph nodes and subsequently to other node groups, including supraclavicular nodes. It can also spread via the blood to the lungs, brain, bone, and suprarenal glands. Lung cancer can invade adjacent structures such as the phrenic nerve, resulting in paralysis of a hemidiaphragm, or the recurrent laryngeal nerve, resulting in hoarseness due to paralysis of the vocal cord.

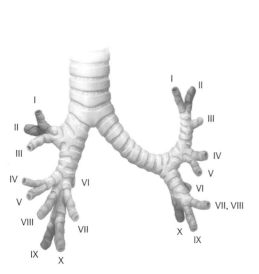

A Trachea with segmental bronchi, anterior view.

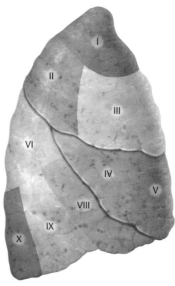

B Right lung, lateral view.

C Right lung, medial view.

D Left lung, lateral view.

E Left lung, medial view.

Fig. 6.7 Segmentation of the lungs

- Each bronchopulmonary segment is an anatomically and functionally independent respiratory unit. This independence allows the surgical resection of individual segments.
- There are 10 bronchopulmonary segments in the right lung and 8 to 10 segments in the left lung.

Right Lung

- Because the dome of the diaphragm is higher on the right side, the right lung is shorter and wider than the left lung.
- Horizontal and oblique fissures divide the right lung into superior, middle, and inferior lobes (see **Fig. 6.5A,B**).
- The root of the lung passes under the arch of the aorta, posterior to the right atrium, and under the arch of the azygos vein (see **Figs. 3.2** and **5.1).**
- The right bronchus and its branches are the most posterior structures within the root of the lung. The pulmonary artery passes anterior to the bronchus, and the pulmonary veins lie anterior and inferior to the artery.

Left Lung

- An oblique fissure divides the left lung into superior and inferior lobes (see **Fig. 6.5C,D**).

- A deep indentation along the anterior border of the superior lobe, called the **cardiac notch,** accommodates the leftward projection of the apex of the heart.
- The **lingula,** a thin tongue of lung tissue from the superior lobe, forms the inferior border of the cardiac notch and moves into and out of the costomediastinal recess during respiration.
- The aortic arch crosses over the left bronchus, and the descending aorta passes behind the root of the lung (see **Fig. 5.1**).
- The left pulmonary artery arches over the left bronchus to become the most superior structure in the root of the lung. Pulmonary veins pass anterior and inferior to the bronchus.

6.3 The Tracheobronchial Tree

The tracheobronchial tree consists of the trachea and the bronchi in the mediastinum, and the bronchial tree (generations of branches formed by successive bifurcations) within the lungs. (The trachea is discussed in Section 5.7.) The tracheobronchial tree has conducting and respiratory components.

- The trachea and its larger proximal branches form the conducting component, a passageway for air exchange between the lung and the external environment **(Figs. 6.8, 6.9, 6.10A)**. All except the most distal of these branches have

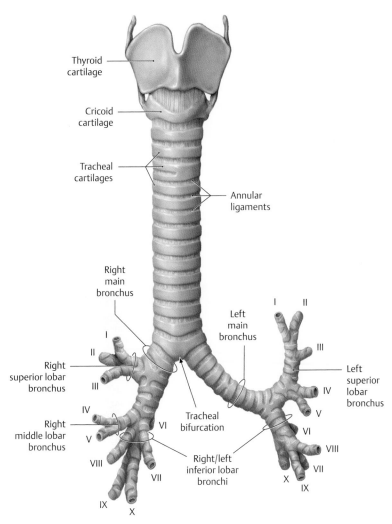

Fig. 6.8 Trachea
Anterior view. The numbers I to IX of the segmental bronchi correspond with bronchopulmonary segments shown in **Fig. 6.7B–D.**

Fig. 6.9 Anteroposterior bronchogram
Anterior view of right lung.

A Divisions of the bronchial tree.

B Respiratory portion of the bronchial tree.

Fig. 6.10 Bronchial tree

cartilaginous rings or plates in their walls. The branches include

- the **right** and **left main** (primary) **bronchi,** formed by the bifurcation of the trachea in the superior mediastinum. One main bronchus enters the hilum of each lung.
- the **lobar** (secondary) **bronchi,** which branch from the main bronchi. One lobar bronchus enters each lobe of the respective lung (three on the right and two on the left).
- the **segmental** (tertiary) **bronchi,** which branch from the lobar bronchi. One segmental bronchus enters each bronchopulmonary segment.
- the **conducting bronchioles,** a network of airways without cartilage that are formed as the segmental bronchi subdivide and decrease in size.
- the **terminal bronchioles,** the last branches of the conducting bronchioles and the final part of the conducting airway.
- The respiratory component (seen only histologically), made up of passages distal to the terminal bronchioles, is involved in air conduction as well as in gas exchange (**Fig. 6.10B**).

- The structures in this part of the bronchial tree include the **respiratory bronchioles, alveolar sacs,** and **alveoli.**
- The single-celled walls of the alveoli are designed for efficient gas exchange.

CLINICAL CORRELATION

ATELECTASIS Atelectasis is the partial or complete collapse of alveoli within the lung and can result from mucus in the airways following surgery (most common), cystic fibrosis, asthma, or obstruction of the airways by a foreign object (e.g., a tumor or blood clot). When severe, it can lead to respiratory failure.

DEVELOPMENT CORRELATION

NEONATAL RESPIRATORY DISTRESS SYNDROME Neonatal respiratory distress syndrome (neonatal RDS), common in preterm infants, results from a deficiency of surfactant, which leads to alveolar collapse (atelectasis). The use of synthetic surfactant and administration of continuous positive airway pressure (CPAP) can help maintain airway patency in these infants.

CHRONIC OBSTRUCTIVE PULMONARY DISEASE Chronic obstructive bronchitis and emphysema, both caused by cigarette smoking, contribute in varying degrees to chronic obstructive pulmonary disease (COPD). Inflammation from chronic bronchitis leads to thickened bronchial tubes, excess mucus production, and a narrowed airway. Emphysema destroys alveolar walls, thereby reducing the capacity for gas exchange, and, as small airways collapse during expiration, air is trapped in the lungs. This chronic hyperinflation of the lungs and the increased work of expiration create a typical barrel chest appearance (increased anteroposterior diameter).

6.4 Mechanics of Respiration

Respiration, the exchange of oxygen and carbon dioxide, requires a continuous flow of air between the lungs and the external environment and is accomplished through the rhythmic change in thoracic volume and corresponding expansion (during **inspiration**) and contraction (during **expiration**) of the lungs (**Figs. 6.11, 6.12, 6.13**).

— Inspiration requires an expansion of the pulmonary cavities and decrease in intrapleural pressure.
  • During quiet respiration, the diaphragm, the chief respiratory muscle, contracts and flattens, increasing the vertical dimension of the cavity.
  • Forced inspiration engages other respiratory muscles (primarily the intercostals, scalenes, and posterior

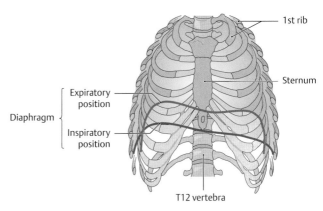

Fig. 6.11 Respiratory changes in thoracic volume
Inspiratory position (red); expiratory position (blue).

serratus) that elevate the ribs and sternum and expand the cavities horizontally.
  • As the cavities expand, the pleural sac is pulled outward, causing an increase in lung volume and a decrease in intrapleural pressure. When the pressure drops below atmospheric pressure (negative pressure), air is pulled into the respiratory passageways.
— Expiration requires a contraction of the pulmonary cavities and increase in intrapleural pressure.
  • Quiet expiration is a passive process. With relaxation of the diaphragm, there is a decrease in thoracic volume and a corresponding contraction of the lungs. As the intrapleural pressure increases, air is expelled.
  • Forced expiration requires the contraction of anterior abdominal and intercostal muscles to decrease thoracic volume.

Inferior border of lung (full expiration)

Inferior border of lung (full inspiration)

Fig. 6.12 Respiratory changes in lung volume

Trachea

Lung (full expiration)

Lung (full inspiration)

Fig. 6.13 Movements of the lung and bronchial tree
As the volume of the lung changes with the volume of the thoracic cavity, the entire bronchial tree moves within the lung. These structural movements are more pronounced in portions of the bronchial tree distant from the pulmonary hilum.

6.5   Neurovasculature of the Lungs and Bronchial Tree

Arteries of the Lungs and Bronchial Tree

— The **pulmonary arteries,** branches of the pulmonary trunk, transport deoxygenated blood to the capillary network surrounding the respiratory alveoli (**Fig. 6.14**). Within the lungs, branches of the arteries follow the branches of the bronchial tree as they ramify within the lobes and bronchopulmonary segments.

— **Bronchial arteries,** branches of the thoracic aorta, supply the bronchial tree, the connective tissue of the lungs, and the visceral pleura. Typically one branch to the right lung and two to the left lung, these bronchial arteries travel along the posterior aspect of the main bronchi and eventually anastomose with distal branches of the pulmonary arteries.

Veins of the Lungs and Bronchial Tree

— **Pulmonary veins** arise from the capillary beds surrounding the alveoli (see **Fig. 6.14**). Arising first as small veins that travel within the intersegmental septa carrying oxygenated blood, they receive veins from adjacent bronchopulmonary segments as well as from the visceral pleura. These veins join to form two pulmonary veins within each lung, which traverse the hilum and enter the left atrium of the heart.

— **Bronchial veins,** one from each lung, drain only the proximal portion of the root and terminate in the azygos and accessory hemiazygos (or superior intercostals) veins.

CLINICAL CORRELATION

PULMONARY EMBOLISM Pulmonary embolism (PE) is the obstruction of a pulmonary artery or its branches by fat emboli, air bubbles, or, most commonly, thromboses (blood clots) that have traveled up from the deep veins of the legs. Large obstructions can impede blood flow into the lung and consequently cause cor pulmonale, right-sided heart failure. Large obstructions are often fatal, but smaller obstructions may affect only a single bronchopulmonary segment and result in a pulmonary infarction.

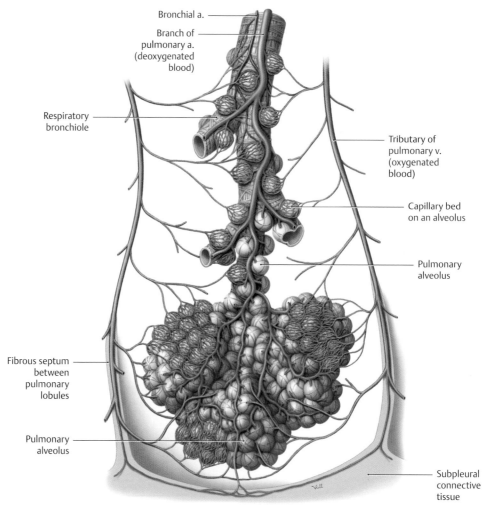

Fig. 6.14 Pulmonary vasculature
Pulmonary arteries *(blue)* carry *deoxygenated* blood and follow the bronchial tree. Pulmonary veins *(red)* are the only veins in the body carrying *oxygenated* blood, which they receive from the alveolar capillaries at the periphery of the lobule.

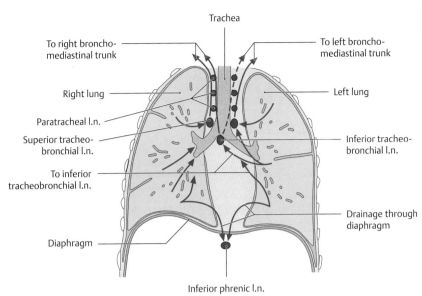

Fig. 6.15 Lymphatic drainage of the pleural cavity
Peribronchial network, coronal section.

Lymphatics of the Lungs and Bronchial Tree

— The **superficial lymphatic plexus** of the lungs, deep to the visceral pleura, drains the pleura and the lung tissue.
— The **deep lymphatic plexus,** within the walls of the bronchi, drains structures associated with the lung root.
— Whereas the superficial and deep plexuses eventually drain to the superior and inferior (carinal) **tracheobronchial nodes,** the deep plexus drains initially to the **bronchopulmonary** nodes along the lobar bronchi **(Fig. 6.15).**
— Lymph from tracheobronchial nodes drains to **paratracheal nodes** and then to the **bronchomediastinal trunks** on either side, which terminate in the junction of the subclavian and jugular veins (jugulosubclavian venous junctions).
— The superior, middle, and inferior lobes of the right lung and the superior lobe of the left lung normally drain along ipsilateral channels. Some lymph from the inferior lobe of the left lung, however, drains to the right tracheobronchial nodes, and from there it continues to follow right-sided channels.

Nerves of the Lungs and Bronchial Tree

— The **pulmonary plexus,** an autonomic nerve plexus that lies anterior and posterior to the root of the lung, innervates the lung, bronchial tree, and visceral pleura **(Table 6.2).**

— Visceral sensory fibers carrying pain from the bronchi and visceral pleura travel with sympathetic splanchnic nerves.
— Visceral sensory fibers from receptors related to cough and stretch reflexes, and receptors for blood pressure and blood gas levels travel with the vagus (parasympathetic) nerve.
— The parietal pleura is innervated by somatic nerves of the thoracic wall, and it is extremely sensitive to pain. Intercostal nerves innervate the costal surface, and phrenic nerves (C3–C5) innervate the mediastinal and diaphragmatic surfaces.
— Irritation of the parietal pleura in the areas supplied by the phrenic nerve is referred to the dermatomes C3–C5 on the neck and shoulder.

Table 6.2 **Autonomic Innervation of the Lungs and Bronchial Tree**

Target Structures	Sympathetic	Parasympathetic
Bronchial muscles	Inhibitory (bronchodilation)	Motor (bronchoconstriction)
Pulmonary vessels	Motor (vasoconstriction)	Inhibitory (bronchodilation)
Secretory cells of alveoli	Secretomotor	Inhibitory

Unit III   Clinical Imaging Basics of the Thorax

Radiographs are always the initial choice for imaging of the thorax. The air-filled lungs are perfectly suited for X-rays, making it easy to identify air space abnormalities such as pneumonia, and provide high contrast to the soft tissues of the heart and mediastinum. When more detail of the heart, mediastinum, or lung parenchyma is required (e.g., evaluation of interstitial lung disease), computed tomography (CT) is used. The value of magnetic resonance imaging (MRI) in cardiac imaging is its ability to acquire dynamic images (heart in motion) without radiation. Ultrasound (echocardiography) also has the utility of dynamic imaging without radiation and without the long scan times and issues of claustrophobia associated with MRI. However, the anatomic detail of ultrasound and the ability to assess the coronary vessels is limited when compared with CT and MRI (**Table 6.3**).

The chest X-ray is the starting point of the vast majority of thoracic imaging. When evaluating a chest X-ray (**Fig. 6.16**), the examiner typically follows the airway from the upper trachea down into both lungs and then views each lung in its entirety, sweeping from side to side. The heart borders are evaluated for size and shape, and the smooth surfaces of each hemidiaphragm and mediastinal border are confirmed. Each rib and vertebra is examined (**Fig. 6.17**), and then attention is given to the chest wall and soft tissues. A similar procedure is used to examine the lateral view.

Computed tomography scans are excellent for showing details of the soft tissues of the thorax and can be examined in different

windows to highlight specific organs (**Fig. 6.18**). MRI, although not well suited for imaging the lungs, provides very good detail of the heart and allows imaging in specific planes (**Fig. 6.19**). An ultrasound of the heart, or echocardiogram, provides a dynamic view of the heart and is best viewed in "real time." However, standard static "snapshots" can provide important information, such as the four-chamber view (**Fig. 6.20**).

Table 6.3 **Suitability of Imaging Modalities for the Thorax**

Modality	Clinical Uses
Radiographs (X-rays)	The mainstay of thoracic imaging and the most common radiologic study performed; excellent for evaluation of the lungs, heart, pulmonary vessels, and pleura
CT (computed tomography)	Exquisite anatomic detail of the lung parenchyma and interstitium
MRI (magnetic resonance imaging)	Best suited for imaging the heart and great vessels; very limited value in evaluating the lungs
Ultrasound	Used primarily for cardiac imaging (echocardiography); provides real-time anatomic and physiologic evaluation of the heart

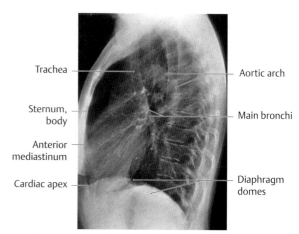

A Anteroposterior (PA) view. On a frontal view the sharp borders created by soft tissue structures, as outlined against the air-filled lungs, can be identified. Note the

— female breast shadows, which can be seen overlying the lower chest, making the lower lungs appear slightly whiter than the upper lungs. The sharp inferior curved margin of the breasts extend to the lateral chest walls.
— tracheal air column, which is well seen in the midline of the upper mediastinum.
— heart borders, mediastinal edges, and domes of the diaphragms, which are well demarcated against the adjacent air-filled lungs.
— stomach, indicated by the "stomach bubble," the air-filled (blacker) structure just under the left hemidiaphragm

B Left lateral view. In the lateral view, right-sided and left-sided structures (e.g., the lungs) are superimposed on each other. Note that the

— hemidiaphragms and the costodiaphragmatic recesses are well demarcated.
— anterior (right ventricle [RV]), posterior (left atrium [LA]) and inferior (left ventricle [LV]) borders of the heart are sharply demarcated against the air-filled lungs. The right atrium is not seen on the lateral view.
— vertebral bodies are rectangular in shape and the disk spaces between vertebra are uniform
— retrosternal space (anterior clear space), seen clearly on the lateral radiograph, is obscured by the sternum on the frontal radiograph.
— breasts can be seen on the anterior chest wall.

Fig. 6.16 Radiograph of the thorax

Fig 6.17 Radiograph of the thorax with the 4th ribs highlighted
Posteroanterior (PA) view.
The ribs extend horizontally from their articulation with the vertebrae and then curve laterally, anteriorly, and inferiorly. When examining a chest radiograph, each rib should be traced over its entire course. Note that the costochondral cartilage is not visible on an X-ray.

A The lung window optimizes details of the lung parenchyma. Subtle lung disease that may be invisible on a chest X-ray can be detected with chest CT.

B The soft tissue widow optimizes the soft tissue structures, but renders the lung parenchyma black (invisible). The soft tissues of the thoracic wall are well delineated. Also note the detail of the aorta and main pulmonary artery as they branch.

Fig. 6.18 CT of the thorax, inferior view.
These images represent the same axial slice from a normal CT scan of the thorax at the level of the main pulmonary artery. This patient received intravenous contrast causing the blood vessels to appear white.

Branchiocephalic trunk

Ascending aorta

Right atrium

Interventricular septum

Right ventricle

Pulmonary a.

Aortic valve

Left ventricle

Fig. 6.19 MRI of the heart showing the left ventricular outflow tract
Coronal view.
Cardiac MRI scans can be obtained in any plane, with several standard planes selected to optimize specific anatomy. In this example, blood in the vessels and chambers is white and the heart muscle is black. This left ventricular outflow tract view positions the left ventricle and the ascending aorta in the same plane so the entire outflow tract is visible on a single image. A complete cardiac MRI would contain slices through the entire heart in this plane as well as several other planes. Additionally, MRI allows for dynamic imaging and can produce "cine" (movie) clips of several cardiac cycles showing chamber, wall, and valve motion. Note that dynamic MRIs cannot be seen in "real time" as with ultrasound.

RV

TV

RA

LV

MV

LA

Fig. 6.20 Echocardiogram (heart ultrasound)
Apical four-chamber view taken with the probe positioned at the cardiac apex.
Both ventricles (RV, LV), both atria (RA, LA), and the mitral and tricuspid valves (MV, TV) are well seen. Although this is a single static image, the true power of echocardiography is the ability to see heart motion with real-time dynamic images. Ventricular wall motion, valve operation, and blood flow can all be seen and analyzed. The displayed echocardiogram allows the imager to synchronize the heart's motion with its electrical activity.

Unit III   Review Questions: Thorax

1. Which of the following nerves contribute to the phrenic nerve?
   A. Anterior rami of C3–C5 spinal nerves
   B. Anterior rami of C5–T1 spinal nerves
   C. Sympathetic fibers from C3–C5 spinal cord segments
   D. Sympathetic fibers from T1–T4 spinal cord segments
   E. Cardiac nerves from the cervical sympathetic trunk

2. Which of the following is true of bronchopulmonary segments?
   A. Each is served by one terminal bronchiole.
   B. There are three in the right lung and two in the left lung.
   C. Each is supplied by one bronchial artery.
   D. Each is an anatomically and functionally distinct respiratory unit of the lung.
   E. They have single-celled walls designed for efficient gas exchange.

3. Which of the following structures is/are found in the right atrium?
   A. Chordae tendineae
   B. Oval fossa
   C. Mitral valve
   D. Papillary muscles
   E. Trabeculae carneae

4. The sternal angle (of Louis) marks the location of the
   A. second costal cartilage
   B. T4–T5 intervertebral disk
   C. origin of the aortic arch
   D. bifurcation of the trachea
   E. All of the above

5. You are studying the CT images of your patient who is being treated for lung cancer. You focus on the scan that shows the carina where you note several enlarged lymph nodes. What other structure is most likely visible in this CT image?
   A. Left atrium
   B. Brachiocephalic artery
   C. Sternal angle
   D. Tricuspid valve
   E. Right pulmonary vein

6. Within hours of arriving home after a 10-hour bus ride, a 77-year-old woman was rushed to the emergency room with shortness of breath, sweating, and nausea. Although she died shortly after being admitted, her workup in the emergency room revealed a pulmonary embolus in her left pulmonary artery. What other findings would you expect in this patient?
   A. Collapse of the left lung
   B. Acute dilation of the right ventricle
   C. A shift of mediastinal structures to the right side
   D. Hypertrophy of the left ventricle
   E. Dilation of the left atrium

7. A malignancy involving the lateral breast would *most* likely metastasize first to which of the following groups of nodes?
   A. Parasternal nodes
   B. Abdominal nodes
   C. Deep pectoral nodes
   D. Axillary nodes
   E. Nodes of the contralateral breast

8. What is the surface landmark on the chest that approximates the position of the apex of the heart?
   A. Sternal angle
   B. Left 3rd intercostal space
   C. Left 5th intercostal space
   D. Right 5th intercostal space
   E. Xiphoid process of the sternum

9. Dr. P. was performing a cardiac bypass on a 53-year-old man whose anterior interventricular artery (also known as the left anterior descending artery, LAD) was narrowed near its origin. Although Dr. P. frequently used a saphenous vein graft for this procedure, he chose to use the left internal thoracic artery instead. Leaving its origin intact, he cut its distal connections and anastomosed it to the LAD beyond the narrowed segment. This successfully restored flow to the anterior part of the heart. What path does the blood take through this diverted route?
   A. Aortic arch to left subclavian artery to internal thoracic artery
   B. Aortic arch to brachiocephalic artery to internal thoracic artery
   C. Aortic arch to internal thoracic artery
   D. Aortic arch to left subclavian artery to pericardiaco-phrenic artery to internal thoracic artery
   E. Aortic arch to axillary artery to internal thoracic artery

10. An elderly man who admits to some dizziness and minor chest palpitations during the past week is finally admitted to the emergency department for chest pain and shortness of breath. Imaging reveals a major blockage of his right coronary artery near the crux of the heart just proximal to the origin of the posterior interventricular artery. Which part of the heart would be affected by the ischemia that results from this blockage?
    A. Sinoatrial (SA) node
    B. Atrioventricular (AV) node
    C. Anterior two thirds of the interventricular septum
    D. Left atrium
    E. Right ventricle

11. A woman who had a recent history of a myocardial infarction (MI) complained to her cardiologist of a sharp, stabbing pain behind her sternum that radiated to her shoulder and was accompanied by shortness of breath, particularly when she was lying down. Her physician noted a pericardial friction rub and treated her for pericarditis, an inflammation of her pericardium caused by the recent MI. Pain from her pericardium was transmitted by the
    A. phrenic nerves
    B. cardiac plexus
    C. pulmonary plexus
    D. intercostal nerves
    E. None of the above

12. The right lymphatic duct drains the lymph from
    A. the entire right side of the body
    B. the right side of the thorax, right upper limb, and right side of the head and neck
    C. only the right side of the thorax
    D. only the right side of the head and neck and right upper limb
    E. the right side of the thorax, the abdomen, and the right lower and the right upper limbs

13. Which of the following features are paired with the correct lung?
    A. Lingula—right lung
    B. Horizontal fissure—left lung
    C. Cardiac notch—left lung
    D. Two lobar bronchi—right lung
    E. Shorter and wider than the contralateral lung—left lung

14. Several weeks after suffering a severe myocardial infarction, a man was rushed to the emergency department but died shortly afterward. It was discovered at autopsy that the muscle anchoring one leaflet of his mitral valve had ruptured, probably as a consequence of his earlier heart attack. Which was the affected muscle?
    A. Papillary muscle
    B. Trabeculae carneae
    C. Pectinate muscle
    D. Terminal crest
    E. Septomarginal trabecula (moderator band)

15. What is the origin of the posterior intercostal arteries?
    A. Aorta
    B. Internal thoracic artery
    C. Lateral thoracic artery
    D. Subclavian artery
    E. Superior epigastric artery

16. A woman with a history of asthma presents to the emergency department with shortness of breath and wheezing. Drugs and oxygen are administered, but her condition worsens. She is transferred to the intensive care unit and put on a ventilator. Twenty-four hours after admission, she dies from complications of asthma. On autopsy it is found that she has severe inflammation, an increase in smooth muscle, and other pathologic changes around a part of the respiratory tree that does not contain cartilage. Which part of the airway was most likely affected in this patient?

    A. Trachea
    B. Main (primary) bronchi
    C. Lobar (secondary) bronchi
    D. Segmental (tertiary) bronchi
    E. Bronchioles

17. During the physical examination of a 28-year-old construction worker, you mention that his heart sounds strong and healthy. He asks you to explain what creates the heart sounds. You tell him that the first heart sound (the "lub") is produced by the
    A. closure of the tricuspid and pulmonary valves
    B. closure of the atrioventricular valves
    C. opening of the semilunar valves
    D. contraction of the ventricles
    E. turbulent flow through the valves

18. All of the following structures are in contact with thoracic vertebral bodies except
    A. Azygos vein
    B. Trachea
    C. Sympathetic trunk
    D. Thoracic duct
    E. Right posterior intercostal artery

19. What is/are the primary muscle(s) used in quiet respiration?
    A. Intercostal muscles
    B. Scalene muscles
    C. Diaphragm
    D. Pectoralis major
    E. Anterior abdominal muscles

20. Which of the following valves is most audible at the right 2nd intercostal space just lateral to the sternum?
    A. Aortic valve
    B. Left atrioventricular valve
    C. Pulmonary valve
    D. Right atrioventricular valve
    E. Valve for the coronary sinus

21. During auscultation of the heart, which of the following relationships is *most* likely to be correct in a normal adult?
    A. The left 4th intercostal space at the midaxillary line is the site of auscultation of the mitral valve.
    B. The left 2nd intercostal space at the sternal border is the site of auscultation of the aortic valve.
    C. The right 3rd intercostal space at the sternal border is the site of auscultation of the pulmonary valve.
    D. The right 2nd intercostal space at the sternal border is the site of auscultation of the aortic valve.
    E. The right 4th intercostal space at the midclavicular line is the site of auscultation of the tricuspid valve.

22. Which of the following events occurs during either quiet or forced expiration?
    A. Collapse of alveolar sacs
    B. Increase in lung volume
    C. Elevation of the ribs
    D. Increase in intrapleural pressure
    E. Temporary collapse of the segmental bronchi

23. During a routine physical exam of a young woman who is training to compete in the Olympic trials, you scrutinize her cardiac rhythm for abnormalities. Which of the following events normally occur during ventricular diastole?

A. Contraction of the ventricles

B. Ejection of blood into the pulmonary trunk

C. Opening of the semilunar valves

D. Filling of the coronary arteries

E. Closure of the atrioventricular valves

Answers and Explanations

1. **A.** The phrenic nerve is a somatic nerve containing C3–C5 anterior rami (Section 3.2).

B. The anterior rami of C5–T1 form the brachial plexus.

C. There are no autonomic nerves that arise from the C3–C5 spinal cord.

D. Sympathetic splanchnic nerves that arise from T1–T4 contribute to the cardiac and pulmonary plexuses.

E. Cardiac branches from the cervical sympathetic trunk contribute to the cardiac plexus and are not related to the phrenic nerve.

2. **D.** Bronchopulmonary segments function independently from other segments and are separated from them by thin septa (Section 6.2).

A. One segmental bronchi enters each bronchopulmonary segment and ramifies into many conducting bronchioles, which in turn divide into many terminal bronchioles.

B. The right lung has 10 bronchopulmonary segments, and the left lung has 8 to 10 segments.

C. Bronchial arteries supply the bronchi and connective tissue of the lungs, including the visceral pleura. Branches of the pulmonary arteries supply the bronchopulmonary segments.

E. Alveoli, the smallest unit of the respiratory tree, have single-celled walls that facilitate gas exchange.

3. **B.** The oval fossa on the interatrial septum is the remnant of the opening between the atria that allows right-to-left shunting in the fetal circulation (Section 5.4).

A. Chordae tendineae are found in the ventricles.

C. The mitral valve separates the left atrium and ventricle.

D. Papillary muscles are found only in the ventricles.

E. Trabeculae carneae are muscular ridges in the walls of the ventricles.

4. **E.** The sternal angle is a palpable bony prominence created at the junction of the body and manubrium of the sternum. It marks the transverse plane that passes through the 2nd costal cartilage, T4–T5 intervertebral disk, origin of the aortic arch, and bifurcation of the trachea (Section 4.2).

5. **C.** The carina, at the bifurcation of the trachea, lies approximately at the T4–T5 vertebral level, which is also the level of the sternal angle (Section 4.2).

A. The left atrium lies approximately at the level of T6–T7, below the carina at the bifurcation of the trachea.

B. The brachiocephalic artery, the first branch of the aortic arch, lies approximately at the level of T3. The carina lies at the level of the sternal angle at T4–T5.

D. The tricuspid valve lies at the level of the 5th costal cartilage. The carina lies at the level of the 2nd costal cartilage and the sternal angle.

E. Pulmonary veins on both sides enter the left atrium, approximately at the level of T6–T7, well below the carina at T4–T5.

6. **B.** Obstruction of the pulmonary artery impedes blood flow into the lung and causes pooling of blood in the right side of the heart. This causes acute dilation of the right atrium and right ventricle (Section 6.5).

A. Collapse of the lung is a symptom of a pneumothorax in which air enters the pleural cavity.

C. The pressure of a tension pneumothorax can cause the heart to shift to the opposite side.

D. Hypertrophy of the left ventricle is the result of a chronic condition that causes the myocardium to work harder in response to a fluid overload or an obstruction in the aortic outflow tract. A pulmonary embolism is usually an acute event that causes a fluid overload in the right ventricle but decreases venous return to the left ventricle.

E. A pulmonary embolism reduces the volume of blood entering the lung from the right side of the heart and therefore results in a diminished venous return to the left side of the heart. The right atria and ventricle may be acutely dilated, but the left atria and ventricle are not.

7. **D.** A malignancy involving the lateral breast would most likely metastasize via the axillary nodes and then on to nodes around the clavicle and the ipsilateral lymphatic duct (Section 4.1).

A. Medial portions of the breast may drain to the parasternal nodes. These nodes also receive lymph from the anterior abdominal wall above the umbilicus, the deeper parts of the anterior portion of the thoracic wall, and the superior surface of the liver.

B. Nodes of the anterior abdominal wall receive lymph from the medial and inferior parts of the breast.

C. Although some lymph from the breast may drain to deep pectoral nodes posterior to the pectoralis muscle, most lymph from the breast drains to axillary nodes.

E. Lymphatic drainage from the medial breast may drain to the contralateral breast, but lymphatic drainage from the lateral breast most abundantly passes to the axillary nodes.

8. **C.** The apex lies at the level of the 5th intercostal space (Section 5.4).

A. The sternal angle is at the level of the 2nd costal cartilages.

B. The 3rd intercostal space is above the level of the heart.

D. The apex of the heart is found at the most inferior and left border of the heart, which lies to the left of the sternum.

E. The xiphoid process lies in the midline, whereas the apex lies to the left side of the sternum.

9. **A.** The internal thoracic artery is a branch of the subclavian artery, the third branch of the aortic arch (Section 3.2).
    B. The internal thoracic artery arises from the subclavian artery.
    C. The internal thoracic artery does not arise directly from the aortic arch. It is a branch of the subclavian artery.
    D. The pericardiacophrenic arteries arise from the internal thoracic arteries to supply the pericardium and diaphragm. They do not contribute to the blood supply of the heart.
    E. The internal thoracic artery arises from the subclavian artery, not the axillary artery.

10. **B.** The AV nodal artery, which branches from the right coronary artery near the origin of the posterior interventricular artery, usually supplies the AV node (Section 5.5).
    A. The SA node is supplied by the SA nodal artery, a branch of the proximal part of the right coronary artery, or by the circumflex branch of the left coronary artery.
    C. The left anterior interventricular artery (LAD) supplies the anterior two thirds of the interventricular septum.
    D. The circumflex branch of the left coronary artery supplies the left atrium.
    E. The marginal branch of the right coronary artery supplies most of the right ventricle. Its origin is well proximal to the crux of the heart and would not be affected by this blockage.

11. **A.** The phrenic nerves (C3–C5) are the primary sensory nerves of the pericardium. Referred pain is often felt in the supraclavicular region, the C3–C5 dermatome (Section 5.3).
    B. The cardiac plexus is a plexus of autonomic fibers that innervate the heart.
    C. The pulmonary plexus, an extension of the cardiac plexus, regulates the constriction and dilation of the pulmonary vessels and bronchial passages.
    D. Intercostal nerves innervate structures of the thoracic and abdominal walls.
    E. Not applicable

12. **B.** The right lymphatic duct drains the lymph from the right side of the thorax, right upper limb, and right side of the head and neck (Section 3.2).
    A. Lymph from all structures below the diaphragm drains to the left lymphatic duct (thoracic duct).
    C. The right side of the head and neck and right upper limb also drain to the right lymphatic duct.
    D. The right side of the thorax also drains to the right lymphatic duct.
    E. Lymph from the abdomen and both lower limbs drains to the thoracic duct (left lymphatic duct).

13. **C.** The cardiac notch is a deep indentation along the anterior border of the superior lobe of the left lung (Section 6.2).
    A. The lingula is a thin tongue of tissue that forms the lower border of the cardiac notch of the superior lobe of the left lung.
    B. The left lung has only an oblique fissure that separates the superior and inferior lobes.
    D. The right lung has three lobes supplied by three lobar bronchi.
    E. The right lung is shorter and wider than the left lung due to the presence of the liver below the right side of the diaphragm.

14. **A.** The papillary muscles of the left ventricle attach to the tendinous cords of the mitral valve leaflets and prevent them from prolapsing during ventricular systole (Section 5.4).
    B. Trabeculae carneae are the thick muscular ridges of the ventricular walls.
    C. Pectinate muscles are found in the right and left auricles.
    D. The terminal crest (crista terminalis) is a muscular ridge within the right atrium that separates its two parts, the venous sinus and the atrium proper.
    E. The interventricular septomarginal trabecula is a muscular band that connects the interventricular septum to the anterior papillary muscle of the right ventricle and carries the right branch of the atrioventricular bundle of the conducting system.

15. **A.** The aorta supplies the posterior intercostal arteries (Section 4.4).
    B. The internal thoracic artery supplies the anterior intercostal arteries.
    C. The lateral thoracic artery originates from the axillary artery and supplies the pectoralis major and minor, and the serratus anterior muscles and the lateral mammary arteries.
    D. The subclavian artery supplies the internal thoracic, vertebral, and axillary arteries, as well as branches to the neck and shoulder.
    E. The superior epigastric artery is a branch of the internal thoracic artery. It supplies the lower anterior intercostal arteries and the anterior abdominal wall.

16. **E.** The bronchioles have no cartilage but do contain a layer of smooth muscle that often hypertrophies (cells increase in size) in severe asthma (Section 6.3).
    A. The trachea contains C-shaped cartilage rings.
    B. The main bronchi contain C-shaped cartilage rings, similar to those in the trachea.
    C. Lobar bronchi contain plates of cartilage.
    D. Segmental bronchi contain plates of cartilage.

17. **B.** Closure of tricuspid and mitral (atrioventricular) valves produces the first ("lub") sound (Section 5.4).
    A. Closure of the tricuspid valve contributes to the first heart sound ("lub"); closure of the pulmonary valve contributes to the second heart sound ("dub").
    C. Opening of the semilunar valves does not produce discernible heart sounds.
    D. Contraction of the ventricles does not produce any sound, although it coincides with the closure of the atrioventricular valves, which produces the first heart sound.
    E. Turbulent flow through the valves, often associated with valvular stenosis and regurgitation, produces a murmur heard on auscultation.

18. **B.** The trachea lies anterior to the esophagus along its entire length and is not in contact with the vertebral bodies (Sections 4.4 and 5.7).
    A. The azygos vein ascends along the anterior surface of the thoracic vertebrae.
    C. The sympathetic trunks lie along the lateral aspects of the thoracic vertebrae.
    D. The thoracic duct ascends along the vertebral bodies between the azygos and hemiazygos veins.
    E. The posterior intercostal arteries arise from the aorta and cross the vertebral bodies to run within the intercostal spaces on the right side.

19. **C.** During quiet respiration the contraction and relaxation of the diaphragm change the volume of the pulmonary cavities and consequently the expansion and contraction of the lungs (Section 6.4).
    A. The intercostal muscles are used to elevate and lower the ribs during forced inspiration and forced expiration.
    B. Scalene muscles are extrinsic muscles of respiration that move the ribs during forced inspiration.
    D. The pectoralis major moves and stabilizes the upper limb but also assists movements of the ribs during deep inspiration.
    E. Anterior abdominal muscles contract during forced expiration.

20. **A.** The aortic valve is most audible at the right 2nd intercostal space just lateral to the sternum (Section 5.4).
    B. Sound from the left atrioventricular (AV) valve is most audible over the left 5th intercostal space on the midclavicular line.
    C. Sound from the pulmonary valve is most audible over the left 2nd intercostal space just lateral to the sternum.
    D. Sound from the right AV valve is most audible from the right lower aspect of the body of the sternum.
    E. There is usually no audible sound from the valve of the coronary sinus.

21. **D.** The right 2nd intercostal space at the sternal border is the site of auscultation of the aortic valve (Section 5.4).
    A. The left 5th intercostal space at the midclavicular line is the site of auscultation of the mitral valve.
    B. The left 2nd intercostal space at the sternal border is the site of auscultation of the aortic valve.

C. The left 2nd intercostal space at the sternal border is the site of auscultation of the pulmonary valve.
    E. The left 5th intercostal space at the sternal border is the site of auscultation of the tricuspid valve.

22. **D.** During expiration, the contraction of the pulmonary cavity causes an increase in intrapleural pressure, which forces air to be expelled from the lung (Section 6.4).
    A. Surfactant lining the walls of the alveoli prevents them from collapsing during expiration.
    B. During inspiration the thoracic cavity expands, pulling the pleural sac outward and causing an increase in lung volume.
    C. The elevation of the ribs increases the size of the thoracic cavity during inspiration.
    E. Incomplete cartilaginous rings in the walls of the bronchi prevent them from collapsing during expiration.

23. **D.** At the beginning of ventricular diastole (relaxation of the ventricles), the semilunar valves close, and backflow in the aorta fills the coronary arteries (Section 5.4).
    A. The ventricles contract during ventricular systole.
    B. Blood from the right ventricle is ejected into the pulmonary trunk during ventricular systole.
    C. The semilunar valves open during ventricular systole to allow blood to flow into the aorta and pulmonary trunk.
    E. During the initial phase of ventricular systole, as ventricular pressure increases, the atrioventricular valves close.

Unit IV   Abdomen

7 The Abdominal Wall and Inguinal Region

The abdomen, the region of the trunk between the thorax and the pelvis, contains the largest portion of the **abdominopelvic cavity,** a peritoneal-lined space that it shares with the pelvis. The abdomen houses the primary organs of the gastrointestinal and urinary systems, although some abdominal viscera (i.e., small intestine) typically overflow the boundaries of the abdomen to occupy pelvic spaces, and pelvic viscera, when distended (i.e., bladder and uterus), can extend superiorly into the abdomen **(Fig. 7.1)**.

The abdominal wall, composed of skin, fascia, and muscles, is supported by its attachments to the ribs, lumbar vertebrae, and bony pelvis. It moves and stabilizes the trunk, supports the abdominal viscera, and creates intra-abdominal pressure that is crucial in digestion and respiration. The muscular abdominal wall provides little protection for underlying viscera, but much of the upper abdominal viscera lies under the dome of the diaphragm, where the viscera are protected by the thoracic skeleton. The bony pelvis protects most viscera in the lower abdomen.

7.1 Regions and Planes of the Abdominal Wall

— In order to describe the location of abdominal viscera, we divide the abdomen into four quadrants or nine regions, using vertical reference lines and standard transverse planes **(Fig. 7.2)**.

— The **transpyloric plane,** a transverse plane at the level of T12-L1, measured halfway between the jugular notch and pubic crest, is a useful horizontal plane that provides orientation to the internal anatomy of the abdomen **(Fig. 7.3;** see also **Fig. 1.4)**. The T12–L1 plane passes through (or very close to)
  • the pylorus of the stomach,
  • the ampulla of the duodenum,
  • the origin of the celiac trunk,
  • the origin of the superior mesenteric artery,
  • the origin of the portal vein,
  • the neck of the pancreas, and
  • the left colic flexure of the large intestine.

Fig. 7.1 Peritoneal relationships
Midsagittal section through male pelvis, viewed from the left side. Peritoneal cavity. The peritoneum is shown *(red)*.

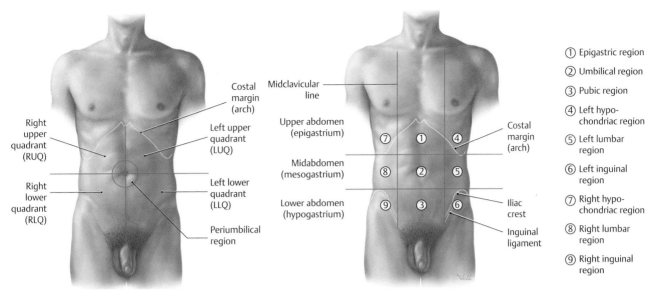

A The abdomen is divided into four quadrants by two perpendicular lines that intersect at the umbilicus.

Fig. 7.2 Criteria for dividing the abdomen into regions

B Coordinate system composed of two vertical and two horizontal lines divide the abdomen into nine regions, each located in either the upper, middle, or lower abdomen. The two vertical lines are the left and right midclavicular lines. One of the two horizontal lines passes through the lowest point of the 10th ribs and the other through the summit of the two iliac crests.

① Epigastric region
② Umbilical region
③ Pubic region
④ Left hypo-chondriac region
⑤ Left lumbar region
⑥ Left inguinal region
⑦ Right hypo-chondriac region
⑧ Right lumbar region
⑨ Right inguinal region

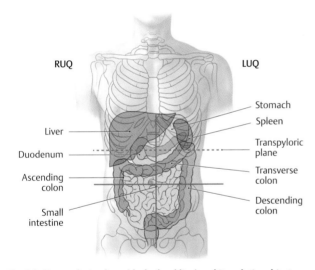

Fig. 7.3 Transpyloric plane (dashed red line) and its relationship to abdominal viscera
Anterior view. RUQ, right upper quadrant; LUQ, left upper quadrant.

7.2 Structure of the Abdominal Wall

Superficial Fascial Layer

- **The superficial fascia** lies deep to the skin and superficial to the muscular layer. It has two components (see **Fig 7.5C**):
  - The **superficial fatty layer (Camper's fascia)**, a subcutaneous layer of fat whose thickness varies among individuals

and that is continuous with the superficial fascia of the thorax, back, and lower limb
  - The **deep membranous layer (Scarpa's fascia)**, a tough fibrous sheet that lies deep to the superficial fatty layer, covers the lower anterior abdominal wall, and extends inferiorly into the perineum, where it is continuous with the **superficial perineal (Colles') fascia.**

Muscular Layer

- Three flat muscles make up most of the muscular layer of the lateral and anterior walls of the abdomen: the **external oblique, internal oblique,** and **transversus abdominis (Table 7.1)**. Their large aponeuroses constitute the most anterior part of the abdominal wall **(Fig. 7.4)**.
  - The thickened inferior edge of the external oblique aponeurosis forms the **inguinal ligament,** which attaches laterally to the **anterior superior iliac spine** and medially to the **pubic tubercle** of the pubis (see **Fig. 10.8A**). Some fibers of the medial end of the ligament reflect downward as the **lacunar ligament** to attach to the superior edge of the pubis (see **Table 7.2**).
  - Inferiorly, the aponeuroses of the internal oblique and transversus abdominis muscles join to form the **conjoined tendon,** where they attach to the pubis.
  - In the anterior midline, the aponeuroses of the three muscles overlap those of the contralateral muscles, forming the **linea alba,** a tendinous raphe (junction) that extends from the xiphoid process to the pubis. The **umbilical ring,** a remnant of the opening for the umbilical cord, interrupts the raphe at its midpoint.

Table 7.1 **Muscles of the Anterolateral and Posterior Abdominal Walls**

Muscle		Origin	Insertion	Innervation	Action
Anterolateral abdominal wall					
External oblique		5th to 12th ribs (outer surface)	Linea alba, pubic tubercle, anterior iliac crest	Intercostal nn. (T7–T11), subcostal n. (T12)	*Unilateral:* bends trunk to same side, rotates trunk to opposite side *Bilateral:* flexes trunk, compresses abdomen, stabilizes pelvis
Internal oblique		Thoracolumbar fascia (deep layer), iliac crest (intermediate line), anterior superior iliac spine, iliopsoas fascia	10th to 12th ribs (lower borders), linea alba (anterior and posterior layers)	Intercostal nn. subcostal n. (T12) iliohypogastric n., ilioinguinal n.	*Unilateral:* bends trunk to same side, rotates trunk to opposite side *Bilateral:* flexes trunk, compresses abdomen, stabilizes pelvis
Transversus abdominis		7th to 12th costal cartilages (inner surfaces), thoracolumbar fascia (deep layer), iliac crest, anterior superior iliac spine (inner lip), iliopsoas fascia	Linea alba, pubic crest	Intercostal nn. (T7–T11), subcostal n. (T12) iliohypogastric n., ilioinguinal n.	*Unilateral:* rotates trunk to same side *Bilateral:* compresses abdomen
Rectus abdominis		*Lateral head:* Crest of pubis to pubic tubercle *Medial head:* Anterior region of pubic symphysis	Cartilages of 5th to 7th ribs, xiphoid process of sternum	Intercostal nn. (T5–T11), subcostal n. (T12)	Flexes trunk, compresses abdomen, stabilizes pelvis
Pyramidalis		Pubis (anterior to rectus abdominis)	Linea alba (runs within the rectus sheath)	Subcostal n.	Tenses linea alba
Posterior abdominal wall					
Psoas major	Superficial layer	T12–L4 vertebral bodies and associated intervertebral disks (lateral surfaces)	Femur (lesser trochanter), joint insertion with iliacus muscle	Lumbar plexus	Hip joint: flexion and external rotation Lumbar spine (with femur fixed): *Unilateral:* contraction bends trunk laterally *Bilateral:* contraction raises trunk from supine position
	Deep layer	L1–L5 (costal processes)			
Psoas minor		T12, L1 vertebrae and intervertebral disk (lateral surfaces)	Pecten pubis, iliopubic ramus, iliac fascia; lowermost fibers may reach inguinal ligament	Lumbar plexus	
Iliacus		Iliac fossa		Femoral n.	Hip joint: flexion and external rotation Lumbar spine (with femur fixed): *Unilateral:* contraction bends trunk laterally *Bilateral:* contraction raises trunk from supine position
Quadratus lumborum		Iliac crest and iliolumbar ligament (not shown)	12th rib, L1–L4 vertebrae (transverse processes)	T12, L1–L4 spinal nn.	*Unilateral:* bends trunk to same side *Bilateral:* bearing down and expiration, stabilizes 12th rib

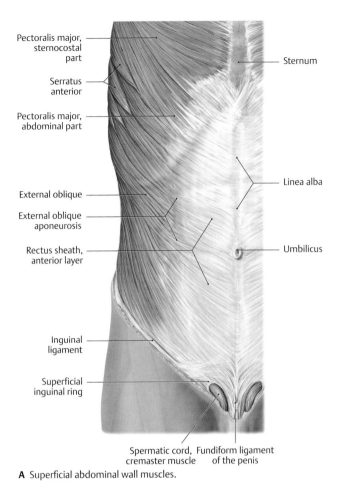

Pectoralis major, sternocostal part

Serratus anterior

Pectoralis major, abdominal part

External oblique

External oblique aponeurosis

Rectus sheath, anterior layer

Inguinal ligament

Superficial inguinal ring

Sternum

Linea alba

Umbilicus

Inguinal ligament

Spermatic cord, cremaster muscle   Fundiform ligament of the penis

A Superficial abdominal wall muscles.

Internal intercostals

External intercostals

Rectus abdominis

External oblique

Internal oblique

Internal oblique aponeurosis

Anterior superior iliac spine

Inguinal ligament

Rectus sheath, anterior layer

Costal cartilage

Sternum

Xiphoid process

Linea alba

Umbilicus

Spermatic cord, cremaster muscle

B *Removed:* External oblique, pectoralis major, and serratus anterior.

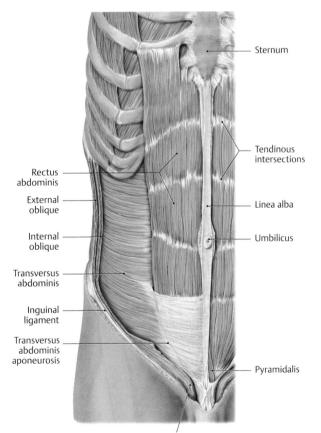

Rectus abdominis

External oblique

Internal oblique

Transversus abdominis

Inguinal ligament

Transversus abdominis aponeurosis

Sternum

Tendinous intersections

Linea alba

Umbilicus

Pyramidalis

Spermatic cord, cremaster muscle

C *Removed:* Internal oblique.

Fig. 7.4 Muscles of the anterior abdominal wall
Right side, anterior view.

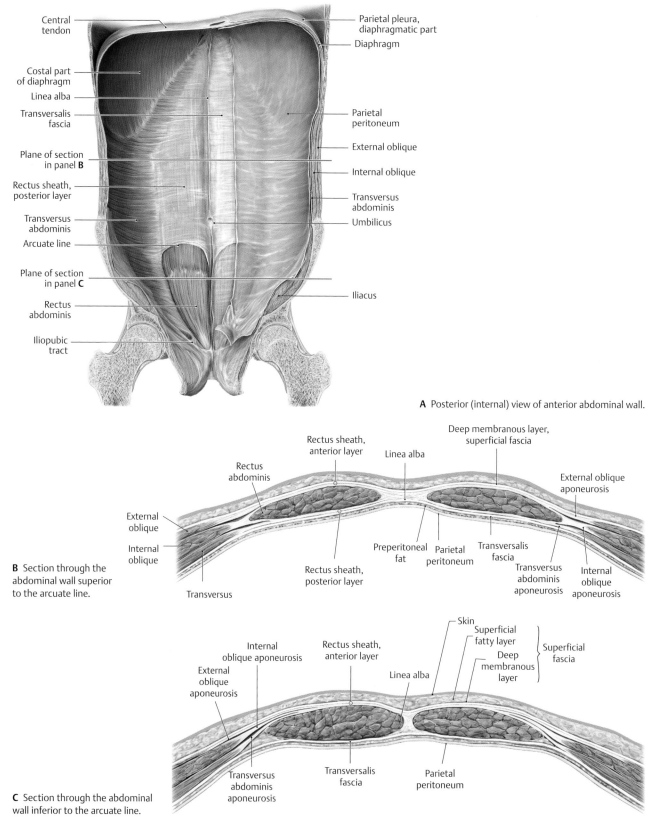

A Posterior (internal) view of anterior abdominal wall.

B Section through the abdominal wall superior to the arcuate line.

C Section through the abdominal wall inferior to the arcuate line.

Fig. 7.5 Anterior abdominal wall and rectus sheath

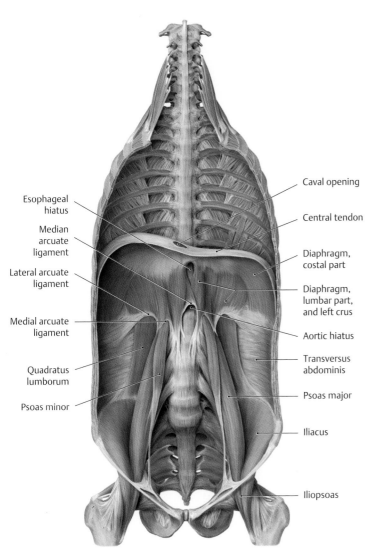

Fig. 7.6 Muscles of the posterior abdominal wall
Coronal section with the diaphragm in the intermediate position, anterior view.

Esophageal hiatus

Median arcuate ligament

Lateral arcuate ligament

Medial arcuate ligament

Quadratus lumborum

Psoas minor

Caval opening

Central tendon

Diaphragm, costal part

Diaphragm, lumbar part, and left crus

Aortic hiatus

Transversus abdominis

Psoas major

Iliacus

Iliopsoas

— **A rectus sheath** encloses the **rectus abdominis** and **pyramidalis muscles** on either side of the anterior midline (**Fig. 7.5**; see also **Fig. 7.4C**).
  • The lateral edges of the sheath are visible externally as the **semilunar lines.**
  • The sheath has anterior and posterior layers, formed by the aponeuroses of the anterolateral muscles as they split to pass around the rectus muscles.
  • The **arcuate line** is the inferior end of the posterior layer of the rectus sheath. Inferior to this, the aponeuroses only pass anterior to the rectus muscles.
— Five muscles form most of the posterior abdominal wall: the **psoas major, psoas minor** (sometimes absent), **quadratus lumborum, iliacus,** and diaphragm (**Fig. 7.6**).
  • The psoas major and iliacus muscles unite to form the **iliopsoas muscle,** which passes into the thigh and acts on the hip joint.
  • The thoracic diaphragm forms part of the superior portion of the posterior abdominal wall.
  • The transversus abdominis muscle contributes to the lateral part of the posterior abdominal wall.
— **Endoabdominal fascia** is a deep fascial layer that lines the internal surface of the abdominal wall muscles. It lies superficial to (outside of) the parietal peritoneum and in

most places is separated from it by a layer of fat called **preperitoneal fat.**
  • Each part of the endoabdominal fascia is named for the muscle it lines: **transversalis fascia** (see **Fig. 7.5B**), **diaphragmatic fascia, psoas fascia.**
  • In the inguinal region (groin), a thickened line of the transversalis fascia, the **iliopubic tract,** attaches to the inner edge of the inguinal ligament, where it supports the posterior wall of the inguinal canal (see **Fig. 7.5A**).

Internal Surface of the Anterior Abdominal Wall

The internal surface of the anterior abdominal wall is lined with transversalis fascia and parietal peritoneum, with a variable amount of intervening preperitoneal fat (**Fig. 7.7**).
— **Peritoneal folds** form where structures tent the peritoneum as they course between it and the transversalis fascia. The folds include
  • the **median umbilical fold,** a single midline fold created by the **median umbilical ligament,** a remnant of the **urachus** (a fetal connection between the bladder and umbilicus);
  • the **medial umbilical folds,** paired folds created by the **medial umbilical ligaments,** remnants of the umbilical arteries in the fetus; and

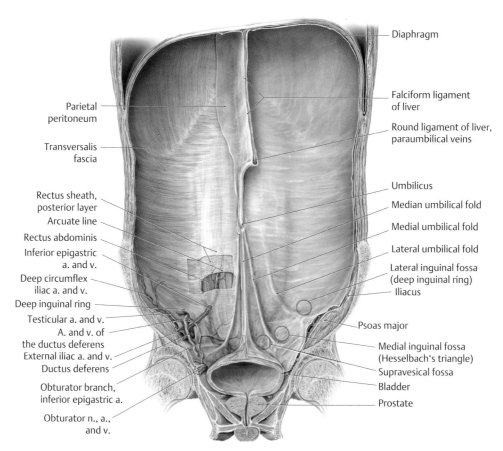

Fig. 7.7 Internal surface anatomy of the anterior abdominal wall in the male
Coronal section through the abdominal and pelvic cavity at the level of the hip joints, posterior view.

- the **lateral umbilical folds,** paired folds created by the **inferior epigastric vessels.**
— **Peritoneal fossae** are formed between the peritoneal folds and are potential sites of herniation (protrusion of viscera through a wall or tissue). The fossae include (**Fig 7.8**)
  - the **supravesical fossa** between the median and medial umbilical folds;
  - the **medial inguinal fossa,** commonly known as the **inguinal triangle of Hesselbach** (Hesselbach's triangle) between the medial and lateral umbilical folds; and
  - the **lateral inguinal fossa,** lateral to the lateral umbilical folds.
— The **falciform ligament** is a double-layered peritoneal reflection between the liver and the anterior abdominal wall that extends superiorly from the umbilicus to the roof of the abdominal cavity. It encloses the round ligament (remnant of the umbilical vein) and paraumbilical veins.

7.3   Neurovasculature of the Abdominal Wall

Arteries of the Abdominal Wall

Arteries of the abdominal wall, which anastomose extensively with one another, arise from the internal thoracic artery, the abdominal aorta, the external iliac artery, and the femoral artery (**Fig. 7.9**).
— The branches of each internal thoracic artery are
  - the musculophrenic artery and

- the superior epigastric artery, which descends within the rectus sheath posterior to the rectus abdominis muscle, where it anastomoses with the inferior epigastric artery.

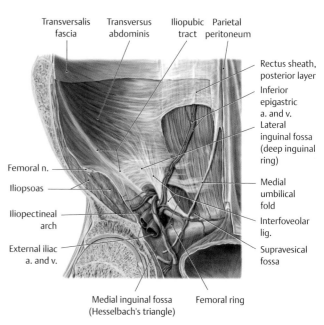

Fig. 7.8 Inferior anterior abdominal wall: structure and fossae
Coronal section, posterior (internal) view of left inferior portion of the anterior abdominal wall.

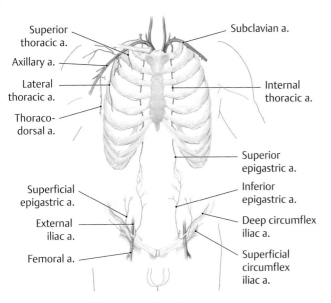

Fig. 7.9 Arteries of the abdominal wall
The superior and inferior epigastric arteries form a potential anastomosis between the subclavian and femoral arteries, which can allow blood to bypass the abdominal aorta.

— The paired segmental branches of the abdominal aorta are
  • the intercostal, subcostal, and lumbar arteries.
— The branches of the external iliac artery are
  • the inferior epigastric artery and deep circumflex iliac artery.
— The branches of the femoral artery in the thigh that supply the abdominal wall are
  • the **superficial epigastric artery** and
  • the **superficial circumflex iliac artery.**

Veins of the Abdominal Wall

— The deep veins of the abdominal wall accompany the arteries of similar name and drain to the superior and inferior venae cavae via the brachiocephalic, azygos, hemiazygos, and common iliac veins (**Fig 7.10**).
— An extensive subcutaneous venous network drains superiorly to the internal thoracic and **lateral thoracic veins** of the thorax and inferiorly to the **inferior** and **superficial epigastric veins.**
— Obstruction of the superior or inferior vena cava may alter the venous flow across the abdominal wall, resulting in the development or enlargement of a superficial anastomosis between the axillary and femoral veins through the thoraco-epigastric vein (see Section 4.4).

Fig. 7.10 Neurovascular structures of the anterior trunk wall
Anterior view.
Left side: superficial dissection. *Right side:* deep dissection. *Removed:* pectoralis major and minor. *Partially removed:* external oblique, internal oblique, transversus abdominis, rectus abdominis, and intercostal muscles.

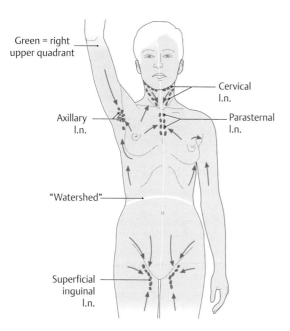

Fig. 7.11 **Lymphatic pathways and regional lymph nodes of the anterior trunk wall**
Anterior view. *Arrows* indicate the direction of lymph flow.

Lymphatic Drainage of the Abdominal Wall

— Lymphatic drainage of the abdominal wall is divided into upper and lower regions by a curved line ("watershed") located between the umbilicus and costal margin **(Fig. 7.11)**.
  • From the upper region, lymph drains superiorly to ipsilateral axillary and parasternal nodes before draining superiorly to the right and left jugulosubclavian junctions (venous angles).
  • From the lower region, lymph drains inferiorly to ipsilateral superficial inguinal nodes. These drain to external iliac and common iliac nodes and eventually to the thoracic duct.

Nerves of the Abdominal Wall

— Nerves of the abdominal wall arise from thoracic and lumbar spinal nerves **(Fig. 7.12)** and include
  • the lower intercostal nerves (T7–T11) and the subcostal nerve (T12) of the thorax, and
  • the iliohypogastric nerve of the lumbar plexus.
— Dermatomes of the abdominal wall follow the slope of the ribs. Landmark dermatomes that correspond to visible surface features of the abdominal wall include T10 at the umbilicus and L1 at the inguinal ligament and top of the pubis.

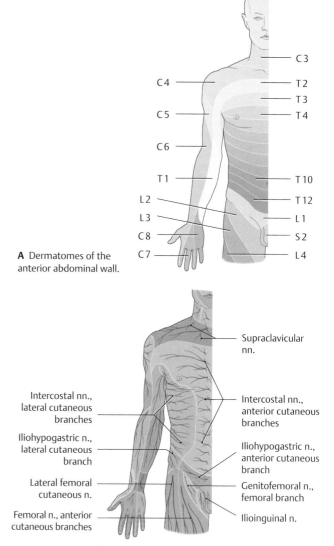

A Dermatomes of the anterior abdominal wall.

B Sensory nerves of the anterior abdominal wall.

Fig. 7.12 **Cutaneous innervation of the anterior abdominal wall**

7.4   The Inguinal Region

The **inguinal region,** or groin, includes the inferolateral region of the anterior abdominal wall **(Fig. 7.13)**.

Inguinal Canal

The inguinal canal is an oblique passage through the abdominal wall that allows structures to pass between the abdominal and

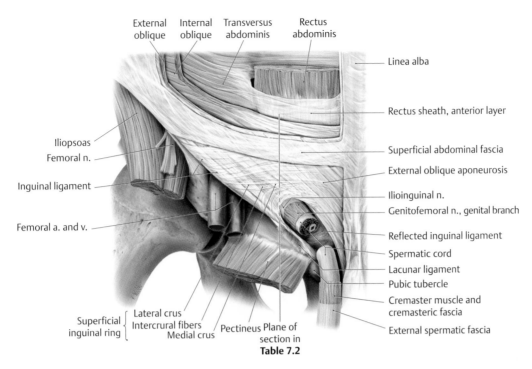

Fig. 7.13 Male inguinal region
Right side, anterior view.

pelvic cavities and the perineum. Deficiencies in the anterolateral abdominal muscles, their aponeuroses, and their deep fascia create the inguinal canal (**Table 7.2**).
— The boundaries of the canal are
  • the anterior wall, formed by the aponeurosis of the external oblique muscle;
  • the posterior wall, formed by transversalis fascia and conjoined tendon;
  • the floor, formed by the inguinal ligament; and
  • the roof, formed by the arching fibers of the aponeuroses of the internal oblique and transversus abdominis muscles.
— The canal has two openings:

  • At the medial end of the canal, fibers of the external oblique aponeurosis split to create an opening known as the **superficial inguinal ring.** This ring lies in the anterior wall of the inguinal triangle of Hesselbach.
  • At the lateral end of the inguinal canal, immediately lateral to the origin of the inferior epigastric vessels, the transversalis fascia evaginates into the canal and creates the **deep inguinal ring.** This ring lies in the lateral inguinal fossa (see **Fig. 7.7**).
— The contents of the inguinal canal include the **spermatic cord** in males and the **round ligament** of the uterus in females (**Fig. 7.14**; also see Section 11.2).

Table 7.2 **Structures of the Inguinal Canal**

Structures		Formed by
Wall	Anterior wall	① External oblique aponeurosis
	Roof	② Internal oblique muscles
		③ Transversus abdominis
	Posterior wall	④ Transversalis fascia
		⑤ Parietal peritoneum
	Floor	⑥ Inguinal ligament (densely interwoven fibers of the lower external oblique aponeurosis and adjacent fascia lata of thigh)
Openings	Superficial inguinal ring	Opening in external oblique aponeurosis; bounded by medial and lateral crus, intercrural fibers, and reflected inguinal ligament
	Deep inguinal ring	Outpouching of the transversalis fascia lateral to the lateral umbilical fold (inferior epigastric vessels)

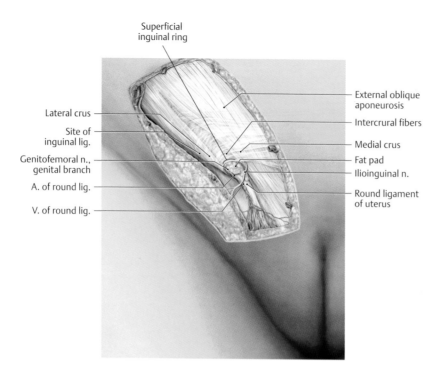

Fig. 7.14 Female inguinal region
Right side, anterior view.

Labels (figure):
- Superficial inguinal ring
- Lateral crus
- Site of inguinal lig.
- Genitofemoral n., genital branch
- A. of round lig.
- V. of round lig.
- External oblique aponeurosis
- Intercrural fibers
- Medial crus
- Fat pad
- Ilioinguinal n.
- Round ligament of uterus

The Spermatic Cord

The spermatic cord forms at the deep inguinal ring, traverses the inguinal canal, and exits through the superficial inguinal ring. It enters the scrotum and descends to the posterior surface of the testis (**Fig. 7.15**).

— The structures in the spermatic cord include
  • the ductus deferens;
  • processus vaginalis;
  • the testicular artery and pampiniform plexus of veins, the artery of the ductus deferens, and the cremasteric artery;
  • lymphatic vessels of the testis and spermatic cord; and
  • sympathetic and parasympathetic fibers of the testicular plexus and the genital branch of the genitofemoral nerve.

— Derivatives of the muscles and fascia of the abdominal wall surround the contents of the spermatic cord as they pass through the inguinal canal. The layers formed by the muscles and fascia are the same as those surrounding the testis (**Table 7.3**):
  • **Internal spermatic fascia** derived from the transversalis fascia
  • **Cremaster muscle** and **cremasteric fascia** derived from the internal oblique muscle and fascia
  • **External spermatic fascia** derived from the external oblique aponeurosis and fascia

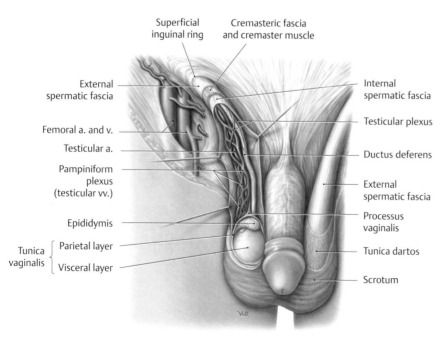

Labels (figure):
- Superficial inguinal ring
- Cremasteric fascia and cremaster muscle
- External spermatic fascia
- Femoral a. and v.
- Testicular a.
- Pampiniform plexus (testicular vv.)
- Epididymis
- Tunica vaginalis { Parietal layer / Visceral layer }
- Internal spermatic fascia
- Testicular plexus
- Ductus deferens
- External spermatic fascia
- Processus vaginalis
- Tunica dartos
- Scrotum

Fig. 7.15 Spermatic cord
Male pelvis, anterior view. *Opened:* Inguinal canal and coverings of the spermatic cord.

Table 7.3 **Coverings of the Testis**

Covering of the Testis	Abdominal Wall Derivative
① Scrotal skin	Abdominal skin
② Tunica dartos	Dartos fascia and muscle
③ External spermatic fascia	External oblique fascia
④ Cremaster muscle and cremasteric fascia	Internal oblique muscle and fascia
⑤ Internal spermatic fascia	Transversalis fascia
⑥ⓐ Tunica vaginalis, parietal layer	Peritoneum
⑥ⓑ Tunica vaginalis, visceral layer	

The transverse abdominis has no contribution to the spermatic cord or covering of the testis.

CLINICAL CORRELATION

INGUINAL HERNIA AND HYDROCELE Inguinal hernias account for the large majority of abdominal wall hernias, and of those, most occur in males. A hernia is the protrusion of a visceral structure into a space that it does not normally occupy. Inguinal hernias involve the protrusion of parietal peritoneum, peritoneal fat, or the small intestine. Of the two types of inguinal hernias, the indirect hernia can be acquired or congenital and is common in young males, whereas the direct hernia is always acquired and results from a weakening of the abdominal wall and generally occurs in middle-aged males **(Fig. 7.16)**.

During development, a tongue of peritoneum, the processus vaginalis, evaginates into the newly formed inguinal canal and accompanies the testis in its descent into the scrotum. Before birth most of the processus vaginalis obliterates, closing the communication between it and the peritoneal cavity. If the processus vaginalis fails to obliterate, however, abdominal contents can herniate (indirect hernia) through its opening at the deep inguinal ring in the lateral inguinal fossa (lateral to the inferior epigastric vessels)

and extend into the scrotum (or labia in females). Herniated viscera travel within the spermatic cord and therefore are covered by the layers of the cord in addition to peritoneum and transversalis fascia.

Direct hernias occur where weakening of the anterior abdominal wall in the medial inguinal triangle (medial to the inferior epigastric vessels) allows viscera to protrude through the medial end of the canal, then through an enlarged superficial ring, and into the scrotum. Since these herniated viscera travel outside the spermatic cord, they are not covered by layers of the spermatic cord but are covered by peritoneum and transversalis fascia of the abdominal wall.

The opening into a persistent processus vaginalis may be small enough to prevent herniation but large enough to form a hydrocele, the accumulation of excess peritoneal fluid. The hydrocele can be confined to the scrotum (hydrocele of the testis) or to the cord (hydrocele of the cord). Ultrasound or transillumination of the scrotum confirms the presence of excess fluid.

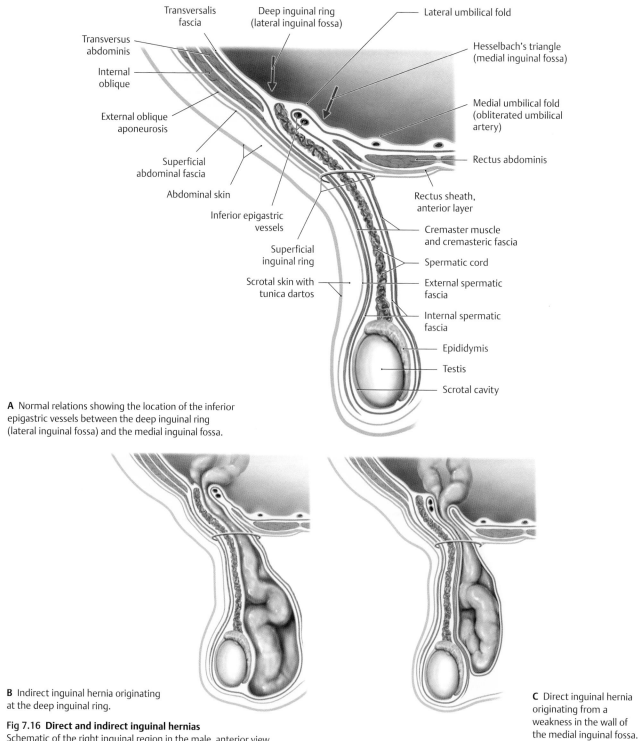

A Normal relations showing the location of the inferior epigastric vessels between the deep inguinal ring (lateral inguinal fossa) and the medial inguinal fossa.

B Indirect inguinal hernia originating at the deep inguinal ring.

C Direct inguinal hernia originating from a weakness in the wall of the medial inguinal fossa.

Fig 7.16 Direct and indirect inguinal hernias
Schematic of the right inguinal region in the male, anterior view.

The Testes

The testes are paired ovoid reproductive organs, 4 to 5 cm long and 3 cm wide, located in separate compartments within the scrotum. They produce spermatozoa and secrete the male hormone testosterone (**Figs. 7.17** and **7.18**; see also **Table 7.3**).

- An extension of the peritoneum known as the **tunica vaginalis** forms a closed sac that folds around the testis, surrounding it on all sides except on its posterior edge. The

tunic has an outer parietal layer and an inner visceral layer that is adherent to the surface of the testis.

- Each testis is enveloped by the **tunica albuginea**, a tough capsule of connective tissue that thickens along the posterior border as the mediastinum of the testis and invaginates to divide the testis into over 200 lobules.

- Sperm are produced in the **seminiferous tubules,** highly coiled tubules within the lobules. They exit the testes through

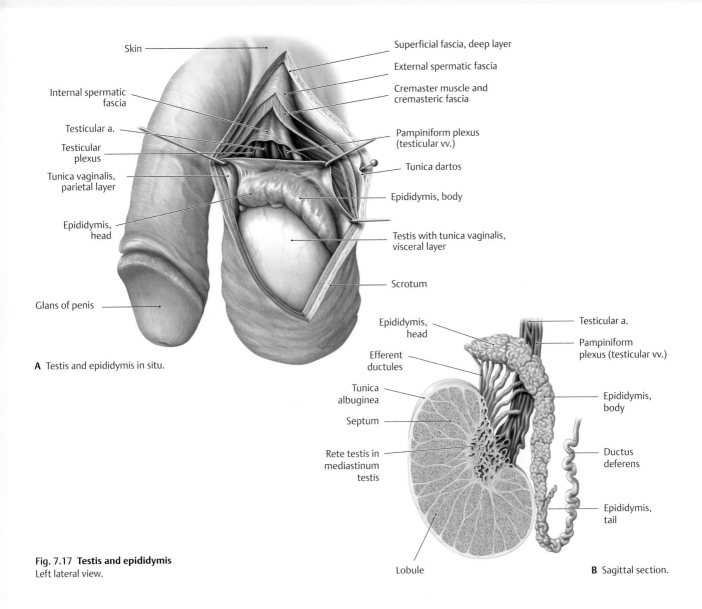

A Testis and epididymis in situ.

Skin

Superficial fascia, deep layer

External spermatic fascia

Cremaster muscle and cremasteric fascia

Internal spermatic fascia

Testicular a.

Pampiniform plexus (testicular vv.)

Testicular plexus

Tunica vaginalis, parietal layer

Tunica dartos

Epididymis, body

Epididymis, head

Testis with tunica vaginalis, visceral layer

Scrotum

Glans of penis

Epididymis, head

Testicular a.

Pampiniform plexus (testicular vv.)

Efferent ductules

Tunica albuginea

Epididymis, body

Septum

Rete testis in mediastinum testis

Ductus deferens

Epididymis, tail

Lobule

Fig. 7.17 Testis and epididymis
Left lateral view.

B Sagittal section.

Pubis

Pubic symphysis

Corpus cavernosum of penis

Spermatic cord

Urethra

Corpus spongiosum of penis

Mediastinum of testis

Tunica albuginea

Testes

Fig 7.18 MRI of the testes
Coronal section, anterior view.

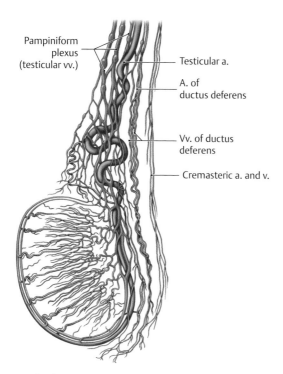

Pampiniform plexus (testicular vv.)

Testicular a.

A. of ductus deferens

Vv. of ductus deferens

Cremasteric a. and v.

Fig. 7.19 Blood vessels of the testis
Left lateral view.

a ductal network, the **rete testis** in the mediastinum, and then pass through **efferent ductules** to the **epididymis.**

— The testicular artery, a branch of the abdominal aorta, supplies the testis. A rich collateral blood supply arises from anastomoses with the artery of the ductus deferens, the **cremasteric artery** (a branch of the inferior epigastric artery), and the **external pudendal artery** (a branch of the femoral artery) **(Fig. 7.19).**

— The **pampiniform plexus** of veins drains the testis and converges to form the testicular vein. The testicular veins drain to the inferior vena cava on the right and to the renal vein on the left.

— The lymph vessels of the testes drain directly to lateral aortic and preaortic lymph nodes.

CLINICAL CORRELATION

VARICOCELE The pampiniform plexus from each testis surrounds the testicular artery and converges to form a testicular vein. If the venous valves become incompetent, the plexus can become dilated and tortuous, forming a varicocele that is often reported to feel like "a bag of worms." Varicoceles are predominantly on the left side. This is generally attributed to the abrupt termination of the left testicular vein at the left renal vein, which may slow venous return.

— The **cremasteric reflex,** initiated by stroking of the inner thigh, contracts the cremaster muscle and elevates the testis. The ilioinguinal nerve provides the sensory limb; the genital branch of the genitofemoral nerve provides the motor limb.

CLINICAL CORRELATION

ABSENT OR REDUCED CREMASTERIC REFLEX An absent or reduced cremasteric reflex that is accompanied by sudden testicular pain, inflammation and elevation of one testis, nausea, and vomiting may indicate testicular torsion (twisting of a testis). Prompt surgery for testicular torsion (to untwist the affected testis and anchor both testes) may prevent loss of a testis.

— The testicular nerve plexus arises from the aortic plexus and travels along with the testicular artery. It contains sympathetic fibers from the T7 spinal cord level, as well as visceral afferent and vagal parasympathetic fibers.

CLINICAL CORRELATION

TESTICULAR CANCER Testicular cancer is the most common cancer in males between 15 and 34 years of age. The vast majority of these cancers are seminomas or germ cell tumors that arise in the germ cells that produce immature sperm. Symptoms include a lump in the affected testis (usually only one testis is affected), a feeling of heaviness in the scrotum, pain in the affected testis or scrotum, a sudden collection of fluid in the scrotum, and the development of excess breast tissue (gynecomastia). Testicular cancer commonly metastasizes via lymph nodes to the lungs or via the bloodstream, commonly to the liver, lungs, brain, and spine.

The Epididymis and Ductus Deferens

The epididymis and ductus deferens are parts of the male ductal system that transport sperm from the testis to the genital structures in the pelvis (see **Fig. 7.17**).

— The epididymis, a highly coiled tubule where sperm are stored and mature, hugs the posterior surface of the testis. Its expanded head contains the lobules with the efferent ductules, its body is made up of a long convoluted duct, and its tail is continuous with the ductus deferens.

— The **ductus deferens** is a muscular tube that transmits sperm from the scrotum to the pelvis.

 • It begins at the tail of the epididymis and continues as part of the spermatic cord through the inguinal canal.

 • At the deep inguinal ring, the ductus deferens descends into the pelvis posterior to the bladder, where, near its termination, it enlarges as the **ampulla of the ductus deferens** (see **Fig. 11.2**).

 • The ampulla joins with the duct of the seminal gland (vesicle) to form the ejaculatory duct (see Section 11.1).

8 The Peritoneal Cavity and Neurovasculature of the Abdomen

8.1 The Peritoneum and Peritoneal Cavity

The **peritoneum**, a thin, transparent serous membrane, lines the abdominopelvic cavity. Parietal and visceral layers of the peritoneum enclose the **peritoneal cavity**, which contains a thin film of serous fluid that facilitates the movement of the viscera during digestion and respiration (see **Fig. 7.1**).

Peritoneal Relations

— Structures in the abdomen are defined with respect to their relationship to the peritoneum (**Table 8.1**; **Figs. 8.1** and **8.2**).
  • **Intraperitoneal** organs, almost completely enclosed by the visceral layer of the peritoneum, are suspended within the peritoneal cavity by **mesenteries**, double layers of peritoneum that attach to the body wall.
  • **Extraperitoneal** structures lie posterior or inferior to the peritoneal cavity.
    ○ **Primarily retroperitoneal** structures lie posterior to the peritoneal cavity, are not suspended by a mesentery, and are covered by peritoneum only on their anterior surface.
    ○ **Secondarily retroperitoneal** structures were previously intraperitoneal structures that became fixed to the posterior abdominal wall when their mesentery fused with the parietal peritoneum of the posterior abdominal wall during development.
    ○ **Subperitoneal structures** include pelvic organs that lie below the peritoneum.
— Organs associated with the gastrointestinal tract are intraperitoneal or secondarily retroperitoneal. Organs of the urinary system are retroperitoneal.

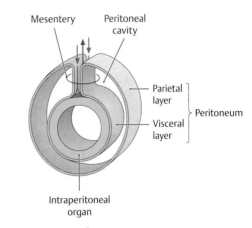

Fig. 8.1 Peritoneum and mesentery
Red and *blue arrows* indicate location of blood vessels.

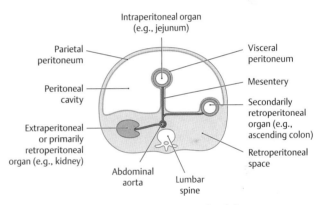

Fig. 8.2 Peritoneal relations of the organs in the abdomen
Transverse section through the abdomen showing the peritoneal relationships of abdominal organs. Viewed from above.

Table 8.1 **Organs of the Abdomen**

Location		Organs
Intraperitoneal organs: These organs have a mesentery and are completely covered by the peritoneum.		
Abdominal peritoneal cavity		• Stomach • Small intestine (jejunum, ileum, some of the superior part of the duodenum) • Spleen • Liver (with the exception of the bare area) • Gallbladder • Cecum with vermiform appendix (portions of variable size may be retroperitoneal) • Large intestine (transverse and sigmoid colons)
Extraperitoneal organs: These organs either have no mesentery or lost it during development.		
Retroperitoneum	Primarily retroperitoneal	• Kidneys • Suprarenal glands
	Secondarily retroperitoneal	• Duodenum (descending, horizontal, and ascending) • Pancreas • Ascending and descending colon

Peritoneal Structures

Most of the abdominal viscera are somewhat mobile during digestion and respiration. Reflections of the peritoneum that connect organs to the body wall or to other organs prevent excessive movement (i.e., twisting), which can compromise normal function. These reflections form mesenteries, omenta, and peritoneal ligaments.

— A **mesentery** is a double layer of peritoneum that connects intraperitoneal organs to the posterior abdominal wall and transmits vessels and nerves (see **Fig. 8.1**). There are three major mesenteries in the abdomen (**Fig. 8.3**):

  • The **mesentery of the small intestine**, or the "mesentery," is a fan-shaped apron of peritoneum that suspends the second and third parts (jejunum and ileum) of the small intestine.
  • The **transverse mesocolon** suspends the transverse section of the large intestine.
  • The **sigmoid mesocolon** suspends the sigmoid colon of the large intestine in the left lower quadrant.

— An **omentum** is a double layer of peritoneum that connects the stomach and duodenum to another organ. There are two omenta (**Figs. 8.4** and **8.5**; see also **Fig. 9.1**):

  • The **greater omentum**, a four-layered apron of peritoneum, originates as a double layer of peritoneum from the greater curvature of the stomach and proximal duodenum. It drapes inferiorly, anterior to the coils of small intestine, before looping upward to its distal attachment on the posterior abdominal wall (**Fig 8.4A**).

    ◦ The **gastrocolic ligament** is a portion of the greater omentum that adheres to the transverse colon (**Fig. 8.6**).
    ◦ The **gastrosplenic ligament** is a lateral extension of the greater omentum that connects the stomach to the spleen and is traversed by branches of the splenic artery (**Fig. 8.7**).

  • The **lesser omentum**, a double layer of peritoneum, extends from the liver to the stomach and proximal duodenum (**Fig 8.4B**). It is formed by

    ◦ the **hepatogastric ligament**, between the liver and stomach, and
    ◦ the **hepatoduodenal ligament**, between the liver and duodenum, which encloses the structures of the **portal triad** (the portal vein, hepatic artery, and **bile duct**) in its free edge.

— **Peritoneal ligaments** are reflections of peritoneum that connect organs to each other or to the body wall. They support the organ in position and may convey their neurovasculature. Individual ligaments are discussed in Sections 9.2 to 9.4 with the specific abdominal organs.

A Transverse mesocolon and small bowel mesentery
Reflected: Greater omentum and transverse colon.

Fig. 8.3 Mesenteries of the peritoneal cavity
Anterior view.

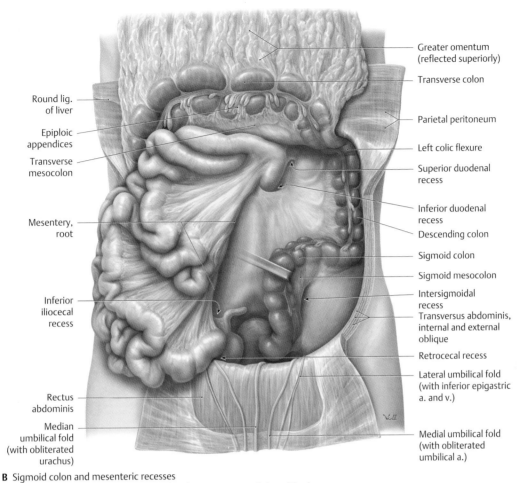

Round lig. of liver

Epiploic appendices

Transverse mesocolon

Mesentery, root

Inferior iliocecal recess

Rectus abdominis

Median umbilical fold (with obliterated urachus)

Greater omentum (reflected superiorly)

Transverse colon

Parietal peritoneum

Left colic flexure

Superior duodenal recess

Inferior duodenal recess

Descending colon

Sigmoid colon

Sigmoid mesocolon

Intersigmoidal recess

Transversus abdominis, internal and external oblique

Retrocecal recess

Lateral umbilical fold (with inferior epigastric a. and v.)

Medial umbilical fold (with obliterated umbilical a.)

B Sigmoid colon and mesenteric recesses
Reflected: Greater omentum, small bowel with mesentery, and sigmoid colon.

Fig. 8.3 (*continued*) **Mesenteries of the peritoneal cavity**

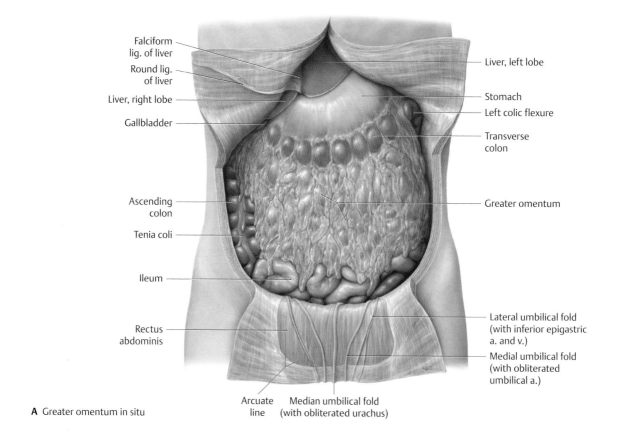

A Greater omentum in situ

B Greater and lesser omenta. *Reflected:* Liver, to expose the lesser omentum. Omental foramen *(arrow)*.

Fig. 8.4 Greater and lesser omenta
Anterior view of the opened abdomen.

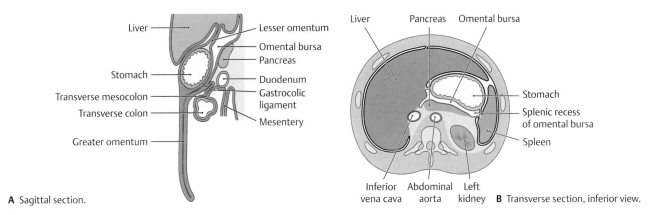

A Sagittal section.

B Transverse section, inferior view.

Fig. 8.5 Peritoneal structures

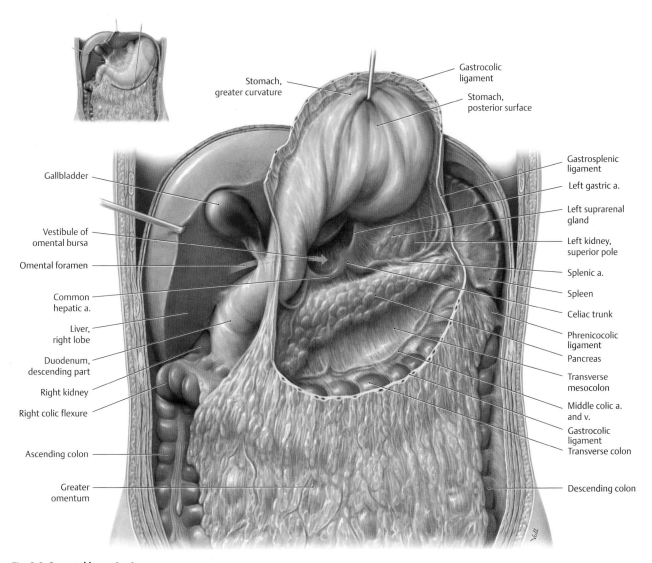

Fig. 8.6 Omental bursa in situ
Anterior view. *Divided:* Gastrocolic ligament. *Retracted:* Liver. *Reflected:* Stomach.

Fig. 8.7 Posterior wall of the peritoneal cavity
Anterior view. *Removed:* All intraperitoneal organs.

Neurovasculature of the Peritoneum

The **parietal** and **visceral layers** of the **peritoneum** derive their blood supply, lymphatic drainage, and innervation from different sources.

— Parietal peritoneum derives its neurovasculature from vessels and nerves of the body wall.
  • Its sensitivity to pain, pressure, and temperature is well localized (felt acutely) through somatic nerves of the overlying muscles and skin.
— Visceral peritoneum derives its neurovasculature from the underlying organs.

• Autonomic nerves mediate sensitivity to stretching and chemical irritation, but the visceral peritoneum lacks sensitivity to touch and temperature.
• Sensation is poorly localized and is usually referred to regions that reflect the embryologic origins of the underlying organ.
  ○ Sensation from foregut structures is referred to the epigastric region.
  ○ Sensation from midgut structures is referred to the umbilical region.
  ○ Sensation from hindgut structures is referred to the pubic region.

Table 8.2 **Boundaries of the Omental Bursa (Lesser Sac)**

Direction	Boundary	Recess
Anterior	Lesser omentum, gastrocolic ligament	–
Inferior	Transverse mesocolon	Inferior recess
Superior	Liver (with caudate lobe)	Superior recess
Posterior	Pancreas, aorta (abdominal part), celiac trunk, splenic a. and v., gastrosplenic fold, left suprarenal gland, left kidney (superior pole)	–
Right	Liver, duodenal bulb	–
Left	Spleen, gastrosplenic ligament	Splenic recess

Subdivisions of the Peritoneal Cavity

— The peritoneal cavity is divided into two spaces:
  • The **greater sac**, which includes the entire peritoneal cavity except that space defined as the lesser sac
  • The **omental bursa (lesser sac)**, which is a small extension of the peritoneal cavity that lies behind the stomach and lesser omentum (**Table 8.2**; see also **Figs. 8.5** and **8.6**). It communicates with the greater sac through a single opening, the **omental (epiploic) foramen** (**Table 8.3**).
— Attachments of the peritoneum to the body wall that form during development of the gastrointestinal tract further subdivide the greater sac. These attachments can influence the flow of fluid within the cavity (**Figs. 8.8 and 8.9**).
  • The **subphrenic recess** between the diaphragm and liver is limited by the coronary ligaments and separated into right and left spaces by the falciform ligament.
  • The **subhepatic space** lies between the liver and the transverse colon. A posterior extension of this space, the

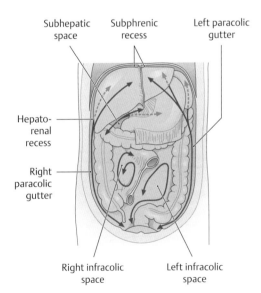

Fig. 8.8 Drainage spaces within the peritoneal cavity
Anterior view.

Labels in figure:
Subhepatic space
Subphrenic recess
Left paracolic gutter
Hepato-renal recess
Right paracolic gutter
Right infracolic space
Left infracolic space

Table 8.3 **Boundaries of the Omental Foramen**

The communication between the greater and lesser sacs is the omental (epiploic) foramen (see arrow in **Figs. 8.4B** and **8.6**).

Direction	Boundary
Anterior	Hepatoduodenal ligament with the portal v., proper hepatic a., and bile duct
Inferior	Duodenum (superior part)
Posterior	Inferior vena cava, diaphragm (right crus)
Superior	Liver (caudate lobe)

hepatorenal recess (hepatorenal pouch, Morison's pouch), lies between the visceral surface of the liver and the right kidney and suprarenal gland. The hepatorenal recess communicates with the right subphrenic recess.
  • The **supracolic** and **infracolic compartments** are defined by the attachment of the transverse mesocolon on the posterior abdominal wall—with the supracolic compartment above the attachment site and the infracolic compartment below it. The root of the mesentery of the small intestine further divides the infracolic compartment into right and left spaces.
  • The **paracolic gutters**, which lie adjacent to the ascending and descending colons, allow communication between the supracolic and infracolic compartments.

CLINICAL CORRELATION

PERITONITIS AND ASCITES Bacterial contamination of the peritoneum following surgery or rupture of an inflamed organ (duodenum, gallbladder, appendix) results in peritonitis, inflammation of the peritoneum. It is accompanied by severe abdominal pain, tenderness, nausea, and fever and can be fatal when generalized throughout the peritoneal cavity. It often results in ascites, the accumulation of excess peritoneal fluid due to a change in concentration gradients that results in loss of capillary fluid. Ascites can also accompany other pathologic conditions, such as metastatic liver cancer and portal hypertension. In these cases, many liters of ascitic fluid can accumulate in the peritoneal cavity. The fluid is aspirated by paracentesis. The needle is carefully inserted into the abdominal wall so as to avoid the urinary bladder and inferior epigastric vessels.

CLINICAL CORRELATION

PERITONEAL INFECTIONS AND ABSCESSES The flow of fluid in the peritoneal cavity can spread intraperitoneal infections and determine the sites of peritoneal abscess formation. Fluid commonly collects in the right and left subphrenic recesses, although abscesses are more likely to form on the right side due to duodenal or appendiceal ruptures. Fluid in the supracolic compartment, such as subphrenic recesses and the omental bursa, can drain to the hepatorenal recess, the lowest part of the abdominal cavity in the supine patient. Therefore, this is a common site of pus accumulation and abscess formation. In the infracolic compartment, the paracolic gutters direct peritoneal fluid and infections toward the pelvis.

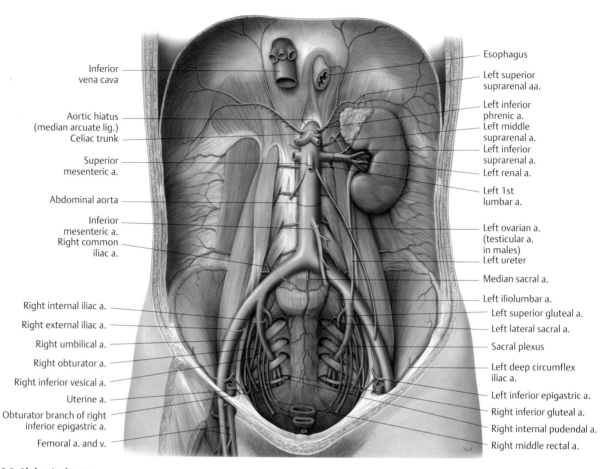

Fig. 8.9 Abdominal aorta
Female abdomen, anterior view. *Removed:* Abdominal organs and peritoneum. The abdominal aorta is the distal continuation of the thoracic aorta. It enters the abdomen at the T12 level and bifurcates into the common iliac arteries at L4.

8.2   Neurovasculature of the Abdomen

Arteries of the Abdomen

— The **abdominal aorta** supplies abdominal viscera and most of the anterior abdominal wall (**Fig. 8.9**).
  • It enters the abdomen at T12 through the aortic hiatus of the diaphragm and descends along the vertebral column to the left of the midline.
  • It terminates at the L4 vertebral level, where it bifurcates into two **common iliac arteries**.
  • A single **median sacral artery** arises near the bifurcation.

CLINICAL CORRELATION

ABDOMINAL AORTIC ANEURYSM Abdominal aortic aneurysms (AAAs) most commonly occur between the renal arteries and the bifurcation of the aorta. When small they can remain asymptomatic, but large aneurysms can be palpated through the abdominal wall to the left of the midline. Ruptured AAAs present with severe abdominal pain that radiates to the abdomen or back. Mortality rates for ruptured aneurysms approach 90% due to overwhelming hemorrhage.

— **Table 8.4** lists major branches of the abdominal aorta.
  • Paired parietal (segmental) branches supply the structures of the posterior abdominal wall. These include the **inferior phrenic** and **lumbar arteries**.

Table 8.4 **Branches of the Abdominal Aorta**

The abdominal aorta gives rise to three major unpaired trunks (bold) and the unpaired median sacral artery, as well as six paired branches.

Branch from Abdominal Aorta	Branches	
Inferior phrenic aa. (paired)	Superior suprarenal aa.	
Celiac trunk	Left gastric a.	
	Splenic a.	
	Common hepatic a.	Proper hepatic a.
		Right gastric a.
		Gastroduodenal a.
Middle suprarenal aa. (paired)		
Superior mesenteric a.		
Renal aa. (paired)	Inferior suprarenal aa.	
Lumbar aa. (1st through 4th, paired)		
Testicular/ovarian aa. (paired)		
Inferior mesenteric a.		
Common iliac aa. (paired)	External iliac a.	
	Internal iliac a.	
Median sacral a.		

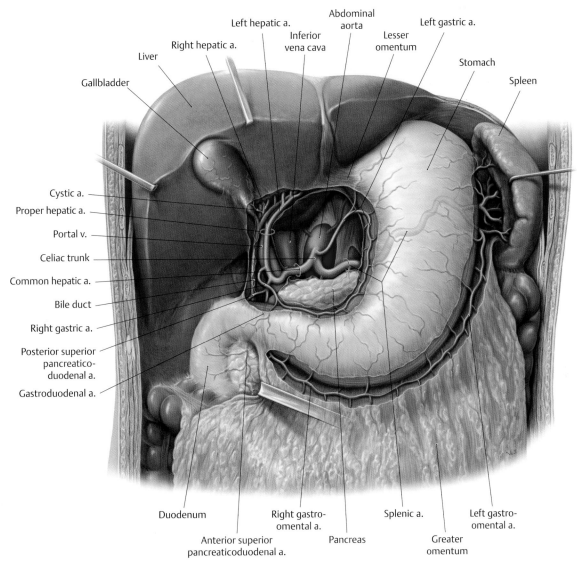

Fig. 8.10 Celiac trunk: Stomach, liver, and gallbladder
Anterior view. *Opened:* Lesser omentum. *Incised:* Greater omentum. The celiac trunk arises from the abdominal aorta at about the level of L1.

- Paired visceral branches supply organs of the retroperitoneum. These are the **middle suprarenal, testicular** or **ovarian**, and **renal arteries**.
- Three unpaired visceral branches supply the intestines and accessory organs of the gastrointestinal tract:
  1. The **celiac trunk**, a short trunk that arises at T12/L1 and supplies the abdominal foregut. Its branches, the **splenic, left gastric**, and **common hepatic arteries**, anastomose extensively with each other (**Figs. 8.10** and **8.11**).
  2. The **superior mesenteric artery** (SMA), which arises at L1, posterior to the neck of the pancreas. It supplies midgut structures, and its major branches include the **inferior pancreaticoduodenal, middle colic, right colic**, and **ileocolic arteries**, as well as a series of **jejunal** and **ileal branches** (**Fig. 8.12**).
  3. The **inferior mesenteric artery** (IMA), which arises at L3 and has the smallest caliber of the three visceral trunks. It supplies the hindgut through its **left colic, sigmoidal**, and **superior rectal** branches (**Fig. 8.13**).
- Common iliac arteries pass along the brim of the pelvis and terminate by bifurcating into two major branches (see **Fig. 8.9**):
  - The **internal iliac artery**, which descends into the pelvis
  - The **external iliac artery**, which gives off the **inferior epigastric** and **deep circumfex iliac arteries** before passing into the lower limb as the **femoral artery**.
- Important anastomoses connect the three unpaired visceral branches of the aorta and provide a collateral blood supply to the intestinal organs (**Fig. 8.14**).
  - The celiac trunk and superior mesenteric artery anastomose in the head of the pancreas through the **pancreaticoduodenal arteries** and in the body and tail of the pancreas through **dorsal pancreatic** and **inferior pancreatic arteries**.

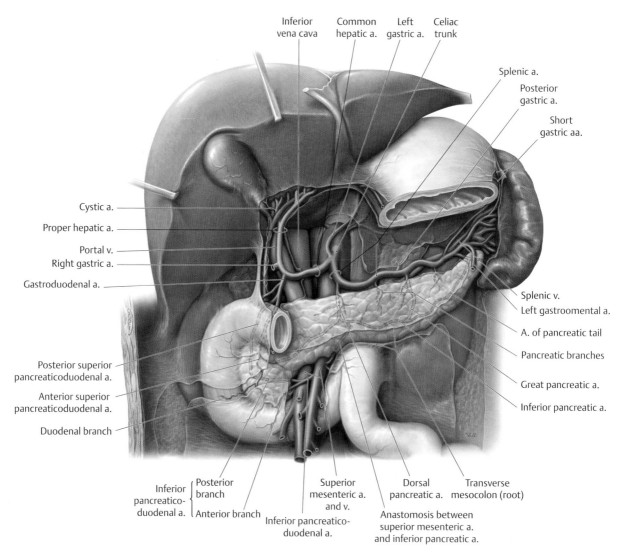

Fig. 8.11 Celiac trunk: Pancreas, duodenum, and spleen
Anterior view. *Removed:* Stomach (body) and lesser omentum.

- The superior mesenteric and inferior mesenteric arteries anastomose near the junction of the transverse and descending colons through the middle and left colic arteries. The **marginal artery** runs along the mesenteric border of the large intestine and connects the ileocolic,

  right colic, middle colic, and left colic arteries (see **Fig. 8.13**).
- The inferior mesenteric artery anastomoses with arteries of the rectum through its **superior rectal artery** (see **Fig. 10.18**).

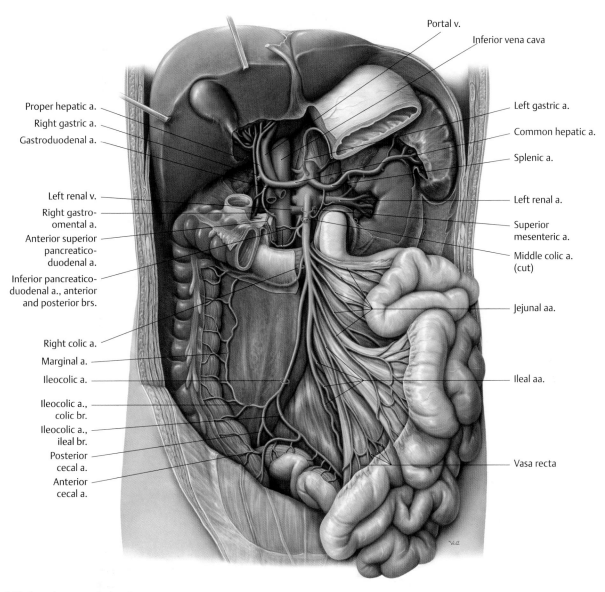

Portal v.
Inferior vena cava
Proper hepatic a.
Right gastric a.
Gastroduodenal a.
Left gastric a.
Common hepatic a.
Splenic a.
Left renal v.
Right gastro-omental a.
Anterior superior pancreatico-duodenal a.
Inferior pancreatico-duodenal a., anterior and posterior brs.
Left renal a.
Superior mesenteric a.
Middle colic a. (cut)
Jejunal aa.
Right colic a.
Marginal a.
Ileocolic a.
Ileal aa.
Ileocolic a., colic br.
Ileocolic a., ileal br.
Posterior cecal a.
Anterior cecal a.
Vasa recta

Fig. 8.12 Superior mesenteric artery
Anterior view. *Partially removed:* Stomach and peritoneum. *Note:* The middle colic artery has been truncated. The superior mesenteric artery arises from the aorta opposite L2.

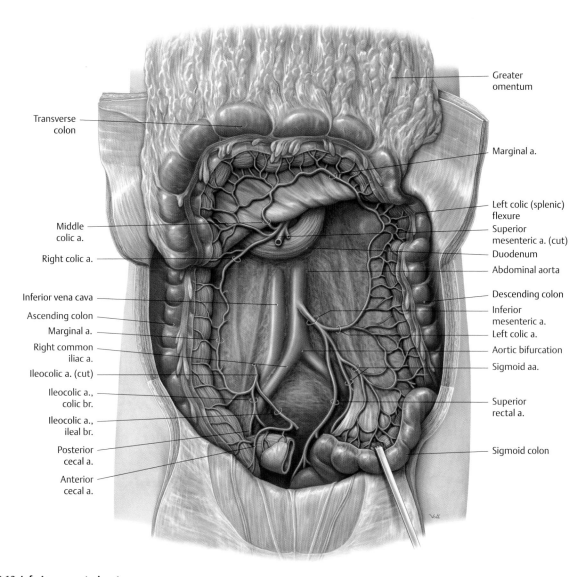

Fig. 8.13 Inferior mesenteric artery

Anterior view. *Removed:* Jejunum and ileum. *Reflected:* Transverse colon. The inferior mesenteric artery arises from the aorta opposite L3.

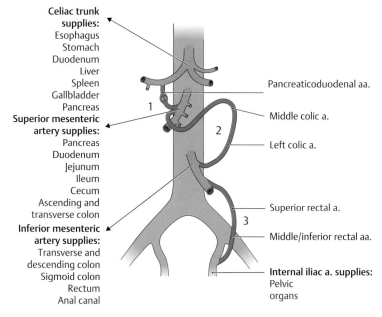

Fig. 8.14 Abdominal arterial anastomoses

Three major anastomoses provide overlap in the arterial supply to ensure adequate blood flow to abdominal areas: *1*, between the celiac trunk and the superior mesenteric artery via the pancreaticoduodenal arteries; *2*, between the superior and inferior mesenteric arteries via the middle and left colic arteries; and *3*, between the inferior mesenteric and internal iliac arteries via the superior and middle or inferior rectal arteries

Veins of the Abdomen

— The **inferior vena cava** (IVC) receives blood from retroperitoneal and pelvic organs, walls of the abdomen and pelvis, and the lower limbs (**Figs. 8.15** and **8.16**).
- It originates at the L5 vertebral level where the **common iliac veins** merge.
- It ascends along the right side of the vertebral column, passes posterior to the liver, and pierces the central tendon of the diaphragm at the T8 vertebral level, where it enters the right atrium of the heart.

— **Table 8.5** lists the direct tributaries of the inferior vena cava.
- Paired common iliac veins drain the **external iliac** and **internal iliac veins.**
- Paired **inferior phrenic** and **lumbar veins** drain the posterior abdominal wall and diaphragm and accompany the arteries of similar name.
- Veins of the retroperitoneal organs include the **right** and **left renal veins**, the right **suprarenal vein**, and the right **testicular** or **ovarian** (gonadal) **vein.** The suprarenal and gonadal veins on the left side drain to the left renal vein.

- Typically three **hepatic veins** enter the IVC from the liver immediately below the diaphragm.

— Paired **ascending lumbar veins** communicate with the lumbar veins and are continuous with the azygos and hemiazygos veins of the thorax. These communications between the lumbar, ascending lumbar, azygos, and hemiazygos veins function as a collateral pathway between the inferior and superior venae cavae (see **Fig. 3.8**).

— The **hepatic portal vein** (usually known as the **portal vein**), part of the **hepatic portal system**, shunts nutrient-rich venous blood from the capillary beds of the gastrointestinal tract and its associated organs to sinusoids of the liver (**Figs. 8.17** and **8.18**). This blood eventually enters the inferior vena cava through the hepatic veins.

— Tributaries of the portal vein are listed in **Table 8.6** and include the following:
- The **splenic vein**, which drains the spleen, and the **superior mesenteric vein**, which drains the small intestine and most of the large intestine. These two veins unite behind the neck of the pancreas to form the hepatic portal vein.

Fig. 8.15 Inferior vena cava
Anterior view. *Removed:* All organs except the kidneys and suprarenal glands.

Fig 8.16 Tributaries of the inferior vena cava
Note the asymmetry of venous drainage from the right and left kidneys, suprarenal glands, gonads, and posterior wall veins.

Table 8.5 **Direct Tributaries of the Inferior Vena Cava**

- Right and left inferior phrenic veins
- Hepatic veins
- Right suprarenal vein
- Right and left renal veins at the L1/L2 level (the left testicular/ovarian vein and left suprarenal vein terminate in the left renal vein)
- Lumbar veins
- Right testicular/ovarian vein
- Common iliac veins (L5 level)
- Median sacral vein (often terminates in the left common iliac vein)

- The **inferior mesenteric vein,** which drains the hindgut portion of the gastrointestinal tract. It usually joins the splenic vein but may empty directly into the portal vein.
- Veins from the lower esophagus, stomach, pancreas, duodenum, and gallbladder
— Normal connections between the systemic (caval) venous system and portal venous system, called **portosystemic pathways (Fig. 8.19)**, can become abnormally dilated when there is an obstruction of the portal or systemic circulations (i.e., cirrhosis of the liver or pregnancy). These dilations are most prominent in
1. **esophageal veins,**
2. **periumbilical veins** through the superior and inferior epigastric veins of the abdominal wall,
3. **colic veins** in the retroperitoneum, and
4. **rectal veins** of the rectum and anal canal.

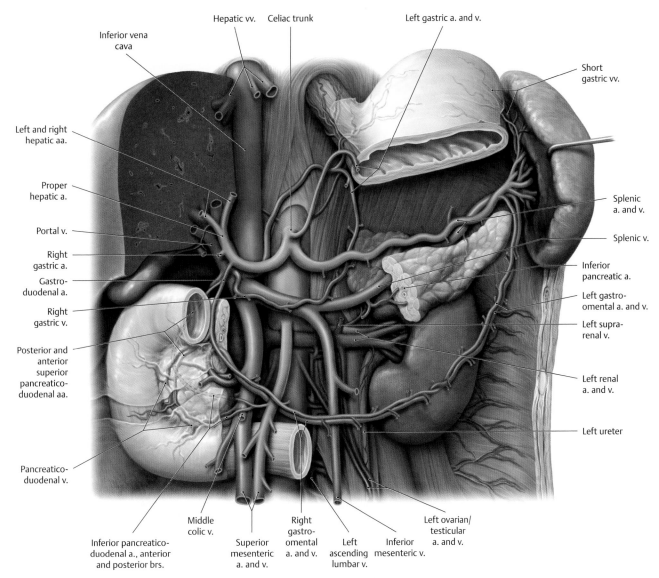

Fig. 8.17 Portal vein: In situ
Anterior view. *Partially removed:* Stomach, pancreas, and peritoneum.

CLINICAL CORRELATION

ESOPHAGEAL VARICES Submucosal veins of the esophagus drain superiorly to the systemic system (through the azygos veins) and inferiorly to the portal system. When flow through the portal vein is obstructed (as in portal hypertension), these portosystemic anastomoses allow blood in the lower esophagus to drain to the systemic veins. The esophageal varices, enlarged veins that result from this increased flow, can rupture, causing severe hemorrhaging.

CLINICAL CORRELATION

PORTAL HYPERTENSION AND SURGICAL PORTOCAVAL SHUNTS Portal hypertension occurs secondary to liver disease (e.g., cirrhosis) or thrombosis of the portal vein. Increased resistance to the flow of blood in the portal system forces portal blood through portocaval anastomoses to the systemic circulation. Symptoms of portal hypertension include ascites, caput medusa (enlargement of periumbilical veins on the anterior abdominal wall), varices of the rectal veins (hemorrhoids), and esophageal varices. Symptoms may be relieved by surgically creating a portocaval shunt between the portal and systemic circulations (portal vein to the inferior vena cava or splenic vein to the left renal vein).

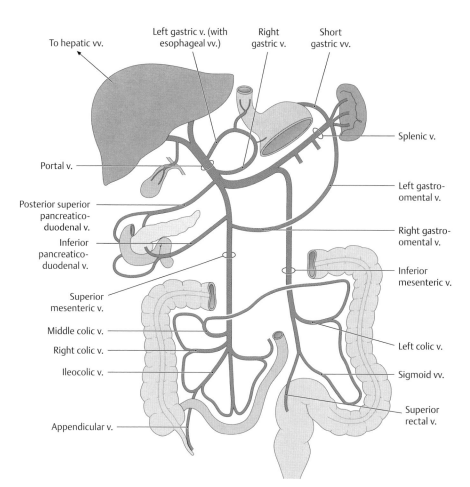

Fig. 8.18 Portal vein distribution
The portal vein drains venous blood from the abdominopelvic organs supplied by the celiac trunk and superior and inferior mesenteric arteries.

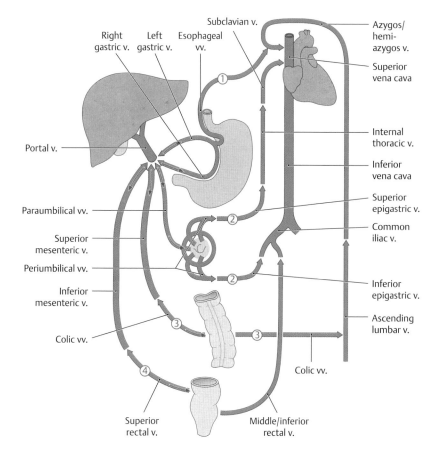

Fig. 8.19 Portosystemic pathways
When the portal system is compromised, the portal vein can divert blood away from the liver back to its supplying veins, which return this nutrient-rich blood to the heart via the venae cavae. *Red arrows* indicate flow reversal in the *(1)* esophageal veins, *(2)* paraumbilical veins, *(3)* colic veins, and *(4)* middle and inferior rectal veins.

Table 8.6 Tributaries of the Portal Vein

- **Superior mesenteric vein** with its tributaries:
  - Pancreaticoduodenal veins
  - Pancreatic veins
  - Right gastro-omental vein
  - Jejunal veins
  - Ileal veins
  - Ileocolic vein
  - Right colic vein
  - Middle colic vein

- **Inferior mesenteric vein** with its tributaries:
  - Left colic vein
  - Sigmoid veins
  - Superior rectal vein

- **Splenic vein** with its tributaries:
  - Left gastro-omental vein
  - Pancreatic veins
  - Short gastric veins

- **Direct tributaries**
  - Cystic vein
  - Left gastric vein with esophageal veins
  - Right gastric vein
  - Posterior superior pancreaticoduodenal vein
  - Prepyloric vein
  - Paraumbilical veins

Lymphatic Drainage of the Abdomen

Lymph from abdominal and pelvic regions drains through lymphatic vessels that usually accompany the arteries supplying those regions. The lymph passes through one or more lymph node groups that can include primary, or regional, nodes and secondary, or collecting, nodes. These latter groups receive lymph from multiple regions and in the abdomen and pelvis and are known as **lumbar lymph nodes**. They surround the aorta and inferior vena cava and are subdivided by location (**Fig. 8.20**). Lymph drains from these nodes into either the **lumbar** or **intestinal lymphatic trunks**, which converge in the upper abdomen to form the **cisterna chyli** and the thoracic duct.

- Groups of lumbar lymph nodes drain all of the abdominal viscera (except a small hepatic segment, which can drain to nodes of the diaphragm) and most of the abdominal wall (**Fig. 8.21; Table 8.7**). They include:
  - **Preaortic nodes**, which lie anterior to the abdominal aorta. They receive lymph from the gastrointestinal tract (as far as the midrectum) and associated organs. Nodes surrounding the base of the major arteries form collecting nodal groups, such as the **superior** and **inferior mesenteric nodes**. These drain to **celiac nodes**, which drain to intestinal lymph trunks.
  - **Right and left lumbar nodes** (lateral aortic and caval nodes), which lie along the medial border of the psoas muscles, the crura of the diaphragm, the aorta, and the inferior vena cava. They drain the abdominal and pelvic

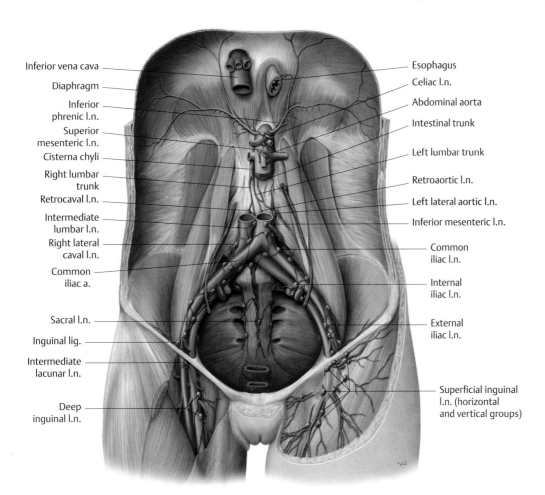

Fig. 8.20 Parietal lymph nodes in the abdomen and pelvis
Anterior view. *Removed*: All visceral structures except vessels

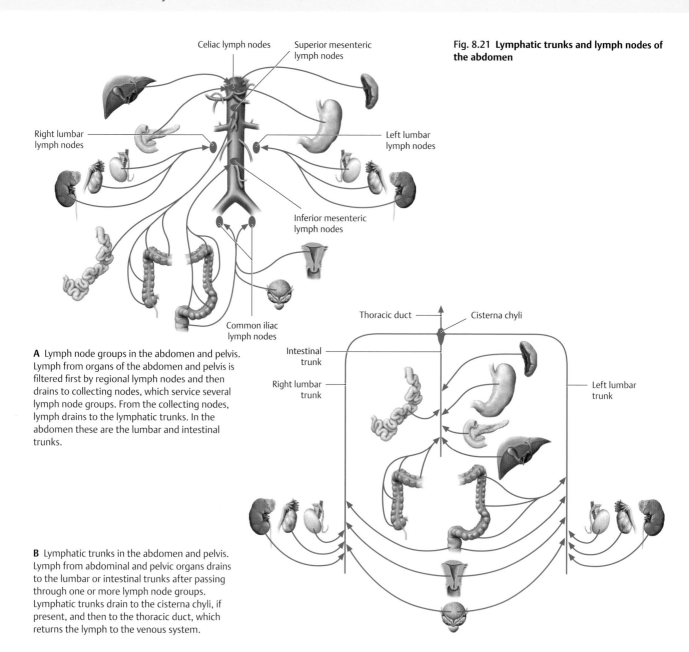

Fig. 8.21 Lymphatic trunks and lymph nodes of the abdomen

A Lymph node groups in the abdomen and pelvis. Lymph from organs of the abdomen and pelvis is filtered first by regional lymph nodes and then drains to collecting nodes, which service several lymph node groups. From the collecting nodes, lymph drains to the lymphatic trunks. In the abdomen these are the lumbar and intestinal trunks.

B Lymphatic trunks in the abdomen and pelvis. Lymph from abdominal and pelvic organs drains to the lumbar or intestinal trunks after passing through one or more lymph node groups. Lymphatic trunks drain to the cisterna chyli, if present, and then to the thoracic duct, which returns the lymph to the venous system.

Table 8.7 **Lymph Node Groups and Tributary Regions**

Lymph Node Groups and Collecting Lymph Nodes	Location	Organs or Organ Segments that Drain to These Lymph Node Groups (Tributary Regions)
Celiac lymph nodes	Around the celiac trunk	Distal third of esophagus, stomach, greater omentum, duodenum (superior and descending parts), pancreas, spleen, liver, and gallbladder
Superior mesenteric lymph nodes	At the origin of the superior mesenteric artery	Second through fourth parts of duodenum, jejunum and ileum, cecum with vermiform appendix, ascending colon, transverse colon (proximal two-thirds)
Inferior mesenteric lymph nodes	At the origin of the inferior mesenteric artery	Transverse colon (distal third), descending colon, sigmoid colon, rectum (proximal part)
Lumbar lymph nodes (right, intermediate, left)	Around the abdominal aorta and inferior vena cava	Diaphragm (abdominal side), kidneys, suprarenal glands, testis and epididymis, ovary, uterine tube, uterine fundus, ureters, retroperitoneum
Iliac lymph nodes	Around the iliac vessels	Rectum (anal end), bladder and urethra, uterus (body and cervix), ductus deferens, seminal vesicle, prostate, external genitalia (via inguinal lymph nodes)

walls and the viscera of the retroperitoneum, including the ovaries and testes. They also receive lymph from the common iliac nodes, which drain the pelvic viscera and the lower limb. Drainage from these lumbar nodes forms a lumbar trunk on each side.

— **Common iliac nodes** drain organs of the pelvis and the lower limbs. Lymph from these nodes drain to the right and left lumbar nodes.

— The cisterna chyli is an elongated, lobulated, thin-walled dilation that, when present, gives rise to the thoracic duct. It lies to the right of the T12 vertebral body and receives the lumbar and intestinal trunks.

Nerves of the Abdomen

— Lower intercostal nerves (T7–T11) and the **subcostal nerve** (T12) continue anteroinferiorly from their position on the thoracic wall to innervate most of the muscles and skin of the anterolateral abdominal wall.

— The nerves of the **lumbar plexus**, a somatic nerve plexus formed by the anterior rami of spinal nerves T12–L4, emerge from the psoas major muscle on the posterior abdominal wall **(Fig. 8.22)**. Most nerves of this plexus innervate the lower limb (see Section 15.4 and **Table 15.1**). Branches that innervate the abdominal wall and inguinal region include

A Lumbar plexus in situ.

B Lumbar plexus dissection.
Windowed: psoas major.

Fig. 8.22 Nerves of the lumbar plexus
Anterior view.

- **iliohypogastric** and **ilioinguinal nerves** (L1), which innervate the skin and muscles of the inferior anterior abdominal wall and the skin over the inguinal and pubic regions;
- **genitofemoral nerve** (L1-L2), whose genital branch innervates the cremaster muscle surrounding the spermatic cord and the skin over the scrotum and labia; and
- short muscular branches (T12–L4) that innervate the muscles of the posterior abdominal wall.

— **Lumbar sympathetic trunks**, the continuations of the sympathetic trunks in the thorax, descend along the lateral aspect of the lumbar vertebral bodies and give off three to four **lumbar splanchnic nerves**, which join the autonomic plexuses of the abdomen.

— Autonomic plexuses form along the aorta and travel with the major abdominal arteries to innervate the abdominal viscera (**Figs. 8.23, 8.24, 8.25, 8.26; Tables 8.8** and **8.9**). The plexuses contain combinations of

- preganglionic sympathetic nerves that synapse in the ganglia associated with the plexuses. (Note that the sympathetic nerves innervating the adrenal medulla are an exception and do not synapse in these ganglia.) The preganglionic sympathetic nerves arise from

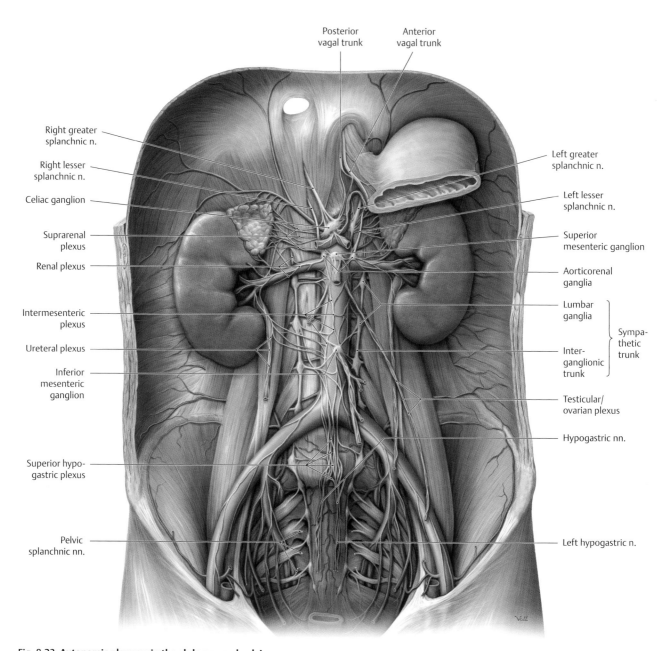

Fig. 8.23 Autonomic plexuses in the abdomen and pelvis
Anterior view of the male abdomen. *Removed:* Peritoneum and majority of the stomach.

- thoracic splanchnic nerves (T5–T12), which contribute to the celiac, superior mesenteric and renal plexuses
- lumbar splanchnic nerves (T11–L2), which contribute to the inferior mesenteric, superior hypogastric, and inferior hypogastric plexuses

• preganglionic parasympathetic nerves, which pass through the plexuses and synapse in ganglia near their target organ. They arise from either

- the vagus nerves (cranial nerve X), which enter the abdomen as anterior and posterior vagal trunks from the esophageal plexus. They supply most of the abdominal viscera, including the digestive tract, except for its most distal segment (the descending colon to the anal canal). They contribute to all of the abdominal plexuses except the inferior mesenteric, superior hypogastric, and inferior hypogastric plexuses.

Or

- the **pelvic splanchnic nerves** (S2–S4), which ascend from the pelvis to innervate the descending and sigmoid colons in the abdomen. They also innervate viscera of the pelvis. These fibers contribute to the inferior hypogastric plexuses.

— Although most abdominal plexuses contain both sympathetic and parasympathetic nerves, the inferior mesenteric and superior hypogastric plexuses contain only sympathetic fibers. Viscera supplied by these plexuses receive parasympathetic innervation via pelvic splanchnic nerves and the inferior hypogastric plexus **(Fig. 8.25A)**.

Table 8.8 **Autonomic Plexuses in the Abdomen and Pelvis**

Ganglia	Subplexus	Distribution	
Celiac plexus			
Celiac ganglia	Hepatic plexus	• Liver, gallbladder	
	Gastric plexus	• Stomach	
	Splenic plexus	• Spleen	
	Pancreatic plexus	• Pancreas	
Superior mesenteric plexus			
Superior mesenteric ganglia	—	• Pancreas (head) • Duodenum • Jejunum • Ileum	• Cecum • Colon (to left colic flexure) • Ovary
Suprarenal and renal plexus			
Aorticorenal ganglion	Ureteral plexus	• Suprarenal gland • Kidney • Proximal ureter	
Ovarian/testicular plexus			
—	—	• Ovary/testis	
Inferior mesenteric plexus			
—	Left colic plexus	• Left colic flexure	
	Superior rectal plexus	• Descending and sigmoid colon • Upper rectum	
Superior hypogastric plexus			
—	Hypogastric nn.	• Pelvic viscera	
Inferior hypogastric plexus			
Pelvic ganglia	Middle and inferior rectal plexus	• Middle and lower rectum	
	Prostatic plexus	• Prostate • Seminal vesicle • Bulbourethral gland	• Ejaculatory duct • Penis • Urethra
	Deferential plexus	• Ductus deferens • Epididymis	
	Uterovaginal plexus	• Uterus • Uterine tube	• Vagina • Ovary
	Vesical plexus	• Urinary bladder	
	Ureteral plexus	• Ureter (ascending from pelvis)	

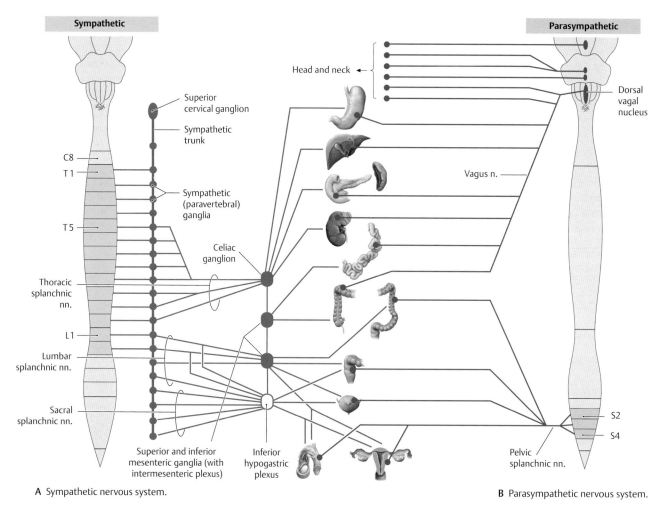

A Sympathetic nervous system.

B Parasympathetic nervous system.

Fig. 8.24 Sympathetic and parasympathetic nervous systems in the abdomen and pelvis

Table 8.9 **Effects of the Autonomic Nervous System in the Abdomen and Pelvis**

Organ (Organ System)		Sympathetic Effect	Parasympathetic Effect
Gastrointestinal tract	Longitudinal and circular muscle fibers	↓ Motility	↑ Motility
	Sphincter muscles	Contraction	Relaxation
	Glands	↓ Secretions	↑ Secretions
Splenic capsule		Contraction	No effect
Liver		↑ Glycogenolysis/gluconeogenesis	
Pancreas	Endocrine pancreas	↓ Insulin secretion	
	Exocrine pancreas	↓ Secretion	↑ Secretion
Urinary bladder	Detrusor vesicae	Relaxation	Contraction
	Functional bladder sphincter	Contraction	Inhibits contraction
Seminal gland and ductus deferens		Contraction (ejaculation)	No effect
Uterus		Contraction or relaxation, depending on hormonal status	
Arteries		Vasoconstriction	Vasodilation of the arteries of the penis and clitoris (erection)
Suprarenal glands (medulla)		Release of adrenalin	No effect
Urinary tract	Kidney	Vasoconstriction (↓ urine formation)	Vasodilation

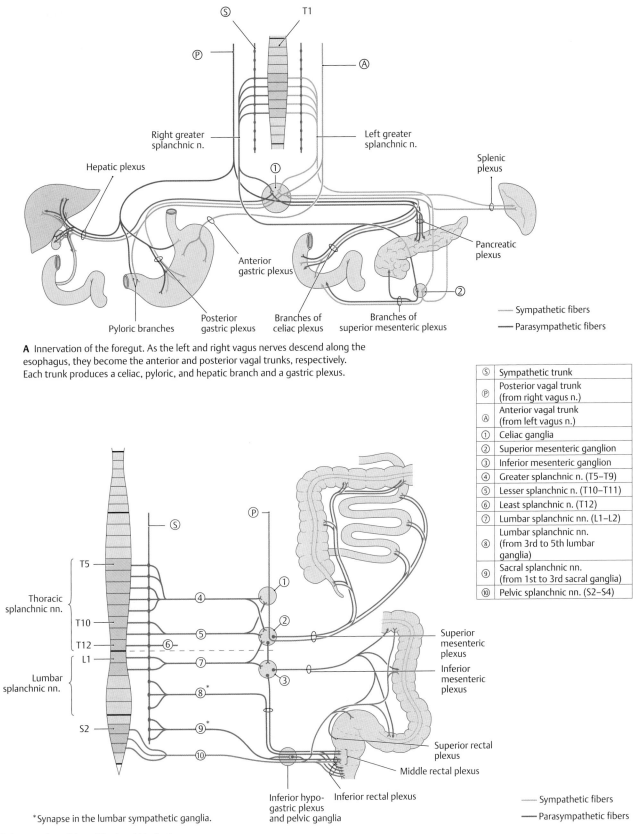

Ⓢ	Sympathetic trunk
Ⓟ	Posterior vagal trunk (from right vagus n.)
Ⓐ	Anterior vagal trunk (from left vagus n.)
①	Celiac ganglia
②	Superior mesenteric ganglion
③	Inferior mesenteric ganglion
④	Greater splanchnic n. (T5–T9)
⑤	Lesser splanchnic n. (T10–T11)
⑥	Least splanchnic n. (T12)
⑦	Lumbar splanchnic nn. (L1–L2)
⑧	Lumbar splanchnic nn. (from 3rd to 5th lumbar ganglia)
⑨	Sacral splanchnic nn. (from 1st to 3rd sacral ganglia)
⑩	Pelvic splanchnic nn. (S2–S4)

A Innervation of the foregut. As the left and right vagus nerves descend along the esophagus, they become the anterior and posterior vagal trunks, respectively. Each trunk produces a celiac, pyloric, and hepatic branch and a gastric plexus.

*Synapse in the lumbar sympathetic ganglia.

B Innervation of the midgut and hindgut.

Fig. 8.25 Autonomic innervation of the intraperitoneal organs

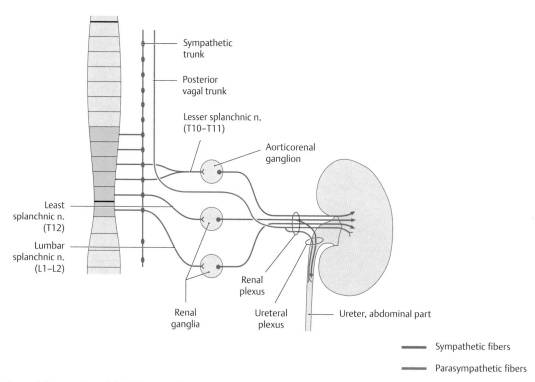

Sympathetic trunk

Posterior vagal trunk

Lesser splanchnic n. (T10–T11)

Aorticorenal ganglion

Least splanchnic n. (T12)

Lumbar splanchnic n. (L1–L2)

Renal ganglia

Renal plexus

Ureteral plexus

Ureter, abdominal part

Sympathetic fibers

Parasympathetic fibers

Fig. 8.26 Autonomic innervation of the kidneys and upper ureters

9 Abdominal Viscera

The peritoneal cavity of the abdomen contains the primary and accessory organs of the gastrointestinal tract. The primary organs are the stomach, small intestine, and large intestine; the accessory organs are the liver, gallbladder, pancreas, and spleen. The kid-neys, proximal ureters, and suprarenal glands are found outside the peritoneal cavity within the retroperitoneum on the posterior abdominal wall (**Fig. 9.1**).

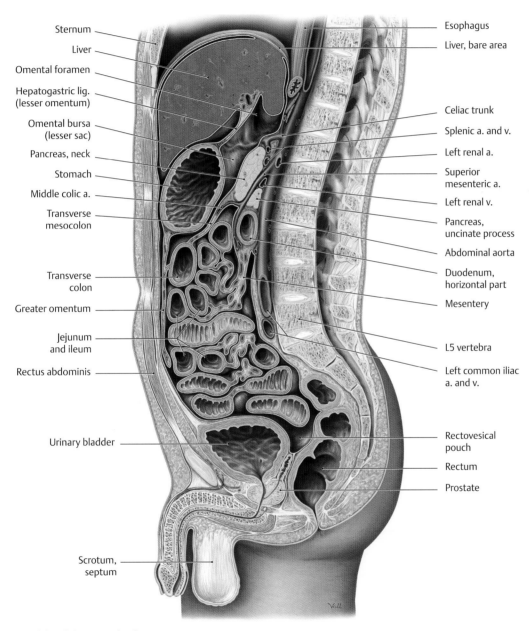

Fig. 9.1 Organs of the abdomen and pelvis
Midsagittal section through male pelvis, viewed from the left side.

9.1   Organs of the Peritoneal Cavity— Gastrointestinal Tract

Divisions of the Gastrointestinal Tract

The three divisions of the embryonic gastrointestinal tract are retained in the adult system and reflected in its blood supply and innervation. These divisions are

— the **foregut**, which consists of the distal esophagus, the stomach, the proximal half of the duodenum, the liver, the gallbladder, and the superior part of the pancreas;
— the **midgut**, which includes the distal half of the duodenum, the jejunum, ileum, cecum, and appendix, and the ascending and proximal two thirds of the transverse colon; and
— the **hindgut**, which includes the distal third of the transverse colon, the descending and sigmoid colons, the rectum, and the upper part of the anal canal.

DEVELOPMENT CORRELATION

ROTATION OF THE MIDGUT TUBE Development of the midgut is characterized by rapid elongation of the gut and its mesentery, resulting in the formation of the primary intestinal loop. The loop is attached anteriorly to the yolk sac by the omphaloenteric duct (yolk stalk) and posteriorly to the posterior abdominal wall by the superior mesenteric artery. As a result of this rapid elongation and expansion of the liver, the abdominal cavity becomes too small to contain all the intestinal loops, and they physiologically herniate into the proximal part of the umbilical cord. Coincident with growth in length, the primary intestinal loop rotates 270 degrees counter-clockwise (if viewed from the front) around the axis established by the attachment of the superior mesenteric artery. Rotation occurs during herniation (approximately 90 degrees) and during the return of the intestinal loops into the abdominal cavity (remaining 180 degrees), which is thought to occur when the relative size of the liver and kidney decreases. Malrotation of the midgut can result in congenital abnormalities such as volvulus (twisting) of the intestine.

DEVELOPMENT CORRELATION

LOCALIZATION OF PAIN FROM FOREGUT, MIDGUT, AND HINDGUT DERIVATIVES Pain from gastrointestinal organs follows pathways determined by embryologic origin. Pain from foregut structures is localized to the epigastric region, pain from structures of the midgut localizes in the periumbilical region, and pain arising from structures of the hindgut localizes in the hypogastric region.

Stomach

The **stomach**, a hollow reservoir that stores, churns, and initiates digestion of food, communicates with the esophagus proximally and the duodenum of the small intestine distally (**Figs 9.2, 9.3, 9.4**).

— It is normally J-shaped and lies in the left upper quadrant, although its shape and position vary among individuals and can change depending on its contents.
— The stomach has four parts:
  1. The **cardia**, which surrounds the opening to the esophagus
  2. The **fundus**, the superior portion that rises above and to the left of the opening between the esophagus and stomach (**cardiac orifice**)
  3. The **body**, the large expanded portion below the fundus
  4. The **pyloric part**, which is the outflow channel made up of the wide **pyloric antrum**, a narrow **pyloric canal**, and the **pyloris** or sphincteric region, which contains a muscular **pyloric sphincter** that surrounds the pyloric orifice into the first part of the duodenum.
— The stomach has a lesser curvature and a greater curvature.
  • The **lesser curvature** makes up the superior concave border. An **angular notch** (or incisure) along the curvature marks the junction of the body and pyloric part.
  • The **greater curvature** makes up the inferior convex border.

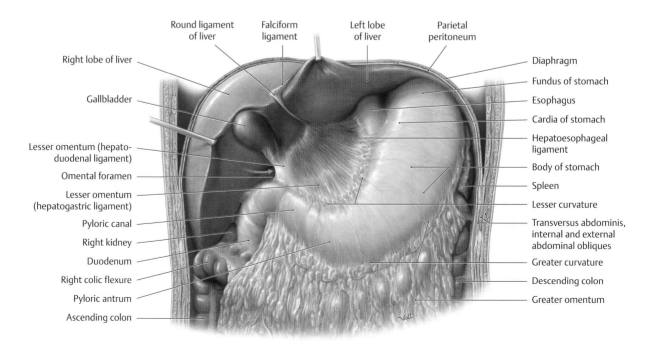

Fig 9.2 Stomach in situ
Anterior view of upper abdomen. The liver has been reflected superiorly to expose the stomach and lesser omentum.

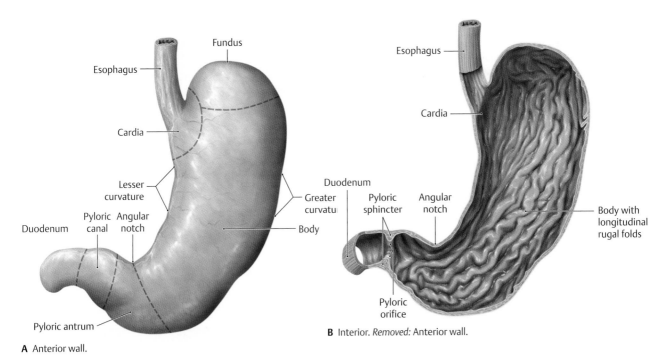

A Anterior wall.

B Interior. *Removed:* Anterior wall.

Fig. 9.3 Stomach
Anterior view.

— The inner surface of the stomach is highly distensible; in adults, the stomach can accommodate 2 to 3 liters. **Rugae** (longitudinal folds) of the gastric mucosa, formed during contraction of the stomach, are most prominent in the pyloric part and along the greater curvature. Gastric filling causes the mucosal folds to disappear.

— The layers of peritoneum on the stomach's anterior and posterior surfaces unite along the lesser curvature to form the lesser omentum; along the greater curvature they unite to form the greater omentum (see **Figs. 9.1** and **9.2**).
— Anteriorly, the stomach is in contact with the abdominal wall, the diaphragm, and the left lobe of the liver. Posteriorly, it forms the anterior wall of the omental bursa.
— When the body is supine, the stomach rests on the pancreas, the spleen, the left kidney, the left suprarenal gland, and the transverse colon and its mesentery.
— Right and left gastric arteries, **right** and **left gastro-omental arteries**, and **short gastric arteries** (all derived from branches of the celiac trunk) supply the stomach (see **Fig. 8.10**).
— Veins that accompany the arteries of the stomach drain to the hepatic portal venous system.
— Lymph vessels drain to gastric and gastro-omental nodes, which drain to the celiac lymph nodes.
— The celiac nerve plexus innervates the stomach.
  • Sympathetic nerves promote vasoconstriction and inhibit peristalsis (see **Fig. 8.25A**).
  • Parasympathetic nerves stimulate gastric secretion.

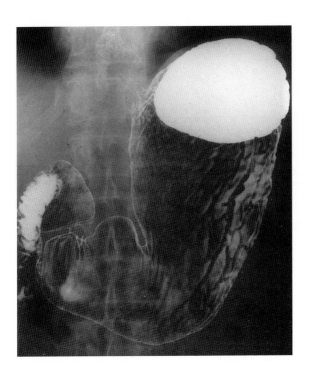

Fig. 9.4 Radiograph of double contrast barium enema of the stomach
Anterior view.

CLINICAL CORRELATION

GASTRIC ULCERS Gastric ulcers are open lesions of the mucosa that are believed to be initiated by increased acid secretion and exacerbated by the presence of the bacterium *Helicobacter pylori*. Gastric ulcers can cause hemorrhaging if they erode into gastric arteries. Posteriorly located ulcers can erode into the pancreas and splenic artery, causing severe hemorrhaging. Patients with chronic ulcers may undergo a vagotomy, the surgical sectioning of the vagus nerve, which may curtail the production of gastric acid.

Small Intestine

The **small intestine** extends from the pyloric orifice of the stomach to the ileocecal orifice at the ileocecal junction and is the primary site of digestion and absorption of digested products. It is made up of three sections, the **duodenum**, which is mostly retroperitoneal, and the **jejunum** and **ileum**, which are suspended by the mesentery of the small intestine.

— The duodenum, the first and shortest section, is in a C-shaped curve around the head of the pancreas and has four parts (**Figs. 9.5, 9.6, 9.7**):

1. The **superior** (first) **part** is at the level of the L1 vertebra.
   ○ The proximal 2-cm segment, called the **duodenal bulb** or ampulla, is suspended from a mesentery.
2. The **descending** (second) **part** extends along the right side of the L1–L3 vertebral bodies.
   ○ This is the site of the junction of the foregut and midgut.
   ○ The **hepatopancreatic duct**, formed by the common bile duct and main pancreatic duct, enters the duodenum through the **major duodenal papilla** on the posteromedial wall. Superior to that, the **accessory pancreatic duct** enters through the **minor duodenal papilla**.
3. The **horizontal** (third) **part** crosses to the left, anterior to the inferior vena cava, the aorta, and the L3 vertebra, along the inferior border of the pancreas.
   ○ The root of the mesentery of the small intestine (mesenteric root) and superior mesenteric vessels cross anteriorly (see **Fig. 8.3**).

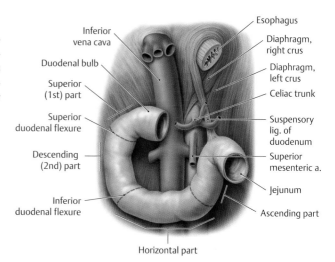

Fig. 9.5 Parts of the duodenum
Anterior view.

CLINICAL CORRELATION

DUODENAL (PEPTIC) ULCERS Duodenal ulcers usually occur within a few centimeters of the pylorus on its posterior wall. Perforation of the duodenum can lead to peritonitis and ulceration of adjacent organs. Severe hemorrhaging results if the ulcer erodes through the gastroduodenal artery, which runs along the posterior side of the duodenum.

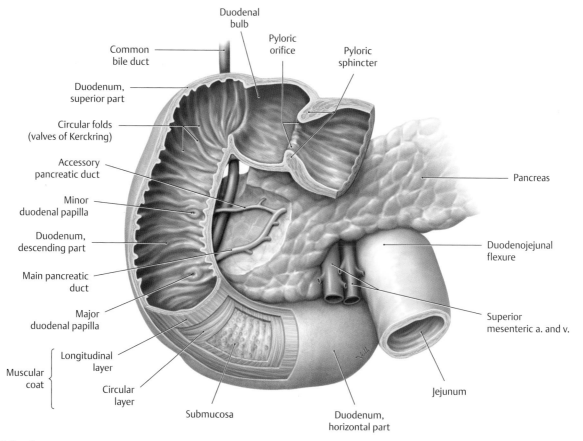

Fig. 9.6 Duodenum
Anterior view with the anterior wall opened.

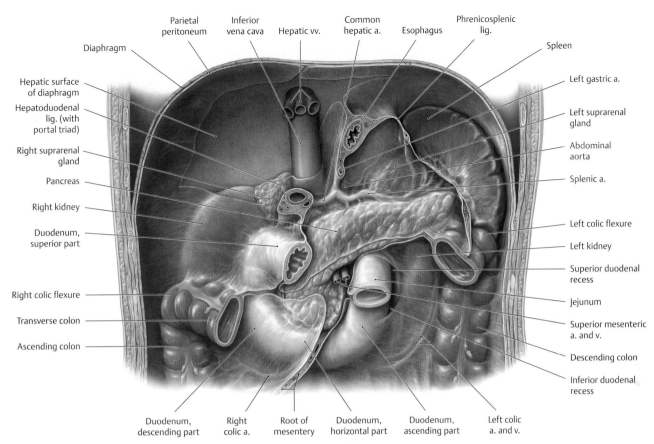

Fig. 9.7 Duodenum in situ
Anterior view. *Removed:* Stomach, liver, small intestine, and large portion of the transverse colon.

4. The **ascending** (fourth) **part** ascends along the left side of the aorta to the level of the L2 vertebra at the inferior border of the pancreas.
   ○ It joins the jejunum at the duodenojejunal flexure, which is suspended from the posterior abdominal wall by the **suspensory ligament** (of Treitz).
— The jejunum, the proximal two fifths of the intraperitoneal portion of the small intestine, is suspended by the small bowel mesentery and is located predominantly in the left upper quadrant (**Figs. 9.8, 9.9, 9.10**; see also **Fig. 8.3**).
   • It is thicker walled and larger in diameter than the ileum.
   • Tall, closely packed **circular folds** (**plicae circulares**) line its inner surface, increasing its surface area for absorption (**Fig. 9.11**).
   • Widely spaced arterial arcades within its mesentery give rise to long, straight arteries, the **vasa recta** (see **Fig. 8.12**).
— The ileum, which makes up the distal three fifths of the intraperitoneal portion of the small intestine, is also suspended by the mesentery of the small intestine. The ileum extends from the end of the jejunum to its junction with the cecum (**ileocecal junction**) and resides in the lower left quadrant and the greater pelvis (see **Figs. 9.9** and **9.10**).
   • It is longer in length than the jejunum.
   • Lymphoid nodules (**Peyer's patches**) bulge outward from the connective tissue layer underlying the epithelium (lamina propria).

• Circular folds (plicae circulares) are low and sparse.
• The ileum has more fat, denser arterial arcades, and shorter vasa recta in its mesentery than the jejunum.

DEVELOPMENT CORRELATION

ILEAL DIVERTICULUM Ileal diverticulum (also known as Meckel's diverticulum), the most common congenital abnormality of the bowel, is an outpouching of the ileum that is a remnant of the omphalomesenteric duct (yolk stalk) that fails to resorb. The diverticulum may be unattached distally or connect to the umbilicus via a fibrous cord or fistula. They are present in ~ 2% of the population, are located ~ 2 feet proximal to the ileocecal junction, and often contain two or more types of mucosa. The diverticulum can contain gastric, pancreatic, jejunal, or colonic tissue. An ileal diverticulum is usually asymptomatic but when inflamed may mimic acute appendicitis.

— The blood supply, lymphatic drainage, and innervation of the parts of the small intestine reflect their development from the embryonic foregut and midgut.
   • The section that extends from the pyloric sphincter to below the major duodenal papilla (foregut) is supplied by the **superior pancreaticoduodenal** branch of the **gastroduodenal artery** (supplied through the celiac trunk) (see **Fig. 8.12**).
   • The midgut (distal part of the descending duodenum, the jejunum, and the ileum) is supplied by the **inferior**

Fig. 9.8 Jejunum and ileum in situ
Anterior view. *Reflected:* Transverse colon and greater omentum.

pancreaticoduodenal, **jejunal**, and **ileal arteries**, branches of the superior mesenteric artery.

- Veins of similar names accompany the arteries and terminate in the hepatic portal system.
- Lymph vessels from the small intestine follow the course of the arteries and drain into the celiac and superior mesenteric nodes.
- The celiac (to foregut) and superior mesenteric (to midgut) plexuses innervate the small intestine (see **Fig.8.25A,B**).
  - Sympathetic innervation inhibits intestinal mobility, secretion, and vasodilation.
  - Parasympathetic innervation restores normal digestive activity following sympathetic stimulation.
  - Visceral sensory fibers transmit feelings of distension (often perceived as cramping), but the intestine is insensitive to most pain stimuli.

CLINICAL CORRELATION

INFLAMMATORY BOWEL DISEASE There are two types of inflammatory bowel disease (IBD): Crohn's disease and ulcerative colitis. Crohn's disease is a chronic inflammatory disease that can affect the entire gastrointestinal (GI) tract but most commonly affects the terminal ileum and colon. It causes ulcers, fistulas (abnormal communications), and granulomata, producing symptoms such as fever, diarrhea, weight loss, and abdominal pain. Ulcerative colitis is a recurrent inflammatory disease of the colon and rectum that produces bloody diarrhea, weight loss, fever, and abdominal pain. These diseases are treated with drugs that reduce the inflammatory response.

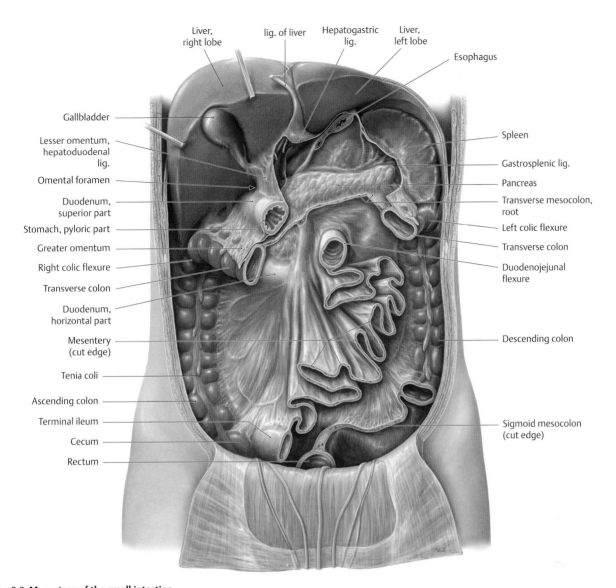

Fig. 9.9 Mesentery of the small intestine
Anterior view. *Removed:* Stomach, jejunum, and ileum. *Reflected:* Liver.

Fig 9.10 Radiograph of double contrast barium enema of the small intestine
Anterior view

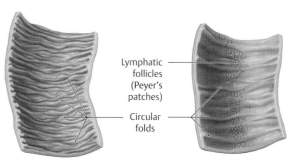

A Wall layers of the small intestine are displayed in a "telescoped" cross section and the mucosal layer has been incised longitudinally and opened.

Fig. 9.11 Wall structure of the small intestine

B,C The jejunum and ileum have wall structures that are similar to those of other hollow organs of the gastrointestinal tract, but local differences can be seen in the circular folds.

Large Intestine

The **large intestine** extends from the cecum to the anal canal (**Figs. 9.12, 9.13, 9.14**). It converts liquid feces to a semisolid state through the absorption of water, electrolytes, and salts. It also stores and lubricates fecal matter. Although it consists of five parts, only the **cecum**, **appendix**, and **colon** reside in the abdo-

men. The **rectum** and **anal canal** are described in Chapter 11, Pelvic Viscera.

— The cecum is a blind pouch located in the right lower quadrant.

  • It is attached proximally in an end-to-side fashion to the terminal ileum and is continuous distally with the ascending colon.

Fig 9.12 Large intestine in situ
Anterior view. *Reflected:* Transverse colon and greater omentum. *Removed:* Intraperitoneal small intestine.

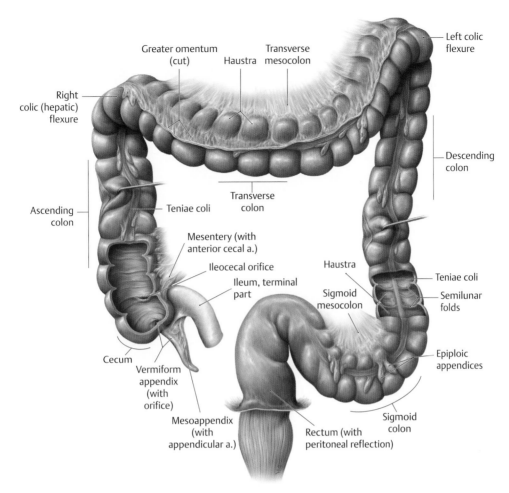

Fig. 9.13 Large intestine
Anterior view.

- It lacks a mesentery but is surrounded by peritoneum and therefore is fairly mobile.
- The (vermiform) appendix is a blind muscular diverticulum (outpouching) that opens into the posteromedial wall of the cecum below the **ileocecal orifice**.
  - Its walls contain large masses of lymphoid tissue.
  - Its mesoappendix (mesentery) suspends it from the ileum.
  - Its position is highly variable, but it is often retrocecal (posterior to the cecum).
- The colon has four parts that frame the abdominal viscera:
  1. The **ascending colon** ascends from the cecum in the right lower quadrant to the **right colic** (hepatic) **flexure** under the liver.
  2. The **transverse colon** crosses the abdomen from the right colic flexure to the left upper quadrant, where it terminates at the **left colic** (splenic) **flexure**.

3. The **descending colon** descends along the left side of the abdomen to the left lower quadrant.
4. The **sigmoid colon** crosses the iliac fossa to join the rectum in the pelvis.
- The appendix, transverse colon, and sigmoid colon are intraperitoneal. Each is suspended by its respective **meso-colon** (mesentery). The left colic flexure is attached to the diaphragm by the **phrenicocolic ligament**.
- The ascending and descending colons are secondarily retroperitoneal and therefore lack mesenteries.
- External features of the colon distinguish it from the small intestine:
  - **Teniae coli**, three longitudinal bands formed by the outer muscular layer
  - **Haustra**, outpouchings of the intestinal wall visible between the teniae coli

Right colic flexure

Transverse colon

Ascending colon

Cecum

Left colic flexure

Colonic haustra

Descending colon

Sacrum

Ilium

Sigmoid colon

Fig. 9.14 Radiograph of double contrast barium enema of the large intestine
Anterior view.

- **Epiploic appendices**, small sacs of fat aligned along the teniae
- The blood supply, lymphatic drainage, and innervation of the parts of the large intestine reflect their development from the embryonic midgut and hindgut.
  - The ileocolic, right colic, and middle colic branches of the superior mesenteric artery supply the cecum, ascending colon, and proximal two thirds of the transverse colon (midgut) (see **Fig. 8.13**).
  - The left colic and sigmoidal branches of the inferior mesenteric artery supply the distal third of the transverse colon, and the descending and sigmoid colons (hindgut). A superior rectal branch supplies the upper rectum in the pelvis.

- The marginal artery runs along the mesenteric border of the large intestine, anastomosing branches of the superior mesenteric artery with those of the inferior mesenteric artery. In turn, the superior rectal artery anastomoses with middle rectal and inferior rectal branches in the pelvis.
- Veins of the colon follow the arteries and drain into the hepatic portal system.
- Lymph vessels follow arterial pathways to drain into superior mesenteric or inferior mesenteric nodes.
- The superior mesenteric (midgut) and inferior mesenteric (hindgut) nerve plexuses innervate the large intestine (see **Fig 8.25A**).

CLINICAL CORRELATION

VOLVULUS OF THE SIGMOID COLON Rotation and twisting of the sigmoid colon on its mesentery can lead to obstruction of the descending and sigmoid colons. Constipation, the primary symptom, may progress to fecal impaction where the bowel becomes obstructed by hardened feces. This may be accompanied by abdominal pain, distension, and vomiting. The volvulus can become ischemic (have a reduced blood supply) and necrotic (tissue death) if not treated. Surgery is required to untwist the affected segment and resect any necrotic bowel.

CLINICAL CORRELATION

APPENDICITIS Inflammation of the appendix is felt initially as vague pain in the periumbilical region, transmitted via visceral fibers from the T10 spinal cord segment. As the inflammation irritates the overlying parietal peritoneum, acute pain is felt in the lower right quadrant and can be elicited by pressure near McBurney's point (located one third of the distance along a line between the anterior superior iliac spine and the umbilicus). Although the attached part of the appendix usually lies deep to this point, its free end is variable and may lie posterior to the cecum (retrocecal) or drape over the pelvic brim.

9.2   Organs of the Peritoneal Cavity— Accessory Organs of the Gastrointestinal Tract

Liver

The **liver** is located in the right upper quadrant under the right hemidiaphragm and extends inferiorly to the costal margin (**Fig. 9.15**). It has a primary role in carbohydrate, protein, and fat metabolism. It also produces and secretes bile and bile pigments; detoxifies substances absorbed by the gastrointestinal tract; and stores vitamins and minerals, such as iron. In the fetus, the liver is the site of hematopoiesis (red blood cell production).

— Externally, ligaments and fissures divide the liver into four anatomic (topographic) lobes: the **right**, **left**, **caudate**, and **quadrate lobes (Fig. 9.16)**.

— The liver's diaphragmatic surface conforms to the shape of the diaphragm and is marked by the **bare area**, which lacks peritoneum and is in direct contact with the diaphragm.

— The liver's visceral (inferior) surface has three prominent fissures:

1. The left sagittal fissure accommodates
   ○ the **round ligament** (ligamentum teres) of the liver anteriorly between the left and quadrate lobes. The round ligament is a remnant of the fetal umbilical vein.
   ○ the **ligamentum venosum** posteriorly between the left and caudate lobes. The ligamentum venosum is a remnant of the fetal ductus venosus.

2. The right sagittal fissure accommodates
   ○ the gallbladder anteriorly between the right and quadrate lobes and

   ○ the inferior vena cava posteriorly between the right and caudate lobes.

3. The transverse fissure accommodates
   ○ the **porta hepatis**, or hilum of the liver. Structures of the **portal triad** [proper hepatic artery, portal vein, and (common) **bile duct**] enter or exit here.

— The liver is intraperitoneal, covered by peritoneum except at the bare area, gallbladder fossa, and porta hepatis. Peritoneal reflections include
- the **coronary** and **triangular ligaments**, single-layered reflections between the liver and diaphragm that surround the bare area;
- the falciform ligament, a double layer of peritoneum, which attaches the liver to the anterior abdominal wall and contains the round ligament in its free edge; and
- the hepatogastric and hepatoduodenal ligaments (both parts of the lesser omentum), which attach the liver to the stomach and proximal duodenum (see **Fig. 8.5**).

— A subperitoneal fibrous capsule, **Glisson's capsule**, covers the surface of the liver.

— Internally, branching of the intrahepatic blood vessels divides the liver into eight functional segments (designated as I through VIII) (**Figs. 9.17**, **Table 9.1**). This segmental arrangement of the blood supply facilitates the resection of individual diseased segments.

— The liver has a dual blood supply: the portal vein and the proper hepatic artery (see **Fig. 8.11**). Both vessels divide to form primary and secondary branches that supply the liver segments.
- The portal vein, carrying nutrient-rich blood from the digestive tract, provides 75 to 80% of the blood volume to the liver.

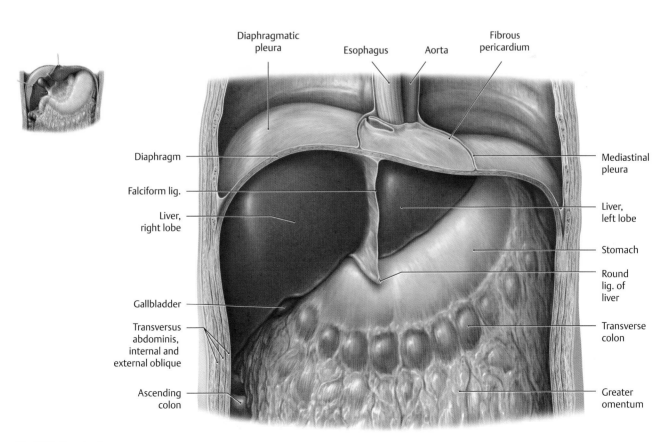

Fig. 9.15 Liver in situ
Anterior view.

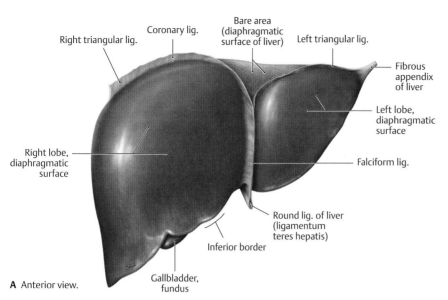

Right triangular lig.

Coronary lig.

Bare area (diaphragmatic surface of liver)

Left triangular lig.

Fibrous appendix of liver

Left lobe, diaphragmatic surface

Right lobe, diaphragmatic surface

Falciform lig.

Round lig. of liver (ligamentum teres hepatis)

Inferior border

Gallbladder, fundus

A Anterior view.

Fig. 9.16 Surfaces of the liver
The liver is divided by its ligaments into four lobes: right, left, caudate, and quadrate.

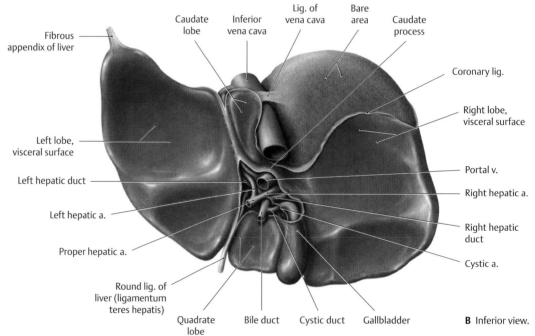

Fibrous appendix of liver

Caudate lobe

Inferior vena cava

Lig. of vena cava

Bare area

Caudate process

Coronary lig.

Right lobe, visceral surface

Left lobe, visceral surface

Left hepatic duct

Left hepatic a.

Proper hepatic a.

Portal v.

Right hepatic a.

Right hepatic duct

Cystic a.

Round lig. of liver (ligamentum teres hepatis)

Quadrate lobe

Bile duct

Cystic duct

Gallbladder

B Inferior view.

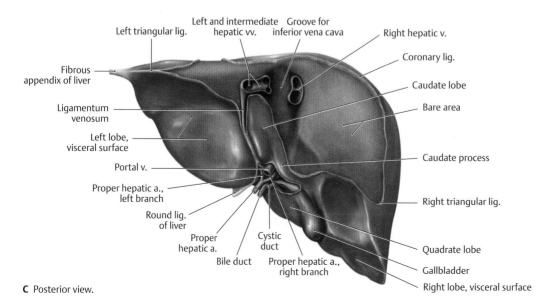

Left triangular lig.

Left and intermediate hepatic vv.

Groove for inferior vena cava

Right hepatic v.

Coronary lig.

Caudate lobe

Fibrous appendix of liver

Ligamentum venosum

Left lobe, visceral surface

Bare area

Caudate process

Portal v.

Proper hepatic a., left branch

Round lig. of liver

Proper hepatic a.

Cystic duct

Bile duct

Proper hepatic a., right branch

Right triangular lig.

Quadrate lobe

Gallbladder

Right lobe, visceral surface

C Posterior view.

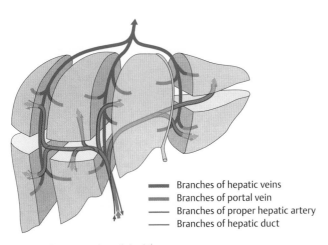

Branches of hepatic veins
Branches of portal vein
Branches of proper hepatic artery
Branches of hepatic duct

Fig. 9.17 Segmentation of the liver
Anterior view. Branches of the hepatic artery, portal vein, and hepatic ducts divide the liver into hepatic segments.

- The proper hepatic artery, supplied by the celiac trunk via the common hepatic artery, contributes 20 to 25% of the blood volume to the liver.
— Right, left, and intermediate (middle) hepatic veins run intersegmentally, draining adjacent segments, and open into the inferior vena cava immediately below the diaphragm.
— The liver has superficial and deep lymphatic drainages.
  - The superficial lymphatic plexus, found within the fibrous capsule, drains the anterior liver surfaces to hepatic nodes (and eventually into the celiac nodes) and drains the posterior surfaces toward the bare area, which flow into phrenic or posterior mediastinal nodes.
  - The deep plexus, which accompanies vessels within the liver segments, drains most of the liver, flowing first into the hepatic nodes in the porta hepatis and lesser omentum, before draining to the celiac nodes.
— The hepatic nerve plexus, a division of the celiac plexus, travels along the vessels of the portal triad to innervate the liver (see **Fig. 8.25A**).

Gallbladder and Extrahepatic Biliary System

The gallbladder is a pear-shaped sac that lies in a fossa on the visceral surface of the liver (**Figs. 9.18** and **9.19**). It stores the bile produced and secreted by the liver and concentrates it by absorbing salts and water. Hormonal or neural stimulation causes the gallbladder to release bile into the **extrahepatic biliary ducts**.
— The gallbladder has four parts (**Fig. 9.20**):
  1. The **fundus**, the expanded distal end that is in contact with the anterior abdominal wall
  2. The **body**, the main portion
  3. The **infundibulum** between the body and neck
  4. The **neck**, the narrow distal segment that joins with the cystic duct
— The extrahepatic biliary system of ducts transports bile from the liver and gallbladder to the duodenum. It consists of
  - the **common hepatic duct** formed by the junction of the right and left hepatic ducts, which drain the liver;
  - the **cystic duct**, which drains the gallbladder and communicates with the common hepatic duct from the liver (a **spiral valve** in the neck of the gallbladder keeps the cystic duct open); and
  - the **bile duct**, formed by the junction of the common hepatic duct and cystic duct, which drains bile into the second part of the duodenum.
— The bile duct passes posterior to the first part of the duodenum and posterior to, or through, the head of the pancreas. It ends at the **hepatopancreatic ampulla** (of Vater), a dilation of the distal end of the duct, where it joins with the **main pancreatic duct** of the pancreas.
— A muscular **sphincter** (of Oddi) surrounds the hepatopancreatic ampulla as it traverses the medial wall of the duodenum through the major duodenal papilla and opens into the descending part of the duodenum (**Fig. 9.21**).

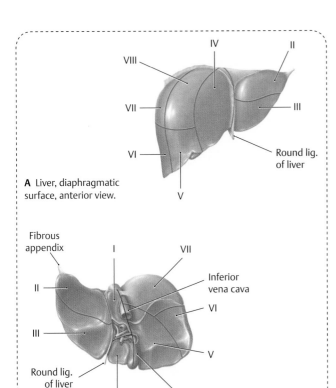

IV
VIII
II
VII
III
VI
V
Round lig.
of liver

A Liver, diaphragmatic surface, anterior view.

Fibrous appendix
I
VII
II
Inferior vena cava
VI
III
V
Round lig.
of liver
IV
Gallbladder

B Liver, visceral surface, inferior view.

Table 9.1 **Hepatic Segments**

Part	Division		Segment
Left part	Posterior part	I	Caudate lobe
	Left lateral division	II	Left posterolateral
		III	Left anterolateral
	Left medial division	IV	Left medial
Right part	Right medial division	V	Right anteromedial
		VI	Right anterolateral
	Right lateral division	VII	Right posterolateral
		VIII	Right posteromedial

— The **cystic artery**, usually a branch of the right hepatic artery, supplies the gallbladder (see **Fig. 8.11**).
— Venous blood from the gallbladder drains into hepatic veins in the liver, which drain into the inferior vena cava.

— The hepatic plexus innervates the gallbladder (see **Fig. 8.25A**).
• Sympathetic stimulation inhibits bile secretion.
• Parasympathetic stimulation causes the gallbladder to contract and release bile.

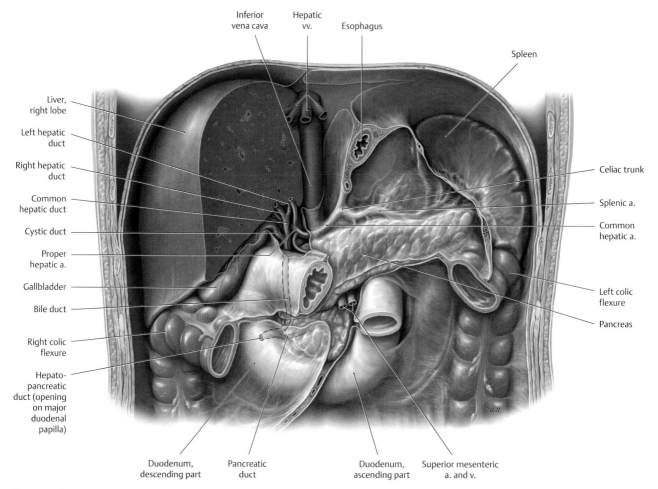

Fig. 9.18 Biliary tract in situ
Anterior view. *Removed:* Stomach, small intestine, transverse colon, and large portions of the liver. The gallbladder is intraperitoneal, covered by visceral peritoneum where it is not attached to the liver.

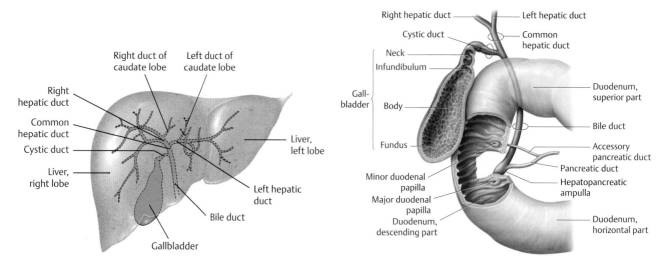

Fig 9.19 Hepatic bile ducts
Projection onto the surface of the liver, anterior view.

Fig. 9.20 Extrahepatic bile ducts
Anterior view. *Opened:* Gallbladder and duodenum.

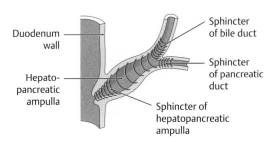

Fig. 9.21 Biliary sphincter system
Sphincters of the pancreatic and bile ducts.

CLINICAL CORRELATION

GALLSTONES Gallstones are concretions of cholesterol crystals that lodge within the biliary tree. They most commonly occur in women over the age of 40. Gallstones can remain asymptomatic, but when they obstruct the hepatopancreatic ampulla, the narrowest part of the biliary tract, they impede the flow of bile and pancreatic secretions to the duodenum. This may cause bile to enter the pancreas, leading to pancreatitis. Gallstones that obstruct the cystic duct cause biliary colic, characterized by severe waves of pain, cholecystitis, and jaundice. Stones that accumulate in the fundus of a diseased gallbladder (also known as Hartmann's pouch) may ulcerate through the wall of the fundus into the transverse colon. These can pass naturally via the rectum, or they may pass into the duodenum and travel through the small intestine, where they are held up at the ileocecal valve, producing an intestinal obstruction (gallstone ileus). Pain arising from gallstones begins in the epigastric region and right hypochondriac region. Pain may also be referred to the posterior thoracic wall or right shoulder due to irritation of the diaphragm.

CLINICAL CORRELATION

CHOLECYSTECTOMY AND THE CYSTOHEPATIC TRIANGLE (OF CALOT) Cholecystectomy (removal of the gallbladder) is usually performed in patients with severe biliary colic. It is important during cholecystectomy to identify the cystohepatic triangle (of Calot) whose borders are defined by the cystic duct (inferiorly), the common hepatic duct (medially), and the inferior surface of the liver (superiorly) and dissect it carefully as the cystic artery arises from the right hepatic artery within the cystohepatic triangle.

CLINICAL CORRELATION

IMPLICATIONS OF THE SHARED EMPTYING OF THE BILE DUCT AND PANCREATIC DUCT The common bile duct and the pancreatic duct both empty into the major duodenal papilla. This has important clinical implications (e.g., a tumor at the head of the pancreas may obstruct the common bile duct, causing biliary reflux into the liver and jaundice). Similarly, a gallstone that lodges in the common bile duct may obstruct the terminal part of the pancreatic duct, causing acute pancreatitis.

Pancreas

The **pancreas** is a lobulated gland that has dual functions. As an exocrine gland it synthesizes digestive enzymes, and as an endocrine gland it produces and secretes the hormones insulin and glucagon.

— It is secondarily retroperitoneal and lies on the posterior wall of the omental bursa (see **Fig. 9.18**).
— It crosses the midline with its head within the "C" of the duodenum and its tail touching the splenic hilum (see **Fig. 9.18**).
— The four parts of the pancreas are the **head** and **uncinate process**, the **neck**, the **body**, and the **tail** (**Figs. 9.22, 9.23** and **9.24**).

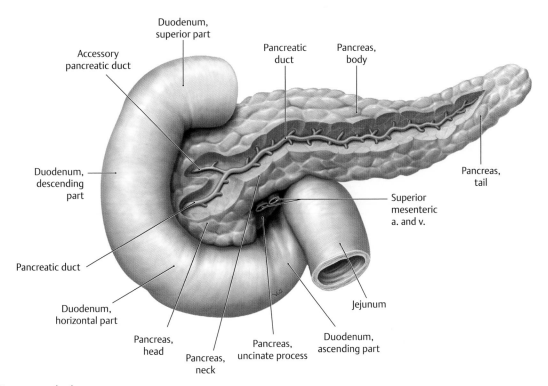

Fig. 9.22 Pancreas and spleen
Transverse section through L1 vertebra, inferior view.

Fig 9.23 CT of the abdomen at the T12-L1 vertebral level.

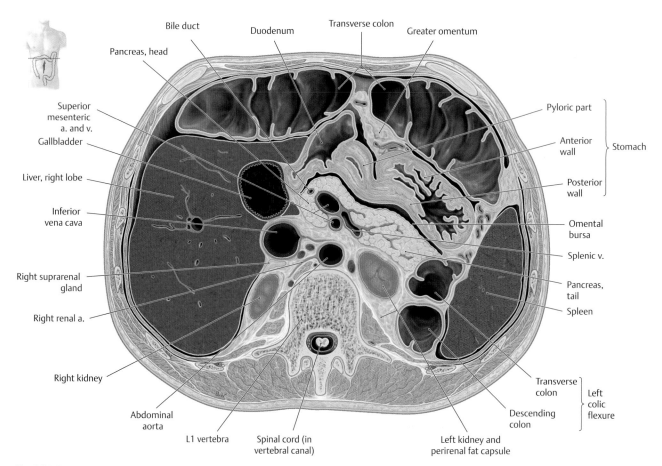

Fig. 9.24 Pancreas
Anterior view with dissection of the pancreatic duct.

— The **main pancreatic duct** (of Wirsung) traverses the length of the gland to join with the common bile duct at the hepatopancreatic ampulla. Together they drain into the descending part of the duodenum at the **major duodenal papilla** (see **Fig. 9.20**).
— When present, an **accessory pancreatic duct** (of Santorini) may drain to the descending part of the duodenum at the **minor duodenal papilla**, 2 cm proximal to the drainage site of the main pancreatic duct.
— Because of its central location in the upper abdomen, the pancreas is related topographically to many of the major abdominal vascular structures (see **Fig. 8.17**):
  • The head lies anterior to the right renal vessels, left renal vein, and inferior vena cava.
  • The neck and body cross anterior to the abdominal aorta, superior mesenteric vessels, and portal vein. The celiac trunk arises from the aorta immediately superior to this.
  • The tail crosses anterior to the left kidney and extends to the hilum of the spleen. The splenic artery runs along its superior border, and the splenic vein courses behind it.
— Branches of the celiac trunk and superior mesenteric artery supply the pancreas (see **Fig. 8.11**).
  • Pancreaticoduodenal branches of the gastroduodenal artery (from the celiac trunk) and superior mesenteric artery supply the head.
  • Branches of the splenic artery supply the neck, body, and tail.
— Venous blood drains into the splenic and superior mesenteric veins, which merge to form the hepatic portal system (see **Fig. 8.17**).
— Lymphatic drainage is as varied as its blood supply but generally follows arterial pathways, ultimately draining into celiac and superior mesenteric nodes.
— The celiac and superior mesenteric plexuses innervate the pancreas (see **Fig. 8.25A**).

CLINICAL CORRELATION

CARCINOMA OF THE PANCREAS Relations of the pancreas are of clinical significance in patients with pancreatic cancer. It metastasizes extensively to deep nodes and adjacent organs. Tumors of the head are most common and can obstruct the drainage of the bile and pancreatic ducts, resulting in obstructive jaundice. Tumors of the neck and body can obstruct the portal vein or inferior vena cava.

Spleen

The **spleen** is an intraperitoneal organ located in the hypochondriac region of the left upper quadrant (**Figs. 9.25, 9.26, 9.27**). It functions as a lymphoid gland and as a filter for old or abnormal red blood cells.

— Nestled under the dome of the diaphragm, the spleen does not normally project below the costal margin and therefore is not palpable on examination.
— The convex surface admits the splenic vessels and nerves at the **splenic hilum**.
— The spleen is connected to adjacent organs by peritoneal ligaments.
  • The **splenorenal ligament**, which contains the branches of the splenic vessels and the tail of the pancreas, connects the spleen to the kidney.

Fig. 9.25 Pancreas and spleen: location
Anterior view. RUQ, right upper quadrant; LUQ, left upper quadrant.

  • The **gastrosplenic ligament**, which contains the short gastric and left gastro-omental vessels, connects the spleen to the stomach.
  • The **splenocolic ligament** connects the spleen to the left colic flexure.
  • The **phrenicosplenic ligament** connects the spleen to the diaphragm.
— Although it is sheltered by the 9th, 10th, and 11th ribs, the spleen is particularly vulnerable to lacerations from fractured ribs, and because of its dense vascularity, it bleeds profusely.
— Accessory spleens are common (20%) and are most often found within the gastrosplenic ligament, near the hilum or tail of the pancreas.
— The splenic artery, a large tortuous branch of the celiac trunk, divides within the splenorenal ligament at the splenic hilum (see **Fig. 8.11**).
— The spleen is vulnerable to infarction (interruption of the blood supply causing tissue death) because the splenic artery has no collateral arteries and is the gland's sole blood supply.
— The splenic vein courses behind the pancreas, where it joins with the superior mesenteric vein to form the portal vein (see **Fig. 8.17**).
— The splenic plexus, a derivative of the celiac plexus, innervates the spleen (see **Fig. 8.25A**).

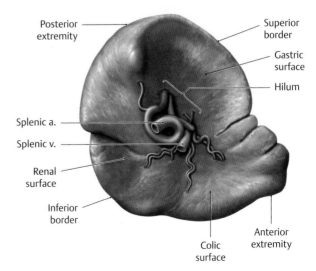

Fig. 9.26 Spleen
Visceral surface.

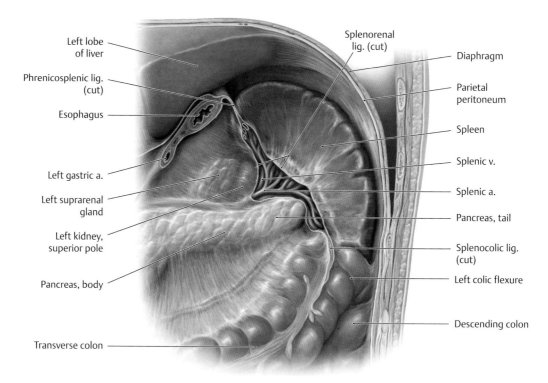

Fig. 9.27 The spleen in situ: peritoneal relationships
Anterior view into the left upper quadrant (LUQ) with the stomach removed.

SPLENIC TRAUMA AND SPLENECTOMY Although the spleen appears to be well protected by the lower ribs on the posterior wall, it is the most frequently injured abdominal organ. It is particularly vulnerable to rupture from left-sided trauma that fractures the lower ribs. An enlarged spleen (splenomegaly) that projects below the costal margin may be vulnerable during blunt abdominal trauma that can rupture the thin splenic capsule. Splenic rupture results in severe hemorrhage and may require a total or partial splenectomy. During a total splenectomy the tail of the pancreas is vulnerable to injury where it passes through the splenorenal ligament with the splenic vessels.

DEVELOPMENT CORRELATION

ACCESSORY SPLEENS Accessory spleens are small nodules of splenic tissue, usually ~ 1 cm in diameter, that form separate from the main spleen. They are usually located at the splenic hilum near the tail of the pancreas, in the gastrosplenic or splenorenal ligament, in the mesentery, or near the ovary or testis.

9.3   Organs of the Retroperitoneum

Kidneys

The **kidneys** are generally smooth-sided, reddish brown organs ~ 11 cm in length. They are retroperitoneal and lie anterior to the quadratus lumborum muscles on each side of the vertebral column between T12 and L3 vertebral levels (**Figs. 9.28** and **9.29**). The kidneys regulate blood pressure and the ionic balance and

water content of the blood; they also eliminate metabolic waste and produce urine.
- The right kidney
  - lies anterior to the 12th rib, slightly lower than the left, because of the presence of the large right lobe of the liver.
  - lies posterior to the right suprarenal gland, liver, descending part of the duodenum, and right colic flexure of the large bowel.

Fig. 9.28 Kidneys and suprarenal glands: location
Posterior view with the trunk wall opened.

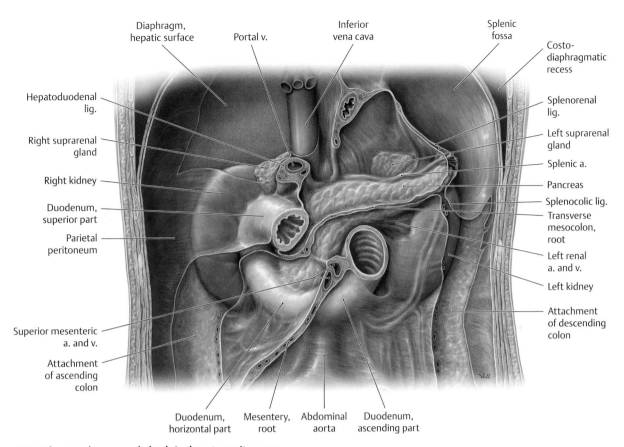

Fig. 9.29 Kidneys and suprarenal glands in the retroperitoneum
Anterior view. Both the kidneys and suprarenal glands are retroperitoneal. *Removed:* Intraperitoneal organs, along with portions of the ascending and descending colon.

— The left kidney
  • lies anterior to ribs 11 and 12.
  • lies posterior to the left suprarenal gland, spleen, tail of the pancreas, and left colic flexure.
— A **renal** (Gerota's) **fascia** surrounds each kidney and its associated suprarenal gland, renal vessels, ureter, and capsule of

perirenal fat (**Fig. 9.30**). Pararenal fat lies outside this space and is thickest posteriorly.
— Deep to the renal fascia, a thin, fibrous **renal capsule** completely invests each kidney (**Fig. 9.31A**).
— The lateral edge of the kidney is smooth and concave; the medial border has a vertical hilum that is pierced by the renal

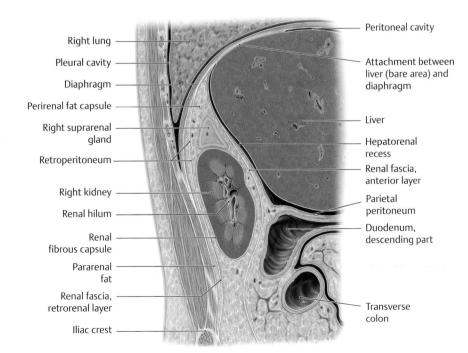

Fig. 9.30 Right kidney in the renal bed
Sagittal section through the right renal bed.

vein, renal artery, and renal pelvis. The hilum expands within the kidney as the **renal sinus**.

— Internally, the kidney consists of cortical and medullary regions that contain up to 2 million nephrons, the renal functional units (**Fig. 9.31B**).

   • The cortex, the outer region, lies deep to the fibrous capsule and extends into the medullary region as **renal columns**.

   • The medulla, the inner region, is arranged in **renal pyramids** with the broad base facing outward and the apex fitting into a cup-shaped **minor calyx**.

   • Up to 11 minor calyces merge to form two or three **major calyces**, which combine to form the **renal pelvis**. At the hilum the renal pelvis narrows to form the ureter.

— A single renal artery, a direct branch of the abdominal aorta at L2, normally supplies each kidney (see **Figs. 8.9** and **8.12**).

   • The right renal artery is longer than the left artery and passes posterior to the inferior vena cava.

   • The artery divides near the hilum to supply anterior and posterior segments of the kidney, which are separated by an avascular longitudinal plane (Brodel's white line).

— A single renal vein from each kidney drains to the inferior vena cava (see **Fig. 8.16**).

   • Both renal veins receive a tributary from the ureter, but only the left renal vein receives the left suprarenal and left testicular or ovarian veins. On the right these veins drain directly into the inferior vena cava.

CLINICAL CORRELATION

RENAL VEIN ENTRAPMENT The left renal vein crosses the midline in the narrow angle between the downwardly directed superior mesenteric artery and the abdominal aorta. Pathologic conditions (atherosclerosis, aneurysms) of the arteries or downward pressure on the superior mesenteric artery can compress the renal vein. This is sometimes called the nutcracker syndrome.

Fig. 9.31 Kidney: structure
Right kidney with suprarenal gland.

A Posterior view

B Posterior view, midsagittal section

COMMON RENAL ANOMALIES Variations in renal vessels are common and usually asymptomatic. Kidneys develop in the pelvis and ascend to their location in the lumbar region between the 6th and 9th fetal weeks. As they ascend, more superior renal arteries and veins replace the inferior renal vessels. In ~ 30% of the population, failure of these inferior vessels to degenerate results in multiple renal arteries and veins.

During ascent, the inferior poles of the kidneys may fuse to form a single U-shaped structure, although they remain functionally separate. These "horseshoe kidneys" get trapped in their ascent under the inferior mesenteric artery and remain at the L3 or L4 level.

- The left renal vein is longer than the right vein and passes anterior to the aorta immediately inferior to the origin of the superior mesenteric artery.

- The longer length of the left renal vein makes the left kidney the preferred choice for organ donation.
- The renal plexus, an extension of the celiac plexus, forms a dense periarterial plexus along the renal arteries (see **Fig. 8.26**).
  - Pain from renal disease is referred along the T12–L2 dermatomes to the lumbar and inguinal regions and the upper part of the anterior thigh.

Ureters

The **ureters** are muscular tubes, 25 to 30 cm in length, that convey urine from the kidneys to the bladder through peristaltic (wavelike) action (**Fig. 9.32**). Both the abdominal and the pelvic parts of the ureters are retroperitoneal along their entire course. The pelvic ureter is discussed further in Chapter 11, Pelvic Viscera.

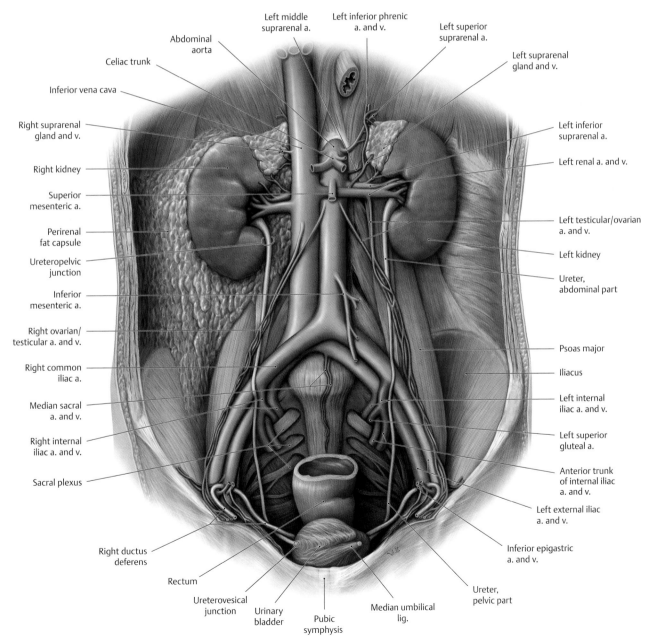

Fig. 9.32 Ureters in situ
Retroperitoneum of male abdomen, anterior view. *Removed:* Nonurinary organs and rectal stump.

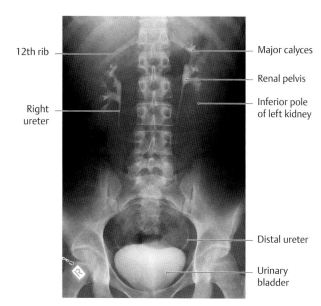

Fig. 9.33 Radiograph of intravenous pyelogram
Anterior view.

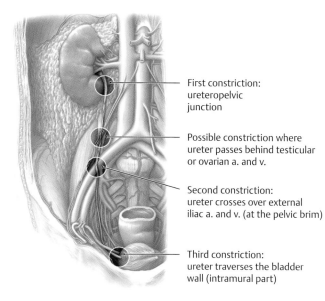

Fig. 9.34 Anatomic constrictions of the ureter
Right side, anterior view.

— Near the hilum of the kidney, the renal pelvis narrows to join with the origin of the ureter at the **ureteropelvic junction** (see **Fig. 9.31**).

— The abdominal part of the ureter descends along the anterior surface of the psoas muscle where it is crossed by the gonadal vessels (**Fig 9.32** and **9.33**).

— The ureter crosses over the pelvic brim to enter the pelvis at the bifurcation of the common iliac artery into internal and external iliac branches.

— The pelvic part of the ureter travels anteriorly along the lateral pelvic wall before it enters the urinary bladder at the **ureterovesical junction**.

— Constrictions of the ureter, caused by ureteral narrowing or compression by adjacent structures, can occur near its origin and along its length (**Fig. 9.34**).

— Branches from several arteries form a delicate anastomosis along the length of the ureter (see **Fig. 8.16**).
  • In the abdomen, this network of vessels usually includes contributions from the abdominal aorta and the renal, gonadal (testicular or ovarian), and common iliac arteries.
  • Branches of the superior vesical, inferior vesical, and uterine arteries supply the pelvic ureter.

— The veins of the ureter accompany the arteries.

— Contributions from the renal, aortic, and superior hypogastric plexuses innervate the abdominal ureter. The inferior hypogastric plexus innervates the pelvic ureter (see Section 10.6).

— Pain from the ureter is relayed along sympathetic routes to spinal cord segments T11–L2 and is referred to the corre-

CLINICAL CORRELATION

CALCULI OF THE KIDNEY AND URETER Calculi (stones) formed in the urine can become lodged in the renal calyces, renal pelvis, or ureter. Calculi lodged in the ureters distend the ureteric walls and cause intense intermittent pain as peristaltic contractions move the calculi inferiorly. As the calculi move toward the pelvis, pain moves from the lumbar to inguinal regions (T11–L2 dermatomes) and may extend into the scrotum and anterior thigh with branches of the genitofemoral nerve.

sponding dermatomes of the lower abdominal wall, inguinal region, and medial aspects of the thigh.

Suprarenal Glands

The paired **suprarenal** (adrenal) **glands** are located in the retroperitoneum, where they cap the superior pole of each kidney and lie anterior to the crura of the diaphragm (see **Fig. 9.32**). The suprarenal glands are neuroendocrine glands that respond to stress.

— Perirenal fat and renal fascia surround both glands; a septum of the fascia separates them from the kidney.

— The right suprarenal gland is pyramidal, and the left is crescent shaped (**Figs. 9.35 and 9.36**).

— The glands are composed of an outer cortex and an inner medulla. Both parts act as endocrine glands (i.e., secrete hormones) but differ from each other developmentally and functionally.

— The **cortex**
  • is derived from mesoderm;
  • is stimulated by hormones such as adrenocorticotropic hormone (ACTH); and
  • secretes hormones (corticosteroids and androgens), which influence blood pressure and blood volume by regulating sodium and water retention in the kidneys.

— The **medulla**
  • is primarily composed of nervous tissue that is derived from neural crest cells (embryonic cells that migrate from the developing neural tube and give rise to a variety of structures associated with the peripheral nervous system);
  • is stimulated by preganglionic sympathetic fibers from the celiac plexus; and
  • contains **chromaffin cells** that function like sympathetic ganglia and secrete hormones (catecholamines) that increase heart rate, blood pressure, blood flow, and respiration.

— Veins and lymphatic vessels exit at the hilum on the anterior surface, but arteries and nerves access the glands at multiple points.

Fig. 9.35 Right kidney and suprarenal gland
Anterior view. *Removed:* Perirenal fat capsule. *Retracted:* Inferior vena cava.

— Each suprarenal gland has multiple superior, middle, and inferior suprarenal arteries, which branch from the inferior phrenic, abdominal aorta, and renal arteries, respectively.
— A single suprarenal vein drains each gland. The right vein drains to the inferior vena cava; the left vein may join with the inferior phrenic vein before draining to the left renal vein.

— Preganglionic sympathetic fibers of the greater splanchnic nerve combine with fibers of the celiac plexus to form the suprarenal plexus, but they do not synapse on the celiac ganglia. These preganglionic fibers, which may be considered homologous with postganglionic sympathetic neurons, terminate directly on the chromaffin cells of the medulla.

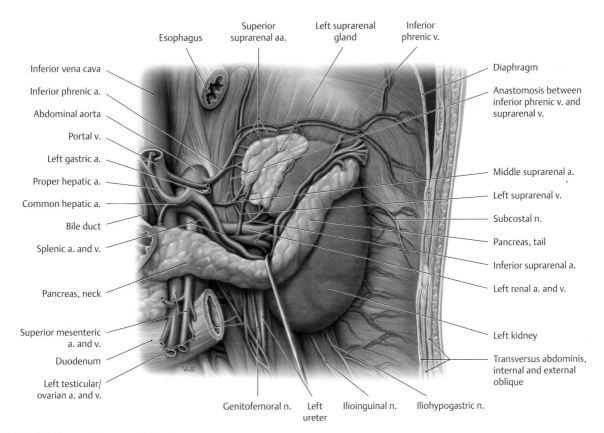

Fig. 9.36 Left kidney and suprarenal gland
Anterior view. *Removed:* Perirenal fat capsule. *Retracted:* Pancreas.

Unit IV   Clinical Imaging Basics of the Abdomen

In patients with acute abdominal pain, radiographs are a quick and inexpensive first imaging step that give an overview of the bowel gas pattern and can identify abdominal emergencies such as a bowel obstruction or a perforated bowel. However, X-rays usually lack the specificity to identify specific pathology.

Computed tomography (CT) on the other hand shows anatomic detail of all of the internal organs and can usually provide a diagnosis of most intra-abdominal pathology. The speed and overall ease of obtaining CT scans make it ideal for emergent conditions. Magnetic resonance imaging (MRI) also shows high detail within the abdomen but is usually reserved for non-emergent situations due to long scanning time. When an abnormality of the biliary system or urinary tract is considered, ultrasound is often the best imaging test. Lack of radiation, easy access and overall low cost of ultrasound make it suitable for both emergent and non-emergent evaluation (**Table 9.2**).

Standard radiographic (X-rays) views of the abdomen include frontal (anteroposterior, AP) views in supine and upright positions (**Fig. 9.37**). Change in position should redistribute bowel gas in a normal patient. When evaluating abdominal radiographs, a systematic approach is important and should include

- evaluating the pattern of gas distribution in the bowel,
- gross estimation of organ size and location, assessment for abnormal calcifications (only the bones should be calcified, i.e., white), and
- assessment for abnormal air (outside of the bowel).

Details of abdominal structures can be enhanced by the use of barium (ingested by the patient), used in fluoroscopic studies (**Fig. 9.38**), and by oral or intravenous contrast used for abdominal CT scans (**Fig. 9.39**). In MRI studies, intra-abdominal fat can act as a natural "contrast agent" by outlining the organs (**Fig. 9.40**). Ultrasound often utilizes adjacent structures to better see specific target organs (**Fig. 9.41**).

Table 9.2 **Suitability of Imaging Modalities for the Abdomen**

Modality	Clinical Uses
Radiographs	
• X-ray	Abdominal X-ray ("KUB": kidneys, ureter, and bladder) is often the first choice in patients with acute abdominal pain to assess for bowel obstruction and/or bowel perforation. Radiography is readily available and a radiograph can be obtained very quickly. Although many patients will require more advanced imaging and/or other testing, the abdominal radiograph can provide crucial information and lead to therapeutic decisions.
• Fluoroscopy	"Real-time" radiography: X-rays viewed dynamically on a computer screen as the image is obtained; most often used to image the gastrointestinal (GI) tract with the aid of intraluminal contrast material (usually barium). The advent of direct visualization with endoscopy has minimized the use of this modality.
CT (computed tomography)	Provides cross-sectional anatomic detail not possible with plain radiographs. Most accurate imaging for evaluation of solid organs, ducts, and blood vessels.
MRI (magnetic resonance imaging)	Very useful for evaluating solid organs and is becoming increasingly more useful for evaluation of the bowel. The drawback of MRI is the long exam time and expense.
Ultrasound	Usually first line of imaging for evaluation of the biliary system and the kidneys.

Liver

Right kidney

Spleen

Pancreas

Left kidney

A The normal positions and sizes of the major abdominal organs are outlined. (Courtesy of Joseph Makris, MD, UMass Memorial Health Care.)

B Upright abdominal radiograph. Note the gas *(blacker area)* in the transverse, descending, and rectosigmoid colon outlining its characteristic haustral pattern. Some gas in the stomach is seen medial to the splenic flexure, but there is no gas in the small bowel. The liver shadow occupies most of the right upper quadrant, although it is difficult to identify its edges. The spleen is hidden by the gas in the splenic flexure of the colon. In this thin patient, there is not enough peritoneal fat to outline the kidneys. (Courtesy of Joseph Makris, MD, UMass Memorial Health Care.)

Fig. 9.37 Abdominal radiographs
Anterior view.

Fig. 9.38 Abdominal radiograph with barium
Anterior view.
The barium has progressed through the bowel, coating its walls, to the level of the ascending colon. Note that the loops of small bowel in the left upper quadrant (jejunum) have many more folds per length of bowel than does the bowel in the lower abdomen (ileum). This beautifully illustrates the physiologic and anatomic properties relating to absorption of nutrients in the proximal and distal small bowel (form follows function). (Courtesy of Joseph Makris, MD, UMass Memorial Health Care.)

Left lobe of liver

Right lobe of liver

Hepatic portal v.

Superior mesenteric a.

Inferior vena cava

Thoracic vertebra

Diaphragm

Splenic v.

Jejunum

Pancreas, tail

Abdominal aorta

Left kidney

Spleen

Fig. 9.39 CT of the abdomen at the level of the upper kidneys
Inferior view.
Oral contrast is used to highlight the bowel *(bright white)*; intravenous contrast is used to enhance the appearance of vessels and organs. This image demonstrates the cortical phase of enhancement; the renal cortex is whiter than the remainder of the kidneys. The full capability of CT is realized when scrolling through a full set of axial images on a computer screen and cross-referencing the axial images with the full data set of sagittal and coronal reformatted images.

Liver

Right kidney

Spleen

Left kidney

Subcutaneous fat

Fig. 9.40 MRI of the abdomen
Coronal section.
In this image fat is *bright,* air is *black,* and the soft tissues are shades of *gray.* Fluid is *darker gray.* Note the architecture of the normal kidney, with darker pyramids (darker because fluid content is greater there than in the cortex). The kidneys are surrounded by retroperitoneal fat. (From Moeller T, et al. Pocket Atlas of Sectional Anatomy, Vol. II: Thorax, Abdomen, Heart, and Pelvis, 3rd ed. Stuttgart: Thieme; 2007.

Liver

Renal cortex

Renal sinus

Psoas muscle

Fig. 9.41 Ultrasound of the right kidney
Sagittal section.
The probe is positioned on the anterior abdominal wall and the liver is used as a "window" to view the kidney. The echogenic *(whiter)* renal sinus is easily seen within the renal cortex. (From Block B. Color Atlas of Ultrasound Anatomy, 2nd ed. New York: Thieme; 2012.)

Unit IV   Review Questions: Abdomen

1. An arteriogram performed on one of your patients revealed significant arterial disease (atherosclerosis) of the proximal 3 cm of the superior mesenteric artery, which narrowed the angle between the artery and the aorta. What structure normally crosses the aorta below the artery and is at risk of compression in this patient?
   A. Left renal vein
   B. Second part of the duodenum
   C. Jejunum
   D. Transverse colon
   E. Pancreas

2. A 12-year-old girl is seen in the emergency department for the suspicion of appendicitis. However, her pain is vague, and she does not complain when you gently press on her abdominal wall in the lower right quadrant. You are undeterred in your diagnosis, however, because you know that pain from an inflamed appendix refers first to another area of the abdomen based on its embryonic origins. Which of the following is true regarding referred pain from the appendix?
   A. As part of the embryonic foregut, pain is referred to the epigastric region.
   B. As part of the embryonic midgut, pain is referred to the epigastric region.
   C. As part of the embryonic midgut, pain is referred to the periumbilical region.
   D. As part of the embryonic hindgut, pain is referred to the hypogastric region.
   E. As part of the embryonic hindgut, pain is referred to the periumbilical region.

3. A renal abscess can irritate the nerves of the posterior abdominal wall. This is often referred to the dermatome that runs just above the inguinal ligament from the iliac crest to the pubis. Which nerves transmit this irritation?
   A. Lateral femoral cutaneous nerve
   B. Ilioinguinal and iliohypogastric nerves
   C. Femoral nerve
   D. Inferior phrenic nerve
   E. T10 intercostal nerve

4. Which of the following is true regarding the renal vessels?
   A. The right renal artery passes posterior to the inferior vena cava.
   B. Both renal veins receive tributaries from the suprarenal glands.
   C. The left renal vein is shorter than the right renal vein.
   D. Renal arteries are the most anterior structure in the renal hilum.
   E. Renal arteries arise from the aorta at the L4 vertebral level.

5. During a colectomy on a patient with colon cancer, you ask a medical student to describe characteristics of the descending colon. Her correct answer would include that it

A. is supplied primarily by branches of the superior mesenteric artery
B. receives parasympathetic innervation by the vagus nerve
C. is marked by three teniae coli on its outer surface
D. is primarily retroperitoneal
E. is derived from the embryonic midgut

6. The external oblique muscle and aponeurosis contribute to the formation of all except which of the following structures?
   A. Umbilical ring
   B. Linea alba
   C. Conjoined tendon
   D. Inguinal ligament
   E. Superficial inguinal ring

7. Which of the following is true regarding the relations of the pancreas?
   A. The splenic artery runs along its inferior border.
   B. The portal vein forms anterior to the neck and body.
   C. The neck crosses the midline slightly superior to the transpyloric plane.
   D. The accessory pancreatic duct drains inferiorly to the horizontal part of the duodenum.
   E. It lies on the posterior wall of the omental bursa.

8. The artery that supplies blood directly to the pyloric region of the stomach is the
   A. left gastric artery
   B. short gastric artery
   C. right gastric artery
   D. left gastro-omental artery
   E. superior pancreaticoduodenal artery

9. Inferior to the arcuate line, the posterior layer of the rectus sheath is composed of the
   A. aponeurosis of the external oblique muscle
   B. aponeurosis of the internal oblique muscle
   C. aponeurosis of the transversus abdominis muscle
   D. transversalis fascia
   E. All of the above

10. One of your elderly patients has lost significant weight and complains of abdominal pain following meals. You know that his inferior mesenteric artery was ligated several years ago as part of an aortic aneurysm repair, and imaging reveals that his superior mesenteric artery is now severely narrowed at its origin. As a result, anastomosing vessels between the celiac trunk and the superior mesenteric artery are enlarged. What vessels are involved in this anastomosis?
    A. Marginal artery
    B. Pancreaticoduodenal arteries
    C. Gastro-omental artery
    D. Proper hepatic arteries
    E. Left gastric artery

11. A 46-year-old woman is admitted to the emergency department with acute abdominal pain due to peritonitis from a ruptured duodenal ulcer. Imaging reveals an abscess in one of the peritoneal recesses. Which of the following is the lowest space within the peritoneal cavity where fluid accumulation and abscess formation are most likely to occur in a bedridden patient?
    A. Omental bursa
    B. Infracolic compartment
    C. Left paracolic gutter
    D. Subphrenic recess
    E. Hepatorenal recess

12. A young mother is determined to get into shape following the birth of her first child. She was humiliated in aerobics class when she could no longer do the required sit-ups. Strengthening which of the following muscles would help her accomplish this exercise?
    A. External oblique
    B. Internal oblique
    C. Rectus abdominis
    D. Psoas major
    E. All of the above

13. Which of the following vessels are involved in the venous drainage of the liver?
    A. Portal vein
    B. Hepatic vein
    C. Ductus venosus
    D. Umbilical vein
    E. All of the above

14. In patients who have conditions that affect the peritoneal cavity, such as an inflammation due to a perforated gastric ulcer, the abdominal wall muscles, in a "defense" reflex, become rigid and can be encountered as such during physical examination. Which of the following nerves contribute sensory and motor branches to this defense mechanism?
    A. Phrenic nerve
    B. Vagus nerve
    C. Intercostal nerves
    D. Lumbar splanchnic nerves
    E. Greater splanchnic nerve

15. A pediatric surgeon is performing an appendectomy on a 10-year-old child, but upon entering the abdomen he finds a healthy appendix. With further exploration he finds an inflamed finger of bowel originating from the ileum ~ 2 feet from the ileocecal valve. It is connected to the umbilicus by a fibrous stalk. What embryonic structure failed to degenerate in this patient?
    A. Ductus venosus
    B. Umbilical vein
    C. Umbilical artery
    D. Omphalomesenteric duct
    E. Urachus

16. One of your patients suffers from multisystem disease as a result of his poor diet and long-term alcoholism. He exhibits many symptoms of chronic portal hypertension, but you suspect that some of his other symptoms have a different underlying cause. Which of the following symptoms are probably not associated with his portal hypertension?
    A. Esophageal varices
    B. Enlarged spleen
    C. Rectal varices
    D. Renal calculi
    E. Ascites (fluid in the peritoneal cavity)

17. A 6-month-old boy underwent surgery for an indirect inguinal hernia. The surgeon opened the superficial inguinal ring and located the hernia sac, which protruded through the abdominal wall
    A. below the inguinal ligament
    B. medial to the inferior epigastric vessels
    C. within the inguinal triangle
    D. at the deep inguinal ring
    E. above the conjoined tendon

18. Which of the following arteries supply branches to the stomach?
    A. Splenic artery
    B. Superior mesenteric artery
    C. Renal artery
    D. Marginal artery
    E. Middle colic artery

19. Your neighbor was recently diagnosed with liver cancer. His doctor explained that, because the primary tumor was in the bare area, it metastasized quickly to the posterior mediastinum and supraclavicular nodes. You recall that, although most lymph from the liver drains toward the celiac nodes and intestinal trunks, the bare area drains to broncho-mediastinal trunks in the thorax. What is the bare area?
    A. An area on the diaphragmatic surface bounded by coronary and triangular ligaments
    B. The area of liver that lines the gallbladder fossa
    C. An area on the visceral surface surrounding the porta hepatis
    D. The space between the leaflets of the falciform ligament
    E. A subperitoneal fibrous capsule that covers the surface of the liver

20. A 58-year-old postal worker complained to his physician that he noticed a swelling in his scrotum that felt similar to "a bag of worms," that was present during the day but disappeared in the morning. On examination you are able to diagnose a varicocele of the pampiniform plexus that drains his left testis. What is the venous drainage of the testes?
    A. The right testis drains to the inferior vena cava; the left testis drains to the left common iliac vein.
    B. The right testis drains to the inferior vena cava; the left testis drains to the left renal vein.
    C. The right testis drains to the right renal vein; the left testis drains to the inferior vena cava.
    D. Both testes drain to ipsilateral renal veins.
    E. Both testes drain to the inferior vena cava.

21. In portal hypertension portocaval anastomoses allow portal blood to divert into the systemic system. These anastomoses might involve the
    A. pancreaticoduodenal vein
    B. periumbilical veins
    C. renal vein
    D. testicular vein
    E. None of the above

22. The bile duct is most often formed by the
  A. right and left hepatic ducts
  B. cystic duct and common hepatic duct
  C. main pancreatic duct and common hepatic duct
  D. hepatopancreatic duct and cystic duct
  E. main pancreatic duct and cystic duct

23. Within the testis, sperm are produced in the
  A. epididymis
  B. tunica albuginea
  C. ductus deferens
  D. rete testis
  E. seminiferous tubules

24. Lateral aortic lymph nodes
  A. drain to intestinal trunks
  B. include superior mesenteric nodes
  C. receive lymph from the ovaries and testes
  D. receive lymph from the pancreas
  E. bypass the cisterna chyli (chyle cistern) and drain directly into the thoracic duct

25. A man presented to his physician's office with the complaint of severe intermittent pain in the upper right quadrant of his abdomen. You recognize his condition as biliary colic due to gallstones lodged at the entrance to the gallbladder. What valve or sphincter maintains the opening of the cystic duct?
  A. Spiral valve
  B. Ileocecal valve
  C. Pyloric sphincter
  D. Sphincter of Oddi
  E. Major duodenal papilla

26. You routinely perform vasectomies at the free clinic in your area. You make a small incision at the top of the scrotum to access the spermatic cord. Ligation of which of the cord structures would be most effective in preventing the transmission of sperm?
  A. Testicular artery
  B. Pampiniform plexus
  C. Urachus
  D. Ductus deferens
  E. Epididymis

27. Sympathetic innervation of abdominal viscera is provided by
  A. pelvic splanchnic nerves
  B. vagus nerve
  C. lumbar splanchnic nerves
  D. subcostal nerve
  E. lumbar plexus

28. Which of the following structures forms as an intraperitoneal organ but becomes secondarily retroperitoneal during later development?
  A. Aorta
  B. Pancreas
  C. Spleen
  D. Transverse colon
  E. Kidney

29. Which of the following are reflections or remnants of peritoneum?
  A. Gerota's fascia
  B. Tunica albuginea
  C. Glisson's capsule
  D. Lesser omentum
  E. Medial umbilical ligament

30. Which of the following are tributaries of the inferior vena cava?
  A. Inferior mesenteric vein
  B. Lumbar vein
  C. Left gastric vein
  D. Left colic vein
  E. Superior rectal vein

Answers and Explanations

1. **A.** The left renal vein passes under the superior mesenteric artery as it crosses the aorta and can be compressed in the narrow angle (Section 9.3).
  B. The second part of the duodenum lies on the right side of the vertebral column and does not cross the aorta.
  C. The jejunum is suspended by the mesentery that contains the superior mesenteric artery.
  D. The transverse colon is suspended from the transverse mesocolon and lies anterior to the superior mesenteric artery.
  E. The pancreas lies anterior to the superior mesenteric artery.

2. **C.** The appendix is derived from the embryonic midgut, which refers pain to the periumbilical region (Section 9.1).
  A. The appendix is derived from the embryonic midgut, not the foregut.
  B. Midgut structures refer pain to the periumbilical region; foregut structures refer pain to the epigastric region.
  D. The appendix is derived from the embryonic midgut, not the hindgut.
  E. Pain from the appendix is referred to the periumbilical region, but it is not part of the embryonic hindgut.

3. **B.** The pain is felt in the L1 dermatome innervated by the ilioinguinal and iliohypogastric nerves (Section 7.2).
  A. The lateral femoral cutaneous nerve transmits sensation from the lateral thigh.
  C. The femoral nerve transmits sensation from the anterior thigh.
  D. The inferior phrenic nerve transmits sensation from the inferior surface of the diaphragm.
  E. The T10 intercostal nerve transmits sensation from the T10 dermatome at the level of the umbilicus.

4. **A.** The right renal artery is longer than the left and passes posterior to the inferior vena cava (Section 9.3).
  B. The left suprarenal gland drains into the left renal vein, but the right suprarenal gland drains into the inferior vena cava.
  C. The left renal vein crosses the aorta and is longer than the right renal vein.
  D. At the renal hilum the renal veins are anterior to the renal arteries. The renal pelvis is the most posterior structure.
  E. Renal arteries arise from the aorta at the L1/L2 vertebral level.

5. C. The teniae coli, three longitudinal bands of muscle, are characteristics of the entire large intestine (Section 9.1).

    A. Branches of the inferior mesenteric artery supply the descending colon.

    B. Pelvic splanchnic nerves provide parasympathetic innervation to the descending colon.

    D. The descending colon forms with the gastrointestinal tract as an intraperitoneal organ and loses its mesentery during later development, becoming secondarily retroperitoneal.

    E. The descending colon is part of the embryonic hindgut.

6. C. The conjoined tendon is formed by the aponeuroses of the internal oblique and transversus abdominis muscles (Section 7.1).

    A. The umbilical ring, a remnant of the opening for the umbilical cord, interrupts the linea alba at the L4 vertebral level.

    B. The linea alba is a tendinous raphe formed in the midline by the aponeuroses of the three anterior abdominal wall muscles.

    D. The lower edge of the external oblique muscle is thickened and curved inward to form the inguinal ligament.

    E. The superficial inguinal ring is a defect in the aponeurosis of the external oblique muscles that allows passage of the spermatic cord.

7. E. The pancreas lies behind the stomach on the posterior wall of the omental bursa (Section 9.2).

    A. The splenic artery runs along the superior border of the pancreas.

    B. The portal vein forms by the union of the splenic and superior mesenteric veins posterior to the neck of the pancreas.

    C. The neck and body cross the midline slightly below the transpyloric plane at approximately the L2 vertebral level.

    D. The accessory pancreatic duct drains into the descending part of the duodenum, superior to the drainage of the main pancreatic duct.

8. C. The right gastric artery, a branch of the proper hepatic artery, supplies the pyloric region (Sections 8.2 and 9.1).

    A. The left gastric artery supplies blood to the cardiac part of the stomach and the gastroesophageal sphincter.

    B. The short gastric arteries supply blood to the fundus of the stomach.

    D. The left gastro-omental artery supplies blood to the greater curvature of the stomach and the greater omentum.

    E. The superior pancreaticoduodenal artery supplies blood to the descending duodenum and the head of the pancreas.

9. D. Inferior to the arcuate line, the posterior wall of the rectus sheath is composed of transversalis fascia (Section 7.1).

    A. The external oblique muscle only contributes to the anterior layer of the rectus sheath.

    B. The internal oblique muscle forms part of the posterior layer of the rectus sheath above the arcuate line and part of the anterior layer of the rectus sheath below the arcuate line.

    C. The transversus abdominis forms part of the anterior layer of the rectus sheath below the arcuate line.

    E. Not applicable.

10. B. The superior pancreaticoduodenal arteries arise from the gastroduodenal artery (a secondary branch of the celiac trunk). The inferior pancreaticoduodenal arteries arise from the superior mesenteric artery. These vessels anastomose within the head of the pancreas and can enlarge significantly to form an effective collateral pathway (Section 8.2).

    A. The marginal artery establishes a collateral circulation between the superior mesenteric and inferior mesenteric arteries but does not communicate directly with branches of the celiac trunk.

    C. The gastro-omental arteries anastomose with the gastroduodenal and splenic arteries but do not communicate with the superior mesenteric artery.

    D. The proper hepatic artery anastomoses with the left gastric artery through its right gastric branch but it does not communicate directly with the superior mesenteric artery.

    E. The left gastric artery anastomoses with the hepatic and splenic arteries but does not communicate directly with the superior mesenteric artery.

11. E. The hepatorenal recess, which is continuous with the subphrenic recess, is the lowest and most gravity-dependent space in the peritoneal cavity. Therefore, it is a common site for fluid collection and abscess formation (Section 8.1).

    A. Fluid from the omental bursa flows into the hepatorenal recess.

    B. The infracolic compartment lies below the transverse mesocolon and is separated into right and left sides by the mesentery of the small intestine. Fluid in this space can drain to the paracolic gutters and the pelvis.

    C. Fluid in the left paracolic gutter would likely drain to the pelvis.

    D. Fluid in the subphrenic recess drains to the more gravity-dependent hepatorenal recess in the supine patient.

12. E. The external oblique, internal oblique, and rectus abdominis muscles flex the trunk when acting bilaterally and help stabilize the pelvis. The psoas major assists in raising the trunk from the supine position (Section 7.1).

    A. The external oblique muscles flex the trunk when acting bilaterally and help stabilize the pelvis. B through D are also correct (E).

    B. The internal oblique muscles flex the trunk when acting bilaterally and help stabilize the pelvis. A, C, and D are also correct (E).

    C. The rectus abdominis flexes the trunk, compresses the abdomen, and stabilizes the pelvis. A, B, and D are also correct (E).

    D. The psoas major flexes the hip and assists in raising the trunk from the supine position. A through C are also correct (E).

13. **B.** Three hepatic veins of the liver drain into the inferior vena cava immediately below the diaphragm (Section 9.2).

A. The portal vein carries blood from the gastrointestinal organs into the liver.

C. During fetal life, the ductus venosus shunts placental blood from the umbilical vein to the inferior vena cava, allowing it to bypass the liver circulation.

D. The umbilical vein is part of the fetal circulation that transports oxygenated blood from the placenta to the ductus venosus in the liver.

E. Only the hepatic veins are involved in venous drainage of the liver.

14. **C.** The intercostal nerves are instrumental in the ability to sense, and react to, abdominal pain as they innervate the parietal peritoneum (sensory branches) and the abdominal wall muscles (motor branches). Inflammation of the parietal peritoneum can cause severe pain. The visceral peritoneum is not very sensitive (Section 8.1).

A. The phrenic nerve innervates the diaphragm but does not contribute to the innervation of the abdominal wall muscles.

B. The vagus nerve innervates neither the peritoneum nor the abdominal wall muscles.

D. Lumbar splanchnic nerves carry sympathetic fibers that innervate abdominal viscera.

E. The greater splanchnic nerve carries only sympathetic fibers, which innervate abdominal viscera.

15. **D.** The omphalomesenteric duct (yolk stalk) has failed to regress and remains as an ileal (Meckel's) diverticulum (Section 9.1).

A. The ductus venosus diverts blood in the umbilical vein into the inferior vena cava in the fetus.

B. The remnant of the umbilical vein, the round ligament (ligamentum teres), runs in the inferior edge of the falciform ligament, which connects the liver to the anterior abdominal wall.

C. The medial umbilical ligament on the anterior abdominal wall is the remnant of the umbilical artery.

E. The urachus, the remnant of the fetal allantois, extends superiorly on the anterior abdominal wall from the apex of the bladder to the umbilicus, as the median umbilical ligament.

16. **D.** Renal calculi form in the kidney from concentrated urine and are associated with inflammatory bowel disease and other pathology but are not a symptom of portal hypertension (Section 9.2).

A. Esophageal veins that drain superiorly to the azygos (systemic) system and inferiorly to the portal system form an important portocaval anastomosis. Varices of these veins are a typical symptom of portal hypertension.

B. In portal hypertension, flow through the splenic vein slows, causing the spleen to enlarge abnormally (splenomegaly).

C. Rectal veins drain superiorly to the portal system and inferiorly to the systemic system. In portal hypertension they enlarge (forming varices) to accommodate the greater flow into the systemic system.

E. Ascites is a typical symptom of portal hypertension due to liver disease.

17. **D.** Indirect inguinal hernias pass through the deep inguinal ring, which is lateral to the inferior epigastric vessels and superior to the inguinal ligament (Section 7.3).

A. Inguinal hernias are located above the inguinal ligament; femoral hernias are located below the ligament.

B. Indirect inguinal hernias are located lateral to the inferior epigastric vessels; direct inguinal hernias are located medial to the vessels.

C. Direct inguinal hernias protrude through the inguinal triangle; indirect inguinal hernias protrude through the deep inguinal ring lateral to the triangle.

E. The aponeuroses of the internal oblique and transversus abdominis muscles form the conjoined tendon where they attach to the pubic ramus. This is not a common site for hernias.

18. **A.** Short gastric and left gastro-omental arteries that supply the wall of the stomach are branches of the splenic artery (Sections 8.2 and 9.1).

B. The superior mesenteric artery supplies the midgut and does not normally supply the stomach.

C. The renal arteries supply no branches to gastrointestinal organs.

D. The marginal artery is an anastomotic connection between branches of the superior mesenteric and inferior mesenteric arteries but has no branches that supply the stomach.

E. The middle colic artery is a branch of the superior mesenteric artery that supplies the transverse colon.

19. **A.** The bare area is an area devoid of peritoneum adjacent to the inferior surface of the diaphragm bounded by the coronary and triangular ligaments (Section 9.2).

B. The fossa of the gallbladder on the visceral surface of the liver is also devoid of peritoneum but is not known as the bare area.

C. Peritoneum covers the surface of the liver around the porta hepatis, the entry site for the structures of the portal triad.

D. The leaflets of the falciform ligament do not contain the bare area, but on the surface of the liver the leaflets separate to form the coronary ligaments, which surround the bare area.

E. The subperitoneal fibrous capsule of the liver is Glisson's capsule, not the bare area.

20. **B.** The right testicular vein drains into the inferior vena cava, but the left vein drains into the left renal vein. The angle at which the left testicular vein enters the left renal vein increases its susceptibility to obstruction. This is probably the reason why varicoceles are most commonly found on the left side (Section 7.3).

A. Neither testis drains to the common iliac vein.

C. The right testis drains to the inferior vena cava, and the left drains to the left renal vein.

D. Although the left testis drains to the ipsilateral renal vein, the right testis drains directly to the inferior vena cava.

E. Although the right testis drains directly to the inferior vena cava, the left testis drains to the ipsilateral renal vein.

21.   **B.** Periumbilical veins anastomose with veins on the anterior abdominal wall and act as a portocaval shunt in severe portal hypertension (Section 8.2).
       A. Pancreaticoduodenal veins drain to the portal vein but do not anastomose with veins of the systemic system.
       C. Renal veins drain into the inferior vena cava and do not connect to the portal system.
       D. Testicular veins drain to the systemic system and do not anastomose with the portal system.
       E. Not applicable.

22.   **B.** The common hepatic duct of the liver joins the cystic duct of the gallbladder to form the bile duct (Section 9.2).
       A. The right and left hepatic ducts join to form the common hepatic duct.
       C. The main pancreatic duct joins the common hepatic duct to form the hepatopancreatic ampulla.
       D. The cystic duct does not join the hepatopancreatic duct. It joins the common hepatic duct to form the common bile duct.
       E. The main pancreatic duct does not join the cystic duct.

23.   **E.** Seminiferous tubules are highly coiled structures within the lobes of the testes where sperm are produced (Section 7.3).
       A. The epididymis is a site of sperm storage and maturation.
       B. The tunica albuginea is the tough connective tissue capsule of the testis.
       C. The ductus deferens transports sperm along the spermatic cord to the deep pelvis.
       D. The rete testis is a network of ducts through which sperm exit the testis.

24.   **C.** Lateral aortic nodes drain the abdominal wall and structures of the retroperitoneum, including the gonads (Section 8.2).
       A. Lateral aortic nodes drain to lumbar trunks. Preaortic nodes drain to intestinal trunks.
       B. Superior mesenteric, inferior mesenteric, and celiac nodes are part of the preaortic group of lymph nodes that drain the gastrointestinal tract.
       D. The pancreas and other organs associated with the gastrointestinal tract drain to preaortic nodes.
       E. Lumbar trunks, which receive lymph from the lateral aortic nodes, drain into the chyle cistern (cisterna chyli) with the intestinal trunks that drain the gastrointestinal tract. If the chyle cistern is absent, the trunks drain directly into the thoracic duct.

25.   **A.** The spiral valve in the neck of the gallbladder maintains the opening of the cystic duct (Section 9.2).
       B. The ileocecal valve is located between the ileum and cecum.
       C. The pyloric sphincter is located between the pylorus of the stomach and the first part of the duodenum.
       D. The sphincter of Oddi surrounds the hepatopancreatic ampulla as it enters the descending part of the duodenum at the major duodenal papilla.
       E. The major duodenal papilla is an elevation on the medial wall of the descending part of the duodenum where the hepatopancreatic ampulla (formed by the union of the bile duct and pancreatic duct) enters.

26.   **D.** The ductus deferens is the structure within the spermatic cord that transmits sperm (Section 7.3).
       A. The testicular artery does not transmit sperm.
       B. The pampiniform plexus is a venous plexus that drains the testis.
       C. The urachus connects the apex of the bladder to the umbilicus and transmits urine in the fetus.
       E. The epididymis is a site for sperm maturation and storage located within the scrotal sac on the posterior surface of the testis.

27.   **C.** Lumbar splanchnic nerves (T11–L2) innervate abdominal viscera (Section 8.2).
       A. Pelvic splanchnic nerves carry only parasympathetic fibers.
       B. The vagus nerve provides parasympathetic innervation to most abdominal viscera (except hindgut structures).
       D. The subcostal nerve is a somatic nerve that innervates part of the abdominal wall.
       E. The lumbar plexus is a somatic plexus whose nerves innervate the lower abdominal wall and lower limb.

28.   **B.** Most of the pancreas is secondarily retroperitoneal. The tail of the pancreas lies within the splenorenal ligament and is considered intraperitoneal (Sections 8.1 and 9.2).
       A. The abdominal aorta is retroperitoneal and lies on the left side of the vertebral bodies.
       C. The spleen is completely intraperitoneal, supported by the gastrosplenic ligament and the splenorenal ligament.
       D. The transverse colon is intraperitoneal, supported by its transverse mesocolon.
       E. The kidney is a primary retroperitoneal organ, surrounded by perirenal fat and covered by peritoneum only on its anterior surface.

29.   **D.** The lesser omentum is a two-layer peritoneal membrane that connects the liver to the stomach and duodenum (Section 8.1).
       A. Gerota's fascia is the renal fascia that surrounds the kidney, suprarenal glands, renal vessels, and perirenal fat.
       B. The tunica albuginea is the tough outer fibrous membrane that surrounds the testis and invaginates to form the testicular lobes.
       C. Glisson's capsule is a subperitoneal fibrous capsule that surrounds the liver.
       E. The medial umbilical ligament is the remnant of the umbilical artery on the anterior abdominal wall.

30.   **B.** The four lumbar veins on each side drain the posterior abdominal wall and terminate in the inferior vena cava (Section 8.2).
       A. The inferior mesenteric vein terminates either in the superior mesenteric or in the splenic veins, which are tributaries of the portal vein.
       C. The left gastric vein drains into the portal vein.
       D. The left colic vein drains to the inferior mesenteric vein, which is a tributary of the portal vein.
       E. The superior rectal vein drains superiorly to the inferior mesenteric vein, which is a tributary of the portal system.

Unit V   Pelvis and Perineum

10 Overview of the Pelvis and Perineum

The pelvic region is the area of the trunk between the abdomen and lower limb. It includes the **pelvic cavity,** the bowl-shaped space enclosed by the bony pelvis, and the **perineum,** the diamond-shaped area inferior to the pelvic floor and between the upper aspects of the thighs.

10.1 General Features

- **Table 10.1** provides an overview of the divisions of the pelvis and perineum.
  - The bony pelvis, or pelvic girdle, encloses the pelvic cavity. Its superior bony landmark is the iliac crest (**Fig. 10.1**).
  - The **pelvic brim** at the plane of the **pelvic inlet** defines the upper border of the bony **true pelvis** (birth canal) and separates it from the **false pelvis** above. A **pelvic outlet** defines the lower border of the true pelvis (**Fig. 10.2**).
  - The muscular floor of the pelvic cavity, the **pelvic diaphragm,** separates the true pelvis from the perineum, which lies below it (**Fig. 10.3**).
  - The diamond-shaped perineum is subdivided into an anterior **urogenital triangle** and a posterior **anal triangle** (**Fig. 10.4**).
  - A membranous **perineal membrane** divides the urogenital triangle into two small spaces, an upper **deep space** and a lower **superficial space** (see **Fig. 10.3**). This membrane is not present in the anal triangle (see **Fig. 11.24**).
- The pelvic inlet and pelvic outlet are apertures of the bony pelvis (**Fig. 10.5**).
  - The pelvic inlet (pelvic brim), the superior aperture, is defined by a line that extends from the promontory of the sacrum, along the arcuate line of the ilium and pectineal line of the pubic bone, to the superior border of the pubic symphysis.
  - The pelvic outlet, the inferior aperture, is defined by a line that connects the coccyx, sacrotuberous ligaments, ischial

tuberosities, ischiopubic rami, and inferior border of the pubic symphysis.
- The cavities of the true pelvis and the false pelvis are continuous with each other but contain different viscera.
  - The **true pelvis** lies below the pelvic brim and is bounded inferiorly by the muscular pelvic floor. In the adult, this space houses the bladder, rectum, and pelvic genital structures.
  - The **false pelvis** is the lower part of the abdominal cavity that lies above the pelvic brim and is bounded on each side by the iliac fossa. It contains the cecum, appendix, sigmoid colon, and loops of the small intestine.
- The peritoneum of the abdominal cavity continues into the pelvic cavity.
  - The peritoneum of the anterior abdominal wall drapes over the bladder, uterus, rectum, and pelvic walls, but it does not extend as far inferiorly as the pelvic floor.
  - Deep pelvic viscera that lie below the peritoneum occupy a **subperitoneal space** that is continuous with the retroperitoneum of the abdomen (see **Fig. 10.3**).

A Female.

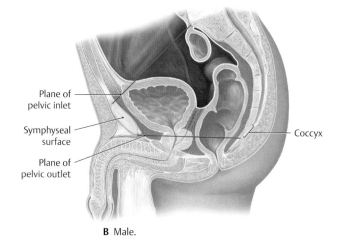

B Male.

Fig. 10.2 True and false pelvis
Midsagittal sections, viewed from the left side.

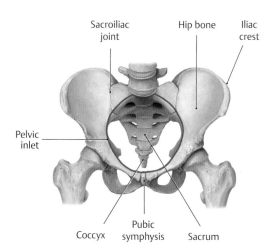

Fig. 10.1 Pelvic girdle
Anterosuperior view. The pelvic girdle consists of the two hip bones and the sacrum.

Table 10.1 **Divisions of the Pelvis and Perineum**

The levels of the pelvis are determined by bony landmarks (iliac alae and pelvic inlet/brim). The contents of the perineum are separated from the true pelvis by the pelvic diaphragm and two fascial layers.

Iliac crest		
Pelvis	**False pelvis**	• Ileum (coils) • Cecum and appendix • Sigmoid colon • Common and external iliac aa. and vv. • Lumbar plexus (branches)
	Pelvic inlet	
	True pelvis	• Distal ureters • Urinary bladder • Rectum • ♀: vagina, uterus, uterine tubes, and ovaries • ♂: ductus deferens, seminal gland, and prostate • Internal iliac a. and v. and branches • Sacral plexus • Inferior hypogastric plexus
Pelvic diaphragm (levator ani and coccygeus)		
Perineum	**Deep pouch**	• Sphincter urethrae and deep transverse perineal mm • Urethra (membranous) • Vagina • Rectum • Bulbourethral gland • Ischioanal fossa • Internal pudendal a. and v., pudendal n. and branches
	Perineal membrane	
	Superficial pouch	• Ischiocavernosus, bulbospongiosus, and superficial transverse perineal mm. • Urethra (spongy) • Clitoris and penis • Internal pudendal a. and v., pudendal n. and branches
	Superficial perineal (Colles') fascia	
	Subcutaneous perineal space	• Fat
Skin		

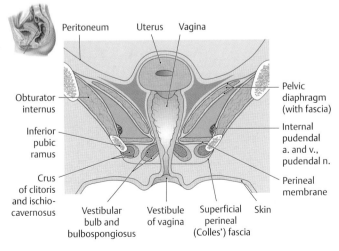

A Female.

B Male.

Fig. 10.3 Pelvis and urogenital triangle of the perineum
Coronal section, anterior view.

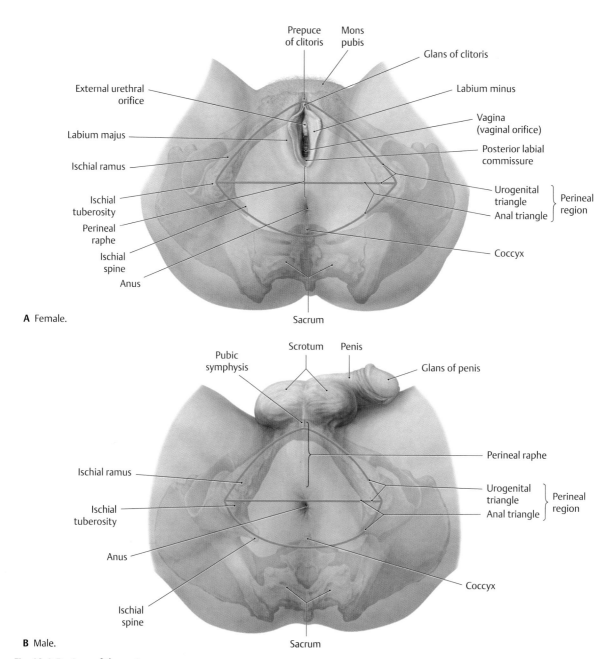

A Female.

B Male.

Fig. 10.4 Regions of the perineum
Lithotomy position, caudal (inferior) view.

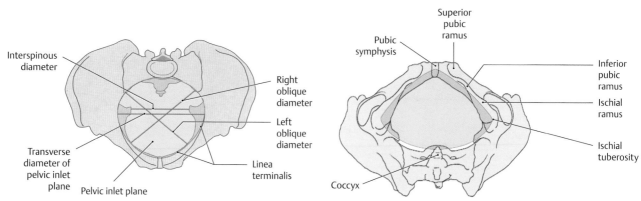

A Female pelvis, superior view. Pelvic inlet outlined in *red*.

B Female pelvis, inferior view. Pelvic outlet outlined in *red*.

Fig. 10.5 Pelvic inlet and outlet

PELVIC DIAMETERS: TRUE CONJUGATE, DIAGONAL CONJUGATE Pelvic measurements are important obstetric predictors of ease of vaginal delivery. The true conjugate, the narrowest anteroposterior diameter of the birth canal, is measured from the upper border of the pubic symphysis to the tip of the sacral promontory (~ 11 cm). Because this distance is difficult to measure accurately, the diagonal conjugate is used to estimate it. This is measured from the lower border of the pubic symphysis to the tip of the sacral promontory (~ 12.5 cm).

— The perineum lies inferior to the pelvic cavity (see **Fig. 10.4**).
  • The pelvic outlet forms the perimeter of the perineum, the pelvic diaphragm forms its roof, and, inferiorly, perineal skin forms its floor.
  • The urogenital triangle of the perineum contains the external genital structures and openings for the urethra and vagina (in females).
  • The anal triangle of the perineum contains the anal opening and anal canal, surrounded by the external anal sphincter.
— The **ischioanal fossae,** wedge-shaped, fat-filled spaces of the anal triangle, lie on either side of the anal canal and extend anteriorly into a small recess of the urogenital triangle (see Section 12.5).

10.2 The Bony Pelvis

The bony pelvis, or **pelvic girdle,** consists of the sacrum, the coccyx, and the two **hip (coxal) bones.** It protects the pelvic viscera, stabilizes the back, and provides an attachment site for the lower limbs. Pelvic joints create the circular configuration of the pelvic girdle, which is maintained by strong pelvic ligaments (see **Fig. 10.1**).
— The sacrum and coccyx, the lowest segments of the vertebral column, constitute the posterior wall of the pelvic girdle.
— Each hip bone, the lateral parts of the pelvic girdle, is formed by the fusion of three bones: the **ilium, ischium,** and **pubis** (**Fig. 10.6**). Features of the hip bones (**Fig. 10.7**) include the following:
  • The **superior** and **inferior pubic rami,** which join anteriorly but diverge laterally around the large **obturator foramen**
  • The **ischial spine** posteriorly, which separates the **greater** and **lesser sciatic notches**
  • The **ischial ramus,** which fuses with the **inferior pubic ramus** anteriorly and ends as the **ischial tuberosity** posteriorly
  • The **iliac wing,** which is concave anteriorly, forming the **iliac fossa.** The superior edge of the iliac wing, the **iliac crest,** ends anteriorly as the **anterior superior iliac spine** and posteriorly as the **posterior superior iliac spine.**
  • **An arcuate line** on the internal surface, which bisects the ilium and continues anteriorly to join with the **pectineal line** of the pubis. Both lines form part of the pelvic inlet.
  • A deep, cup-shaped depression, the **acetabulum,** on the lateral surface, which articulates with the femur of the lower limb

— The joints of the pelvic girdle include the following (see **Fig. 10.1**):
  • The paired **sacroiliac joints,** which are synovial joints between the auricular surfaces of the sacrum and the hip bones
  • The **pubic symphysis,** an immobile cartilaginous joint in the anterior midline that joins the pubic portions of the hip bones with an intervening fibrocartilaginous disk
— Ligaments that support pelvic joints (**Fig. 10.8**) include the following:
  • The strong **anterior, posterior,** and **interosseous sacroiliac ligaments** that support the sacroiliac joints
  • The **iliolumbar ligaments** that stabilize the junction between the lumbar spine and sacrum
  • Two pairs of posterior ligaments that secure the sacrum and hip bone articulations and resist posterior displacement of the sacrum
    1. The **sacrotuberous ligaments** originate on the sacrum and insert on the ischial tuberosities.
    2. The **sacrospinous ligaments** originate on the sacrum and insert on the ischial spines.
— The pelvic bones and ligaments form openings that allow pelvic vessels, nerves, and muscles to connect to adjacent regions (**Fig. 10.9**).
  • The **greater sciatic foramen** is a posterior opening that connects the pelvis to the gluteal region (the buttocks).
  • The **lesser sciatic foramen** is a passageway between the sacrotuberous and sacrospinous ligaments that connects the gluteal region and perineum.
  • An **obturator membrane** covers most of the bony obturator foramen, leaving a small **obturator canal** through which the obturator nerve and vessels pass into the thigh.

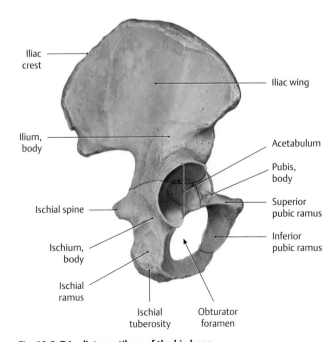

Fig. 10.6 Triradiate cartilage of the hip bone
Right hip bone, lateral view. The hip bone consists of the ilium, ischium, and pubis.

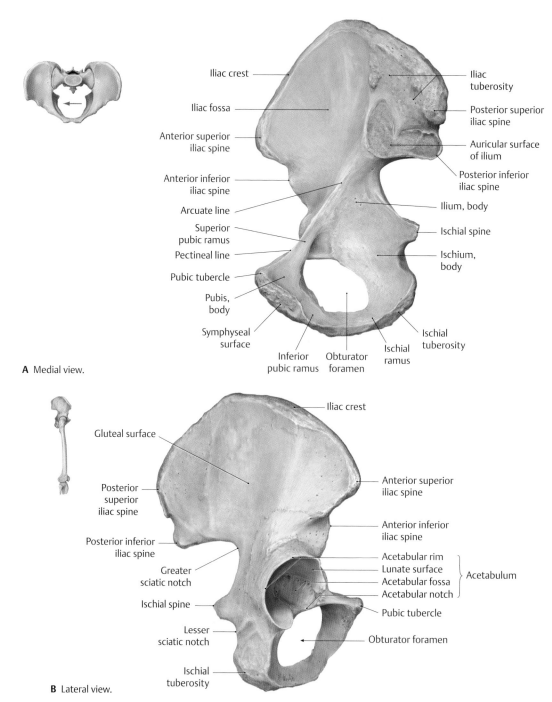

A Medial view.

Iliac crest

Iliac fossa

Anterior superior iliac spine

Anterior inferior iliac spine

Arcuate line

Superior pubic ramus

Pectineal line

Pubic tubercle

Pubis, body

Symphyseal surface

Inferior pubic ramus

Obturator foramen

Ischial ramus

Iliac tuberosity

Posterior superior iliac spine

Auricular surface of ilium

Posterior inferior iliac spine

Ilium, body

Ischial spine

Ischium, body

Ischial tuberosity

B Lateral view.

Gluteal surface

Posterior superior iliac spine

Posterior inferior iliac spine

Greater sciatic notch

Ischial spine

Lesser sciatic notch

Ischial tuberosity

Iliac crest

Anterior superior iliac spine

Anterior inferior iliac spine

Acetabular rim

Lunate surface

Acetabular fossa

Acetabular notch

Acetabulum

Pubic tubercle

Obturator foramen

Fig. 10.7 Hipbone
Right hip bone (male).

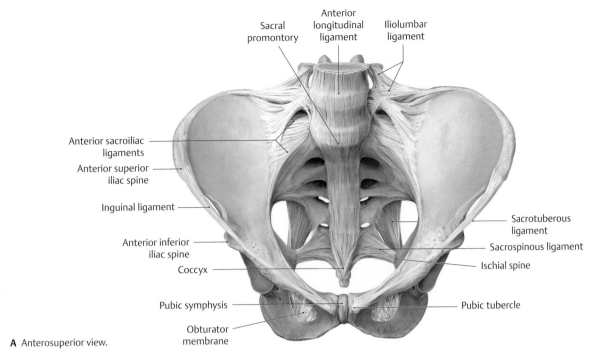

Sacral promontory

Anterior longitudinal ligament

Iliolumbar ligament

Anterior sacroiliac ligaments

Anterior superior iliac spine

Inguinal ligament

Anterior inferior iliac spine

Coccyx

Pubic symphysis

Obturator membrane

Sacrotuberous ligament

Sacrospinous ligament

Ischial spine

Pubic tubercle

A Anterosuperior view.

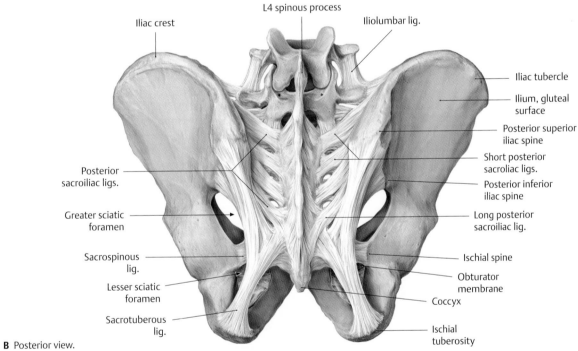

L4 spinous process

Iliac crest

Iliolumbar lig.

Iliac tubercle

Ilium, gluteal surface

Posterior superior iliac spine

Short posterior sacroiliac ligs.

Posterior inferior iliac spine

Long posterior sacroiliac lig.

Ischial spine

Obturator membrane

Coccyx

Ischial tuberosity

Posterior sacroiliac ligs.

Greater sciatic foramen

Sacrospinous lig.

Lesser sciatic foramen

Sacrotuberous lig.

B Posterior view.

Fig. 10.8 Ligaments of the pelvis
Male pelvis.

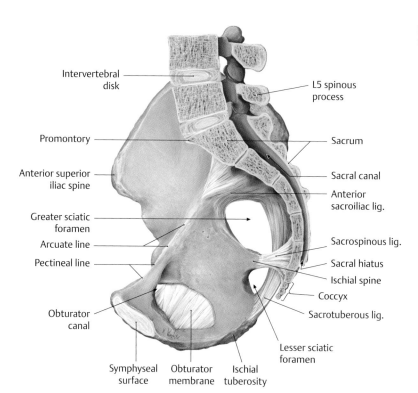

Fig. 10.9 Pelvic openings
Right half of male pelvis, medial view.

Labels (top to bottom, left side):
Intervertebral disk
Promontory
Anterior superior iliac spine
Greater sciatic foramen
Arcuate line
Pectineal line
Obturator canal
Symphyseal surface
Obturator membrane
Ischial tuberosity

Labels (right side):
L5 spinous process
Sacrum
Sacral canal
Anterior sacroiliac lig.
Sacrospinous lig.
Sacral hiatus
Ischial spine
Coccyx
Sacrotuberous lig.
Lesser sciatic foramen

10.3   Pelvic Walls and Floor (Table 10.2; Fig. 10.10)

— The muscles that line the pelvic walls pass into the gluteal region, where they attach to the femur (thigh bone) and act on the hip joint.
  • The **piriformis** lines the posterior wall of the pelvis.
    ○ It passes from the pelvis to the gluteal region through the greater sciatic foramen.

○ It forms the bed for the sacral plexus and internal iliac vessels on the posterior pelvic wall.
• The **obturator internus,** covered by an overlying **obturator fascia,** lines the sidewall of the pelvis and perineum.
  ○ Its tendon passes from the perineum to the gluteal region through the lesser sciatic foramen.
  ○ A thickening of the obturator fascia, the **tendinous arch of the levator ani,** runs from the body of the pubis to the ischial spine.

Table 10.2 **Muscles of the Pelvic Floor**

Muscle		Origin	Insertion	Innervation	Action
Muscles of the pelvic diaphragm					
Levator ani	Puborectalis	Superior pubic ramus (both sides of pubic symphysis)	Anococcygeal ligament	Direct branches of sacral plexus (S4), inferior anal n.	Pelvic diaphragm: Supports pelvic viscera
	Pubococcygeus	Pubis (lateral to origin of puborectalis)	Anococcygeal ligament, coccyx		
	Iliococcygeus	Internal obturator fascia of levator ani (tendinous arch)			
Coccygeus		Sacrum (inferior end)	Ischial spine	Direct branches from sacral plexus (S4–S5)	Supports pelvic viscera, flexes coccyx
Muscles of the pelvic wall (parietal muscles)					
Piriformis		Sacrum (pelvic surface)	Femur (apex of greater trochanter)	Direct branches from sacral plexus (S1–S2)	Hip joint: external rotation, stabilization, and abduction of flexed hip
Obturator internus		Obturator membrane and bony boundaries (inner surface)	Femur (greater trochanter, medial surface)	Direct branches from sacral plexus (L5–S1)	Hip joint: External rotation and abduction of flexed hip

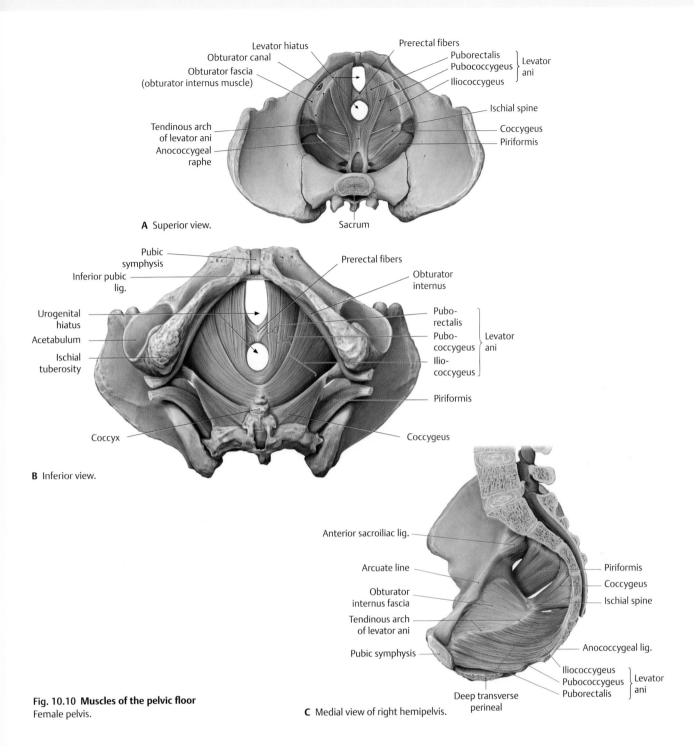

A Superior view.

B Inferior view.

C Medial view of right hemipelvis.

Fig. 10.10 Muscles of the pelvic floor
Female pelvis.

— The funnel-shaped pelvic floor is composed of muscles, collectively known as the **pelvic diaphragm**, that support the pelvic viscera and resist intra-abdominal pressure (i.e., pressure created during coughing, sneezing, forced expiration, defecating, and parturition). The pelvic diaphragm is composed of the **levator ani** and the **coccygeus muscles.**

- The levator ani forms the largest part of the pelvic floor. The three muscles of the levator ani arise from the superior pubic ramus and the tendinous arch. They insert in the midline on the coccyx and along a tendinous raphe, called the **anococcygeal ligament (levator plate).**
  ○ The **pubococcygeus** forms the anterior part of the levator ani.

  ○ The **iliococcygeus** forms the middle part of the levator ani.
  ○ The **puborectalis** forms a muscular sling that loops around the anorectum. Normal tone of the muscle maintains the anterior angle of the anorectum where it passes through the pelvic diaphragm. The muscle relaxes during defecation.
- The coccygeus muscle forms the posterior part of the pelvic diaphragm; it attaches to the sacrum and ischial spine and tightly adheres to the sacrospinous ligament along its entire length.

— The **levator** (or **genital) hiatus,** a gap between the puborectalis muscles on either side, allows the passage of the urethra, vagina, and rectum into the perineum.

— The inferior gluteal, superior gluteal, and lateral sacral branches of the internal iliac arteries and the median sacral branch of the abdominal aorta supply most muscles of the pelvic walls and floor (see **Fig. 10.14A**).

— Veins that accompany the arteries and drain the pelvic floor and walls ultimately drain to the internal iliac veins, although the lateral sacral veins may also drain to the internal vertebral venous plexus.

10.4   Pelvic Fascia

Pelvic fascia is a connective tissue layer located between the viscera and the muscular walls and floor of the pelvis. There are two types, **membranous fascia** and **endopelvic fascia** (**Figs. 10.11** and **10.12**; see also **Fig. 10.3**).

— Membranous pelvic fascia, usually a thin layer that adheres to the pelvic walls and viscera, has visceral and parietal layers.

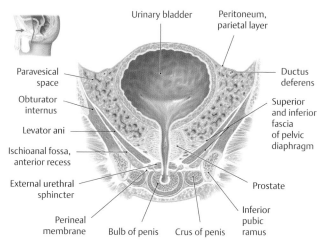

Fig. 10.11 Pelvic fascia
Male pelvis in coronal section, anterior view.

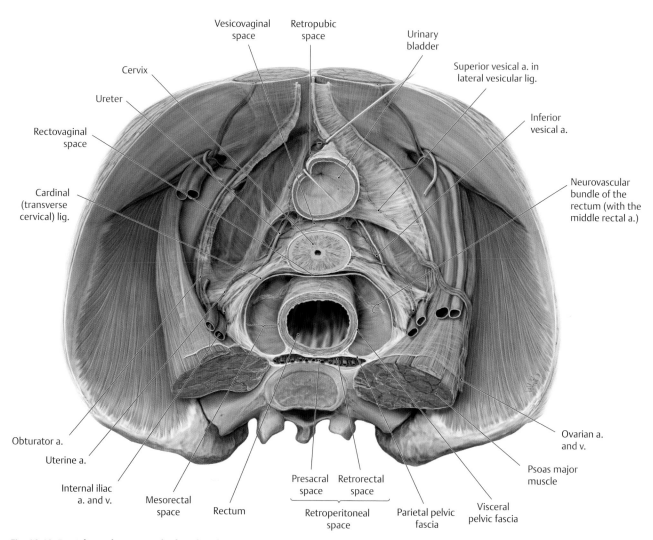

Fig. 10.12 Fascial attachments in the female pelvis
Transverse section through the cervix, superior view.

- The **visceral pelvic fascia** surrounds the individual organs, and when in contact with the peritoneum it lies between the visceral peritoneum and the organ wall.
- The **parietal pelvic fascia** lines the inner surface of the muscles of the pelvic walls and floor. It is continuous with the transversalis fascia and psoas fascia of the abdomen and is named regionally for the muscle it covers (i.e., obturator fascia).
- Where the pelvic viscera pierce the pelvic diaphragm, the parietal and visceral layers merge to form a **tendinous arch of the pelvic fascia.** This arch runs from the pubis to the sacrum on either side of the pelvic floor and attaches to, and supports, pelvic viscera.
— **Endopelvic fascia** forms a loose connective tissue matrix that fills the subperitoneal space between the visceral and parietal layers of the membranous fascia.
- Much of this fascia has a cotton candy–like consistency that pads the subperitoneal space but allows for distension of the pelvic viscera (e.g., vagina, rectum).
- Large supporting columns of this connective tissue extend from the pelvic walls to the rectum as the **lateral ligaments of the rectum,** and from the pelvic wall to the bladder as the **lateral ligaments of the bladder.**
- In some areas, the endopelvic fascia forms fibrous condensations [e.g., cardinal (transverse cervical) ligament] that support the pelvic viscera and their vascular and nerve plexuses.

10.5 Pelvic Spaces

The peritoneum of the abdominal wall covers the superior surface of the bladder, the anterior and posterior surfaces of the uterus, and the anterolateral surfaces of the rectum. Because the peritoneum does not descend to the pelvic floor, spaces are created above the peritoneum, within the peritoneal cavity, and below the peritoneum in the subperitoneal space (**Fig. 10.13**).
— **Peritoneal recesses,** intraperitoneal spaces that are continuous with the peritoneal cavity of the abdomen and lined by the visceral peritoneum of the pelvic organs, are normally occupied by loops of small intestine and peritoneal fluid.
- In males, a **rectovesical pouch** between the bladder and rectum is the lowest point in the male peritoneal cavity.
- In females, a **vesicouterine pouch** forms between the bladder and uterus, and a **rectouterine pouch** (of Douglas) forms between the uterus and rectum. The rectouterine pouch is the lowest point of the female peritoneal cavity.
— **Subperitoneal recesses** are extraperitoneal spaces that are continuous with the retroperitoneum of the abdomen and are filled with endopelvic fascia.
- The **retropubic space** (prevesical space, space of Retzius) lies between the pubic symphysis and the bladder.
- The **rectorectal space** (presacral space) lies between the rectum and sacrum.
— A double-layered peritoneal septum descends from the rectovesical (or rectouterine) pouch to the perineum.
- In males, this **rectovesical septum** separates the rectum from the seminal glands and prostate. Its lower part is often referred to as the **rectoprostatic fascia.**
- In females, the **rectovaginal septum** separates the rectum from the vagina.

A Female.

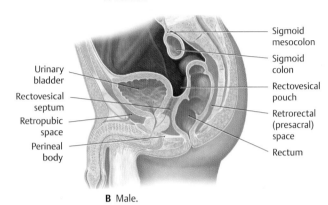

B Male.

Fig. 10.13 Peritoneal and subperitoneal spaces in the pelvis
Midsagittal section, viewed from the left side. Subperitoneal spaces shown in *green.*

10.6 Neurovasculature of the Pelvis and Perineum

Arteries of the Pelvis and Perineum (Fig. 10.14)

Pelvic viscera are well vascularized, primarily by branches of the internal iliac artery, with abundant ipsilateral and contralateral communications. The superior rectal artery and paired ovarian arteries in females that arise in the abdomen provide an important collateral blood supply.
— The **right** and **left common iliac arteries** descend along the pelvic brim before bifurcating into the external and internal iliac arteries at the level of the L5–S1 intervertebral disk.
— Each **external iliac artery** continues along the pelvic brim, lateral to the accompanying vein, and enters the lower limb without contributing branches to pelvic viscera.
— Each **internal iliac artery** descends into the lesser pelvis along the lateral wall before branching into two divisions (**Table 10.3**)
1. The anterior division supplies most of the pelvic viscera, structures of the perineum, and some muscles in the gluteal region and thigh.
2. The posterior division contributes only parietal branches that supply muscles of the posterior abdominal wall, lower back, and gluteal region, as well as spinal branches that supply the meninges of the sacral spinal roots.
— The **internal pudendal artery,** a branch of the internal iliac artery, supplies most structures in the perineum. It exits the pelvis through the greater sciatic foramen and then passes through the lesser sciatic foramen into the perineum where it

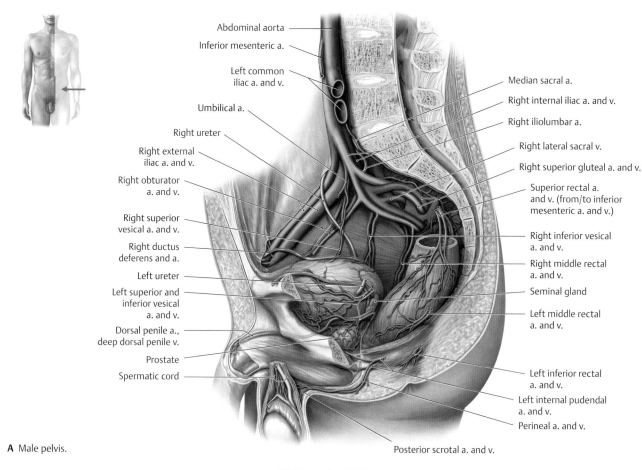

Abdominal aorta

Inferior mesenteric a.

Left common
iliac a. and v.

Median sacral a.

Right internal iliac a. and v.

Right iliolumbar a.

Right lateral sacral v.

Umbilical a.

Right superior gluteal a. and v.

Right ureter

Right external
iliac a. and v.

Superior rectal a.
and v. (from/to inferior
mesenteric a. and v.)

Right obturator
a. and v.

Right inferior vesical
a. and v.

Right superior
vesical a. and v.

Right middle rectal
a. and v.

Right ductus
deferens and a.

Seminal gland

Left ureter

Left middle rectal
a. and v.

Left superior and
inferior vesical
a. and v.

Dorsal penile a.,
deep dorsal penile v.

Prostate

Left inferior rectal
a. and v.

Spermatic cord

Left internal pudendal
a. and v.

Perineal a. and v.

A Male pelvis.

Posterior scrotal a. and v.

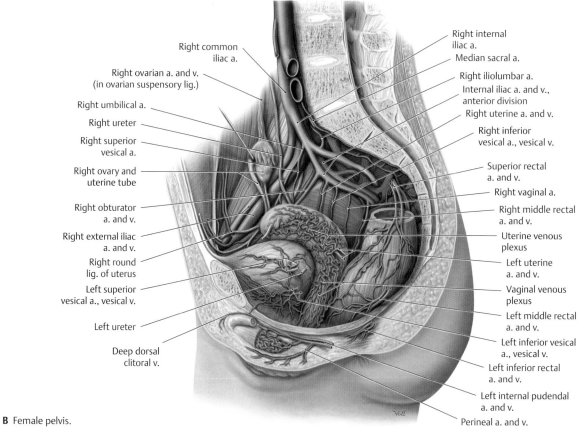

Right common
iliac a.

Right internal
iliac a.

Median sacral a.

Right ovarian a. and v.
(in ovarian suspensory lig.)

Right iliolumbar a.

Internal iliac a. and v.,
anterior division

Right umbilical a.

Right uterine a. and v.

Right ureter

Right inferior
vesical a., vesical v.

Right superior
vesical a.

Right ovary and
uterine tube

Superior rectal
a. and v.

Right vaginal a.

Right obturator
a. and v.

Right middle rectal
a. and v.

Right external iliac
a. and v.

Uterine venous
plexus

Right round
lig. of uterus

Left uterine
a. and v.

Left superior
vesical a., vesical v.

Vaginal venous
plexus

Left middle rectal
a. and v.

Left ureter

Left inferior vesical
a., vesical v.

Deep dorsal
clitoral v.

Left inferior rectal
a. and v.

Left internal pudendal
a. and v.

B Female pelvis.

Perineal a. and v.

Fig. 10.14 Blood vessels of the pelvis
Idealized right hemipelvis, left lateral view.

Table 10.3 Branches of the Internal Iliac Artery

Anterior Division		Posterior Division
Visceral branches	Parietal branches	Parietal branches
Umbilical—superior vesical*	Obturator	Iliolumbar
Uterine (female)	Inferior gluteal	Lateral sacral
Vaginal (female)		Superior gluteal
Inferior vesical (male)		
Middle rectal		
Internal pudendal		

*After birth, the distal portion of the umbilical artery obliterates, but its remnant remains as the medial umbilical ligament on the anterior abdominal wall; the proximal portion remains as the superior vesical artery to the bladder.

runs along the lateral wall of the anal triangle to the perineal membrane. Its major branches (**Figs. 10.15** and **10.16**) include the following:

- The **inferior rectal artery,** which supplies the external anal sphincter and skin around the anus
- The **perineal artery,** which supplies the structures of the superficial perineal pouch through posterior scrotal or posterior labial branches
- The **dorsal penile** or **clitoral artery,** which supplies structures in the deep perineal pouch and the glans of the penis or clitoris
— The **external pudendal artery,** a branch of the femoral artery in the thigh, supplies superficial tissues of the perineum.
— The **ovarian artery** in females arises from the abdominal aorta at L2 and descends along the posterior abdominal wall. It crosses the pelvic brim and enters the pelvis within the **suspensory ligament of the ovary.** The ovarian artery supplies the ovary and uterine tube and anastomoses with the uterine artery (**Fig. 10.17**).
- The testicular artery passes through the inguinal canal as part of the spermatic cord to supply the testis and therefore is not a vessel of the pelvis (**Fig 10.18**).
— The **superior rectal artery,** a branch of the inferior mesenteric artery, supplies the upper rectum and anal canal and anastomoses with middle and inferior rectal arteries in the pelvis and perineum (**Fig. 10.19**).

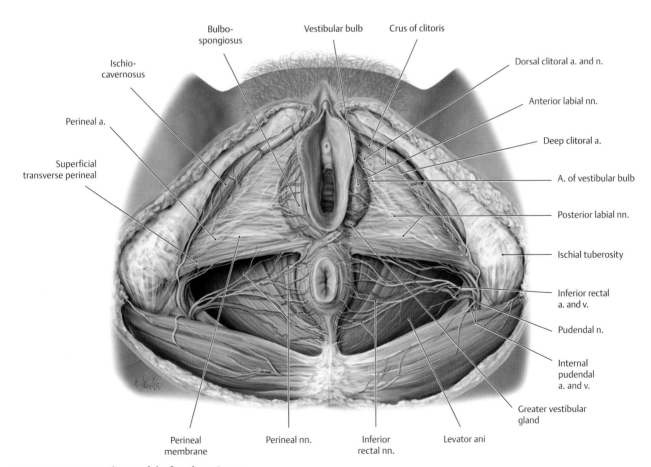

Fig. 10.15 Neurovasculature of the female perineum
Lithotomy position. *Removed:* Perineal membrane and left bulbospongiosus and ischiocavernosus muscles.

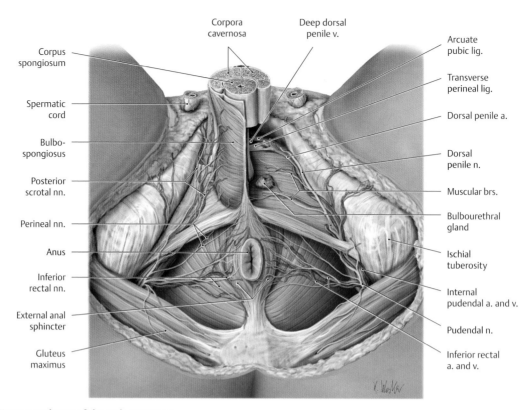

Fig. 10.16 Neurovasculature of the male perineum
Lithotomy position. *Removed from left side:* Perineal membrane, bulbospongiosus muscle, and root of penis.

Fig. 10.17 Blood vessels of the female genitalia
Anterior view. *Removed from left side:* Peritoneum. *Displaced:* Uterus.

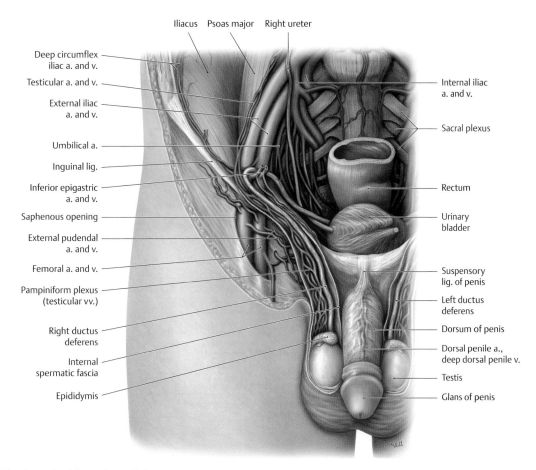

Fig. 10.18 Blood vessels of the male genitalia
Anterior view. *Opened:* Inguinal canal and coverings of the spermatic cord.

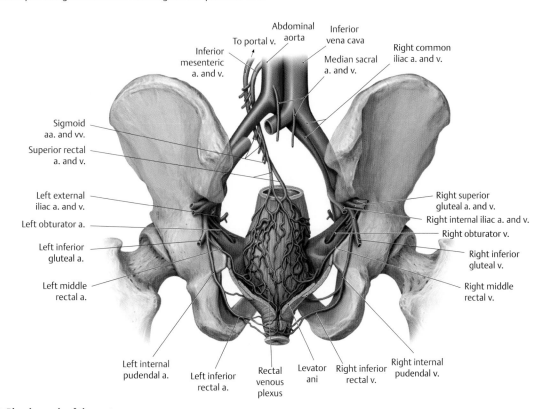

Fig. 10.19 Blood vessels of the rectum
Posterior view. The main blood supply to the rectum is from the superior rectal artery; the middle rectal arteries serve as an anastomosis between the superior and inferior rectal arteries.

Veins of the Pelvis and Perineum

Blood from most pelvic viscera drains to a venous plexus contained either within the visceral fascia surrounding the organ (bladder, prostate) or within the organ wall (rectum).

— The visceral venous plexuses in the pelvis communicate freely, and most drain to the inferior vena caval system through tributaries of the internal iliac veins that accompany the arteries of similar name and vascular territory (area supplied by a vessel) (see **Fig. 10.14**).
— The **internal pudendal vein** accompanies the internal pudendal artery and drains most structures of the perineum. However, erectile tissues in the urogenital triangle drain through **deep dorsal veins** that pass under the pubic symphysis to join with visceral venous plexuses in the pelvis.
— The **internal iliac veins** ascend from the pelvis to join with the **external iliac veins.** These join to form the **right** and **left common iliac veins,** which converge to form the inferior vena cava at the L5 vertebral level.
— There are three alternate venous drainages from pelvic viscera:
  1. Ovarian veins drain directly into the inferior vena cava on the right and into the renal vein on the left, but they also communicate with other pelvic venous plexuses (uterine, vaginal), which drain to the internal iliac veins (see **Fig. 10.17**).
  2. The superior rectal vein drains to the hepatic portal system through the inferior mesenteric vein. This drainage establishes an anastomosis between the portal and caval venous systems (a portosystemic anastomosis) with the middle and inferior rectal veins, which are tributaries of the internal iliac veins (see **Figs. 10.19** and **8.19**).
  3. The vertebral venous plexus, which drains into the azygos system, communicates with pelvic visceral plexuses through tributaries of the internal iliac veins (see **Fig. 2.19B**).

Lymphatics of the Pelvis and Perineum

Lymph from the pelvis and perineum travels through one or more groups of lymph nodes, all of which ultimately drain into the thoracic duct (**Table 10.4**). The groups of nodes tend to be interconnected but vary in size and number.

There are several general drainage patterns.

— Within the pelvis, lymph drainage usually follows venous pathways, although structures that drain to the external iliac nodes do not follow this pattern.
— External iliac nodes receive lymph from the superior parts of the anterior pelvic viscera.
— Internal iliac nodes receive lymph from deep pelvic and deep perineal structures.
— Sacral nodes receive lymph from deep posterior pelvic viscera.
— Superficial and deep inguinal nodes drain most structures of the perineum.
— Inguinal nodes drain to external iliac nodes.
— External iliac, internal iliac, and sacral nodes drain to common iliac nodes, which in turn drain to lateral aortic nodes and lumbar trunks.

Table 10.4 **Lymph Nodes (l.n.s) of the Pelvis**

Preaortic l.n.	① Superior mesenteric l.n.	
	② Inferior mesenteric l.n.	
③ Left lumbar l.n. (lateral aortic l.n.)		
④ Right lumbar l.n. (lateral aortic or caval l.n.)		
⑤ Common iliac l.n.		
⑥ Internal iliac l.n.		
⑦ External iliac l.n.		
⑧ Superficial inguinal l.n.	Horizontal group	
	Vertical group	
⑨ Deep inguinal l.n.		
⑩ Sacral l.n.		

Nerves of the Pelvis and Perineum

Nerves of the pelvis and perineum include branches from somatic nerve (lumbar and sacral) plexuses as well as autonomic (superior hypogastric and inferior hypogastric) plexuses (**Figs. 10.20** and **10.21**).

— The obturator nerve (L2–L4), a branch of the lumbar plexus, passes along the sidewall of the pelvis and exits through the obturator canal. It does not innervate structures of the pelvis but can be injured during pelvic surgery.
— The **sacral plexus** forms on the posterior wall of the pelvis from the anterior rami of L4–S4. Except for short branches to pelvic floor muscles, branches of the plexus exit the pelvis through the greater sciatic foramen, where they innervate structures in the perineum, gluteal region, and lower limb (see Section 15.4).
— The **pudendal nerve** (S2–S4), a branch of the sacral plexus, is the primary nerve of the perineum. It passes through the greater sciatic foramen close to the ischial spine and then into the perineum through the lesser sciatic foramen, where it courses anteriorly with the internal pudendal vessels (**Figs. 10.21, 10.22, 10.23**). The pudendal nerve is a mixed somatic nerve (motor and sensory) but also carries postganglionic sympathetic fibers to perineal structures. Its major branches include the following:
  • The **inferior rectal nerve,** which innervates the external anal sphincter

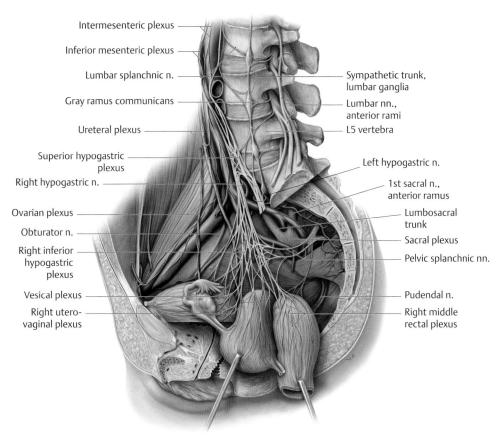

Intermesenteric plexus

Inferior mesenteric plexus

Lumbar splanchnic n.

Gray ramus communicans

Ureteral plexus

Superior hypogastric plexus

Right hypogastric n.

Ovarian plexus

Obturator n.

Right inferior hypogastric plexus

Vesical plexus

Right utero-vaginal plexus

Sympathetic trunk, lumbar ganglia

Lumbar nn., anterior rami

L5 vertebra

Left hypogastric n.

1st sacral n., anterior ramus

Lumbosacral trunk

Sacral plexus

Pelvic splanchnic nn.

Pudendal n.

Right middle rectal plexus

Fig. 10.20 Innervation of the female pelvis
Right pelvis, left lateral view.
Reflected: Uterus and rectum.

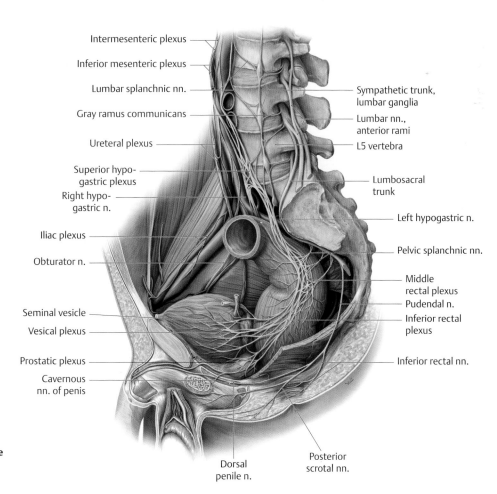

Intermesenteric plexus

Inferior mesenteric plexus

Lumbar splanchnic nn.

Gray ramus communicans

Ureteral plexus

Superior hypo-gastric plexus

Right hypo-gastric n.

Iliac plexus

Obturator n.

Seminal vesicle

Vesical plexus

Prostatic plexus

Cavernous nn. of penis

Sympathetic trunk, lumbar ganglia

Lumbar nn., anterior rami

L5 vertebra

Lumbosacral trunk

Left hypogastric n.

Pelvic splanchnic nn.

Middle rectal plexus

Pudendal n.

Inferior rectal plexus

Inferior rectal nn.

Posterior scrotal nn.

Dorsal penile n.

Fig. 10.21 Innervation of the male pelvis
Right pelvis, left lateral view.

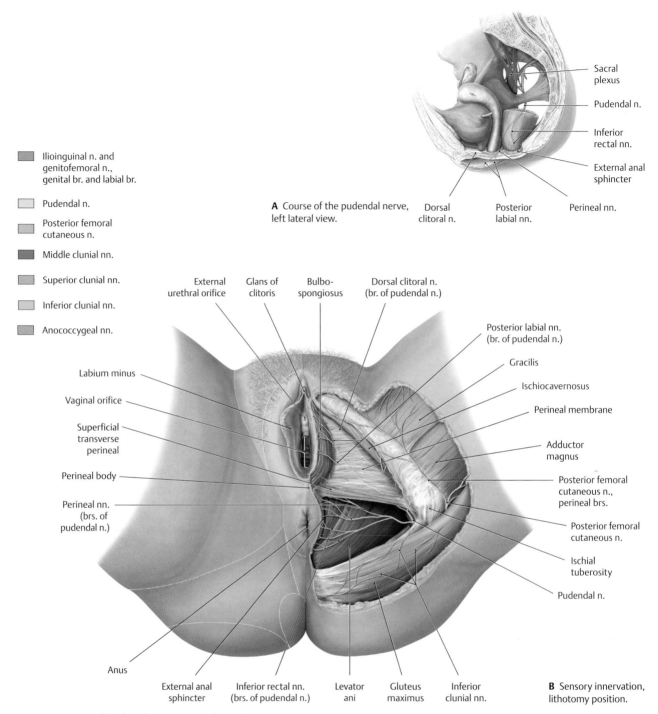

Ilioinguinal n. and genitofemoral n., genital br. and labial br.

Pudendal n.

Posterior femoral cutaneous n.

Middle clunial nn.

Superior clunial nn.

Inferior clunial nn.

Anococcygeal nn.

A Course of the pudendal nerve, left lateral view.

Sacral plexus

Pudendal n.

Inferior rectal nn.

External anal sphincter

Perineal nn.

Dorsal clitoral n.

Posterior labial nn.

External urethral orifice

Glans of clitoris

Bulbo-spongiosus

Dorsal clitoral n. (br. of pudendal n.)

Posterior labial nn. (br. of pudendal n.)

Gracilis

Ischiocavernosus

Perineal membrane

Adductor magnus

Posterior femoral cutaneous n., perineal brs.

Posterior femoral cutaneous n.

Ischial tuberosity

Pudendal n.

Labium minus

Vaginal orifice

Superficial transverse perineal

Perineal body

Perineal nn. (brs. of pudendal n.)

Anus

External anal sphincter

Inferior rectal nn. (brs. of pudendal n.)

Levator ani

Gluteus maximus

Inferior clunial nn.

B Sensory innervation, lithotomy position.

Fig. 10.22 Nerves of the female perineum and genitalia

- The **perineal nerve,** which supplies cutaneous branches to the scrotum and labia and motor branches to the muscles of the deep and superficial perineal pouches
- The **dorsal penile (clitoral) nerve,** which is the primary sensory nerve to the penis and clitoris, especially to the glans
— **Sacral sympathetic trunks,** the continuations of the lumbar sympathetic trunks, provide postganglionic fibers to pelvic plexuses and to lower limb branches of the sacral plexus. The trunks descend along the anterior surface of the sacrum to the coccyx, where they merge to form a small ganglion, the ganglion impar.

CLINICAL CORRELATION

PUDENDAL NERVE BLOCK During labor, anesthesia of the pudendal nerve can ease perineal pain of delivery. A pudendal block can be administered through the posterior wall of the vagina, with the surgeon aiming the needle toward the ischial spine. The block can also be administered externally, inserting the needle through the skin medial to the ischial tuberosity. Since the pudendal nerve innervates only the perineum, the superior vagina and cervix are not affected by the block, and the mother continues to feel the uterine contractions.

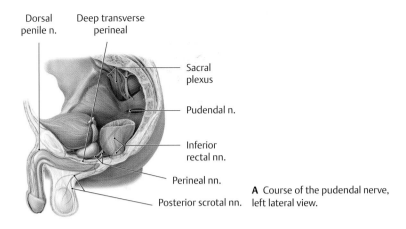

A Course of the pudendal nerve, left lateral view.

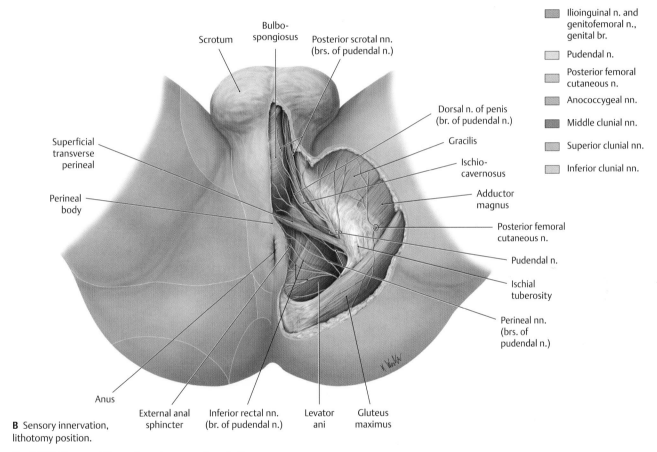

B Sensory innervation, lithotomy position.

Fig. 10.23 Nerves of the male perineum and genitalia

— The superior hypogastric plexus, a continuation of the intermesenteric plexus in the abdomen, receives additional contributions from the two lower lumbar splanchnic nerves (sympathetic). It drapes over the bifurcation of the aorta and branches into right and left **hypogastric nerves,** which pass into the pelvis.
— The pelvic splanchnic nerves, the pelvic component of the parasympathetic nervous system, originate from the sacral spinal cord and enter the pelvis with the S2–S4 anterior rami.
— The hypogastric nerves, joined by sacral splanchnic nerves

(sympathetic) nerves and pelvic splanchnic nerves (parasympathetic), form right and left **inferior hypogastric** (pelvic) **plexuses.**
— **Vesical, prostatic** (in males), **uterovaginal** (in females), and **rectal plexuses** are derived from the inferior hypogastric plexus and surround individual pelvic organs (**Figs. 10.24, 10.25, 10.26**).
— **Cavernous nerves** from the inferior hypogastric plexus pass through the genital hiatus carrying parasympathetic nerves to perineal structures. They are responsible for erection of the penis and clitoris.

— Visceral sensory fibers from most structures in the pelvis travel with sympathetic or parasympathetic nerves depending on the relationship of the viscera to the peritoneum.
  • From pelvic viscera in contact with the peritoneum, sensory fibers travel with sympathetic nerves to the superior hypogastric plexus and thoracic spinal cord.

• From pelvic viscera below the peritoneum, sensory fibers travel with parasympathetic pelvic splanchnic nerves to the sacral spinal cord.
• Although the rectum is in contact with the peritoneum on most of its surfaces, its visceral sensory fibers also travel with pelvic splanchnic nerves.

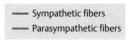

| —— | Sympathetic fibers |
| —— | Parasympathetic fibers |

Ⓢ	Sympathetic trunk
Ⓟ	Posterior vagal trunk (from right vagus n.)
③	Inferior mesenteric ganglion
⑤	Lesser splanchnic n. (T10–T11)
⑥	Least splanchnic n. (T12)
⑦	Lumbar splanchnic nn. (L1–L2)
⑨	Sacral splanchnic nn. (from 1st to 3rd sacral ganglia)
⑩	Pelvic splanchnic nn. (S2–S4)
⑪	Renal ganglia
⑫	Superior hypogastric plexus
⑬	Inferior hypogastric plexus

Fig. 10.24 Autonomic innervation of the urinary organs

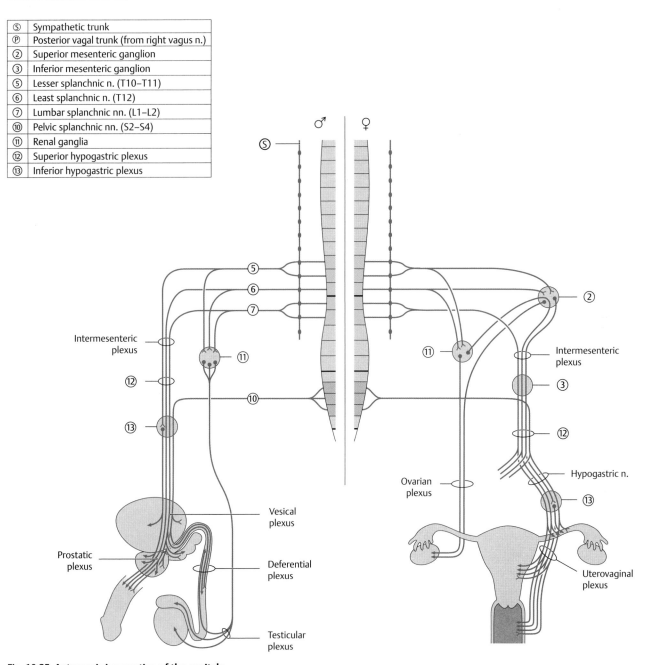

Fig. 10.25 Autonomic innervation of the genitals

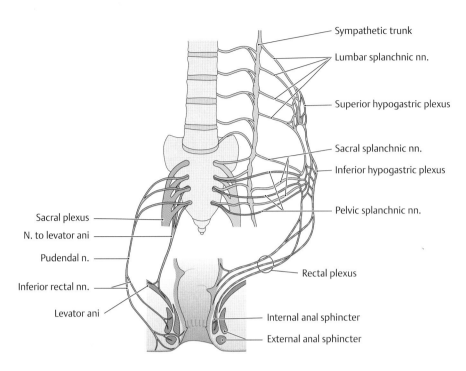

Sympathetic trunk

Lumbar splanchnic nn.

Superior hypogastric plexus

Sacral splanchnic nn.

Inferior hypogastric plexus

Pelvic splanchnic nn.

Sacral plexus

N. to levator ani

Pudendal n.

Inferior rectal nn.

Levator ani

Rectal plexus

Internal anal sphincter

External anal sphincter

Fig. 10.26 Innervation of the rectum
Left side of image shows somatic nn.; right side of image shows autonomic nn.

11 Pelvic Viscera

The pelvic cavity contains the male or female genital organs, the pelvic urinary organs, and the rectum. These organs normally reside in the true pelvis, although when enlarged the bladder and uterus can extend into the abdominal cavity.

11.1 Male Genital Structures

The male gonad, the testis, is located in the inguinal region and is discussed in Chapter 7. The seminal glands (vesicles) and prostate gland are male accessory reproductive structures found in the pelvis (**Fig. 11.1**).

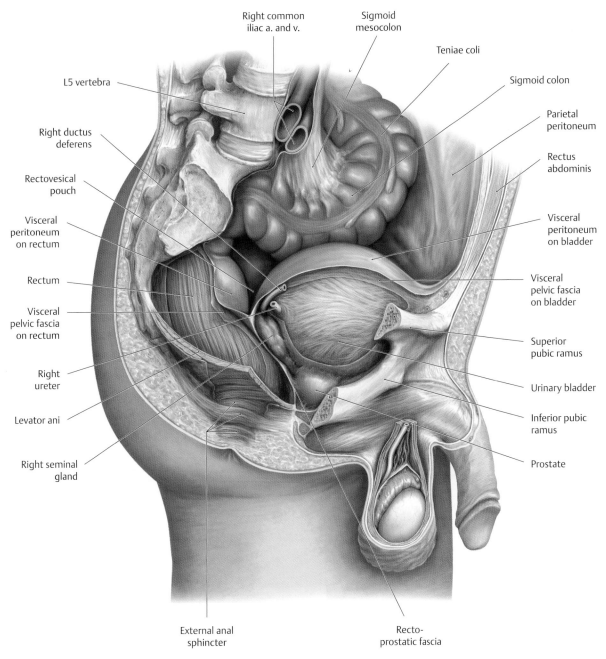

Fig. 11.1 Male pelvis
Parasagittal section, viewed from the right side.

Seminal Glands (Vesicles)

The **seminal glands** are paired convoluted tubules that produce 70% of the seminal fluid (**Figs. 11.2** and **11.3**).

— They lie superior to the prostate, between the urinary bladder and the rectum.

— The seminal glands are subperitoneal, located immediately below the peritoneum of the rectovesical pouch.

— The duct of each seminal gland joins with the ampulla of the ductus deferens to form the **ejaculatory ducts,** which pierce the prostate and drain into the **prostatic urethra.**

— The middle rectal and inferior vesical arteries supply the seminal glands. Veins of similar names accompany the arteries.

— Branches from the pelvic plexus innervate the seminal glands.

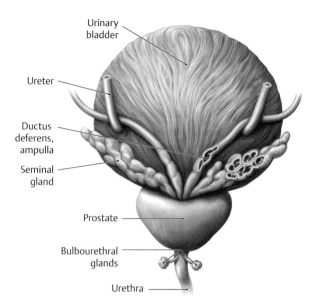

Fig. 11.2 Accessory sex glands
The bladder, prostate, seminal glands, and bulbourethral glands, posterior view.

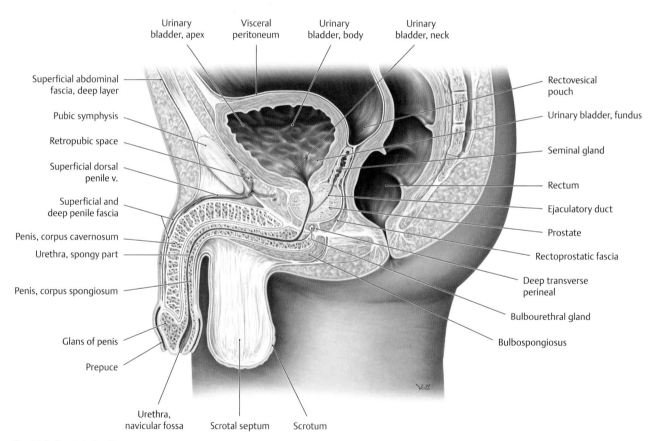

Fig. 11.3 Prostate in situ
Sagittal section through the male pelvis, left lateral view.

The Prostate

The **prostate** is an accessory reproductive gland that produces ~ 25% of the seminal fluid (**Fig. 11.4;** see also **Figs. 11.2** and **11.3**).

— The base, or superior surface, sits directly below the bladder. The apex points inferiorly and is in contact with the external urethral sphincter.

— It is posterior to the lower part of the pubic symphysis and anterior to the **rectovesical septum,** which separates it from the rectum.

— The prostate surrounds the proximal (prostatic) part of the urethra. Secretions from prostatic glands drain into the urethra through numerous prostatic ductules.

— A fibromuscular capsule surrounds the prostate. The prostatic capsule is separated from the outer prostatic sheath (derived from endopelvic fascia) by the prostatic venous plexus.

— **Puboprostatic ligaments,** anterior extensions of the tendinous arch of the pelvic fascia, attach the apex of the prostate (and neck of the bladder) to the pubis (see **Fig. 11.18**). Posterior extensions of the tendinous arch secure it to the sacrum.

— The anatomic lobes of the prostate include the following:
  • A fibromuscular isthmus anterior to the urethra
  • Right and left lateral lobes that are subdivided into lobules
  • The lower posterior lobule (sometimes referred to as the posterior lobe), which lies posterior to the urethra and inferior to the ejaculatory ducts, is palpable by digital exam.
  • A poorly defined middle lobe that sits above the lateral lobes between the urethra and ejaculatory ducts and is in close contact with the neck of the bladder

— For clinical purposes, the prostate is divided into three major zones determined by their proximity to the urethra: **periure-thral, central** (comparable to the anatomic middle lobe), and **peripheral.** A small **transition zone** consists of two lobes that account for approximately 5% of the glandular prostatic tissue (**Fig 11.5**).

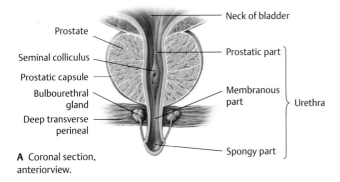

A Coronal section, anterior view.

Labels: Prostate, Seminal colliculus, Prostatic capsule, Bulbourethral gland, Deep transverse perineal, Neck of bladder, Prostatic part, Membranous part, Spongy part, Urethra

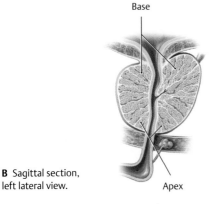

B Sagittal section, left lateral view.

Labels: Base, Apex

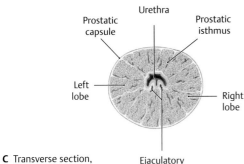

C Transverse section, superior view.

Labels: Urethra, Prostatic capsule, Prostatic isthmus, Left lobe, Right lobe, Ejaculatory duct orifices

Fig. 11.4 Prostate

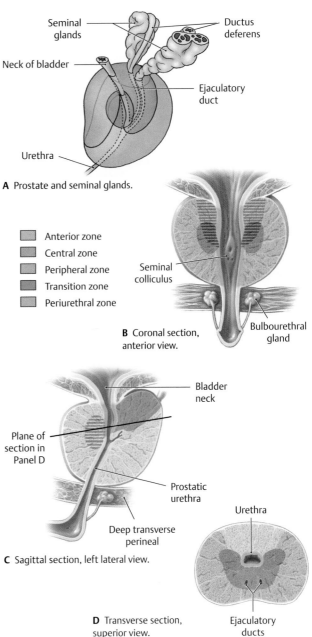

A Prostate and seminal glands.

Labels: Seminal glands, Neck of bladder, Urethra, Ductus deferens, Ejaculatory duct

Legend:
- Anterior zone
- Central zone
- Peripheral zone
- Transition zone
- Periurethral zone

B Coronal section, anterior view.

Labels: Seminal colliculus, Bulbourethral gland

C Sagittal section, left lateral view.

Labels: Plane of section in Panel D, Bladder neck, Prostatic urethra, Deep transverse perineal

D Transverse section, superior view.

Labels: Urethra, Ejaculatory ducts

Fig. 11.5 Clinical divisions of the prostate

— Prostatic arteries are usually branches of the inferior vesical arteries. Middle rectal arteries also contribute to the prostatic blood supply (see **Fig. 10.14A**).

— The prostatic venous plexus, continuous with the vesical venous plexus of the bladder, drains to internal iliac veins. The prostatic plexus also communicates with the vertebral venous plexus (see **Fig. 2.1**).

— The lymph vessels of the prostate follow venous pathways to the internal iliac nodes.

— The prostatic nerve plexus is a derivative of the inferior hypogastric plexus. The role of parasympathetic innervation is unclear, but sympathetic nerves cause the smooth muscle of the gland to contract, expelling prostatic secretion into the prostatic urethra during ejaculation.

CLINICAL CORRELATION

PROSTATECTOMY Prostatectomy is the surgical removal of the prostate gland. Open radical prostatectomy involves removal of the prostate along with the seminal glands, ductus deferens, and pelvic lymph nodes via a retropubic or perineal incision. Transurethral resection of the prostate (TURP) is performed using a cystoscope that is advanced through the urethra to resect the prostate. Cavernous nerves carrying parasympathetic fibers that are responsible for penile erection run alongside the prostate and are particularly at risk during these procedures.

CLINICAL CORRELATION

BENIGN PROSTATIC HYPERTROPHY (HYPERPLASIA) Benign prostatic hypertrophy (more accurately called hyperplasia) is the benign enlargement of the prostate gland that results from the proliferation of the epithelial and stromal tissues, particularly in the periurethral area **(Fig. 11.6)**. Although it is common in men of middle age, the incidence increases in later years and is thought to be due to the greater conversion of testosterone to the more active form, dihydrotestosterone (DHT), in the aging prostate gland. The hyperplasia constricts the internal urethral orifice, causing dysuria (difficult or painful urination), nocturia (excessive urination at night), and urgency (sudden desire to urinate). It is treated with a 5α-reductase inhibitor that blocks the conversion of testosterone to DHT by inhibiting the enzyme 5α-reductase. This may be used in combination with α-blockers that relax the muscles in the prostate and in the neck of the bladder, making urination easier. In severe cases, transurethral resection of the prostate may be necessary.

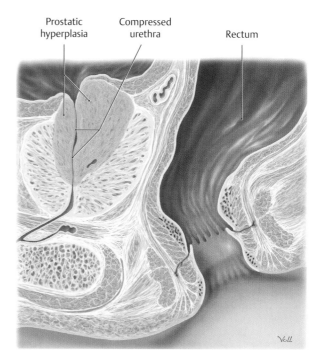

Fig. 11.6 **Benign prostatic hypertrophy**

CLINICAL CORRELATION

CARCINOMA OF THE PROSTATE Carcinoma of the prostate is a slow-growing cancer affecting elderly men that commonly arises in the posterior lobe of the prostate. It metastasizes to the bony pelvis, vertebral column, skull, and brain via the vertebral venous plexus but also to the heart and lungs via drainage through the internal iliac veins and inferior vena cava. Symptoms include hesitancy (difficulty in beginning the flow of urination), frequency, and dribbling on urination (collectively known as prostatism). It can be diagnosed by digital examination of the rectum, ultrasonography, or prostate-specific antigen (PSA) levels. A PSA value greater than 4.0 ng/mL indicates disease activity.

11.2   Female Genital Structures

Female genital structures, which include the ovaries, uterine tubes, uterus, and vagina, are located in the middle of the pelvis between the bladder anteriorly and the rectum posteriorly **(Figs. 11.7 and 11.8)**.

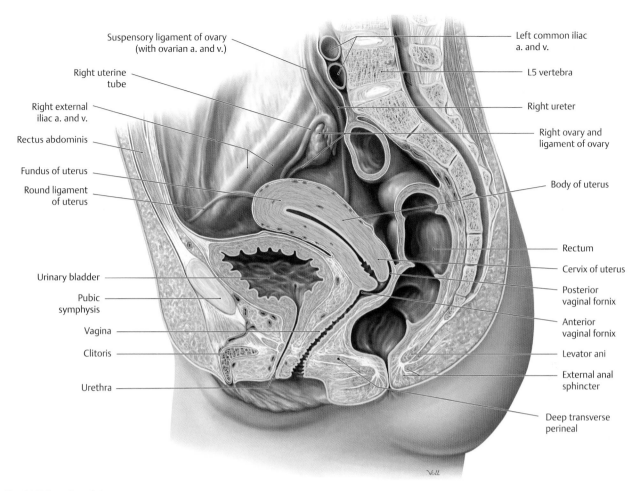

Suspensory ligament of ovary
(with ovarian a. and v.)

Right uterine tube

Right external iliac a. and v.

Rectus abdominis

Fundus of uterus

Round ligament of uterus

Urinary bladder

Pubic symphysis

Vagina

Clitoris

Urethra

Left common iliac a. and v.

L5 vertebra

Right ureter

Right ovary and ligament of ovary

Body of uterus

Rectum

Cervix of uterus

Posterior vaginal fornix

Anterior vaginal fornix

Levator ani

External anal sphincter

Deep transverse perineal

Fig. 11.7 Female pelvis
Sagittal section viewed from the left side.

Myometrium

Cervical canal

Endometrium

Bladder

Pubic symphysis

Rectum

Coccyx

Levator ani

External anal sphincter

Urethra

Vagina

Fig. 11.8 MRI of the female pelvis
Sagittal section, left lateral view
The uterus in the first half of the menstrual cycle (proliferative phase) with narrow endometrium and relatively low-signal intensity of the myometrium.
(From Hamm B, et al. MRT von Abdomen und Becken, 2. Aufl. Stuttgart: Thieme; 2006).

The Ovary

The **ovary** is the female gonad, an ovoid structure that produces eggs and reproductive hormones and resides in the lateral wall of the pelvis **(Fig. 11.9)**.

— The **ligament of the ovary** attaches the ovary to the supralateral aspect of the uterus.

— The **suspensory ligament of the ovary** is a fold of peritoneum that encloses the ovarian vessels and nerves as they pass over the pelvic brim to the ovary.

— The **mesovarium** suspends the ovary from the posterior part of the broad ligament.

— The ovarian artery, a branch of the abdominal aorta at L2, supplies the ovary (see **Fig. 10.17**).

— A pampiniform plexus, which may converge to form a single ovarian vein, drains the ovary. The right ovarian vein is a direct tributary of the inferior vena cava; the left ovarian vein is a tributary of the left renal vein.

— Lymphatic vessels follow the ovarian vessels superiorly to the lateral aortic nodes.

— Both the ovarian nerve plexus, which follows the ovarian vessels, and the pelvic nerve plexus, which follows the uterine vessels, innervate the ovary.

The Uterine Tubes

The **uterine tubes** (fallopian tubes, oviducts), paired muscular tubes that extend laterally from the horns (supralateral corners) of the uterus, transmit ova from the ovary and sperm from the uterine cavity (see **Fig. 11.9**).

— The uterine tubes are the normal sites of fertilization and are also the most common sites of ectopic pregnancies (implantation of a fertilized ovum outside the uterus).

— The uterine tube has four parts:
   1. The uterine (intramural) part, the segment that passes through the wall of the uterus

A Posterosuperior view.

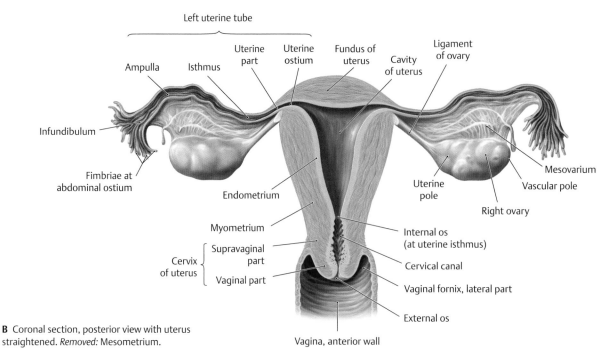

B Coronal section, posterior view with uterus straightened. *Removed:* Mesometrium.

Fig. 11.9 Uterus and uterine tube

2. The isthmus, the narrowest part
3. The ampulla, the longest and widest part and normally the site of fertilization
4. The infundibulum, the trumpet-shaped terminal part that is open to the peritoneal cavity, with fingerlike fimbriae that surround the ovary

— The uterine tube is ensheathed in the upper edge of the broad ligament, where it is supported by its mesosalpinx.
— The uterine tube is supplied by the anastomosing ovarian and uterine arteries and drained by accompanying veins.
— Lymph vessels follow the ovarian veins to the lateral aortic nodes.
— The ovarian and uterine plexuses innervate the uterine tubes.

CLINICAL CORRELATION

ECTOPIC PREGNANCY Implantation of a fertilized ovum outside the uterus can occur anywhere, but the ampulla of the uterine tube is the most common site. Often the tube has been partially blocked by inflammation (salpingitis), preventing the blastocyst from completing its journey to the uterus. If not diagnosed early in the pregnancy, rupture of the uterine tube with consequent hemorrhage into the peritoneal cavity can result in a life-threatening situation for the mother. A ruptured ectopic pregnancy on the right side may be misdiagnosed as a ruptured appendix because both conditions irritate the parietal peritoneum and have similar presentations.

The Uterus

The **uterus** is a pear-shaped muscular organ located in the center of the pelvis, posterior to the bladder and anterior to the rectum (see **Figs. 11.7** and **11.8**). It is the site of implantation of the fertilized egg, subsequent development of the embryo, and parturition of the fetus.

— The uterus (see **Fig. 11.9**) has two parts:
1. The **body** is the superior two thirds of the uterus and includes
   ◦ the **fundus,** the uppermost part above the openings of the uterine tubes, and

◦ the uterine **isthmus,** a narrow inferior segment that extends into the cervix.
2. The **cervix** is the narrow inferior third of the uterus and its least mobile part.
   ◦ A supravaginal part sits above the vagina.
   ◦ A vaginal part protrudes into the upper vagina and is surrounded by the vaginal fornices (upper recesses).

— The **uterine cavity,** a narrow space within the uterine body,
• communicates with the lumen of the uterine tubes where they enter at the uterine horns, and
• extends inferiorly through the **internal os** (orifice) to the **cervical canal** and terminates where the **external os** opens into the vagina.

DEVELOPMENT CORRELATION

BICORNUATE UTERUS The embryonic uterus is formed from the fusion of two paramesonephric ducts. When these ducts fail to fuse properly, a bicornuate uterus results in which the upper part of the uterus is bifurcated. The caudal part of the uterus is usually normal. Although a normal pregnancy is possible with this malformation, there is a greater risk of recurrent pregnancy loss, preterm birth, and malpresentation of the baby (e.g., the baby may be in a breech or transverse position).

— Although the body of the uterus is mobile, its position changes with the fullness of the bladder and rectum. Its normal position is anteflexed and anteverted (**Fig. 11.10**).
• **Flexion** describes the angle between the long axis of the upper uterine cavity and the isthmus and cervical canal. In an anteflexed uterus, the long axis of the uterine body is tipped anteriorly; a **retroflexed** uterus is tipped posteriorly.
• **Version** describes the angle between the cervix and vagina. In an anteverted uterus, the axis of the cervix is bent anteriorly; in a **retroverted** uterus, the cervix is bent posteriorly.

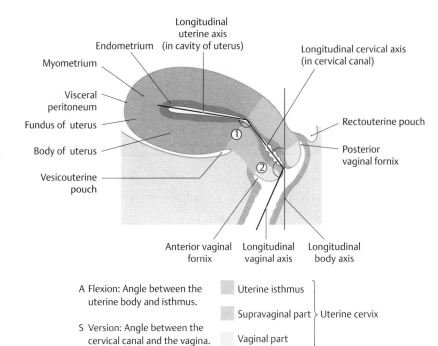

A Flexion: Angle between the uterine body and isthmus.

S Version: Angle between the cervical canal and the vagina.

Uterine isthmus
Supravaginal part } Uterine cervix
Vaginal part

Fig. 11.10 Curvature of the uterus
Midsagittal section, left lateral view. The position of the uterus can be described in terms of flexion *(1)* and version *(2)*.

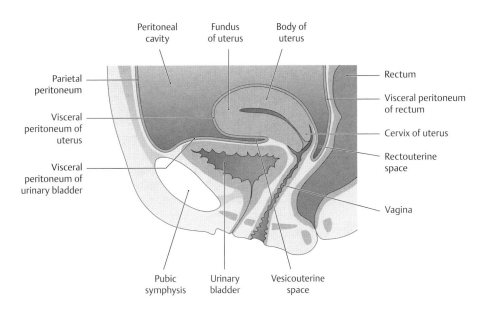

Fig. 11.11 Peritoneum in the female pelvis

— Peritoneum covers the body of the uterus, extending as far inferiorly as the cervix on its posterior surface. The uterus is flanked anteriorly by the vesicouterine space and posteriorly by the rectouterine space (pouch) **(Fig. 11.11)**.

— Uterine ligaments that arise from the uterine body include the broad ligament and the round ligaments of the uterus **(Fig. 11.12;** see also **Fig. 11.9A)**.

• The **broad ligament** is a double fold of peritoneum that extends laterally from each side of the uterus to the sidewalls of the pelvis. The parts of the broad ligament **(Fig. 11.13)** are

  ○ the **mesosalpinx,** which ensheaths the uterine tube;

  ○ the **mesovarium,** a posterior extension, which suspends the ovary; and

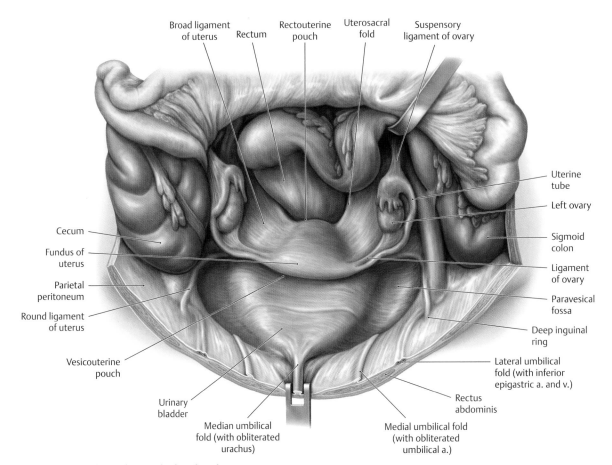

Fig. 11.12 Peritoneal relationships in the female pelvis
Lesser pelvis, anterosuperior view. *Retracted:* Small intestine loops and colon (portions).

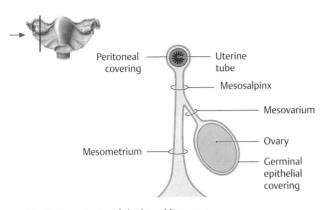

Fig. 11.13 Mesenteries of the broad ligament
Sagittal section. The broad ligament of the uterus is a combination of the mesosalpinx, mesovarium, and mesometrium.

- the **mesometrium,** which extends from the uterine body below the mesovarium to the sidewall of the pelvis.
- The paired **round ligaments of the uterus,** which originate near the fundus from each side of the uterus, pass through the deep inguinal rings, traverse the inguinal canals, and insert in the labia majora of the perineum.

— Uterine ligaments that arise from the cervix include the transverse cervical ligaments and the uterosacral ligaments (**Fig. 11.14** and **11.15**).
  - The paired **cardinal** (transverse cervical) **ligaments** are thickenings of endopelvic fascia that connect the uterine cervix to the pelvic sidewall. They are located at the base of the broad ligament and transmit the uterine vessels.
  - The paired **uterosacral ligaments** are thickenings of endopelvic fascia that connect the uterine cervix to the sacrum and help to maintain the anteverted position of the uterus.
— The uterine artery, the primary blood supply to the uterus (see **Fig. 10.17**), traverses the cardinal ligament and anastomoses superiorly with the ovarian artery and inferiorly with the vaginal artery.
— A uterine venous plexus receives the uterine veins and drains to the internal iliac vein.
— Lymphatic drainage of the uterus is complex but generally follows the uterine veins or the uterine ligaments (see **Table 10.4**).
  - The uterine fundus drains to para-aortic nodes via the ovarian veins.
  - The supralateral part of the uterus drains to superficial inguinal nodes via the round ligament.
  - The uterine body drains to external iliac nodes via the broad ligament.

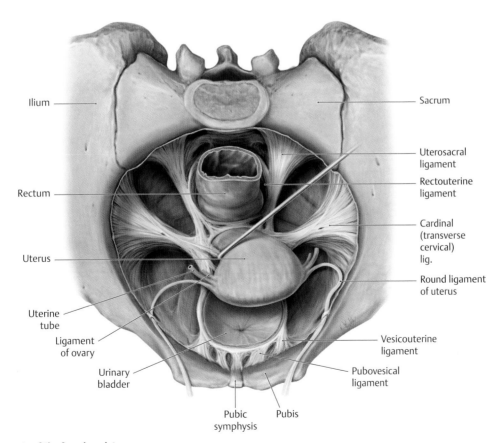

Fig. 11.14 Ligaments of the female pelvis
Superior view. *Removed:* Peritoneum, neurovasculature, and superior portion of bladder to demonstrate only the fascial condensations. Deep pelvic ligaments support the uterus within the pelvic cavity and prevent uterine prolapse, the downward displacement of the uterus into the vagina.

Piriformis

Rectum

Fascia over
obturator internus

Tendinous arch
of levator ani

Tendinous arch
of pelvic fascia

Levator ani

Lateral lig. of
the bladder

Pubovesical lig.

Uterosacral lig.

Cardinal (transverse
cervical) lig.

Cervix

Paracolpium

Fascia over
anterior vagina

Obturator canal

Urethra

Pubic symphysis

Fig. 11.15 Ligaments of the deep pelvis in the female
Superior view. Uterosacral ligaments and paracolpium support and maintain the position of the cervix and vagina in the pelvis.

- The cervix drains to internal iliac and sacral nodes via
  the cardinal and uterosacral ligaments.
- The uterovaginal nerve plexus, derived from the inferior
  hypogastric plexus, innervates the uterus (see **Figs. 10.20**
  and **10.25**).

The Vagina

The **vagina** is a fibromuscular tube that extends from the cervix of
the uterus to the vaginal orifice in the perineum (**Figs. 11.16** and
11.17). It serves as the inferior part of the birth canal and the con-

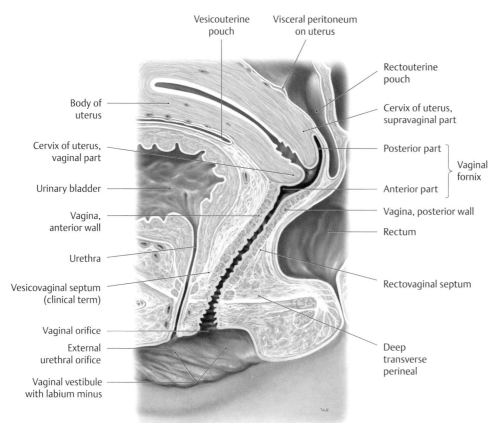

Vesicouterine
pouch

Visceral peritoneum
on uterus

Body of
uterus

Cervix of uterus,
vaginal part

Urinary bladder

Vagina,
anterior wall

Urethra

Vesicovaginal septum
(clinical term)

Vaginal orifice

External
urethral orifice

Vaginal vestibule
with labium minus

Rectouterine
pouch

Cervix of uterus,
supravaginal part

Posterior part

Anterior part

Vaginal
fornix

Vagina, posterior wall

Rectum

Rectovaginal septum

Deep
transverse
perineal

Fig. 11.16 Vagina
Midsagittal section, left lateral
view.

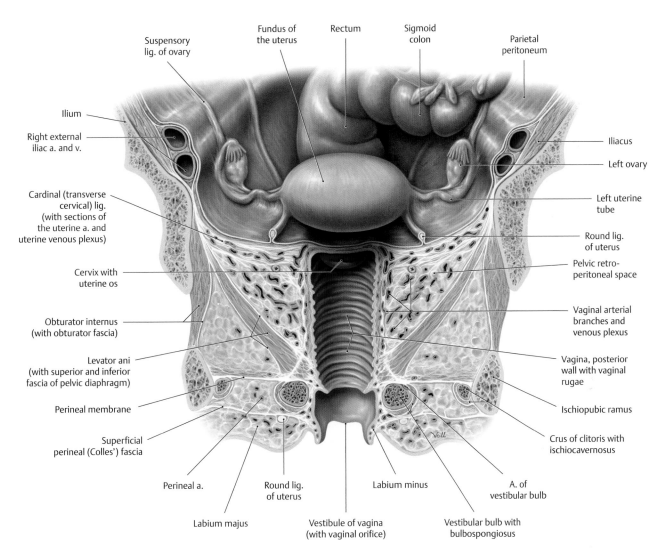

Fig. 11.17 Female pelvis
Coronal section, anterior view.

duit for menstrual fluid, and it accommodates the penis during sexual intercourse.

— The vagina is posterior to the bladder and urethra and anterior to the rectum.
— It is normally flattened with its anterior and posterior walls in contact.
— Connections to the sacrum via the uterosacral ligaments and to the tendinous arch of the pelvic fascia on the side wall of the pelvis via the **paracolpium** stabilize the vagina, especially during childbirth (see **Fig 11.15**).
— The vaginal fornix, which has anterior, lateral, and posterior parts, is a recess that surrounds the lower cervix as it protrudes into the upper vagina (see **Figs. 11.7** and **11.9B**).
  • The posterior fornix is in contact with the rectouterine pouch, thereby providing access to the peritoneal cavity. The anterior fornix is shorter and lies against the posterior wall of the bladder.
— The internal iliac artery supplies the vagina through its uterine, vaginal, and internal pudendal branches (see **Figs. 10.14B** and **10.17**).
— Veins of the vagina contribute to the uterovaginal venous plexus, which drains to the internal iliac vein.

— Lymphatic vessels of the vagina drain to several groups of nodes.
  • The superior part of the vagina drains to external or internal iliac nodes.
  • The inferior part of the vagina drains to sacral and common iliac nodes.
  • The vaginal orifice drains to superficial inguinal nodes.
— The uterovaginal nerve plexus, an extension of the inferior hypogastric plexus, innervates the superior three fourths of the vagina (see **Fig. 10.20**).
— A deep perineal branch of the pudendal nerve, a branch of the sacral plexus, innervates the lowest vaginal segment (see **Fig. 10.15**). This somatically innervated segment is the only part of the vagina that is sensitive to touch.

CLINICAL CORRELATION

CULDOCENTESIS Culdocentesis is a procedure in which peritoneal fluid is extracted from the rectouterine pouch by needle aspiration. The needle is advanced through the posterior fornix of the vagina. No fluid or a small amount of clear fluid is normal, but purulent fluid is suggestive of pelvic inflammatory disease (PID). The presence of blood is an indication for emergency surgery.

11.3 Pelvic Urinary Organs

The pelvic urinary organs include the distal ureters, the urinary bladder, and the urethra.

The Ureters

Each ureter crosses over the brim of the pelvis at the bifurcation of the common iliac artery and descends along the lateral wall near the ischial spine. It runs anteriorly and enters the posterolateral wall of the bladder.

— In males, the ureter passes under the pelvic portion of the ductus deferens and enters the bladder lateral and superior to the free ends of the seminal glands (**Fig. 11.18**; see also **Fig. 11.2**).

— In females, the ureter passes inferior to the uterine arteries within the cardinal ligament, ~ 2 cm lateral to the vaginal part of the cervix (**Fig. 11.19**).

— The most reliable blood supply to the pelvic part of the ureter is the uterine artery in females and the inferior

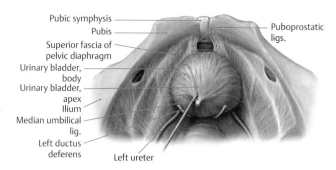

Fig. 11.18 Ureter and bladder in the male pelvis
Superior view.

vesical artery in males. Veins of similar names accompany the arteries.

— The pelvic part of the ureter derives its innervation from the inferior hypogastric plexuses.

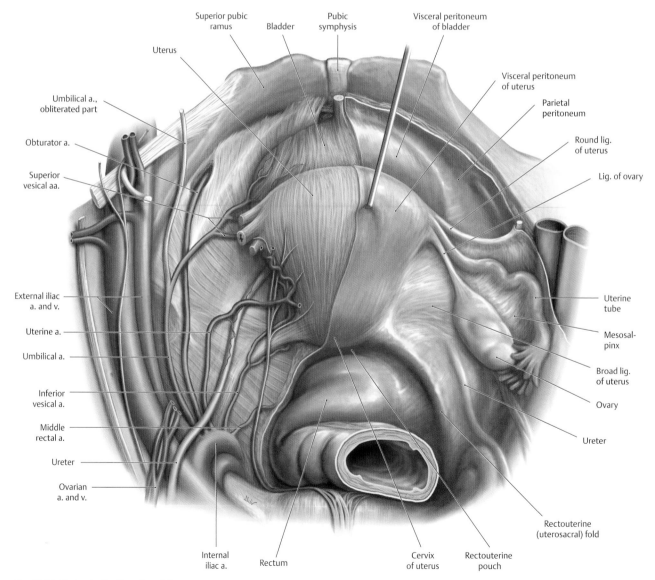

Fig. 11.19 Ureter in the female pelvis
Superior view. *Removed from right side:* Peritoneum and broad ligament of uterus.

— Visceral sensory fibers follow sympathetic nerves to spinal cord levels T11–L2; therefore, ureteric pain is usually felt in the ipsilateral inguinal region.

The Urinary Bladder

The bladder is a muscular reservoir for the temporary storage of urine. Although normally located in the true pelvis, when full it may extend superiorly into the abdomen.

— It lies directly posterior to the pubic symphysis, separated from it by the retropubic space. Posteriorly, it is related to the rectum in the male (see **Fig. 11.1**) and the upper vagina in the female (see **Fig. 11.7**).

— It is covered by peritoneum only on its superior surface.

— The bladder is tetrahedral with superior, posterior, and two inferolateral surfaces (**Fig. 11.20**). It has four parts:
  1. The **apex** points toward the pubic symphysis. The median umbilical ligament extends from the apex to the umbilicus.
  2. The **fundus** forms the bladder base, or posterior wall.
  3. The **body** makes up most of the bladder.
  4. The **neck** is the lowest and least mobile region.

— The neck of the bladder is firmly attached to
  • the pubis by anterior extensions of the tendinous arch of the pelvic fascia, the **pubovesical ligaments** in females, and puboprostatic ligaments in males (see **Figs. 11.14** and **11.18**); and
  • the lateral pelvic walls by condensations of endopelvic fascia, the **lateral ligaments of the bladder** (see **Fig. 10.12**).

— The walls are made up of bundles of smooth muscle fibers. In the male, the muscle fibers near the bladder neck, which form the internal urethral sphincter, contract during ejaculation.

— The internal surface of the base of the bladder is marked by the **trigone**, a smooth triangular region (**Fig. 11.21**). The corners of the triangle are formed posterolaterally by the slitlike openings of the right and left ureters and anteriorly by the urethral orifice.

— The bladder is highly distensible and in most individuals may hold up to 600 to 800 mL (painfully), although micturition

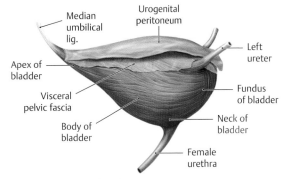

A Female bladder and urethra

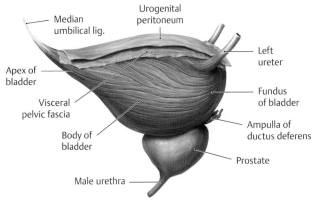

B Male bladder with prostate and proximal urethra

Fig. 11.20 Structure of the bladder
Left lateral view

(urination) usually occurs at a much smaller volume. Normally, no urine remains in the bladder after voiding.

— The superior vesical arteries, with contributions from the inferior vesical arteries (in males) and vaginal arteries (in females), supply the bladder (see **Fig. 10.14**).

— The vesical venous plexus surrounds the inferolateral surfaces of the bladder and drains to the internal iliac veins. The plexus communicates with the prostatic plexus in males, with the

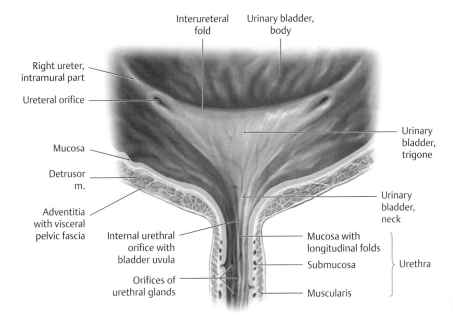

Fig. 11.21 Trigone of the bladder
Coronal section, anterior view.

uterovaginal plexus in females, and with the vertebral venous plexus in both sexes.
— Lymph from the bladder drains to internal and external iliac nodes.
— The vesical nerve plexus of the bladder is a derivative of the inferior hypogastric plexus (see **Figs. 10.20** and **10.24**).
  • Sympathetic stimulation relaxes the detrusor muscle and contracts the internal sphincter, thus inhibiting micturition.
  • Parasympathetic nerves stimulate the detrusor muscle to contract while inhibiting the internal sphincter, thereby facilitating micturition.
  • Visceral sensory fibers carrying pain from the inferior bladder follow parasympathetic routes. Pain fibers from the superior bladder follow sympathetic routes.

The Urethra

The urethra is the muscular conduit for urine in the female and for urine and semen in the male. It extends from the internal urethral orifice at the bladder neck to the external urethral orifice in the perineum.
— The male urethra extends 18 to 22 cm from the urinary bladder to the tip of the glans penis (**Fig. 11.22**). The male urethra has four parts. Although all are mentioned here, the membranous and spongy parts are located in the perineum and are discussed further in Chapter 12.
  1. The **preprostatic** part at the neck of the bladder contains the internal urethral orifice. Sympathetic nerves of the superior hypogastric plexus control closure of the **internal urethral sphincter** during ejaculation.

  2. The **prostatic** part is surrounded by the prostate gland and characterized by
     ∘ the **urethral crest,** a vertical ridge on the posterior wall that contains a central eminence, the **seminal colliculus;** and
     ∘ ejaculatory ducts that open onto the urethral crest, and prostatic ductules from the prostate that open into recesses on either side of the crest.
  3. The **membranous** part passes through the perineal membrane in the urogenital triangle and is surrounded by the external urethral sphincter.
  4. The **spongy** part passes through the corpus spongiosum, one of the vascular erectile bodies of the penis.
— The female urethra extends 4 cm from the internal urethral orifice at the bladder neck to the external urethral orifice in the perineum (**Fig. 11.23**).
  • Within the pelvis it lies anterior to the vagina, forming an elevation within the anterior vaginal wall.
  • It passes through the genital hiatus of the pelvic diaphragm, the external urethral sphincter (there is no organized internal urethral sphincter), and the perineal membrane.
  • In the perineum, the urethra opens within the vestibule of the vagina directly anterior to the vaginal orifice (see **Fig. 12.9**).
— Branches of the pudendal artery, as well as the inferior vesical artery in the male and vaginal artery in the female, supply the urethra. In both sexes, a venous plexus that accompanies the arteries drains the urethra.
— The female urethra and proximal parts of the male urethra (preprostatic, prostatic, and membranous) drain to the internal iliac nodes. The spongy urethra of the male (the perineal part) drains to deep inguinal nodes.
— Nerves to the urethra arise from the prostatic nerve plexus in the male and comparable vesical nerve plexus in the female. Sympathetic nerves control the closure of the external urethral sphincter in males.
— Visceral sensory fibers from the pelvic urethra travel with pelvic splanchnic nerves; somatic sensory fibers from the perineal urethra travel with the pudendal nerve.

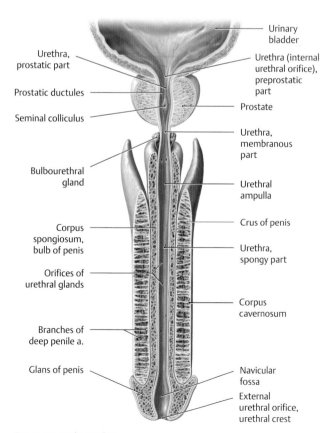

Urinary bladder

Urethra, prostatic part

Urethra (internal urethral orifice), preprostatic part

Prostatic ductules

Prostate

Seminal colliculus

Urethra, membranous part

Bulbourethral gland

Urethral ampulla

Crus of penis

Corpus spongiosum, bulb of penis

Urethra, spongy part

Orifices of urethral glands

Corpus cavernosum

Branches of deep penile a.

Glans of penis

Navicular fossa

External urethral orifice, urethral crest

Fig. 11.22 Male urethra
Longitudinal section, anterior view.

CLINICAL CORRELATION

URETHRAL RUPTURE IN MALES Fractures of the pelvic girdle may be accompanied by a rupture of the membranous part of the urethra. This allows the extravasation (escape) of urine and blood into the deep perineal space and superiorly through the genital hiatus to the subperitoneal spaces around the prostate and bladder. Rupture of the bulbous part of the spongy urethra may occur from a straddle injury in which there is a forceful blow to the perineum, or from the false passage of a transurethral catheter. In this case urine can leak into the superficial peritoneal space, which is continuous with the scrotal sac, the space around the penis, and the space on the inferior anterior abdominal wall between the abdominal muscles and the membranous layer of the superficial fascia. The attachment of the superficial perineal fascia to the fascia lata (fascia enclosing the thigh muscles) prevents urine from spreading laterally into the thighs. Similarly, it is prevented from spreading into the anal triangle by the attachment of the fascia to the deep perineal fascia and perineal membrane.

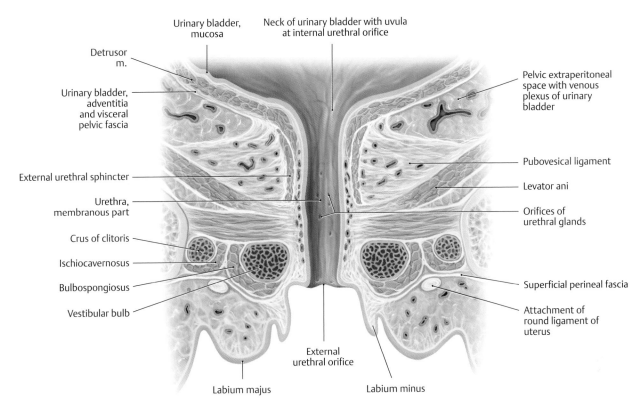

Fig. 11.23 Female urethra
Coronal section tilted slightly posterior, anterior view.

11.4   The Rectum

The rectum is the continuation of the gastrointestinal tract in the pelvis and functions as a temporary storage site for fecal matter. It is continuous with the sigmoid colon superiorly and the anal canal inferiorly (**Figs. 11.24** and **11.25;** see Section 12.5).

— It lies anterior to the lower sacrum and coccyx and rests on the anococcygeal ligament of the pelvic floor.
— Anteriorly, the rectum is related to the bladder, seminal glands, and prostate in males and to the vagina in females. A rectovesical or rectovaginal septum separates the rectum from these anterior structures.
— The rectum has no mesentery. Its superior two thirds are retroperitoneal and form the posterior surface of the rectovesical and rectouterine pouches. The distal third is subperitoneal.
— Unlike the colon, the rectum lacks taeniae coli, haustra, and epiploic appendices.
— The rectum begins at the **rectosigmoid junction,** the point at which the teniae coli disappear. At this junction, muscle fibers of the bands spread out evenly over the surface of the rectum. This junction usually occurs anterior to the S3 vertebra.
— The rectum terminates at the **anorectal junction** (its junction with the anal canal), where it passes through the pelvic diaphragm adjacent to the tip of the coccyx.
— The internal wall of the rectum has three transverse **rectal folds,** one on the right and two on the left, which create lateral flexures that are visible externally.
— The **ampulla,** the most distal segment of the rectum, stores accumulating fecal material until defecation and has an important role in fecal continence. It narrows abruptly as

it joins with the anal canal and passes through the pelvic diaphragm.
— The rectum has a dual blood supply:
   • The superior rectal artery, the unpaired terminal branch of the inferior mesenteric artery, supplies the upper rectum (see **Fig. 10.19**).
   • Right and left middle rectal arteries, branches of the internal iliac arteries, supply the lower rectum.
— The rectal veins drain a submucosal rectal venous plexus, which has internal and external (subcutaneous) components.
   • The external plexus communicates with other visceral venous plexuses in the pelvis.
   • The internal plexus communicates with branches from the rectal arteries (an arteriovenous anastomosis), forming a thickened vascular tissue **(hemorrhoidal plexus)** that surrounds the anorectal junction. This tissue forms prominent anal cushions in the left lateral, right antero-lateral, and right posterolateral positions.

CLINICAL CORRELATION

RECTAL EXAMINATION A rectal examination is performed by inserting a gloved, lubricated finger into the rectum, while the other hand is used to press on the lower abdomen or pelvic region. Palpable structures include the prostate, seminal glands, ampulla of the ductus deferens, bladder, uterus, cervix, and ovaries. Pathologic anomalies such as hemorrhoids, tumors, enlargements, and changes in consistency of the tissues can be felt. The tonicity of the anal sphincter, mediated by the pudendal nerve (S2–S4), can also be assessed.

Fig. 11.24 Rectum in situ
Female pelvis, coronal section, anterior view.

— Venous blood from the rectum drains into the portal and caval (systemic) venous systems (see **Fig. 10.19**).
  • A superior rectal vein, which drains the upper rectum, is a tributary of the portal system via the inferior mesenteric vein.
  • The paired middle and inferior rectal veins that drain the lower rectum (and anal canal) are tributaries of the inferior vena cava via the internal iliac veins.
  • Communications between the superior, middle, and inferior rectal veins form clinically important portocaval anastomoses that enlarge in portal hypertension.
— Lymphatic drainage follows vascular pathways.
  • The upper rectum drains to inferior mesenteric nodes along the course of the superior rectal vessels. It eventually drains to lumbar nodes, although some lymph may drain first to sacral nodes.
  • The lower rectum drains primarily to sacral nodes or directly to internal iliac nodes.
— Sympathetic innervation to the rectum is carried by lumbar splanchnic nerves to the hypogastric plexuses, as well as by

CLINICAL CORRELATION

HEMORRHOIDS External hemorrhoids are thrombosed veins of the external venous plexus, commonly associated with pregnancy or chronic constipation. They lie below the dentate line and are covered by skin. Because they are somatically innervated, they are more painful than internal hemorrhoids.

Internal hemorrhoids contain dilated veins of the internal rectal plexus. With a breakdown of the muscularis layer, these vascular cushions prolapse into the anal canal and may become ulcerated. Because they lie above the dentate line and are viscerally innervated, these hemorrhoids are painless. They are generally not associated with portal hypertension, but bleeding is characteristically bright red due to the anastomoses between the venous plexus and branches of the rectal arteries.

nerves of the inferior mesenteric nerve plexus traveling along the superior rectal artery (see **Figs. 10.20, 10.21, 10.26**).
— Parasympathetic innervation originates in pelvic splanchnic nerves, which also carry visceral sensory fibers.

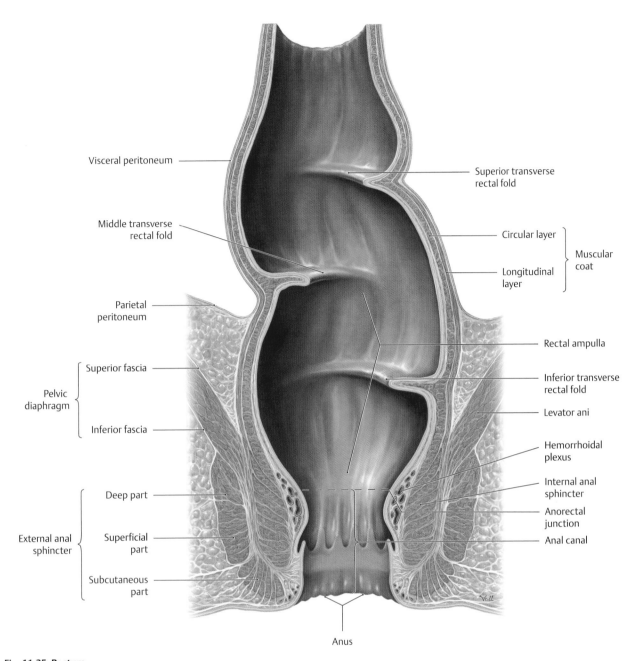

Visceral peritoneum

Middle transverse rectal fold

Parietal peritoneum

Pelvic diaphragm
  Superior fascia
  Inferior fascia

External anal sphincter
  Deep part
  Superficial part
  Subcutaneous part

Superior transverse rectal fold

Circular layer

Longitudinal layer

Muscular coat

Rectal ampulla

Inferior transverse rectal fold

Levator ani

Hemorrhoidal plexus

Internal anal sphincter

Anorectal junction

Anal canal

Anus

Fig. 11.25 Rectum
Coronal section, anterior view.

12 The Perineum

The perineum is the space inferior to the pelvic floor, which is divided into a urogenital triangle and an anal triangle. The urogenital triangle contains the male and female external genital structures, and the anal triangle contains the anal canal and anus.

12.1 Perineal Spaces

— The boundaries of the diamond-shaped perineum (**Figs. 12.1** and **12.2**; see also **Fig. 10.4**) are
  • the pelvic outlet (pubic symphysis, ischiopubic rami, sacrotuberous ligaments, and coccyx), which forms the perimeter;
  • the lower parts of the obturator internus muscles and their obturator fasciae, which line the lateral walls;
  • the inferior surface of the pelvic diaphragm, which forms the roof; and
  • the skin of the perineum, which forms the floor.
— A line connecting the ischial tuberosities separates the perineum into an anterior urogenital triangle and a posterior anal triangle
— The **perineal membrane,** a tough, fibrous sheet, stretches between the ischiopubic rami, extending anteriorly almost to the pubic symphysis and posteriorly to the ischial tuberosities.
  • It separates the urogenital triangle into the **deep perineal** and **superficial perineal spaces** (see **Fig. 10.3**).
  • It forms a platform for the attachment of the cavernous bodies (which become engorged during arousal) of the external genitalia.

— The superficial perineal space is a potential space bounded above by the perineal membrane and below by the **superficial perineal fascia** (Colles' fascia), the extension of the membranous layer of superficial fascia (Scarpa's fascia) on the abdominal wall.
  • In both sexes it contains
    ◦ the **bulbospongiosus, ischiocavernosus,** and **superficial transverse perineal muscles** (see Section 12.2) and
    ◦ the **deep perineal branches** of the internal pudendal vessels and pudendal nerve.
  • In males (see Section 12.3) it also contains
    ◦ the **root** of the penis and
    ◦ the proximal portion of the spongy (penile) urethra.
  • In females (see Section 12.4) it also contains
    ◦ the **clitoris** and associated muscles,
    ◦ the **vestibular bulb,** and
    ◦ the **greater vestibular glands.**
— The deep perineal space is bounded inferiorly by the perineal membrane and superiorly by the pelvic diaphragm.
  • In both sexes it contains
    ◦ part of the urethra and inferior part of the **external urethral sphincter,**
    ◦ the anterior recesses of the **ischioanal fat pads,** and
    ◦ neurovascular structures to the penis or clitoris.
  • In males it also contains
    ◦ the membranous part of the urethra,
    ◦ the **bulbourethral glands,** and
    ◦ the **deep transverse perineal muscles.**

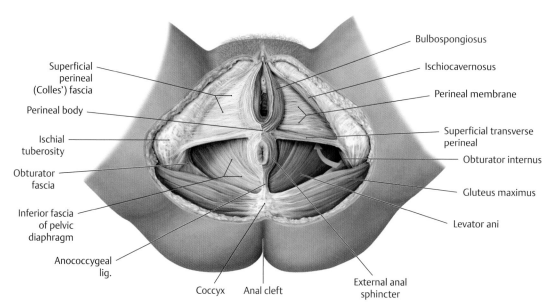

Fig. 12.1 Muscles and fascia of the female perineum
Lithotomy position, caudal (inferior) view. The *green arrow* is pointing forward to the anterior recess of the ischioanal fossa.

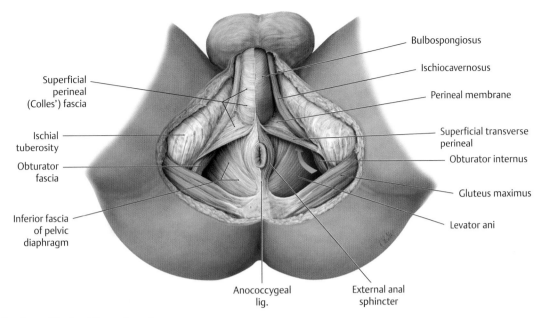

Fig. 12.2 Muscles and fascia of the male perineum
Lithotomy position, caudal (inferior) view. The *green arrow* is pointing forward to the anterior recess of the ischioanal fossa.

- In females it also contains
  ◦ compressor urethrae and urethrovaginal sphincter,
  ◦ the proximal part of the urethra, and
  ◦ associated with the **perineal body.**

12.2   Muscles of the Perineum

— Muscles of the perineum support the pelvic floor, surround the orifices of the urethra and anus, and assist in the erection of genital structures (**Table 12.1; Fig. 12.3**).
— The **perineal body** is an irregular subcutaneous mass of fibro-muscular tissue formed by converging fibers of the levator ani, the deep transverse perineal and bulbospongiosus muscles, and the external anal sphincter.
  - It lies between the rectum and bulb of the penis in males and between the rectum and vagina in females.
  - It supports the pelvic diaphragm and pelvic viscera.
— **Perineal branches** of the internal pudendal artery supply muscles of the perineum. Venous blood drains to the internal pudendal vein and the internal iliac vein.
— The pudendal nerve (S2–S4) innervates the muscles of the perineum.

CLINICAL CORRELATION

EPISIOTOMY During vaginal delivery, pressure on the perineum risks tearing the perineal muscles. A clean incision through the posterior vaginal orifice into the perineal body, known as an episiotomy, is often performed to enlarge the opening and prevent damage to perineal muscles. A median episiotomy extends only into the perineal body, but if further traumatic tearing occurs to extend the cut, it can damage the external anal sphincter (resulting in fecal incontinence) or create an anovaginal fistula. Mediolateral episiotomies often replace the midline incisions. These extend laterally from the vaginal orifice to the superficial perineal muscles, thus avoiding the perineal body and the possible sequelae from extensive tearing.

CLINICAL CORRELATION

PROLAPSE OF PELVIC ORGANS The pelvic diaphragm, pelvic ligaments, and perineal body provide important structural support for the pelvic viscera. Stretching or disruption of these tissues often occurs during childbirth and results in prolapse of the uterus into the vagina. A widening of the genital hiatus from an atrophic pelvic floor or a weakened perineal body can allow the bladder (cystocele), rectum (rectocele), or rectovesical pouch (enterocele) to bulge into the vaginal wall.

Table 12.1 **Muscles of the Perineum**

Muscle	Origin	Insertion	Innervation	Action
Deep perineal space				
External urethral sphincter		Encircles urethra	Pudendal n. (S2–S4)	Compresses urethra
Compressor urethrae (females)	Ischiopubic ramus	Part of external urethral sphincter		
Urethrovaginal sphincter (females)	Anterior urethra	Interdigitates with opposite side posterior to vagina		Compresses urethra and vagina
Deep transverse perineal (often replaced by smooth muscle in females)	Inferior pubic ramus, ischial ramus	Wall of vagina or prostate, perineal body		Supports the prostate
Superficial perineal space				
Bulbospongiosus	Runs anteriorly from perineal body to clitoris (female) or		Pudendal n. (S2–S4)	Females: compresses greater vestibular gland Males: assists in erection
Ischiocavernosus	Ischial ramus	Crus of clitoris or penis	Pudendal n. (S2–S4)	Maintains erection by squeezing blood into the corpus cavernosum of the clitoris or penis
Superficial transverse perineal	Ischial ramus	Perineal body	Pudendal n. (S2–S4)	Stabilizes the perineal body
Anal triangle				
External anal sphincter		Encircles anus (runs posteriorly from perineal body to anococcygeal ligament)	Pudendal n. (S2–S4)	Closes the anus

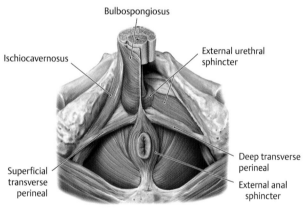

A Superficial and deep perineal muscles in the male.

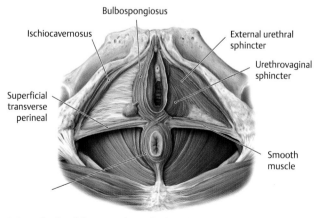

B Superficial and deep muscles in the female.

Fig. 12.3 Muscles of the perineum
Inferior view.

12.3   Male Urogenital Triangle

The male urogenital triangle contains the scrotum, penis, bulbourethral glands, perineal muscles, and associated neurovasculature (see **Fig. 11.3**).

The Scrotum

— The **scrotum** is a saccular extension of the anterior abdominal wall that encloses the testes and spermatic cord (see Section 7.3).
— The subcutaneous layer of the skin over the scrotum is devoid of fat, but the **dartos fascia** that underlies the skin is continuous with the deep membranous layer of the superficial fascia (Scarpa's fascia) of the abdomen and with the superficial perineal fascia (Colles' fascia) of the perineum.
— An extension of the dartos fascia divides the scrotum into right and left compartments and is visible externally as the **scrotal raphe.**
— Scrotal branches of the internal pudendal and external pudendal arteries, and cremasteric branches of the inferior epigastric artery supply the scrotum. Veins of similar names accompany the arteries (**Figs. 12.4** and **12.5**).
— Lymph from the scrotum drains to superficial inguinal nodes. Recall that lymph from the contents within the scrotum (i.e., the testis and epididymis) drains directly to the para-aortic nodes.
— Innervation of the scrotum (see **Fig. 10.23B**) is supplied by
   • the ilioinguinal and genitofemoral (genital branch) nerves, which innervate the anterior scrotum, and
   • the pudendal and posterior femoral cutaneous nerves of the thigh, which innervate the posterior scrotum.

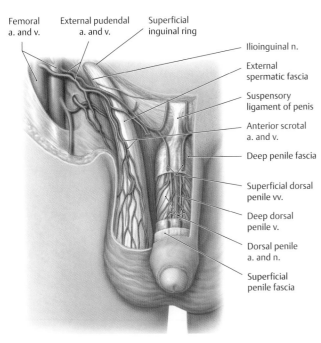

Fig. 12.4 **Neurovasculature of the penis and scrotum**
Anterior view. *Partially removed:* Skin and fascia.

A Arterial supply.

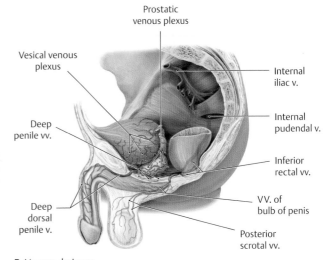

B Venous drainage.

Fig. 12.5 **Blood vessels of the male genitalia**
Left lateral view.

The Penis

The **penis** serves both copulatory and urinary functions. It contains three cylindrical bodies of erectile tissue, one of which surrounds the spongy urethra that transmits urine from the bladder as well as semen during sexual intercourse (**Figs. 12.6** and **12.7**).

— The penis has three parts:

1. The **root,** the most proximal part, is attached to the perineal membrane and is covered by muscles. It is composed of
   ◦ right and left **crura** that are attached to the ischiopubic rami on either side and are covered by the ischiocavernosus muscles, and
   ◦ the **bulb of the penis,** which is attached to the perineal membrane and covered by the bulbospongiosus muscle. The spongy (penile) urethra enters on its dorsal surface.

2. The **body,** pendulous and not covered by muscle, is made up of three cylindrical bodies of erectile tissue. A **tunica albuginea,** a dense fibrous coat, surrounds each erectile body, and distally a **deep penile fascia** (Buck's fascia) binds the three bodies together. The three erectile bodies include
   ◦ two **corpora cavernosa,** continuations of the crura, which lie side by side on the dorsum of the penis, and
   ◦ one **corpus spongiosum,** a continuation of the bulb of the penis, which lies ventral to the two corpora cavernosa and is traversed by the spongy (penile) urethra.

3. The **glans penis** (also known as the **glans**), an expansion of the distal end of the corpus spongiosum, is characterized by
   ◦ the **corona,** which overhangs the distal ends of the corpora cavernosa, and
   ◦ the **external urethral orifice** at its tip.

— External pudendal arteries supply the skin and subcutaneous tissue of the penis. Venous drainage of this tissue passes

through the **superficial dorsal veins,** which drain to the external pudendal veins (see **Fig. 12.4**).

— Internal pudendal arteries supply the deep penile structures. Their branches (**Fig. 12.8;** see also **Fig. 12.6B**) include
   • the **artery of the bulb of the penis,** which supplies the bulb of the penis, the urethra within the bulb, and the bulbourethral glands;
   • the **dorsal penile artery,** which runs between the deep penile fascia and tunica albuginea to supply the penile fascia and skin and the glans; and
   • the **deep penile artery,** which runs within the corpus cavernosum and gives off **helicine arteries** that supply the erectile tissue and are responsible for engorgement of the corpora during erection.

— The erectile bodies are drained by venous plexuses that empty into the single **deep dorsal vein,** which passes under the pubic symphysis to join the prostatic venous plexus in the pelvis.

— Lymphatic drainage areas of the penis include
   • the erectile bodies of the penis, which drain to internal iliac nodes;

A Inferior (ventral) view.

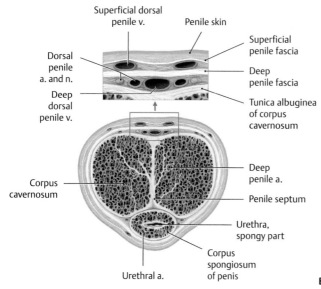

B Cross section through the body of the penis.

Fig. 12.6 Penis

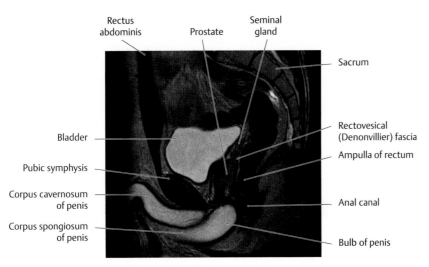

Fig. 12.7 MRI of the male pelvis
Sagittal section, left lateral view.

Labels: Rectus abdominis, Prostate, Seminal gland, Sacrum, Rectovesical (Denonvillier) fascia, Ampulla of rectum, Bladder, Pubic symphysis, Corpus cavernosum of penis, Corpus spongiosum of penis, Anal canal, Bulb of penis

- the glans penis, which drains to deep inguinal nodes; and
- the urethra, which drains to internal iliac and deep inguinal nodes.
— The glans of the penis is richly innervated by sensory fibers via the **dorsal penile nerve,** a branch of the pudendal nerve.

Sympathetic fibers from the hypogastric nerve plexus are also carried along this route.
— Parasympathetic fibers carried by the cavernous nerves derived from the prostatic plexus innervate the helicine arteries within the erectile tissue and are responsible for penile erection.

Bulbourethral Glands

The bulbourethral glands are paired mucus-secreting glands (see **Figs. 11.2** and **11.3**).
— They lie on either side of the urethra below the prostate, surrounded by the urethral sphincter.
— Their ducts open into the proximal part of the spongy urethra.
— They are active during sexual arousal.

Erection, Emission, and Ejaculation

The sexual responses of **erection, emission,** and **ejaculation** involve sympathetic, parasympathetic, and somatic (via the pudendal nerve) pathways.
— During erection
  • constriction of the helicine arteries, normally maintained by sympathetic innervation, is inhibited by parasympathetic stimulation. As the arteries relax, the cavernous spaces within the erectile bodies dilate and become engorged;
  • contractions of the bulbocavernosus and ischiocavernosus muscles, innervated by the pudendal nerve, impede venous outflow and maintain the erection.
— During emission
  • parasympathetic stimulation mediates the secretion of seminal fluid from the seminal glands, bulbourethral glands, and prostate gland, and

Fig. 12.8 Neurovasculature on the dorsum of the penis
Superior (dorsal) view. *Removed:* Skin.

Labels: External pudendal a. and v., Deep dorsal penile v., Dorsal penile a. and n., Tunica albuginea, Superficial dorsal penile vv., Deep penile fascia, Corona of glans, Glans of penis

- sympathetic stimulation mediates emission (the movement of seminal fluid through the ducts) by initiating peristalsis of the ductus deferens and seminal glands. This propels the seminal fluid into the prostatic urethra, where additional fluid is added as the prostate contracts.
- During ejaculation
  - sympathetic stimulation constricts the internal urethral sphincter, which prevents the seminal fluid from entering the bladder (retrograde ejaculation);
  - parasympathetic stimulation contracts the urethral muscles; and
  - the pudendal nerve contracts the bulbospongiosus muscle.

CLINICAL CORRELATION

RETROGRADE EJACULATION Relaxation of the detrusor muscle and contraction of the internal urethral sphincter in males are controlled by sympathetic fibers from the superior hypogastric plexus. Closure of the sphincter occurs during ejaculation, preventing the retrograde flow of semen into the bladder. Disruption of the sympathetic nerves can result in retrograde ejaculation. This can occur during the repair of an abdominal aortic aneurysm, for example, if the aneurysm involves the bifurcation of the aorta.

12.4   Female Urogenital Triangle

As in the male perineum, the female perineum contains erectile bodies, secretory glands, and their associated neurovasculature. In addition, it contains paired folds of skin that surround the urethral and vaginal orifices. These external genitalia are known collectively as the **vulva (Figs. 12.9, 12.10, 12.11).**

- **The mons pubis,** a superficial mound of fatty subcutaneous tissue that is continuous with the superficial fatty layer of the abdominal wall, lies anterior to the pubic symphysis and is continuous with the **labia majora.**

- **Labia majora,** bilateral folds of fatty subcutaneous tissue, flank the **pudendal cleft,** the opening between the labia. The labia join anteriorly at the **anterior commissure** and posteriorly at the **posterior commissure.** Pigmented skin and coarse pubic hair cover the labia's outer surface; the inner surface is smooth and hairless.
- **Labia minora,** bilateral folds of hairless skin within the pudendal cleft, flank the vestibule of the vagina.
- The **clitoris,** a highly sensitive erectile organ, is located at the anterior junction of the paired labia minora.
  - Paired erectile bodies, the **corpora cavernosa,** make up the crura, which join to form the **body** of the clitoris. The **prepuce** (hood) covers the body.
  - The **glans** at the tip of the clitoris is its most sensitive part.
- The **vestibule** of the vagina is a space surrounded by the two labia minora. It contains the urethral and vaginal orifices and the openings of the ducts of the greater vestibular and lesser vestibular glands.
- **Vestibular bulbs** are paired masses of erectile tissue that lie deep to the labia minora and are covered by the bulbospongiosus muscles.
- **Greater vestibular** (Bartholin's) **glands,** small glands that lie under the posterior end of the vestibular bulbs, help to lubricate the vestibule during sexual arousal.
- Small **lesser vestibular glands** lie on each side of the vestibule and secrete mucus to moisten the labia and vestibule.
- The external pudendal arteries supply the skin over the mons pubis and labia majora. Similar to those in the male, these superficial structures drain to the external pudendal veins.
- The internal pudendal arteries supply most of the external genitalia through branches that are similar to those in the male perineum **(Fig. 12.12A).**
  - The **perineal arteries** supply perineal muscles and labia minora.

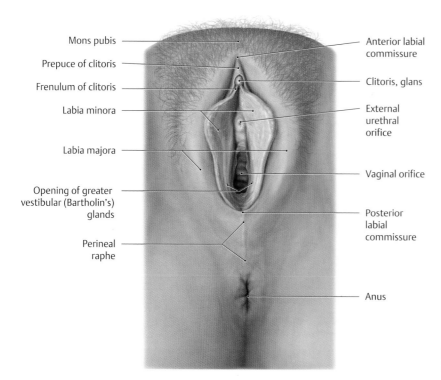

Mons pubis

Prepuce of clitoris

Frenulum of clitoris

Labia minora

Labia majora

Opening of greater vestibular (Bartholin's) glands

Perineal raphe

Anterior labial commissure

Clitoris, glans

External urethral orifice

Vaginal orifice

Posterior labial commissure

Anus

Fig. 12.9 Female external genitalia
Lithotomy position with labia minora separated.

Fig. 12.10 Vestibule and vestibular glands
Lithotomy position with labia separated.

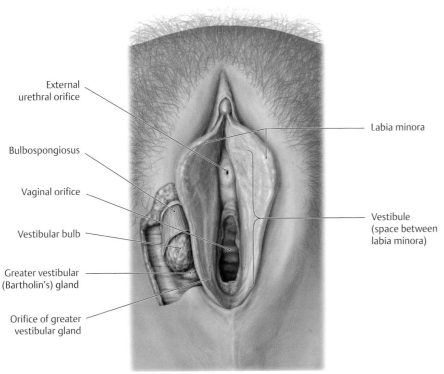

External
urethral orifice

Bulbospongiosus

Vaginal orifice

Vestibular bulb

Greater vestibular
(Bartholin's) gland

Orifice of greater
vestibular gland

Labia minora

Vestibule
(space between
labia minora)

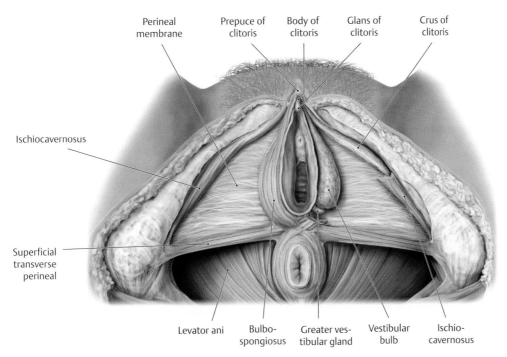

Perineal
membrane

Prepuce of
clitoris

Body of
clitoris

Glans of
clitoris

Crus of
clitoris

Ischiocavernosus

Superficial
transverse
perineal

Levator ani

Bulbo-
spongiosus

Greater ves-
tibular gland

Vestibular
bulb

Ischio-
cavernosus

Fig. 12.11 Erectile muscles and tissue of the female genitalia
Lithotomy position. *Removed:* Labia, skin, and perineal membrane. *Removed from leftside:* Ischiocavernosus and bulbospongiosus muscles; greater vestibular (Bartholin's) gland.

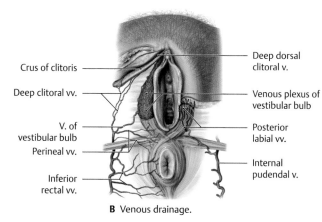

A Arterial supply.

Deep clitoral a.
A. of vestibular bulb
Posterior labial branches
Internal pudendal a.
Dorsal clitoral a.
Vestibular bulb
Superficial transverse perineal
Perineal a.
Inferior rectal a.

Crus of clitoris
Deep clitoral vv.
V. of vestibular bulb
Perineal vv.
Inferior rectal vv.
Deep dorsal clitoral v.
Venous plexus of vestibular bulb
Posterior labial vv.
Internal pudendal v.

B Venous drainage.

Fig. 12.12 Blood vessels of the female external genitalia
Inferior view.

- The **arteries of the vestibular bulb** supply the bulbs of the vestibule and greater vestibular glands.
- The **dorsal clitoral arteries** supply the glans of the clitoris.
- The **deep clitoral arteries** supply the corpora cavernosa and are responsible for engorgement during arousal.
— Tributaries of the internal pudendal veins drain most perineal structures and accompany the arteries. A single **deep dorsal clitoral vein** drains the venous plexuses of the erectile tissue and passes under the pubic symphysis to join the venous plexuses in the pelvis (**Fig. 12.12B**).
— Most lymph from the female perineum drains to superficial inguinal lymph nodes. Exceptions include
  - the clitoris, bulbs of the vestibule, and anterior labia, which drain to deep inguinal or internal iliac nodes; and
  - the urethra, which drains to sacral or internal iliac nodes.
— The right and left pudendal nerves are the primary nerves of the perineum (see **Fig. 10.22B**). They supply
  - **perineal nerves** to the vaginal orifice and superficial perineal muscles;
  - **dorsal clitoral nerves** to deep perineal muscles and sensation from the clitoris, especially the glans; and
  - **posterior labial nerves** to the posterior vulva.
— Similar to the innervation of the male scrotum, the anterior vulva receives sensory innervation (see **Fig. 10.22B**) from
  - the ilioinguinal nerves and genital branch of the genitofemoral nerves, which supply branches to the mons pubis and anterior labia; and
  - posterior femoral cutaneous nerves, which supply the posterolateral vulva.

— Sympathetic fibers to the perineum travel with the hypogastric nerve plexes; parasympathetic fibers travel with cavernous nerves of the uterovaginal plexus. Both innervate the erectile tissue of the clitoris and bulbs of the vestibule.

12.5   Anal Triangle

The anal triangle contains the anal canal and ischioanal fossae.

The Anal Canal

The **anal canal,** the terminal part of the gastrointestinal tract, controls fecal continence and the defecation response. It extends from the anorectal junction at the pelvic diaphragm to the **anus** (**Fig. 12.13**).
— The puborectalis muscle forms a sling around the anorectal junction, pulling it anteriorly and creating the **perineal flexure** (**Fig. 12.14**). From this angle the anal canal descends inferiorly and posteriorly between the anococcygeal ligament (levator plate) and the perineal body (see **Fig. 12.1**).
— Two sphincters surround the anal canal:
  1. The **internal anal sphincter** is a thickening of the circular muscular layer that surrounds the upper part of the anal canal.
     ○ It is an involuntary sphincter.
     ○ It remains contracted via sympathetic innervation except in response to distension of the rectal ampulla. Parasympathetic innervation relaxes the sphincter.
  2. The **external anal sphincter** is a broad band of muscle that extends anteriorly to merge with the perineal body, posteriorly to attach to the coccyx (through the anococcygeal ligament), and superiorly to merge with the puborectalis muscle of the pelvic floor (see also **Figs. 11.1, 12.1, 12.2**). Although it is described as having deep, superficial, and subcutaneous parts, they are functionally, and often anatomically, indistinct.
     ○ It is a voluntary sphincter.
     ○ The inferior rectal nerve, a branch of the pudendal nerve, innervates this sphincter.
— The inner surface of the anal canal is characterized by
  - **anal columns,** vertical ridges formed by underlying branches of the superior rectal vessels;
  - **anal valves** that connect the inferior edges of the anal columns; and
  - **anal sinuses,** recesses at the base of the anal columns that secrete mucus to facilitate defecation.
— **The dentate (pectinate) line** is an irregular ridge at the base of the anal columns.

CLINICAL CORRELATION

ANAL FISSURES Anal fissures are tears in the mucosa around the anus (usually in the posterior midline) that are caused by the passing of hard or large stools. Because they are below the pectinate line and innervated by the inferior rectal nerves, these lesions are painful. Most anal fissures heal spontaneously within a few weeks if care is taken to prevent constipation. Perianal abscesses that develop from the fissures can spread into the adjacent ischioanal fossae.

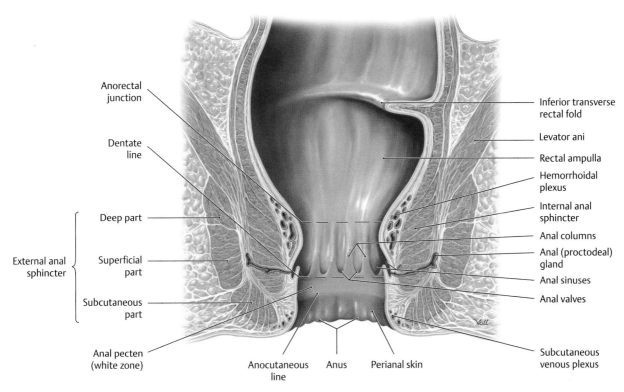

Anorectal junction

Dentate line

External anal sphincter
- Deep part
- Superficial part
- Subcutaneous part

Anal pecten (white zone)

Anocutaneous line

Anus

Perianal skin

Inferior transverse rectal fold

Levator ani

Rectal ampulla

Hemorrhoidal plexus

Internal anal sphincter

Anal columns

Anal (proctodeal) gland

Anal sinuses

Anal valves

Subcutaneous venous plexus

Fig. 12.13 Anal canal
Coronal section, anterior view.

- It divides the anal canal into a superior part derived from the endoderm of the embryonic hindgut and an inferior part derived from the embryonic ectoderm.
- It divides the anal canal in its blood supply, lymphatic drainage, and innervation.
— Below the dentate line, a smooth lining devoid of glands and hair, the **anal pecten,** extends down to the **anocutaneous line,** or intersphincteric groove.
— Below the anocutaneous line, the anal canal is lined by hair-bearing skin that is continuous with **perianal skin** that surrounds the anus.
— Above the dentate line the neurovasculature of the anal canal is similar to that of the distal gastrointestinal tract (see **Figs. 10.19** and **10.21**).

- It receives its blood supply from the superior rectal artery, a branch of the inferior mesenteric artery.
- The rectal venous plexus drains through the superior rectal vein into the portal venous system.
- Lymph drains to the internal iliac nodes.
- Visceral innervation is transmitted via rectal plexuses to the inferior hypogastric plexus.
  ◦ Sympathetic stimulation maintains the tone of the sphincter.
  ◦ Parasympathetic innervation relaxes the sphincter and stimulates peristalsis of the rectum.
  ◦ Visceral sensory fibers travel with pelvic splanchnic (parasympathetic) nerves and convey only sensation of stretching (no sensitivity to pain).
— Below the dentate line the neurovasculature of the anal canal is similar to that of the perineum (see **Figs. 10.15** and **10.16**).
- It receives its blood supply from the right and left **inferior rectal arteries,** branches of the internal iliac arteries.
- The rectal venous plexus drains into **inferior rectal veins,** which in turn drain to internal iliac veins of the venae caval system.
- Lymph drains to superficial inguinal nodes.
- Somatic innervation is transmitted via the **inferior rectal nerve,** a branch of the pudendal nerve.
  ◦ Somatic motor fibers stimulate contraction of the external anal sphincter.
  ◦ Somatic sensory fibers transmit pain, touch, and temperature.

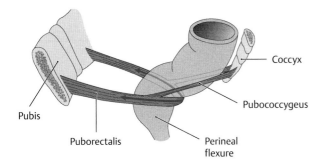

Coccyx

Pubococcygeus

Pubis

Puborectalis

Perineal flexure

Fig. 12.14 Closure of the rectum
Left lateral view.
The puborectalis acts as a muscular sling that kinks the anorectal junction. It functions in the maintenance of fecal continence.

Ischioanal Fossae and Pudendal Canal

— The ischioanal fossae are paired wedge-shaped spaces on either side of the anal canal bounded by the pelvic diaphragm superiorly and the skin of the anal region inferiorly (see **Fig. 11.24**).

- Fat and loose connective tissue, strengthened by strong fibrous bands, fill the fossae. These tissues support the anal canal but can be displaced readily when the anal canal distends with feces.
- The inferior rectal vessels and nerve, branches of the internal pudendal vessels and pudendal nerve, traverse the fossae.
- The ischioanal fossae extend anteriorly into the urogenital triangle superior to the perineal membrane.

— The pudendal canal is a passageway formed by the splitting of the fascia of the obturator internus muscle on the lateral wall of the ischioanal fossa.

- The internal pudendal artery and vein and the pudendal nerve enter the canal after exiting the lesser sciatic foramen and giving off inferior rectal branches.

Unit V   Clinical Imaging Basics of the Pelvis and Perineum

Radiography of the pelvis is used in the evaluation of trauma patients and for a quick first-line assessment of the hip joints. If greater detail of the soft tissues is required, magnetic resonance imaging (MRI) is the next step. For evaluation of pelvic contents in female patients, ultrasound provides superb images quickly and inexpensively and without exposing the gonads to radiation. Therefore, ultrasound is very useful in emergent situations (e.g., acute pelvic pain). MRI also shows excellent detail of the pelvis, but because it takes longer to acquire the images, it is less useful in emergencies (**Table 12.2**).

Standard radiographic views of the bony pelvis include an anteroposterior (AP) projection showing both hip joints (**Fig. 12.15**). In patients with pelvic fractures, different obliquities are often used to assess alignment. There are several approaches to imaging the contents of the pelvis. As in the abdomen, computed tomography (CT) is often used with oral or intravenous contrast to enhance the pelvic organs (**Fig. 12.16**), but in non-emergent conditions, MRI provides the best anatomic detail (**Fig. 12.17**). In comparison, ultrasound offers less detail, but because it is safer and faster, it is usually the first choice for imaging female pelvic organs (**Figs. 12.18** and **12.19**).

Table 12.2 **Suitability of Imaging Modalities for the Pelvis**

Modality	Clinical Uses
Radiographs (X-rays)	Used primarily to evaluate the pelvic bones
CT (computed tomography)	Provides excellent anatomic detail, but at the expense of radiation
MRI (magnetic resonance imaging)	Ideal for evaluation of the pelvic bones and surrounding muscles and soft tissues; also useful as an adjunct to ultrasound for the female pelvis
Ultrasound	The primary imaging modality for evaluation of the female pelvis, specifically the uterus and ovaries; in men, the mainstay of imaging of the scrotum and testicles

Fig. 12.15 Radiograph of the pelvis in an adult.
Anterior view.
Note that the rounded femoral heads sit uniformly in each acetabulum, and the sacroiliac joints and pubic symphysis are sharply seen. The lower part of the sacrum is partially obscured by gas and stool in the rectum (irregular dark and light gray shapes in the mid-pelvis). The iliac crests can be traced along their edges to the acetabulum and into the ischium and pubic symphysis. The edges of the bones should curve smoothly and be sharply defined.

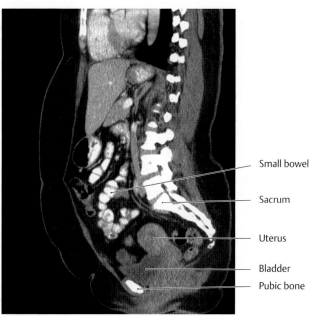

Fig. 12.16 CT of the female pelvis
Left lateral view.
This CT reconstruction, shown in the "soft tissue window," highlights the relationships of the pelvic organs. Oral contrast causes the bowel to appear white; intravenous contrast enhances the vascularized soft tissues (light gray). The urine filled bladder has a water density of dark gray. The uterus is enhanced by the intravenous contrast and is easily seen against the bladder anteriorly and fat superiorly. The endometrium is barely seen within the uterus. It is difficult to precisely define the plane between the uterus and the adjacent rectum.

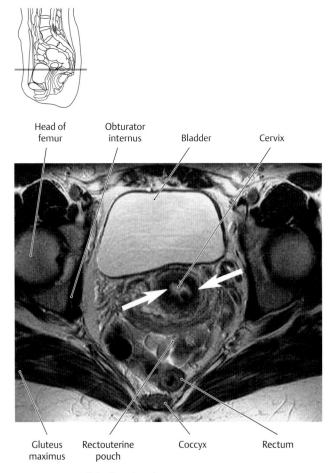

Head of femur   Obturator internus   Bladder   Cervix

Gluteus maximus   Rectouterine pouch   Coccyx   Rectum

Fig. 12.17 MRI of the female pelvis
Transverse section through the level of the cervix.
In this MRI sequence, fluid is white, muscle is black, and other soft tissues are gray. Soft tissue detail seen on MRI is superior to that seen on CT and ultrasound. Note the dark *(black)* cervical stroma *(arrows)* that surrounds the white fluid in the cervical canal. Because MRI is very sensitive in differentiating tissue types, it is easy to distinguish the pelvic organs from each other and from the adjacent bowel. The bright fat planes between structures provide good contrast.

A Midsagittal (longitudinal) section.

B Transverse section.

Fig. 12.18 Transabdominal ultrasound of the uterus and ovaries
With transabdominal imaging of the pelvis, the ultrasound probe is placed on the lower abdominal wall anterior to the bladder. A full bladder provides an acoustic "window" to better visualize the uterus and related structures. (Patients are required to drink plenty of fluid prior to the exam.) The urine in the bladder is anechoic *(black)*. The muscular and vascular structure of the uterus and follicular and vascular structure of the ovaries make these structures hypoechoic *(dark gray)*. The ovaries should appear relatively symmetric in size and shape.
1, urine filled bladder; *2,* uterus; *3,* cervix; *4,* vagina; *5,* rectum.

Fig. 12.19 Transvaginal ultrasound of the right ovary
An empty bladder (patient is asked to urinate immediately before the exam) positions the uterus and associated structures for optimal visualization. The tip of the ultrasound probe is positioned directly against the cervix and pointed toward the side of interest until the ovary is found. The close proximity of the tip of the ultrasound probe to the pelvic structures provides significantly improved image detail over transabdominal images. This patient has enlarged ovaries due to polycystic ovarian syndrome. Note the detail of the numerous small ovarian follicles *(black, since they are fluid filled).*

Unit V   Review Questions: Pelvis and Perineum

1. During a practice match, a heavyweight prizefighter endured an illegal hit to the left flank. Following the match, a focused assessment with sonography for trauma (FAST) exam revealed that blood from a renal laceration had tracked inferiorly and accumulated in the groove between the psoas major and iliacus muscles. What nerve would you expect to be irritated by blood in this location?
   A. Sciatic
   B. Femoral
   C. Obturator
   D. Superior gluteal
   E. Lateral femoral cutaneous

2. Which one of the following statements best describes the muscles of the pelvis?
   A. The obturator internus muscle leaves the pelvis through the greater sciatic foramen.
   B. The levator ani muscle is composed of the pubococcygeus, puborectalis, and iliococcygeus.
   C. The pelvic diaphragm is a sling of muscle that separates the true pelvis from the false pelvis.
   D. The piriformis muscle forms the lateral wall of the pelvis.
   E. The coccygeus muscle attaches to the sacrotuberous ligament.

3. Typically, the posterior division of the internal iliac artery supplies
   A. structures of the perineum
   B. muscles of the medial thigh
   C. meninges of the sacral spinal roots
   D. uterus and uterine tubes
   E. prostate

4. The components of the pelvic splanchnic nerves are most similar to the components of the
   A. lumbar splanchnic nerves
   B. sacral splanchnic nerves
   C. pudendal nerve
   D. vagus nerve
   E. hypogastric nerves

5. Carcinoma of the prostate can metastasize to bone and the brain through its connections with the vertebral venous plexus. Which other structures communicate with this venous plexus?
   A. Breast
   B. Spinal cord
   C. Intercostal muscles
   D. Esophagus
   E. All of the above

6. Although branches of the uterine artery anastomose extensively throughout the pelvis, the main stem of the vessel travels within the
   A. proper ovarian ligament
   B. cardinal ligament
   C. uterosacral ligament
   D. ovarian suspensory ligament
   E. round ligament

7. Which of the following statements accurately describes the relations of the ureter?
   A. It is crossed anteriorly by the gonadal vessels on the posterior abdominal wall.
   B. It crosses the brim of the pelvis at the bifurcation of the common iliac artery.
   C. In females it passes under the uterine artery ~ 2 cm lateral to the cervix.
   D. It enters the bladder at the posterolateral aspect of the trigone.
   E. All of the above

8. During a routine physical exam on a male patient, you test the integrity of the external anal sphincter. What spinal cord segments are involved in this?
   A. T12–L1
   B. L2–L4
   C. L4–L5
   D. S1–S2
   E. S2–S4

9. The superficial perineal fascia is continuous with the
   A. perineal membrane
   B. dartos fascia
   C. deep penile fascia
   D. tunica albuginea of the penis
   E. endopelvic fascia

10. The boundary of the pelvic inlet
    A. provides the attachment site for the pelvic diaphragm
    B. includes the iliac crests
    C. includes the ramus of the ischium
    D. is crossed by the ovarian and testicular arteries
    E. separates the cavity of the true pelvis from the abdominal cavity

11. Several years after delivering a twin boys, a woman experienced mild uterine prolapse and urinary incontinence. Her gynecologist was able to confirm that the angle of her anococcygeal ligament had changed, suggesting a laxity in her pelvic floor muscles. Which muscles insert on the anococcygeal ligament?
    A. Coccygeus
    B. Iliococcygeus
    C. Piriformis
    D. Deep transverse perineal
    E. Obturator internus

12. Tumors that metastasize via the bloodstream often form metastases in the first capillary bed that the cells reach after they enter the bloodstream. Based on their venous drainage, tumors in which of the following locations are likely to reach the lung before they reach the liver?
    A. Ascending colon
    B. Sigmoid colon
    C. Pancreas
    D. Superior (proximal) rectum
    E. Inferior (distal) rectum

13. Which one of the following structures passes through the genital hiatus?
A. Ductus deferens
B. Cavernous nerves
C. Round ligament
D. Obturator nerve
E. External iliac artery

14. A 44-year-old woman undergoes a total hysterectomy for painful fibroids. The ovaries will not be removed during the procedure. Which of the following ligaments must be preserved?
A. Suspensory ligament
B. Ovarian ligament
C. Uterosacral ligament
D. Transverse cervical ligament
E. Round ligament

15. Which of the following statements best describes the uterine cervix?
A. In a normally anteflexed uterus, the cervix is tilted posteriorly.
B. Vaginal fornices surround its supravaginal part.
C. It is the attachment site for the round ligament.
D. It makes up the inferior third of the uterus.
E. It communicates with the uterine cavity through the external os.

16. A 53-year-old man had an aortic aneurysm that extended through his aortic bifurcation into his common iliac arteries. During the open repair, the surgeon opened the vessels longitudinally and fixed a synthetic graft to the walls of the vessels above and below the aneurysm. Following surgery, the man experienced retrograde ejaculation because of damage to nerves that innervated his internal urethral sphincter. Which nerves were damaged?
A. Sympathetic nerves of the superior hypogastric plexus
B. Parasympathetic nerves of the superior hypogastric plexus
C. Somatic nerves of the sacral plexus
D. Pelvic splanchnic nerves
E. Sympathetic trunk

17. You are treating a 34-year-old woman for hemorrhoids. Although she does not complain of pain, the hemorrhoids protrude into her anal canal and are becoming ulcerated. There is no evidence of portal hypertension, but blood from the ulcers is bright red. Based on her brief history, what can you surmise about her condition?
A. The prolapsed tissue contains the dilated veins of the external rectal plexus.
B. The hemorrhoids originate from below the dentate line.
C. The dilated veins in the hemorrhoids drain to the inferior rectal veins.
D. The dilated veins communicate with the rectal arteries to form an arteriovenous hemorrhoidal plexus.
E. All of the above

18. During a robotic prostatectomy on a 41-year-old man, the cavernous nerves were inadvertently damaged. What symptoms would you expect in this patient?

A. Loss of tone in his external anal sphincter
B. Urinary incontinence
C. Inability to ejaculate
D. Inability to form an erection
E. Loss of sensation at the tip of the penis

19. Structures that pass through the greater sciatic foramen include the
A. obturator internus
B. coccygeus
C. iliopsoas
D. piriformis
E. obturator nerve

20. The tendinous arch of the pelvic fascia
A. is a condensation of endopelvic fascia
B. includes the lateral ligaments of the rectum
C. supports the pelvic viscera
D. provides an attachment site for the pelvic diaphragm
E. All of the above

21. Structures that drain (directly or indirectly) into the deep inguinal lymph nodes include the
A. glans of the penis
B. perianal skin
C. supralateral part of the uterus via the round ligament
D. scrotum
E. All of the above

22. During the national championships an Olympic gymnast fell backward off the balance beam, fracturing the tip of her coccyx and subluxing (dislocating) her sacroiliac joint. The team physician was concerned about damage to her sacral plexus and its branches that exit the pelvis. Nerves of the sacral plexus pass through the
A. posterior sacral foramina
B. obturator canal
C. greater sciatic foramen
D. superficial inguinal ring
E. deep inguinal ring

23. A young, pregnant woman in her third trimester was alarmed when she experienced a sharp pain in the anterior part of her labia majora when she stood up. Her obstetrician assured her that this was a common problem in late pregnancy and was most likely caused by
A. stretching of the round ligament
B. tightening of the inguinal ligament
C. pressure on the obturator nerve
D. irritation of the perineal branch of the pudendal nerve
E. stretching of the iliohypogastric nerve

24. A vascular surgeon is repairing an aneurysm of the aortic bifurcation that extends along the right common iliac artery to its division into internal iliac and external iliac branches. What structure does the surgeon encounter that is at risk as it crosses over the pelvic brim at this distal end of the aneurysm?
A. Ureter
B. Testicular artery
C. Lumbosacral trunk
D. Sciatic nerve
E. Ductus deferens

25. Similar to other sections of the large intestine, the rectum is characterized by
  A. teniae coli
  B. haustra
  C. a mesentery
  D. epiploic appendices
  E. None of the above

26. Which of the following are found within the superficial perineal space?
  A. Bulbourethral glands
  B. External urethral sphincter
  C. Bulbospongiosus muscle
  D. Anterior extension of ischioanal fat pad
  E. Inferior rectal nerve

Answers and Explanations

1. **B.** The femoral nerve runs in the groove between the psoas and iliacus muscles (Sections 10.1 and 15.4).
  A. The blood accumulated above the pelvic brim in a muscular pocket of the false pelvis. The sciatic nerve does not pass through the false pelvis.
  C. The obturator nerve passes medial to the psoas muscle and not in the groove between the psoas and iliacus muscles.
  D. The superior gluteal nerve is a branch of the sacral plexus and does not pass through the false pelvis where the blood accumulated.
  E. The lateral femoral cutaneous nerve crosses the iliacus muscle in the iliac fossa and passes under the inguinal ligament close to the anterior superior iliac spine to innervate the skin of the lateral thigh.

2. **B.** The levator ani muscle is composed of the pubococcygeus, puborectalis, and iliococcygeus muscles (Section 10.3).
  A. The obturator internus muscle covers the sidewall of the pelvis and perineum. Its tendon passes from the perineum to the gluteal region through the lesser sciatic foramen.
  C. The pelvic diaphragm separates the true pelvis from the perineum, which lies below it.
  D. The piriformis muscle forms the posterior muscular wall of the pelvis.
  E. The coccygeus muscle attaches to the sacrospinous ligament along its entire length.

3. **C.** The posterior division supplies parietal branches to the posterior abdominal wall, some gluteal muscles, and the meninges of the sacral spinal roots (Section 10.6).
  A. The internal pudendal artery, a branch of the anterior division of the internal iliac artery, supplies most structures of the perineum.
  B. The obturator artery, a branch of the anterior division of the internal iliac artery, supplies muscles of the medial thigh.
  D. The uterine artery, a branch of the anterior division of the internal iliac artery, supplies the uterus and uterine tubes.
  E. The prostatic arteries, usually branches of the inferior vesical arteries, are derived from the anterior division of the internal iliac artery.

4. **D.** The pelvic splanchnic nerves represent the sacral component of the parasympathetic system; the vagus nerve represents the cranial component of the parasympathetic system (Section 10.6).
  A. Lumbar splanchnic nerves arise from the lumbar sympathetic trunk and carry postganglionic sympathetic fibers.
  B. Sacral splanchnic nerves arise from the sacral sympathetic trunk and carry postganglionic sympathetic fibers.
  C. The pudendal nerve arises from the sacral plexus and carries somatic sensory and motor fibers.
  E. Hypogastric nerves derive from the superior hypogastric plexus carrying postganglionic sympathetic fibers to the pelvic plexus.

5. **E.** The vertebral venous system is a tributary of the azygos system. The breast, intercostal muscles, and esophagus drain via intercostal veins to the azygos system, and the spinal cord drains directly into the vertebral venous plexus (Section 11.1 and Unit III, Thorax).
  A. Blood from the breast drains to intercostal veins and the azygos system, which communicates with the vertebral venous plexus. B through D are also correct (E).
  B. The veins of the spinal cord drain to the vertebral venous plexus. A, C, and D are also correct (E).
  C. The intercostal veins that drain intercostal muscles terminate in the azygos system, which also receives the vertebral venous plexus. A, B, and D are also correct (E).
  D. Veins of the lower esophagus drain to the portal system, but in the thorax esophageal veins drain to the azygos system, which also receives the vertebral venous plexus. A through C are also correct (E).

6. **B.** The uterine artery and vein travel within the cardinal ligament at the base of the broad ligament (Section 11.2).
  A. The proper ovarian ligament connects the ovary to the uterus and does not contain any major vessels.
  C. The uterosacral ligament is a thickening of endopelvic fascia that connects the cervix of the uterus to the sacrum. It does not contain any major vessels.
  D. The ovarian suspensory ligament is a fold of peritoneum that contains the ovarian vessels as they cross over the pelvic brim.
  E. The round ligament extends from the uterus through the inguinal canal to the labia majora. Although it is accompanied by small vessels, it does not contain any major arteries.

7. **E.** All are correct (Section 11.3).
  A. The gonadal vessels cross anterior to the ureter as it descends along the posterior abdominal wall. B through D are also correct (E).
  B. The bifurcation of the common iliac artery is a useful landmark for locating the ureter as it crosses the pelvic brim. A, C, and D are also correct (E).
  C. The ureter passes under the uterine artery lateral to the uterine cervix and therefore is at risk of injury during a hysterectomy. A, B, and D are also correct (E).
  D. The ureteral openings posterolaterally and the urethral opening in the anterior midline define the apexes of the trigone. A through C are also correct (E).

8. **E.** The pudendal nerve (S2–S4) provides motor innervation to the external sphincter (Sections 11.4 and 10.6).
   A. T12–L1 nerve roots contribute to the subcostal, iliohypogastric, and ilioinguinal nerves, which innervate muscles of the anterior abdominal wall.
   B. The L2–L4 nerve roots form the femoral and obturator nerves, which innervate muscles of the anterior and medial thigh.
   C. Nerves from L4–L5 spinal cord segments form the lumbosacral trunk, which joins the sacral plexus to innervate muscles of the lower limb.
   D. S1–S2 nerve roots contribute to the sacral plexus, which innervates muscles of the lower limb.

9. **B.** The superficial perineal fascia is continuous with the dartos fascia that lines the scrotum and with the membranous layer (Scarpa's fascia) of the superficial fascia of the abdominal wall (Section 12.1).
   A. The perineal membrane is a fibrous sheet that forms the roof of the superficial perineal space.
   C. Deep penile fascia is a fibrous layer that binds the three erectile bodies of the penis.
   D. Each of the three erectile bodies of the penis is surrounded by the dense, fibrous tunica albuginea.
   E. Endopelvic fascia is the loose connective tissue matrix that fills the subperitoneal spaces of the pelvis.

10. **E.** The pelvic inlet separates the true pelvis from the false pelvis. The cavity of the false pelvis is the lower part of the abdominal cavity and contains abdominal viscera (Section 10.1).
   A. The pelvic diaphragm attaches to the superior pubic ramus, tendinous arch of the levator ani, and sacrospinous ligament.
   B. The iliac crests form the upper boundary of the false pelvis. The pelvic inlet forms its lower boundary.
   C. The ramus of the ischium forms part of the pelvic outlet but not the pelvic inlet.
   D. The ovarian arteries cross the pelvic inlet, but the testicular arteries pass along the brim of the pelvis (pelvic inlet) to the deep inguinal ring, where they enter the inguinal canal as part of the spermatic cord.

11. **B.** The anococcygeal ligament (also known as the levator plate) is a midline raphe between the anus and coccyx that serves as the insertion for the pubococcygeus and iliococcygeus muscles (Section 10.3).
   A. The coccygeus inserts on the ischial spine.
   C. The piriformis inserts on the greater trochanter of the femur.
   D. Deep transverse perineal muscles insert on the vagina (or prostate) and perineal body.
   E. The obturator internus inserts on the greater trochanter of the femur.

12. **E.** The inferior rectal veins drain through the caval system (via the internal iliac vein and inferior vena cava) back to the heart and pulmonary circulation. All other choices are tributaries of the portal system, which drains through the liver before returning to the heart (Sections 8.2 and 11.4).
   A. Veins of the ascending colon are tributaries of the portal system. Therefore, blood passes through the liver before returning to the heart and pulmonary circulation.
   B. Veins of the sigmoid colon, and all parts of the gastrointestinal tract, are tributaries of the portal system.

Therefore, blood passes through the liver before returning to the heart and pulmonary circulation.
   C. Veins of the pancreas are tributaries of the portal system. Therefore, blood from the pancreas drains through the liver before returning to the heart and pulmonary circulation.
   D. The superior rectal vein that drains the superior rectum is a tributary of the portal system. Therefore, this blood passes through the liver before returning to the heart and pulmonary circulation.

13. **B.** The cavernous nerves carry parasympathetic innervation from the pelvic plexus to the perineum by passing through the genital hiatus (Section 10.6).
   A. The ductus deferens passes through the deep inguinal ring and inguinal canal of the male.
   C. The round ligament traverses the female inguinal canal and terminates in the labia majora.
   D. The obturator nerve passes through the obturator canal into the medial thigh.
   E. The external iliac artery passes below the inguinal ligament into the anterior thigh.

14. **A.** The suspensory ligament contains the ovarian vessels and is removed only during the removal of the ovary (Section 11.2).
   B. The ovarian ligament attaches the ovary to the uterus and must be ligated to extract the uterus.
   C. The uterosacral ligament connects the cervix to the sacrum.
   D. The transverse cervical ligament contains the uterine arteries, which are ligated during a hysterectomy.
   E. The round ligament passes through the inguinal canal and connects the uterus to the labia majora.

15. **D.** The uterus comprises a body that forms the superior two thirds and a cervix that forms the inferior one third (Section 11.2).
   A. In an anteflexed uterus, the cervix is tilted anteriorly.
   B. The vaginal part of the cervix is surrounded by the vaginal fornices.
   C. The round ligaments arise from the upper part of the uterus.
   E. The cervix communicates with the body of the uterus through the internal os.

16. **A.** The superior hypogastric plexus, a sympathetic nerve plexus, drapes over the aortic bifurcation as it enters the pelvis. It is frequently cut during surgery for the repair of an aneurysm at the location. The sympathetic nerves stimulate closure of the internal urethral sphincter during ejaculation, preventing the retrograde flow of seminal fluid into the bladder. Damage to these nerves can result in retrograde ejaculation (Sections 10.6 and 12.3).
   B. The superior hypogastric plexus is a sympathetic nerve plexus derived from the intermesenteric plexus and lumbar splanchnic nerves.
   C. Somatic nerves do not stimulate visceral responses such as closure of the sphincter.
   D. Pelvic splanchnic nerves do not innervate the internal urethral sphincter.
   E. The paired sympathetic trunks run along the vertebral bodies on either side and would not be damaged in this procedure.

17.   **D.** The submucosal venous plexus of the anorectal region communicates with branches of the rectal arteries in an arteriovenous anastomosis, creating a thickened vascular tissue known as the hemorrhoidal plexus. As a result of these anastomoses, bleeding from the internal rectal plexus appears bright red (Section 11.4).
  A. Prolapsed internal hemorrhoids contain the dilated veins of the internal rectal plexus and are painless. External hemorrhoids, containing the external rectal plexus, are covered by skin and sensitive to pain.
  B. External hemorrhoids that occur below the dentate line are somatically innervated and therefore very painful, but internal hemorrhoids are viscerally innervated and painless.
  C. Veins of painless internal hemorrhoids lie above the dentate line and therefore drain to the superior rectal vein, a tributary of the portal system.
  E. A, B, and C are incorrect.

18.   **D.** The cavernous nerves carry parasympathetic nerves that are responsible for engorgement of the erectile tissue of the penis (Sections 10.6 and 12.3).
  A. The external anal sphincter is innervated by the pudendal nerve, a branch of the sacral plexus.
  B. The external urethral sphincter that regulates urinary continence is innervated by the pudendal nerve, a branch of the sacral plexus.
  C. Ejaculation is a sympathetically mediated response. The cavernous nerves carry parasympathetic nerves from the inferior hypogastric plexus.
  E. The pudendal nerve carries sensation from perineal structures such as the tip of the penis.

19.   **D.** The piriformis passes through the greater sciatic foramen to insert on the trochanter of the femur (Section 10.3).
  A. The tendon of the obturator internus muscle passes through the lesser sciatic foramen from the perineum to the gluteal region.
  B. The coccygeus muscle lies along the sacrospinous ligament and forms the lower border of the greater sciatic foramen.
  C. The iliopsoas muscle passes under the inguinal ligament into the thigh.
  E. The obturator nerve passes along the sidewall of the pelvis and through the obturator canal into the thigh.

20.   **C.** The tendinous arch of the pelvic fascia is a thickening of the membranous fascia on the floor of the pelvis where visceral and parietal fascial layers meet. It provides support for pelvic viscera (Section 10.4).
  A. The tendinous arch of the pelvic fascia is a thickening of the membranous fascia, which lines the pelvic walls and viscera. Endopelvic fascia is a loose connective tissue layer that fills the subperitoneal spaces.
  B. The lateral ligaments of the rectum, like the lateral ligaments of the bladder, are supporting columns of endopelvic fascia that connect the viscera to the pelvic walls.
  D. The tendinous arch of the levator ani, a condensation of the fascia over the obturator internus muscle, is the attachment site for the levator ani part of the pelvic diaphragm.
  E. A, B, and D are incorrect.

21.   **E.** The superficial and deep inguinal nodes drain most structures of the perineum, including the glans of the penis, perianal skin, and scrotum. The supralateral parts of the uterus drain along the round ligaments (which terminate in the labia majora) to superficial inguinal nodes. These nodes drain to the deep inguinal nodes (Section 10.6).
  A. Lymph from the glans of the penis drains to deep inguinal nodes. B through D are also correct (E).
  B. Lymph from perianal skin, like all skin of the perineum, drains to superficial inguinal nodes, which drain to deep inguinal nodes. A, C, and D are also correct (E).
  C. Lymph from the supralateral parts of the uterus drain along the round ligaments (which terminate in the labia majora) to superficial inguinal nodes. These nodes drain to the deep inguinal nodes. A, B, and D are also correct (E).
  D. Lymph from the scrotum drains to superficial inguinal nodes, which drain to deep inguinal nodes. A through C are also correct (E).

22.   **C.** Most nerves of the sacral plexus pass through the greater sciatic foramen to innervate muscles of the gluteal region and lower limb.
  A. Only posterior rami of sacral spinal nerves pass through the posterior sacral foramina. The sacral plexus is formed by anterior rami of sacral spinal nerves.
  B. The obturator nerve, which passes through the obturator canal, is a branch of the lumbar plexus.
  D. The ilioinguinal and genitofemoral nerves, which pass through the superficial inguinal ring, are branches of the lumbar plexus.
  E. The genitofemoral nerve, a branch of the lumbar plexus, passes through the deep inguinal ring.

23.   **A.** The round ligament originates on the superior aspect of the anterolateral uterus and inserts in the labia majora. As the uterus enlarges and stretches the ligament, pain is felt in the labia (Section 11.2).
  B. During late pregnancy pelvic ligaments are more relaxed in preparation for the passage of the child through the birth canal.
  C. Pressure on the obturator nerve would be felt on the medial thigh.
  D. The anterior part of the labia majora is innervated by the labial branches of the genitofemoral nerve, not the pudendal nerve.
  E. The iliohypogastric nerve innervates the skin above the pubic crest and does not extend inferiorly to the labia.

24.   **A.** The ureter crosses the pelvic brim at the bifurcation of the common iliac artery into its internal iliac and external iliac branches (Section 11.3).
  B. The testicular artery does not cross the pelvic brim but enters the deep inguinal ring.
  C. The lumbosacral trunk crosses the pelvic brim posterior to the common iliac vessels and anterior to the sacroiliac joint. It enters the pelvis to join the sacral plexus.
  D. The sciatic nerve passes through the greater sciatic foramen and does not cross the pelvic brim.
  E. The ductus deferens courses around the inferior epigastric vessels and over the distal end of the external iliac vessels to descend into the pelvis.

25. **E.** The rectum is devoid of teniae coli, haustra, a mesentery, and epiploic appendices (Section 11.4).

   A. The teniae coli of the large intestine converge to form a uniform layer surrounding the rectum.

   B. The haustra of the large intestine disappear at the rectosigmoid junction.

   C. The rectum has no mesentery. The upper rectum is covered anteriorly by peritoneum, but the lower rectum lies in the subperitoneal space.

   D. Epiploic appendices are not present in the rectum.

26. **C.** The bulbospongiosus muscle is found within the superficial perineal space (Section 12.1).

   A. The bulbourethral glands are found in the deep perineal space.

   B. The external urethral sphincter is located in the deep perineal space.

   D. The anterior extensions of the ischioanal fat pads are found in the deep perineal space.

   E. The inferior rectal nerve is found in the anal triangle, not the deep perineal or the superficial perineal spaces of the urogenital triangle.

Unit VI Upper Limb

13 Overview of the Upper Limb

The upper limb is designed for mobility and dexterity. Actions at the shoulder and elbow joints that allow positioning of the limb complement fine movements of the hands and fingers. Some stability is sacrificed for this extensive mobility, particularly in the shoulder, which makes the upper limb vulnerable to injury.

13.1 General Features

— In the anatomic position, the upper limbs hang vertically with the elbow joint pointing posteriorly and the palm of the hand facing anteriorly.
— The major regions of the upper limb **(Fig. 13.1)** are
  • the **shoulder region,** which includes the **pectoral, scapular, deltoid,** and **lateral cervical regions** and overlies the **pectoral (shoulder) girdle;**
  • the **axilla (axillary region),** the armpit;
  • the **arm (brachial region),** between the shoulder and elbow;
  • the **cubital region,** at the elbow;
  • the **forearm (antebrachial region),** between the elbow and wrist;
  • the **carpal region,** at the wrist; and
  • the **hand,** which has palmar and dorsal surfaces.
— Movements at joints of the upper limb include
  • **flexion,** bending the joint;
  • **extension,** straightening the joint;
  • **abduction,** movement away from a central axis;

- **adduction,** movement toward a central axis;
- **external (lateral) rotation,** outward rotation around a longitudinal axis;
- **internal (medial) rotation,** inward rotation around a longitudinal axis;
- **circumduction,** circular motion around the point of articulation;
- **supination,** turning the palm up;
- **pronation,** turning the palm down;
- **radial** or **ulnar deviation,** angling the wrist toward the radius or ulnar side (also abduction or adduction of the wrist); and
- **opposition,** movement of the thumb or 5th digit to oppose the other fingers.
— Muscles of the upper limb are categorized as
  • **intrinsic muscles,** whose origin and insertion are near the joint (e.g., intrinsic muscles of the hand originate and insert on bones of the wrist and hand), and
  • **extrinsic muscles,** whose origin is distant from the area of movement but insert near the joint via a long tendon (e.g., forearm muscles that flex the fingers are extrinsic muscles of the hand).
    ∘ The tendons of extrinsic muscles are often referred to as **long flexor** (or **extensor**) **tendons.**
    ∘ **Synovial tendon sheaths,** which surround tendons of extrinsic muscles at the wrist and fingers, provide a lubricated surface that facilitates movement of these tendons across the joint.

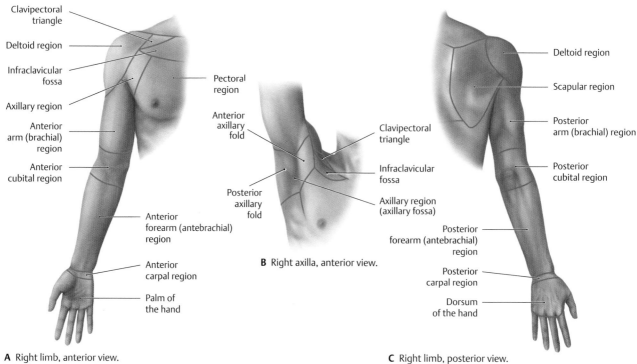

A Right limb, anterior view.

B Right axilla, anterior view.

C Right limb, posterior view.

Fig. 13.1 Regions of the upper limb

13.2 Bones of the Upper Limb

Bones of the upper limb include the clavicle and scapula that make up the pectoral girdle, the humerus of the arm, the radius and ulna of the forearm, the carpal bones of the wrist, and the meta-carpal bones and phalanges of the hand (**Fig. 13.2**).

— The **clavicle** is an S-shaped bone that forms the anterior part of the pectoral girdle (**Fig. 13.3**).

• It articulates with the clavicular notch of the manubrium medially and the acromion of the scapula laterally.

• It is palpable along its entire length.

CLINICAL CORRELATION

CLAVICULAR FRACTURES Fractures of the clavicle are common, particularly in children. A midclavicular fracture may be displaced by the upward pull of the proximal segment by the sternocleido-mastoid muscle and the downward pull of the distal fragment by the weight of the upper limb. Distal clavicular fractures may disrupt the acromioclavicular joint or the coracoclavicular ligaments.

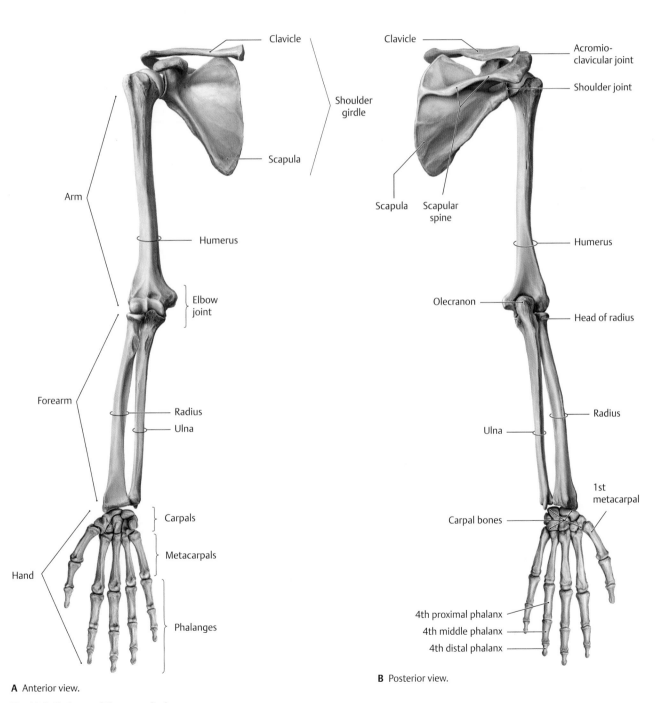

A Anterior view.

B Posterior view.

Fig. 13.2 Skeleton of the upper limb
Right limb. The upper limb is subdivided into three regions: arm, forearm, and hand. The pectoral (shoulder) girdle (clavicle and scapula) joins the upper limb to the thorax at the sternoclavicular joint.

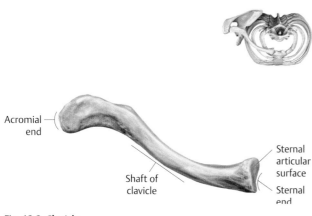

— The **scapula** is a flat triangular bone that forms the posterior part of the pectoral girdle (**Figs. 13.4** and **13.5**).
  • It overlies the 2nd to 7th ribs on the posterior thoracic wall.
  • It has medial, lateral, and superior borders and a superior and inferior angle.
  • Laterally, a shallow depression, the **glenoid cavity,** articulates with the humerus.
  • A narrow **neck** separates the glenoid cavity from the large body of the scapula.
  • A **subscapular fossa** lies on the anterior surface against the rib cage.
  • The **spine** of the scapula on the posterior surface separates the **supraspinous** and **infraspinous fossae.** Laterally, the spine expands to form the **acromion.**
  • **A coracoid process** extends anteriorly and superiorly over the glenoid cavity.

Fig. 13.3 Clavicle
Right clavicle.
Superior view

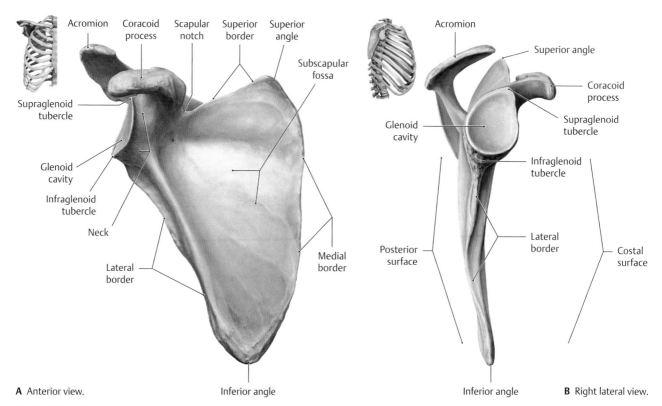

A Anterior view.

Fig. 13.4 Scapula
Right scapula.

B Right lateral view.

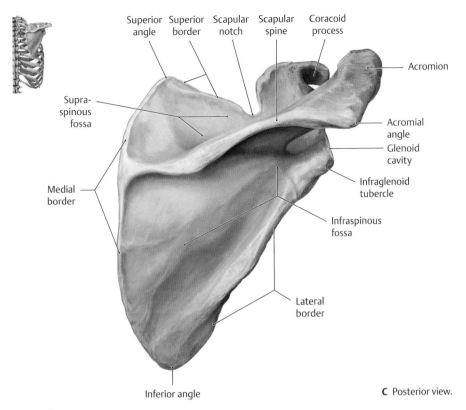

Fig. 13.4 *(continued)* **Scapula**

C Posterior view.

— The **humerus** is the long bone of the arm (**Fig. 13.6**).
  • Proximally, the **head** articulates with the glenoid cavity of the scapula.
  • Anteriorly, an **intertubercular groove** separates the **greater** and **lesser tubercles.**
  • **An anatomic neck** separates the head from the greater and lesser tubercles. The **surgical neck** is the narrow part of the shaft immediately distal to the head and tubercles.

CLINICAL CORRELATION

HUMERAL FRACTURES Fractures of the humerus are very common and are often associated with injury to blood vessels and nerves. A proximal fracture at the anatomic neck can damage the posterior circumflex artery and axillary nerve, at the midshaft the radial nerve may be injured in the radial groove, and distally the median and ulnar nerves are vulnerable in supracondylar fractures.

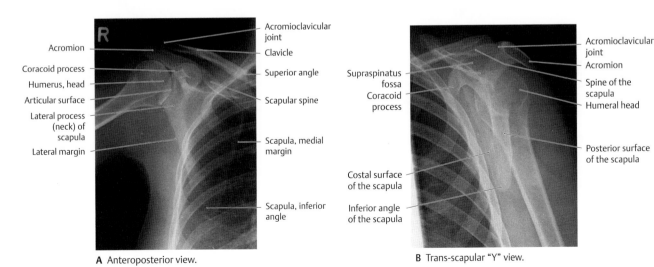

A Anteroposterior view.

B Trans-scapular "Y" view.

Fig. 13.5 **Radiograph of the scapula**

Fig. 13.6 Humerus

Right humerus. The head of the humerus articulates with the scapula at the glenohumeral joint. The capitulum and trochlea of the humerus articulate with the radius and ulna, respectively, at the elbow (cubital) joint.

- A **deltoid tuberosity** on the midshaft is a site for attachment of the deltoid muscle.
- A **radial groove** runs obliquely around the posterior and lateral surfaces.
- Distally, the humerus articulates with the radius at the **capitulum** and with the ulna at the **trochlea.**
- A large **medial epicondyle** and smaller **lateral epicondyle** are attachment sites for muscles.
- An **ulnar groove** separates the medial epicondyle and trochlea.

— The **ulna** is the medial bone of the forearm (**Fig. 13.7**).
- A C-shaped **trochlear notch,** formed by the **olecranon** posteriorly and the **coronoid process** anteriorly, articulates with the trochlea of the humerus.
- The ulna articulates with the radius at the **radial notch.**
- **An interosseous membrane** joins the shafts of the radius and ulna.
- An **ulnar styloid process** projects from its distal end.

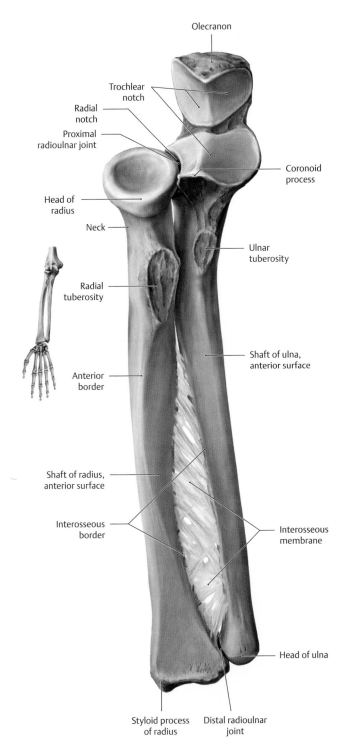

Olecranon

Trochlear notch

Radial notch

Proximal radioulnar joint

Head of radius

Neck

Radial tuberosity

Anterior border

Shaft of radius, anterior surface

Interosseous border

Coronoid process

Ulnar tuberosity

Shaft of ulna, anterior surface

Interosseous membrane

Head of ulna

Styloid process of radius

Distal radioulnar joint

Fig. 13.7 Radius and ulna
Right forearm, anterosuperior view.

— The **radius** is the lateral bone of the forearm (see **Fig. 13.7**).
  • A round **radial head** articulates with the humerus and ulna and sits on top of a narrow **neck.**
  • **A radial tuberosity** on the anterior surface provides attachments for the biceps brachii muscle.
  • Distally, the radius is triangular in cross section with a flattened anterior surface.
  • The radius articulates with the ulna proximally at the elbow and distally at the wrist. The interosseous membrane attaches the radius to the shaft of the ulna.
  • A **radial styloid process** projects from the distal end and extends farther than the styloid process of the ulna.
  • The radius articulates with carpal bones at the wrist.

CLINICAL CORRELATION

COLLES' FRACTURES A Colles' fracture, a transverse fracture through the distal 2 cm of the radius, is the most common forearm fracture and results from a fall on an outstretched hand. The distal segment of bone is displaced dorsally and proximally, and with shortening of the radius, the styloid process appears proximal to the styloid of the ulna. The resulting appearance is referred to as the "dinner fork" deformity.

— The **carpal bones** consist of eight short bones that are arranged in two curved rows at the wrist (**Figs. 13.8**, **13.9, 13.10**). From lateral to medial, they are
  • in the proximal row, the **scaphoid, lunate, triquetrum, and pisiform;** and,
  • in the distal row, the **trapezium, trapezoid, capitate, and hamate.**

CLINICAL CORRELATION

LUNATE DISLOCATION The lunate is the most commonly displaced of the carpal bones. Normally located in the floor of the carpal tunnel, a displaced bone moves toward the palmar surface and can compress structures of the carpal tunnel.

CLINICAL CORRELATION

SCAPHOID FRACTURES Scaphoid fractures are the most common carpal bone fractures, generally occurring at the narrow waist between the proximal and distal poles. Because the blood supply to the bone is transmitted via the distal segment, fractures at the waist can compromise the supply to the proximal segment, often resulting in nonunion and avascular necrosis.

— The **metacarpal bones** consist of five long bones that form the hand.
  • Proximally, their **bases** articulate with the carpal bones.
  • Distally, their **heads,** the knuckles of the hand, articulate with the proximal phalanges.
— The **phalanges** are small long bones that form the fingers.
  • They are designated as proximal, middle, and distal in each finger except in the thumb, which has only a proximal and a distal phalanx.
— Fingers and their corresponding metacarpals and phalanges are designated as 1st through 5th, with the thumb as the 1st digit and the little finger as the 5th digit.

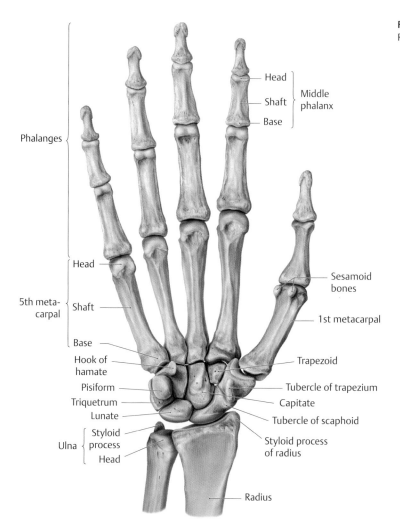

Fig. 13.8 Bones of the hand
Right hand, palmar view.

Phalanges

Head
Shaft — Middle
Base — phalanx

Head

5th meta-
carpal — Shaft

Base

Hook of
hamate

Pisiform

Triquetrum

Lunate

Ulna — Styloid
process

Head

Sesamoid
bones

1st metacarpal

Trapezoid

Tubercle of trapezium

Capitate

Tubercle of scaphoid

Styloid process
of radius

Radius

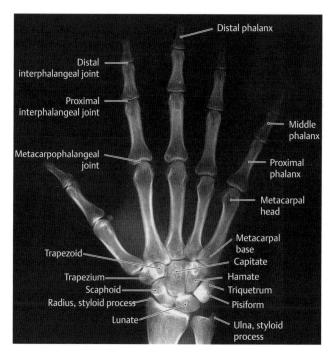

Distal phalanx

Distal
interphalangeal joint

Proximal
interphalangeal joint

Metacarpophalangeal
joint

Middle
phalanx

Proximal
phalanx

Metacarpal
head

Trapezoid

Trapezium

Scaphoid

Radius, styloid process

Lunate

Metacarpal
base

Capitate

Hamate

Triquetrum

Pisiform

Ulna, styloid
process

Fig. 13.9 Radiograph of the hand

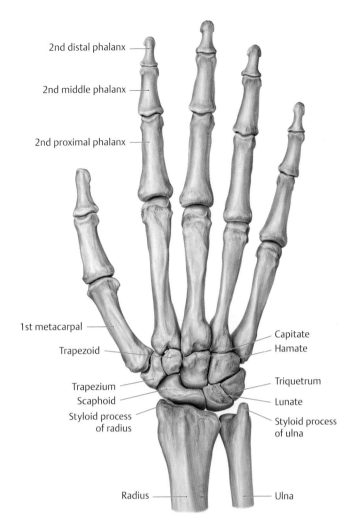

Fig. 13.10 **Bones of the hand**
Right hand, dorsal view.

13.3 Fascia and Compartments of the Upper Limb

— Deep fascia snugly encloses muscles of the upper limb. It is continuous over the pectoral girdle, the axilla, and the upper limb but has regional designations.
  • **Pectoral fascia** invests the pectoralis major muscle.
  • **Clavipectoral fascia** invests the subclavius and pectoralis minor muscles.
  • **Axillary fascia** forms the floor of the **axilla.**
  • **Brachial fascia** invests muscles of the arm.
  • **Antebrachial fascia** invests muscles of the forearm and extends onto the wrist as transverse thickened bands, the **flexor** and **extensor retinacula.**
  • Fascia of the hand is continuous over the dorsum and palm, but in the center of the palm it forms a thickened fibrous sheet, the **palmar aponeurosis.**
  • **Digital fibrous sheaths,** extensions of the palmar aponeurosis onto the fingers, surround the flexor tendons.
— Intermuscular septa arising from the deep fascia attach to the bones of the arm, forearm, and hand, separating the limb musculature into discrete compartments. The muscles within each compartment usually share a similar function, innervation, and blood supply. The compartments of the upper limb (see **Figs. 14.39** and **14.40**) are
  • the **anterior** and **posterior compartments** of the arm;
  • the **anterior** and **posterior compartments** of the forearm; and
  • the **thenar, hypothenar, central, adductor,** and **inter-osseous compartments** of the palm of the hand.

13.4 Neurovasculature of the Upper Limb

Arteries of the Upper Limb

— The **subclavian artery** and its branches supply structures in the neck, part of the thoracic wall, and the entire upper limb (**Fig. 13.11**).
  • The right subclavian artery is a branch of the brachiocephalic trunk, which arises from the aortic arch. The left subclavian artery arises directly from the aortic arch.

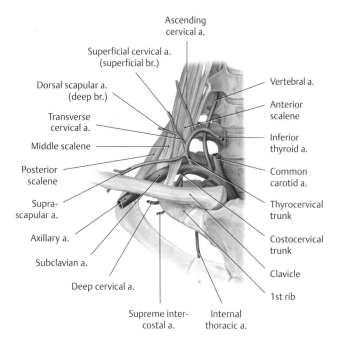

Fig. 13.11 Branches of the subclavian artery
Right side, anterior view.

- The subclavian arteries enter the neck through the superior thoracic aperture, pass laterally toward the shoulder, and terminate as they pass over the 1st rib.
- The subclavian artery branches that supply the neck and thoracic wall (discussed further in Section 17.3) include
    ○ the **vertebral artery;**
    ○ the internal thoracic artery; and
    ○ the **thyrocervical trunk,** whose branches are the **suprascapular, ascending cervical, inferior thyroid,** and **transverse cervical arteries.**
- The branches of the thyrocervical trunk that supply muscles and skin of the scapular region include
    ○ the transverse cervical artery and its **dorsal scapular branch** and
    ○ the suprascapular artery.
— The **axillary artery,** the continuation of the subclavian artery, begins at the lateral edge of the 1st rib and terminates at the lateral border of the axilla (the lower border of the teres major muscle).
— Within the axilla, the **pectoralis minor** muscle lies anterior to the middle third of the axillary artery. Branches of the axillary artery, therefore, are described as arising from its proximal, middle, or distal thirds (**Fig. 13.12**).
    - The proximal third has one branch:
        ○ The **superior thoracic** branch supplies the muscles of the first intercostal space.
    - The middle third has two branches:
        ○ The **thoracoacromial artery** divides into deltoid, pectoral, clavicular, and acromial branches.
        ○ The **lateral thoracic artery** supplies the lateral thoracic wall, including the serratus anterior muscle and the breast.

- The distal third has three branches:
    ○ The **subscapular artery** further divides into a **thoracodorsal artery,** supplying the latissimus dorsi muscle, and a **circumflex scapular artery,** supplying muscles of the scapula.
    ○ The **anterior circumflex humeral artery.**
    ○ The **posterior circumflex humeral artery.** These circumflex arteries encircle the humeral neck to supply the deltoid region
— A **scapular arcade,** formed by the anastomoses of the dorsal scapular and suprascapular branches of the subclavian artery, and the circumflex scapular and thoracodorsal branches of the axillary artery provide an important collateral circulation to the scapular region when the axillary artery is injured or ligated (**Fig. 13.13**).
— The **brachial artery,** the continuation of the axillary artery, begins after the lateral border of the axilla (the lower margin of the tendon of the teres major), runs superficially along the medial border of the **biceps brachii muscle,** and terminates at its bifurcation in the cubital fossa (anterior elbow region). Its branches (see **Fig. 13.12**) include
    - the **deep artery of the arm** (deep brachial artery, profunda brachii), which arises proximally, descends on the posterior surface of the humerus, and supplies muscles of the posterior arm;
    - the **superior** and **inferior ulnar collateral arteries,** distal branches, which anastomose with the deep artery of the arm and arteries of the forearm to supply the elbow joint; and
    - the **radial** and **ulnar arteries,** the terminal branches of the brachial artery, which supply the forearm and hand.
— The ulnar artery originates in the cubital fossa, descends along the medial side of the forearm, and crosses through a narrow space at the wrist, the **ulnar canal.** It terminates as the **superficial palmar arch** of the hand. The major branches of the ulnar artery in the forearm (see **Fig. 13.12**) are
    - the **ulnar recurrent artery,** which anastomoses with ulnar collateral arteries to supply the elbow joint, and
    - the **common interosseous artery,** which arises in the proximal forearm and branches into anterior and **posterior interosseous arteries.** These interosseous branches descend on either side of the interosseous membrane and supply the anterior and posterior muscle compartments of the forearm.
— The radial artery, the smaller lateral branch of the brachial artery, descends from the cubital fossa along the lateral side of the forearm to the wrist. It crosses the wrist through the **anatomic snuffbox** on the dorsal side, pierces the muscles between the 1st and 2nd digits, and enters the palm of the hand, where it ends as the **deep palmar arch.** Its branches (see **Fig. 13.12**) include
    - the **radial recurrent artery,** which anastomoses with collateral branches of the deep artery of the arm to supply the elbow joint, and
    - the **palmar** and **dorsal carpal arteries,** which anastomose with branches of the ulnar artery in the wrist and hand.

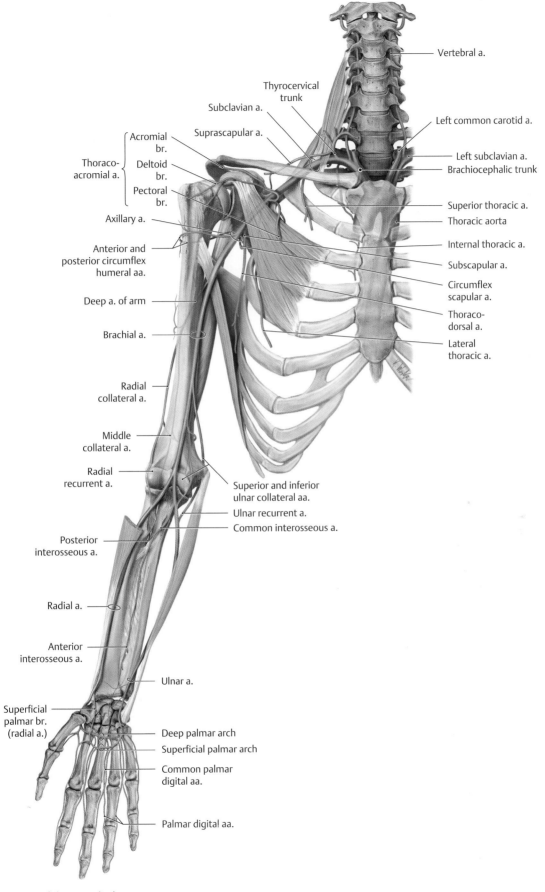

Fig. 13.12 Arteries of the upper limb
Right limb, anterior view.

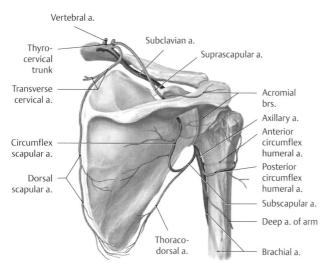

Fig. 13.13 Scapular arcade
Right side, posterior view.

— Arteries of the wrist and hand **(Fig. 13.14)** include
   • the **palmar** and **dorsal carpal networks,** which form by contributions from radial, ulnar, and anterior interosseous arteries;
   • the superficial and deep palmar arches, which arise from the ulnar and radial arteries, respectively. A **deep palmar branch** of the ulnar artery connects the two palmer arches;
   • the **princeps pollicis artery,** a branch of the radial artery, which follows the ulnar surface of the 1st metatarsal to the base of the thumb, where it divides into two digital branches;
   • the **radialis indicis,** which arises from the princeps pollicis or radial artery and courses along the radial side of the index finger;
   • the **palmar metacarpal** and **digital arteries,** which arise from the superficial and deep palmar arches in the palm of the hand; and
   • the **dorsal metacarpal** and **digital arteries,** which arise from the dorsal carpal arch on the dorsum of the hand.

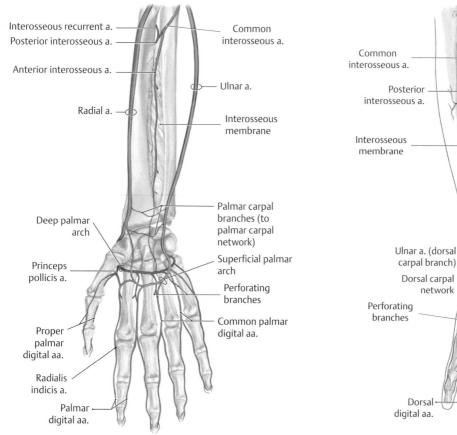

A Anterior (palmar) view.

B Posterior (dorsal) view.

Fig. 13.14 Arteries of the forearm and hand
Right limb. The ulnar and radial arteries are interconnected by the superficial and deep palmar arches, the perforating branches, and the dorsal carpal network.

Veins of the Upper Limb

— Veins of the limbs, similar to veins of the trunk, are more variable than the arteries, and they often form anastomoses that surround the arteries they accompany. Veins of the limbs have unidirectional valves that prevent pooling of blood in the extremities and facilitate the movement of blood back to the heart. The limbs have both deep and superficial veins.

— Deep veins accompany the major arteries and their branches and have similar names (**Fig. 13.15**).

  • In the distal limb, the deep veins, referred to as **accompanying veins** (venae comitantes), are paired and surround the artery. Proximally, the pairs merge to form a single vessel.

  • The **axillary vein** drains the shoulder, arm, forearm, and hand and receives additional contributions from
    ◦ the lateral chest wall, including the breast, and
    ◦ the thoracoepigastric vein of the anterolateral abdominal wall.

  • The **subclavian vein,** the continuation of the axillary vein, also receives the venous drainage from the scapular region.

— The superficial veins are found in the subcutaneous tissue and drain into the deep venous system via **perforating** (connecting) **veins (Fig. 13.16)**.

  • The **dorsal venous network** on the dorsum of the hand drains into two large superficial veins, the **cephalic** and **basilic veins.**

  • The **cephalic vein** originates on the lateral side of the dorsum of the hand and ascends on the lateral side of the forearm and arm. In the shoulder, it passes through the **deltopectoral groove** (formed by the borders of the deltoid and pectoralis major muscles) before emptying into the axillary vein.

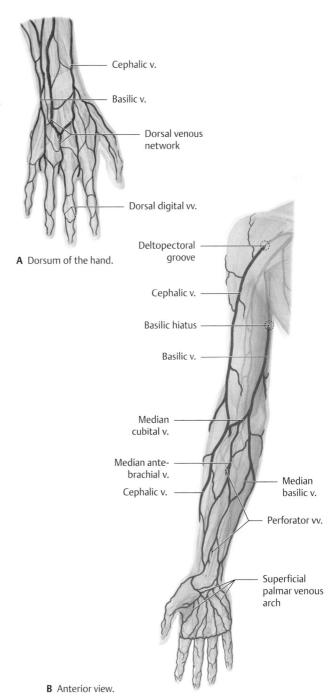

A Dorsum of the hand.

B Anterior view.

Fig. 13.16 Superficial veins of the upper limb
Right limb.

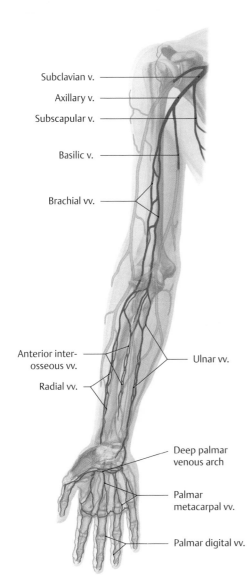

Fig. 13.15 Deep veins of the upper limb
Right limb, anterior view.

- The **basilic vein** arises on the medial side of the dorsum of the hand and runs posteromedially to pass anterior to the medial epicondyle of the humerus. In the arm, it pierces the brachial fascia (at the **basilic hiatus**) and joins the paired **deep brachial veins** to form the axillary vein.
- The **median cubital vein** connects the cephalic and basilic veins anterior to the cubital fossa.
- The **median antebrachial vein** arises from the venous network of the palm, ascends on the anterior forearm, and terminates in the basilic or median cubital vein.

Lymphatic Drainage of the Upper Limb

Lymphatic vessels of the upper limb drain toward the axilla. They usually accompany the veins of the superficial system (cephalic and basilic veins), although there are numerous connections between the deep and superficial drainages.

— Axillary lymph node groups, each containing four to seven large nodes, are described in relation to the pectoralis minor muscle (**Fig. 13.17**).
- The lower axillary group lies lateral and deep to the pectoralis minor.
    ◦ **Pectoral** (anterior) **nodes** on the anterior wall of the axilla drain the anterior thoracic wall, including the breast (75% of lymph from the breast drains to axillary nodes).
    ◦ **Subscapular nodes** along the posterior axillary fold drain the posterior thoracic wall and scapular region.
    ◦ **Humeral** (posterior) **nodes** lie medial and posterior to the axillary vein and receive lymphatic vessels that accompany the basilic vein and the deep veins of the arm.
    ◦ **Central nodes** lie deep to the pectoralis minor muscle and receive lymph from the pectoral, subscapular, and humeral nodes.
- The middle axillary group lies on the surface of the pectoralis minor muscle.
    ◦ **Interpectoral nodes** lie between the pectoralis major and pectoralis minor muscles and drain to the apical nodes.
- The upper axillary group lies medial to the pectoralis minor muscle.
    ◦ **Apical nodes** lie along the axillary vein adjacent to the first part of the axillary artery in the apex of the axilla. They receive lymph from the central nodes as well as from lymphatic vessels traveling along the cephalic vein.
— Apical lymph vessels unite to form the subclavian lymph trunks, which usually drain to the right lymphatic trunk and the thoracic duct (left lymphatic duct).

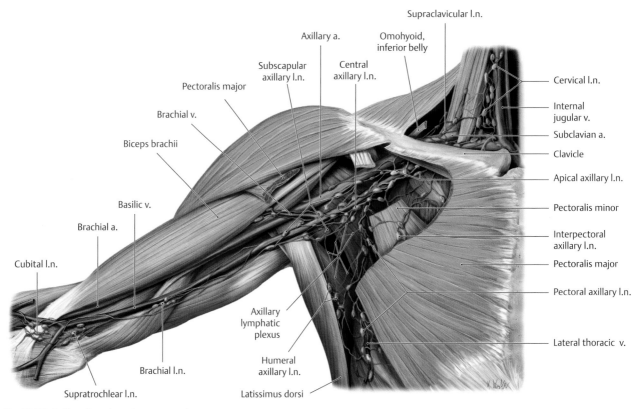

Fig. 13.17 Axillary lymph nodes
Anterior view.

Nerves of the Upper Limb: The Brachial Plexus

The upper limb is innervated almost entirely by the nerves of the **brachial plexus,** which originates from the lower cervical and upper thoracic spinal cord **(Table 13.1; Figs. 13.18, 13.19, 13.20, 13.21, 13.22).** (One exception, the intercostobrachial nerve, formed by the anterior rami of T1 and T2, is sensory to the medial arm but is not part of the plexus.)

— Roots of the brachial plexus emerge from the vertebral column between the anterior and middle scalene muscles (interscalene groove) in the neck.

— Formation of the plexus begins in the neck **(supraclavicular part),** where it accompanies the subclavian artery, and continues into the axilla **(infraclavicular part),** where it accompanies the axillary artery.

— The roots, trunks, and divisions of the plexus are **supraclavicular** (above the clavicle); the cords form at the level of the clavicle, and their branches are **infraclavicular** (below the clavicle).

— **Fig. 13.18** shows the architecture of the brachial plexus.
  • Anterior rami of spinal nerves C5–T1 form five **roots.**
    ○ Within the plexus, upper roots form nerves that innervate muscles of the proximal limb; lower roots form nerves that innervate muscles of the distal limb.
    ○ The terms **pre-fixed** or **post-fixed plexus** indicate that the plexus includes anterior rami from one spinal level above (C4) or below (T2) the normal levels, respectively.

  • Roots C5 to T1 combine to form three **trunks:**
    1. C5 and C6 form the **upper trunk.**
    2. C7 forms the **middle trunk.**
    3. C8 and T1 form the **lower trunk.**

  • Anterior and posterior divisions (components of the anterior rami of all spinal nerves), which are bundled together in the roots and trunks of the plexus, separate to form three **cords:**
    1. Anterior divisions of the upper and middle trunk (C5–C7) form the **lateral cord.**
    2. Anterior divisions of the lower trunk (C8–T1) form the **medial cord.**
    3. Posterior divisions of all trunks (C5–T1) form the **posterior cord.**

  • The three cords divide to form the five **terminal nerves** of the plexus.
    ○ Medial and lateral cords form the **musculocutaneous, median,** and **ulnar nerves,** which innervate the anterior muscles of the arm and forearm, and all muscles of the palm.
    ○ The posterior cord forms the **axillary** and **radial nerves,** which innervate muscles of the scapular and deltoid regions and posterior muscles of the arm and forearm.

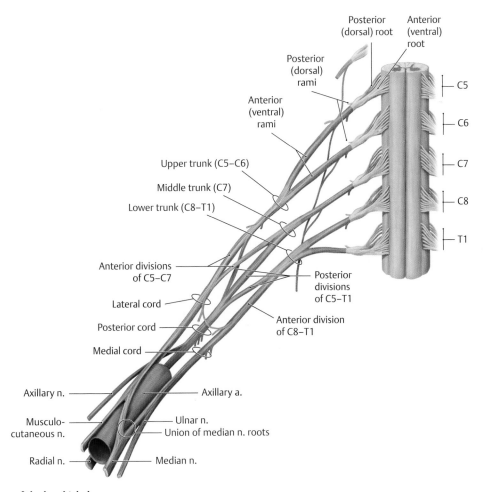

Fig. 13.18 Structure of the brachial plexus
Right side, anterior view.

Table 13.1 **Nerves of the Brachial Plexus**

Nerve			Level	Area of Innervation
Supraclavicular part				
Direct branches from the anterior rami or plexus trunks				
● Dorsal scapular n.			C4–C5	Levator scapulae, rhomboid major and minor
Suprascapular n.			C4–C6	Supraspinatus, infraspinatus
N. to the subclavius			C5–C6	Subclavius m.
Long thoracic n.			C5–C7	Serratus anterior
Infraclavicular part				
Short and long branches from the plexus cords				
● **Lateral cord**	Lateral pectoral n.		C5–C7	Pectoralis major
	Musculocutaneous n.			Coracobrachialis, biceps brachii, brachialis; skin of lateral forearm
●	Median n.	Lateral root	C6–C7	Pronator teres, flexor carpi radialis, palmaris longus, flexor digitorum superficialis, pronator quadratus, flexor pollicis longus, flexor digitorum profundus (radial half), abductor pollicis brevis, flexor pollicis brevis (superficial head), opponens pollicis, 1st and 2nd lumbricals; skin of radial half of palm and palmar surface and distal dorsal segment of 2nd and 3rd digits and half of 4th digit
Medial cord		Medial root	C8–T1	
●	Medial pectoral n.			Pectoralis major and minor
	Medial antebrachial cutaneous n.			Skin of medial forearm
	Medial brachial cutaneous n.		T1	Skin of medial arm
	Ulnar n.		C7–T1	Flexor carpi ulnaris, flexor digitorum profundus (ulnar half), palmaris brevis, abductor digiti minimi, flexor digiti minimi, opponens digiti minimi, 3rd and 4th lumbricals, interossei, adductor pollicis, flexor pollicis brevis (deep head); skin of ulnar half of the dorsum and palm of the hand, dorsum and palmar surface of the 4th and 5th digits and half of the 3rd digit
● **Posterior cord**	Upper subscapular n.		C5–C6	Subscapularis (upper part)
	Thoracodorsal n.		C6–C8	Latissimus dorsi
	Lower subscapular n.		C5–C6	Subscapularis (lower part), teres major
	Axillary n.			Deltoid, teres minor; skin of lower deltoid region
	Radial n.		C5–T1	Muscles of posterior arm and forearm; skin of posterior and inferolateral arm, posterior forearm, radial half of dorsum of hand, dorsum of 1st, 2nd, 3rd digits and half of 4th digit

— The musculocutaneous nerve (C5–C7) pierces and innervates the coracobrachialis muscle of the arm as it leaves the axilla and then descends within the anterior compartment of the arm between the biceps brachii and brachialis muscles.
  • In the arm, its **muscular branches** innervate the muscles of the anterior compartment, the biceps brachii and the brachialis muscles.
  • It enters the forearm at the lateral edge of the cubital fossa as the **lateral antebrachial cutaneous nerve** to supply the skin of the lateral forearm.

CLINICAL CORRELATION

MUSCULOCUTANEOUS NERVE INJURY The musculocutaneous nerve is protected on the medial side of the arm, and isolated injuries are uncommon, but they would affect the coracobrachialis, biceps brachii, and brachialis muscles. Flexion and supination at the elbow would be weakened but not absent because the brachioradialis and supinator muscles, which are innervated by the radial nerve, also provide those movements.

— The median nerve (C6–T1) is formed by contributions from the medial and lateral cords.
  • In the arm, the median nerve descends with the brachial vessels, medial to the biceps brachii, but it does not innervate any arm muscles.
  • In the forearm, it travels deep within the anterior compartment but becomes superficial at the wrist before passing through the carpal tunnel into the hand. It innervates most muscles in the anterior forearm (except the flexor carpi ulnaris and the medial half of the flexor digitorum profundus).
    ○ Its largest branch in the forearm is the **anterior antebrachial interosseous nerve.**
    ○ **A palmar branch** arises distally and crosses the wrist superficial to the carpal tunnel to supply the skin of the palm.

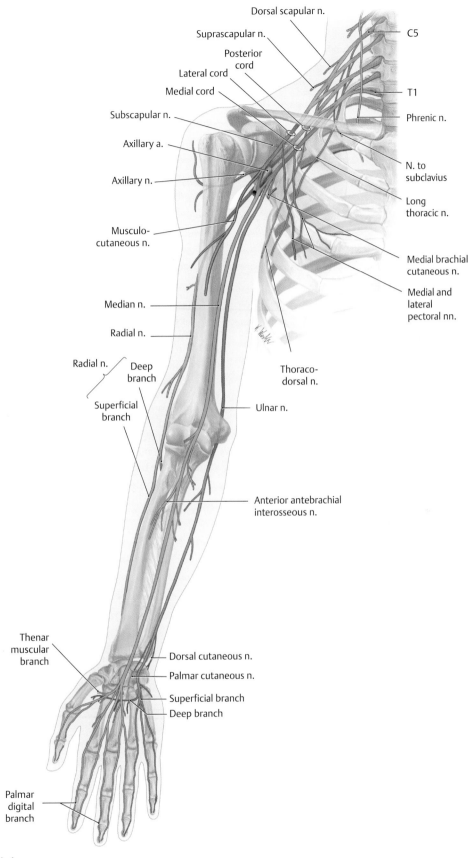

Fig. 13.19 Brachial plexus
Right side, anterior view.

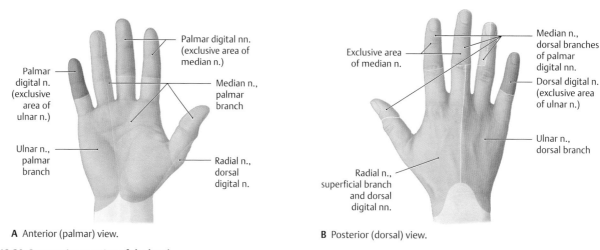

A Anterior (palmar) view.

B Posterior (dorsal) view.

Fig. 13.20 Sensory innervation of the hand

Right hand. Extensive overlap exists between adjacent areas. Exclusive nerve territories indicated with darker shading.

- In the hand, the median nerve has motor and sensory functions.
  - A thenar muscular branch, the **recurrent nerve,** innervates most muscles of the thenar compartment (intrinsic muscles of the thumb).
  - **Palmar digital branches** innervate the lateral two lumbricals (intrinsic muscles of the central compartment) and the skin of the 1st through 3rd fingers and lateral half of the 4th finger.
— The ulnar nerve [(C7) C8, T1] is a branch of the medial cord.
  - In the arm, it descends on the medial side with the brachial artery. At the mid-arm, it pierces the intermuscular septum to enter the posterior compartment. It crosses the elbow joint behind the medial epicondyle, where it is subcutaneous and vulnerable to injury. It does not innervate any muscles in the arm.

- In the forearm, it runs deep to the flexor muscles but becomes superficial just proximal to the wrist.
  - Its **muscular branches** innervate the flexors on the medial side (flexor carpi ulnaris and medial half of the flexor digitorum profundus).
  - **Palmar** and **dorsal cutaneous nerves** arise in the wrist but are distributed to the skin of the medial half of the hand, proximal parts of the 5th digit, and medial half of the 4th digit.
- It crosses the wrist with the ulnar artery within a narrow space, the **ulnar canal,** where it splits into deep and superficial branches.
  - Its **deep branch** supplies most of the intrinsic muscles of the palm (except two of the thenar muscles and the 1st and 2nd lumbricals).

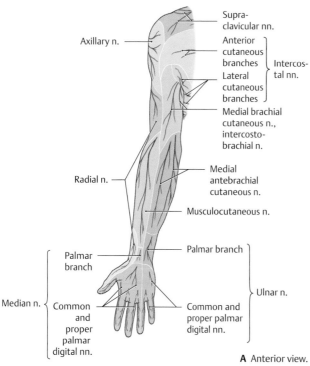

A Anterior view.

B Posterior view.

Fig. 13.21 Cutaneous innervation of the upper limb

A Anterior view. **B** Posterior view.

Fig. 13.22 Dermatomes of the upper limb

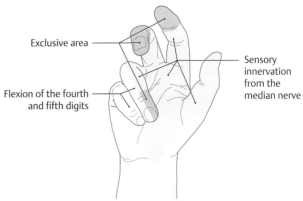

A "Hand of benediction" following a proximal median nerve injury.

In a healthy hand, the thumb can be abducted to fully grasp a cylindrical object

With a proximal median nerve lesion, the thumb cannot be fully abducted

B Positive "bottle sign" due to loss or weakness of finger flexion and thumb abduction.

Fig. 13.23 Median nerve injury

- Its **superficial branch** innervates a small superficial muscle of the palm (palmaris brevis) and contributes to sensory innervation of the 4th and 5th digits.

CLINICAL CORRELATION

MEDIAN NERVE INJURY Injury at the distal humerus is often caused by a supracondylar fracture **(Fig. 13.23)** and results in

- loss of sensation in the palm and palmar surface of the lateral three and a half digits,
- loss of flexion of the 1st to 3rd digits,
- positive "bottle sign" due to loss of thumb abduction (with proximal nerve lesion)
- weakened flexion of the 4th and 5th digits,
- loss of thenar opposition,
- loss of pronation,
- an "ape hand" produced by flattening of the thenar eminence, and
- the "hand of benediction" produced by flexing the hand in a fist (the 2nd and 3rd digits remain partly extended).

CLINICAL CORRELATION

ULNAR NERVE INJURY The ulnar nerve may be injured at the elbow by a fracture of the medial epicondyle, compressed in the cubital fossa between the two heads of the flexor carpi ulnaris, or compressed in the ulnar canal at the wrist. These injuries **(Fig. 13.24)** result in the following:

- Paresthesia of the palmar and dorsal side of the medial hand and the medial one and a half digits
- Loss of thumb adduction
- Hyperextension of the metacarpophalangeal (MCP) joints
- Loss of extension of interphalangeal (IP) joints
- Weakened adduction and flexion of the wrist (for lesions at the elbow)
- Inability to form a fist due to "claw hand" deformity

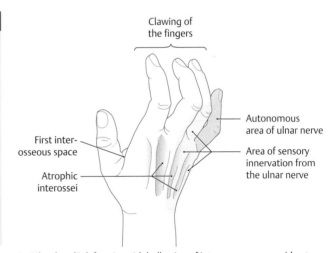

A "Claw hand" deformity with hollowing of interosseous spaces (due to atrophy of interossei).

Strong adduction of the thumb in the healthy hand

The thumb is flexed at the interphalangeal joint, signifying an ulnar nerve lesion

B Positive "Froment sign" indicating palsy of the adductor pollicis muscle.

Fig. 13.24 Ulnar nerve injury

— The axillary nerve (C5–C6), a branch of the posterior cord, passes to the posterior shoulder region with the posterior circumflex humeral vessels.
  • In the shoulder region, it innervates scapular and deltoid muscles and skin of the deltoid region.

CLINICAL CORRELATION

AXILLARY NERVE INJURY The axillary nerve is most vulnerable as it courses around the neck of the humerus and can be injured by fractures at the surgical neck or dislocation of the glenohumeral joint. Denervation of the deltoid results in substantial functional weakness of shoulder movements including:
• Weakened flexion and extension at the shoulder joint
• Inability to abduct the shoulder even to the horizontal position
• Loss of sensation over the deltoid region
• A flattened shoulder contour

— The radial nerve (C5–T1) forms from the posterior cord.
  • In the arm, it runs posteriorly around the humerus in the radial groove with the deep brachial artery and descends within the posterior compartment.
    ◦ Its **muscular branches** innervate all of the muscles of the posterior arm, the triceps brachii and anconeus muscles.
    ◦ Its sensory branches of the arm include the **posterior brachial cutaneous** and **inferior lateral brachial cutaneous nerves.**
    ◦ **A posterior antebrachial cutaneous nerve** arises in the arm but innervates skin over the posterior forearm.
  • In the cubital region, it passes through the lateral intermuscular septum into the anterior compartment, where it runs anterior to the medial epicondyle. As it enters the proximal forearm, it splits into deep and superficial branches.

CLINICAL CORRELATION

RADIAL NERVE INJURY The radial nerve is most vulnerable to injury from a midhumeral fracture where the nerve courses along the radial groove. Because radial branches to the triceps brachii are usually proximal to the injury, elbow flexion is unaffected. Other effects **(Fig. 13.25)** include the following:
• Loss of wrist extension
• Loss of extension at the metacarpophalangeal (MCP) joints
• Weakened pronation
• Flexed wrist and fingers producing the "wrist drop" position

---

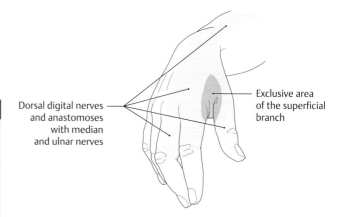

Dorsal digital nerves and anastomoses with median and ulnar nerves

Exclusive area of the superficial branch

Fig. 13.25 Radial nerve injury
"Wrist drop" resulting from loss of wrist extensors.

  ◦ The deep branch becomes the **posterior interosseous nerve** as it circles around the radius into the posterior forearm compartment. It innervates all muscles of this compartment.
  ◦ The **superficial branch** descends along the lateral forearm to the wrist.
  • In the hand, the radial nerve has no motor branches.
    ◦ At the wrist, the superficial branch runs posteriorly to innervate the skin on the dorsum of the hand and proximal segments of the 1st through 3rd digits and half of the 4th digit.

CLINICAL CORRELATION

BRACHIAL PLEXUS INJURIES Injuries to the proximal segments of the brachial plexus, involving the avulsion of the roots or stretching or compression of the trunks, have classic presentations that represent the distribution of the affected nerves.

Upper plexus injuries (Erb-Duchenne palsy) involve the C5 and C6 roots or the upper trunk and are usually caused by trauma that forcefully separates the head and shoulder. The resulting deformity includes an adducted shoulder and medially rotated limb that is extended at the elbow.

Injuries of the lower plexus (Klumpke's palsy) are far less common than those of the upper plexus, but a violent upward pull of the limb can avulse the C8 and T1 roots or damage the lower trunk. This affects the intrinsic muscles of the hand and creates a "claw hand" deformity. Because C8 and T1 are the superiormost contributions to the sympathetic trunk, avulsion of these nerve roots also affects the sympathetic innervation in the head. The manifestation of this is known as Horner's syndrome (see Section 20.1).

14 Functional Anatomy of the Upper Limb

The upper limb is characterized by its wide range of movement and fine motor ability. Coordinated movements at the pectoral girdle, as well as the shoulder, elbow, radioulnar, and wrist joints, position the hand for performing work as vital as eating and as complicated as playing a violin.

Schematics of upper limb muscles accompany the muscle tables (origin, attachment, innervation, and action) in the appropriate chapter sections. To see the muscles in situ, view the gallery of topographic images in Section 14.7 at the end of this chapter.

14.1 The Pectoral Girdle

The **pectoral girdle,** formed by the clavicle and scapula, attaches the upper limb to the trunk (**Fig. 14.1**). The clavicle, acting as a strut, holds the scapula and humerus away from the trunk, allowing the free range of motion necessary for upper limb function.

Joints of the Pectoral Girdle

The joints of the pectoral girdle include articulations of the clavicle with the sternum and scapula, and a nonosseous joint that permits gliding movement between muscles of the trunk and scapula.

— The **sternoclavicular joint** is a strong but highly mobile synovial joint between the sternal end of the clavicle and the manubrium and 1st costal cartilage (**Fig. 14.2**).
- It is the only bony articulation between the upper limb and the trunk.
- An articular disk separates the articulating surfaces.

- **Anterior** and **posterior sternoclavicular, costoclavicular,** and **interclavicular ligaments** strengthen the joint.
- The joint allows the clavicle to elevate and rotate in conjunction with limb movements.

— The **acromioclavicular joint** is a plane type of synovial joint between the acromion of the scapula and acromial end of the clavicle (**Fig. 14.3**).
- An articular disk separates the articulating surfaces.
- An **acromioclavicular ligament** supports the joint superiorly.
- The **coracoclavicular ligament**, an extrinsic ligament (distant from the joint), strengthens the joint by anchoring the clavicle to the coracoid process. Its two parts are the **conoid** and **trapezoid ligaments.**

— The **scapulothoracic joint** is not a bony articulation but a functional relationship between the serratus anterior and subscapularis muscles that allows the scapula to glide and pivot on the chest wall (**Fig. 14.4**).

CLINICAL CORRELATION

INJURY TO THE LONG THORACIC NERVE The superficial course of the long thoracic nerve (C5–C7) along the medial wall of the axilla puts it at risk of injury during regional surgeries such as axillary node dissection. Nerve damage results in the inability of the serratus anterior to laterally rotate the scapula, which is necessary to abduct the arm above the horizontal plane. The serratus anterior is also unable to support the scapula against the thoracic wall, which creates a "winged" scapula, especially noticeable when the subject presses the outstretched arm against a hard surface.

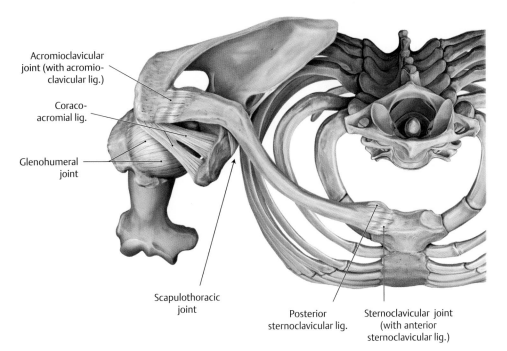

Acromioclavicular joint (with acromio-clavicular lig.)

Coraco-acromial lig.

Glenohumeral joint

Scapulothoracic joint

Posterior sternoclavicular lig.

Sternoclavicular joint (with anterior sternoclavicular lig.)

Fig. 14.1 Joints of the shoulder girdle
Right side, superior view.

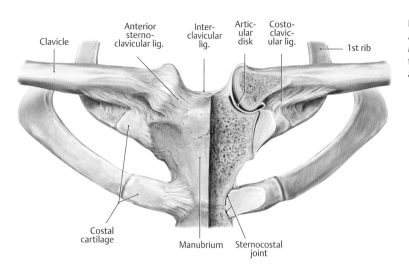

Fig. 14.2 Sternoclavicular joint
Anterior view with sternum coronally sectioned (left).
Note: A fibrocartilaginous articular disk compensates for the mismatch of surfaces between the two saddle-shaped articular facets of the clavicle and the manubrium.

Fig. 14.3 Acromioclavicular joint
Anterior view. The acromioclavicular joint is a plane joint. Because the articulating surfaces are flat, they must be held in place by strong ligaments, greatly limiting the mobility of the joint.

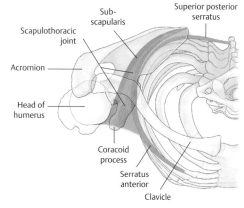

Fig. 14.4 Scapulothoracic joint
Right side, superior view. In all movements of the shoulder girdle, the scapula glides on a curved surface of loose connective tissue between the serratus anterior and the subscapularis muscles. This surface can be considered a scapulothoracic joint.

Muscles of the Pectoral Girdle

Muscles of the pectoral girdle attach the upper limb to the trunk and move and stabilize the pectoral girdle in response to movements of the glenohumeral joint at the shoulder (**Table 14.1**).
— Anterior muscles of the pectoral girdle, which lie on the anterior and lateral thoracic wall,
   • include the **subclavius, pectoralis minor,** and **serratus anterior,** and
   • are anchored to the ribs, as well as to the bones of the pectoral girdle.
— Posterior muscles of the pectoral girdle, which are part of the superficial muscular layer of the back,
   • include the **trapezius, levator scapulae, rhomboid major,** and **rhomboid minor,** and
   • arise from cervical and thoracic vertebrae and insert on the scapula.
— Movements of the pectoral girdle and the muscles that provide them are listed in **Table 14.2.**

A Subclavius and pectoralis minor, right, anterior view.

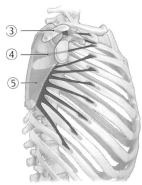

B Serratus anterior, right lateral view.

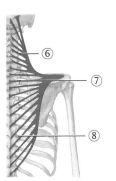

C Trapezius, right posterior view.

D Levator scapulae with rhomboids major and minor, right posterior view.

Table 14.1 **Pectoral Girdle Muscles**

Muscle		Origin	Insertion	Innervation	Action
① Subclavius		1st rib	Clavicle (inferior surface)	N. to subclavius (C5, C6)	Steadies the clavicle in the sternoclavicular joint
② Pectoralis minor		3rd to 5th ribs	Coracoid process	Medial pectoral n. (C8, T1)	Draws scapula downward, causing inferior angle to move posteromedially; rotates glenoid inferiorly; assists in respiration
Serratus anterior	③ Superior part	1st to 9th ribs	Scapula (costal and dorsal surfaces of superior angle)	Long thoracic n. (C5–C7)	Superior part: lowers the raised arm
	④ Intermediate part		Scapula (costal surface of medial border)		Entire muscle: draws scapula laterally forward; elevates ribs when shoulder is fixed
	⑤ Inferior part		Scapula (costal surface of medial border and costal and dorsal surfaces of inferior angle)		Inferior part: rotates inferior angle of scapula laterally forward (allows elevation of arm above 90 degrees)
Trapezius	⑥ Descending part	Occipital bone; spinous process of C1–C7	Clavicle (lateral one third)	Accessory n. (CN XI); C3–C4 of the cervical plexus	Draws scapula obliquely upward; rotates glenoid cavity superiorly; tilts head to same side and rotates it to opposite
	⑦ Transverse part	Aponeurosis at T1–T4 spinous processes	Acromion		Draws scapula medially
	⑧ Ascending part	Spinous processes of T5–T12	Scapular spine		Draws scapula medially downward
					Entire muscle: steadies scapula on thorax
⑨ Levator scapulae		Transverse processes of C1–C4	Scapula (superior angle)	Dorsal scapular n. and cervical spinal nn. (C3–C4)	Draws scapula medially upward while moving inferior angle medially; inclines neck to same side
⑩ Rhomboid minor		Spinous process of C6, C7	Medial border of scapula above (minor) and below (major) scapular spine	Dorsal scapular n. (C4–C5)	Steadies scapula; draws scapula medially upward
⑪ Rhomboid major		Spinous process of T1–T4 vertebrae			

Abbreviation: CN, cranial nerve.

A Elevation and depression during elevation and depression of the shoulder girdle.

B Abduction and adduction during protraction and retraction of the shoulder girdle.

Antero-posterior axis of motion

C Lateral rotation of the inferior angle during abduction or elevation of the arm.

Table 14.2 **Movements of the Pectoral Girdle**

Action	Primary Muscles
Elevation	Trapezius (descending part) Levator scapulae
Depression	Pectoralis minor Trapezius (ascending part)
Protraction	Pectoralis minor Serratus anterior
Retraction	Trapezius (transverse part) Rhomboid minor Rhomboid major
Lateral rotation	Serratus anterior (inferior part) Trapezius (descending part)
Medial rotation	Levator scapulae Rhomboid minor Rhomboid major

14.2   The Shoulder Region

The shoulder region includes the axilla, a passageway for neurovascular structures between the trunk and upper limb, and the glenohumeral joint, the largest joint of the upper limb. Muscles of the pectoral, scapular, and deltoid regions support the joint.

The Axilla

The **axilla** is a four-sided pyramidally shaped region between the upper parts of the arm and lateral thoracic wall (**Fig. 14.5;** see also **Fig. 13.1A,C**).

— Its boundaries are
  • the **cervicoaxillary canal,** the narrow space between the clavicle and 1st rib, which forms the apex;
  • the axillary fascia and axillary skin between the upper arm and the lateral thoracic wall, which form the base, or floor;
  • the pectoralis major and pectoralis minor muscles, which form the anterior axillary wall (the lower edge of the pectoralis major forms a prominent ridge called the **anterior axillary fold**);
  • the subscapularis, latissimus dorsi, and teres major muscles, which form the posterior axillary wall (the lower edge of the latissimus dorsi and teres major form a prominent ridge called the **posterior axillary fold**); and
  • the lateral thoracic wall and the humerus of the arm, which form the medial and lateral walls, respectively.

— The contents of the axilla (**Fig. 14.6**), which are embedded in axillary fat, include
  • the axillary artery and its branches,
  • the axillary vein and its tributaries,
  • axillary lymph nodes and vessels, and
  • the cords and terminal nerves of the brachial plexus.

— An extension of the fascia of the neck forms a sleevelike **axillary sheath** that encloses the axillary vessels and the brachial plexus.

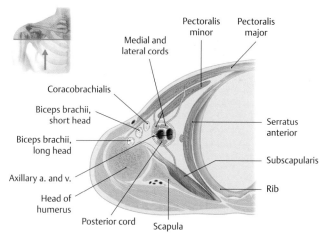

Fig. 14.5 Walls of the axilla
Right side, inferior view.

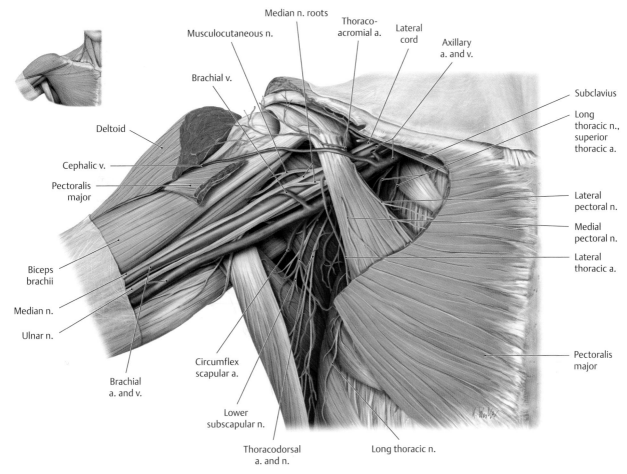

Fig. 14.6 Dissection of the axilla
Right shoulder, anterior view. *Removed*: Pectoralis major and clavipectoral fascia.

The Glenohumeral (Shoulder) Joint

The **glenohumeral joint** is a ball-and-socket type of synovial joint between the shallow glenoid cavity of the scapula and the large head of the humerus (**Figs. 14.7** and **14.8**).

— The **glenoid labrum,** a rim of fibrocartilage attached to the glenoid cavity, deepens the articular surface.

CLINICAL CORRELATION

GLENOHUMERAL DISLOCATION The glenohumeral joint is the most mobile but least stable joint of the body, and dislocations are frequent. Rotator cuff muscles provide the greatest stability, supporting the joint anteriorly, posteriorly, and superiorly, but inferior support is lacking. The coracoacromial arch, coracohumeral ligament, and capsular glenohumeral ligaments add further support. The majority of dislocations (90%) occur inferiorly, although most are labeled "anterior" dislocations based on the position of the displaced humeral head relative to the glenoid. These injuries can damage the axillary nerve and lead to a flattened shoulder profile. Posterior dislocations are rare and most often associated with seizures or electrocutions.

— A fibrous capsule, lined by a synovial membrane, surrounds the joint (**Fig. 14.9**). Ligaments that support the joint capsule include
  • anteriorly, three thickenings of the capsule, the **superior, middle,** and **inferior glenohumeral ligaments,** and

• superiorly, a **coracohumeral ligament,** that extends between the coracoid process of the scapula and lesser tubercle of the humerus.

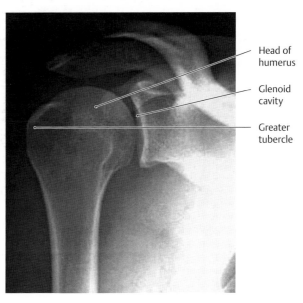

Fig. 14.7 Radiograph of the right shoulder
Anteroposterior view.

A Anterior view.

B Posterior view.

Fig. 14.8 Glenohumeral joint: bony elements
Right shoulder, anterior view.

— A synovial membrane lines the joint space (synovial cavity) **(Fig. 14.10)**.
  • It forms a tubular sheath around the tendon of the biceps brachii as the tendon passes through the joint space.
  • The synovial cavity communicates with a bursa under the subscapularis tendon (subtendinous bursa of the subscapularis).

— The **coracoacromial ligament** between the coracoid process and acromion prevents superior dislocation of the humerus.
— Three large bursae are associated with the glenohumeral joint **(Fig. 14.11)**:
  1. Anteriorly, the **subtendinous bursa of the subscapularis,** which lies between the tendon of the subscapularis and

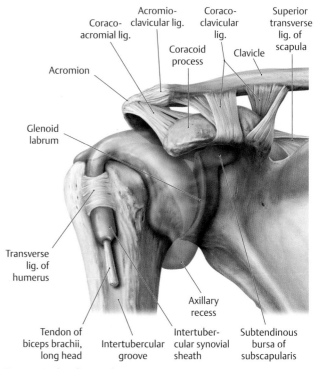

Fig. 14.9 Glenohumeral joint: capsule and ligaments
Right shoulder, anterior view.

Fig. 14.10 Glenohumeral joint cavity
Right shoulder, anterior view.

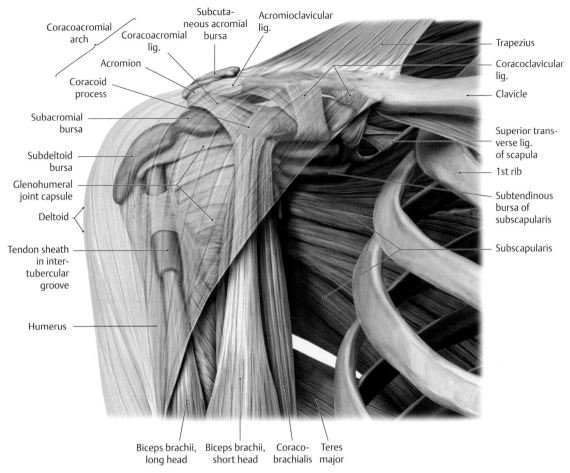

Fig. 14.11 Bursae of the shoulder region
Right shoulder, anterior view.

the neck of the scapula, communicates with the synovial cavity of the joint.

2. Superiorly, the **subacromial bursa** lies under the coracoacromial ligament and above the supraspinatus tendon and glenohumeral joint capsule.

3. Laterally, the **subdeltoid bursa** lies deep to the deltoid muscle and above the subscapularis tendon. It communicates with the subacromial bursa.

Muscles of the Shoulder Region

Muscles that cross the glenohumeral joint stabilize the head of the humerus in the glenoid cavity and assist in movements of the arm (**Tables 14.3** and **14.4**).

— Two muscles of the trunk, the **pectoralis major** and **latissimus dorsi,** extend from the axial skeleton to the humerus and together provide strong adduction and medial rotation of the arm.
  • The pectoralis major is a strong flexor of the arm.
  • The latissimus dorsi is a strong extensor of the arm.
— Scapulohumeral muscles attach the humerus to the scapula and provide stability for the glenohumeral joint.
  • The **deltoid,** which forms the rounded contour of the shoulder, abducts, flexes, and extends the arm.
  • The **teres major** adducts and medially rotates the arm.

• The **supraspinatus** initiates abduction of the arm and assists the deltoid in the first 15 degrees of movement.
• The **infraspinatus** externally rotates the arm.
• The **teres minor** externally rotates the arm.
• The **subscapularis** on the anterior surface of the scapula internally rotates the arm.

— A musculotendinous **rotator cuff** around the glenohumeral joint includes four of the scapulohumeral muscles, which are the important dynamic stabilizers of the joint.
  • The rotator cuff muscles include the **supraspinatus, infraspinatus, teres minor,** and **subscapularis.**
  • Their tendons insert on, and reinforce, the fibrous capsule of the joint, forming a supportive cuff around the anterior, posterior, and superior aspects of the joint.

CLINICAL CORRELATION

ROTATOR CUFF TEARS Rotator cuff tears can occur at any age but are most common in the older patient and usually involve the supraspinatus tendon. Degenerative changes and chronic inflammation from repetitive use (baseball pitchers are a good example) can cause the tendon to fray and rupture. When the subacromial and subdeltoid bursae tear in conjunction with the ruptured tendon, they become continuous with the cavity of the glenohumeral joint (**Fig. 14.12**).

A Pectoralis major and coracobrachialis, right side, anterior view.

B Latissimus dorsi, right side, posterior view.

C Teres major, right side, posterior view.

Table 14.3 **Shoulder Muscles**

Muscle		Origin	Insertion	Innervation	Action
Pectoralis major	① Clavicular part	Clavicle (medial half)	Humerus (crest of greater tubercle)	Medial and lateral pectoral nn. (C5–T1)	Entire muscle: adduction, internal rotation
	② Sternocostal part	Sternum and costal cartilages 1–6			Clavicular and sternocostal parts: flexion; assist in respiration when shoulder is fixed
	③ Abdominal part	Rectus sheath (anterior layer)			
④ Coracobrachialis		Scapula (coracoid process)	Humerus (in line with crest of lesser tubercle)	Musculocutaneous n. (C5–C7)	Flexion, adduction, internal rotation
Latissimus dorsi	⑤ Vertebral part	Spinous processes of T7–T12 vertebrae; thoracolumbar fascia	Floor of the intertubercular groove of the humerus	Thoracodorsal n. (C6–C8)	Internal rotation, adduction, extension, respiration ("cough muscle")
	⑥ Scapular part	Scapula (inferior angle)			
	⑦ Costal part	9th to 12th ribs			
	⑧ Iliac part	Iliac crest (posterior one third)			
⑨ Teres major		Scapula (inferior angle)	Crest of lesser tubercle of the humerus (anterior angle)	Lower subscapular n. (C5–C7)	Internal rotation, adduction, extension

— A few muscles of the arm cross the glenohumeral joint and support its movements (see **Table 14.6**).
   • The tendon of the long head of the **biceps brachii** passes through the intertubercular groove of the humerus and enters the joint cavity, where it is ensheathed by the synovial layer of the capsule. It prevents dislocation of the humerus during abduction and flexion.

   • The short head of the biceps brachii and the **coracobrachialis** muscles cross the joint anteriorly and assist in flexion of the arm.
   • The long head of the **triceps brachii** crosses the joint posteriorly and assists in adduction and extension.
— Movements at the glenohumeral joint and the muscles that provide them are listed in **Table 14.5.**

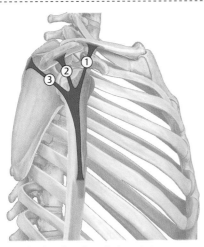

A Deltoid, right side, right lateral view.

B Rotator cuff (supraspinatus, infraspinatus, and teres minor), right shoulder, posterior view.

C Rotator cuff (subscapularis), right shoulder, anterior view.

Table 14.4 **Deltoid and Rotator Cuff Muscles**

Muscle		Origin	Insertion	Innervation	Action
Deltoid	① Clavicular part	Lateral one third of clavicle	Humerus (deltoid tuberosity)	Axillary n. (C5–C6)	Flexion, internal rotation, adduction
	② Acromial part	Acromion			Abduction
	③ Spinal part	Scapular spine			Extension, external rotation, adduction
④ Supraspinatus	Scapula	Supraspinous fossa	Humerus (greater tubercle)	Suprascapular n. (C4–C6)	Abduction
⑤ Infraspinatus		Infraspinous fossa			External rotation
⑥ Teres minor		Lateral border		Axillary n. (C5, C6)	External rotation, weak adduction
⑦ Subscapularis		Subscapular fossa	Humerus (lesser tubercle)	Subscapular n. (C5, C6)	Internal rotation

Labels on figure:
- Skin
- Subcutaneous tissue
- Trapezius
- Acromion
- Subacromial bursa
- Supraspinatus tendon
- Supraspinatus
- Head of humerus
- Glenoid cavity
- Subdeltoid bursa
- Scapula
- Subscapularis
- Glenoid labrum
- Axillary recess
- Deltoid
- Teres major
- Latissimus dorsi
- Humerus

Fig. 14.12 Coronal section through the right shoulder
Anterior view. The *arrows* are pointing at the supraspinatus tendon, which is frequently injured in a "rotator cuff tear."

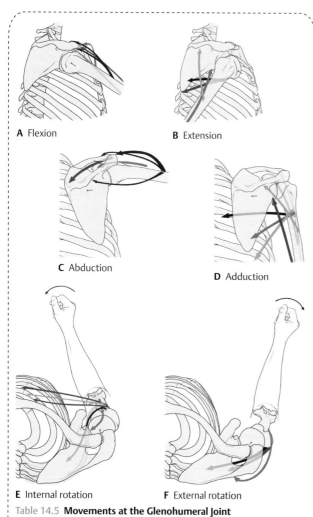

A Flexion

B Extension

C Abduction

D Adduction

E Internal rotation

F External rotation

Table 14.5 **Movements at the Glenohumeral Joint**

Action	Primary Muscles
Flexion	Deltoid (clavicular part)
	Pectoralis major (clavicular and sternocostal parts)
	Coracobrachialis
	Biceps brachii (short head)
Extension	Deltoid (spinal part)
	Latissimus dorsi
	Teres major
	Triceps brachii (long head)
Abduction	Deltoid (acromial part)
	Supraspinatus
Adduction	Deltoid (clavicular and spinal parts)
	Pectoralis major
	Latissimus dorsi
	Teres major
	Triceps brachii (long head)
Internal rotation	Deltoid (clavicular part)
	Pectoralis major (clavicular part)
	Latissimus dorsi
	Teres major
	Subscapularis
External rotation	Deltoid (spinal part)
	Infraspinatus
	Teres minor

Spaces of the Posterior Shoulder Region

Spaces formed between muscles of the shoulder and the scapula allow nerves and vessels to pass between the axilla and the posterior scapular and humeral regions (**Fig. 14.13**).

— The **scapular notch,** limited superiorly by the superior transverse scapular ligament, lies deep to the supraspinatus muscle. The suprascapular nerve passes below the ligament, and the suprascapular artery passes above it.

— The **quadrangular space,** bounded by the long head of the triceps, the humerus, and the teres major and teres minor muscles, transmits the posterior circumflex humeral artery and axillary nerve.

— The **triangular space,** bounded by the long head of the triceps and the teres major and teres minor muscles, transmits the circumflex scapular artery.

— The **triceps hiatus,** between the long and lateral heads of the triceps and below the teres major muscle, transmits the radial nerve and deep brachial artery.

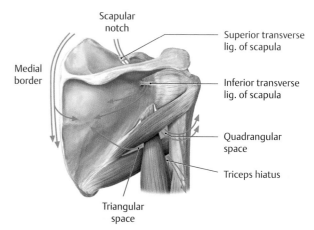

A Schematic. The course of arteries and nerves through the spaces are shown by *red* and *yellow arrows.*

Fig. 14.13 **Spaces of the posterior shoulder region**
Right shoulder, posterior view.

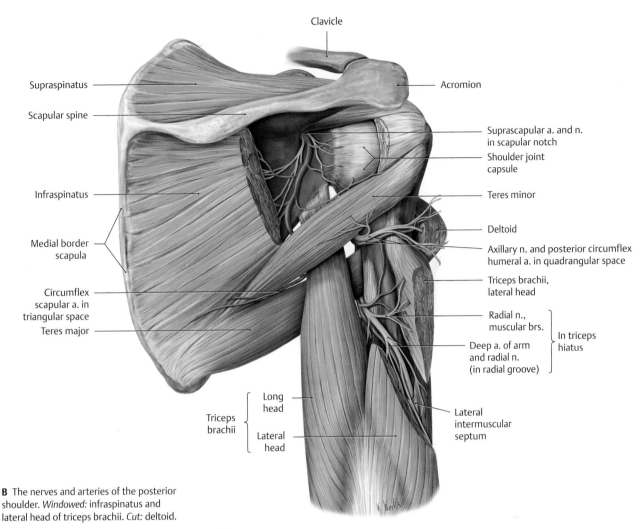

Clavicle

Supraspinatus

Scapular spine

Acromion

Suprascapular a. and n. in scapular notch

Shoulder joint capsule

Infraspinatus

Teres minor

Medial border scapula

Deltoid

Axillary n. and posterior circumflex humeral a. in quadrangular space

Triceps brachii, lateral head

Circumflex scapular a. in triangular space

Teres major

Radial n., muscular brs.

In triceps hiatus

Deep a. of arm and radial n. (in radial groove)

Long head

Lateral intermuscular septum

Triceps brachii

Lateral head

B The nerves and arteries of the posterior shoulder. *Windowed:* infraspinatus and lateral head of triceps brachii. *Cut:* deltoid.

Fig. 14.13 (*continued*) **Spaces of the posterior shoulder region**

14.3 The Arm and Cubital Region

The arm (brachial region) extends from the shoulder to the elbow and contains the humerus and muscles of the arm. The cubital region contains the cubital fossa and the elbow joint.

Muscles of the Arm

Muscles of the arm move the shoulder and elbow joints. Brachial fascia that surrounds the arm divides these muscles into anterior and posterior compartments (**Table 14.6**).

— The anterior compartment contains
  • muscles that flex the glenohumeral and elbow joints and supinate the radioulnar joint,
  • the musculocutaneous nerve, and
  • the brachial artery and vein.
— The posterior compartment contains
  • muscles that extend the glenohumeral and elbow joints,
  • the radial nerve, and
  • the deep brachial artery and vein.
— The median and ulnar nerves descend along the medial side of the arm between the anterior and posterior compartments but do not innervate muscles of the arm.

A Biceps brachii, brachialis, and corachobrachialis, right arm, anterior view.

B Triceps brachii and anconeus, right arm, posterior view.

Table 14.6 **Arm Muscles, Anterior and Posterior Compartments**

Muscle		Origin	Insertion	Innervation	Action
Anterior Compartment					
Biceps brachii	① Long head	Supraglenoid tubercle of scapula	Radial tuberosity and bicipital aponeurosis	Musculocutaneous n. (C5–C6)	Elbow joint: flexion; supination* Shoulder joint: flexion; stabilization of humeral head during deltoid contraction; abduction and internal rotation of the humerus
	② Short head	Coracoid process of scapula			
③ Brachialis		Humerus (distal half of anterior surface)	Ulnar tuberosity	Musculocutaneous n. (C5–C6) and radial n. (C7, minor)	Flexion at the elbow joint
Posterior compartment					
Triceps brachii	④ Long head	Scapula (infraglenoid tubercle)	Olecranon of ulna	Radial n. (C6–C8)	Elbow joint: extension Shoulder joint, long head: extension and adduction
	⑤ Medial head	Posterior humerus, distal to radial groove; medial intermuscular septum			
	⑥ Lateral head	Posterior humerus, proximal to radial groove; lateral intermuscular septum			
⑦ Anconeus		Lateral epicondyle of humerus (variance: posterior joint capsule)	Olecranon of ulna (radial surface)		Extends the elbow and tightens its joint

*Note: When the elbow is flexed, the biceps brachii acts as a powerful supinator because the lever arm is almost perpendicular to the axis of pronation/supination.

The Cubital Fossa

The **cubital fossa** is a shallow depression anterior to the elbow joint (**Fig. 14.14**).
— Its boundaries are,
  • medially, the pronator teres;
  • laterally, the brachioradialis; and
  • superiorly, a line that connects the medial and lateral epicondyles of the humerus.
— The cubital fossa contains

• the tendon of the biceps brachii,
• the brachial artery and vein,
• the proximal part of radial and ulnar arteries and veins, and
• the median and radial nerves and the cutaneous branch of the musculocutaneous nerve (lateral antebrachial cutaneous nerve).

— The **bicipital aponeurosis,** a fascial extension of the biceps brachii, forms the root of the fossa, and the medial cubital vein crosses the fossa superficially.

A Superficial cubital fossa. *Removed:* Fasciae and epifascial neurovascular structures.

B Deep cubital fossa. *Removed:* Biceps brachii (distal muscle belly). *Retracted:* Brachioradialis.

Fig. 14.14 Cubital region
Right elbow, anterior view.

The Elbow Joint

The elbow joint is made up of three separate synovial joints contained within a single joint capsule (**Figs. 14.15, 14.16, 14.17**).

— The hinge-type **humeroulnar joint** is an articulation between the trochlea of the humerus and the trochlear notch of the ulna.

• The **ulnar** (medial) **collateral ligament,** which supports the joint medially, connects the coronoid process and olecranon with the medial epicondyle of the humerus.

— The hinge-type **humeroradial joint** is an articulation between the capitullum of the humerus and the head of the radius.

A Anterior view.

B Posterior view.

Fig. 14.15 Elbow (cubital) joint
Right elbow in extension. The elbow consists of three articulations: the humeroulnar, humeroradial, and proximal radioulnar.

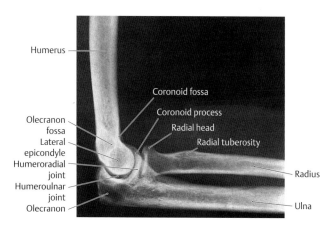

Fig. 14.16 Radiograph of the elbow
Lateral view.

- • The **radial** (lateral) **collateral ligament,** which supports the joint laterally, extends from the lateral epicondyle of the humerus to the **annular ligament** of the radius that encircles the radial neck.
- — The proximal radioulnar joint, the articulation between the head of the radius and the radial notch of the ulna, is discussed further with the radioulnar joints of the forearm.
- — Movements at the humeroulnar and humeroradial joints and the muscles that provide them are listed in **Table 14.7.**

Fig. 14.17 Joint capsule of the elbow
Right elbow in extension, anterior view.

A Flexion

B Extension

Table 14.7 **Movements at the Humeroulnar and Humeroradial Joints**

Action	Primary Muscles
Flexion	Biceps brachii
	Brachialis
	Brachioradialis
Extension	Triceps brachii

14.4   The Forearm

The forearm (antebrachial region) extends from the elbow to the wrist and contains the radius and ulna and the muscles of the forearm.

Radioulnar Joints

The radioulnar joints connect the bones of the forearm proximally at the elbow and distally at the wrist. Movement at these joints allows rotation of the distal radius around the ulna, causing supination (palm up) and pronation (palm down) of the hand (**Figs. 14.18** and **14.19**). These movements and the muscles of the arm and forearm that provide them are listed in **Table 14.8.**

- — The **proximal radioulnar joint** is a synovial joint that allows rotation of the radial head within the cuff formed by the anular ligament and the radial notch of the ulna. This articulation is contained within the elbow joint capsule.
- — The **distal radioulnar joint** has an L-shaped joint cavity with a triangular articular disk that separates the radioulnar joint from the cavity of the wrist joint. It is supported by palmar and dorsal radioulnar ligaments.
- — An **interosseous membrane** connects the shafts of the radius and ulna and transfers energy absorbed by the distal radius to the proximal ulna.

Fig. 14.18 Forearm in supination
Right forearm, anterior view.

Fig. 14.19 Forearm in pronation
Right forearm, anterior view.

A Supination   B Pronation

Table 14.8 **Movements at the Radioulnar Joints**

Action	Primary Muscles
Supination	Supinator
	Biceps brachii
Pronation	Pronator teres
	Pronator quadratus

A The upward pull on a child's arm can cause the immature head of the radius to slip under the anular ligament.

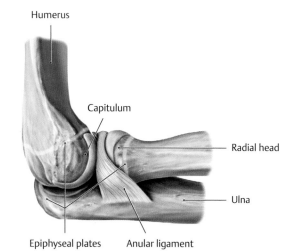

Humerus

Capitulum

Radial head

Ulna

Epiphyseal plates   Anular ligament

B The anular ligament caught between the radius and capitulum.

Fig. 14.20 Nursemaid's elbow

Muscles of the Forearm

Muscles of the forearm move joints of the elbow, wrist, and hand. Most forearm flexors and extensors have long tendons that cross the wrist and extend into the fingers. Intermuscular septa and the interosseous membrane create anterior and posterior muscular compartments.

— The anterior forearm compartment **(Table 14.9)** contains
  • muscles that flex and pronate joints of the elbow, wrist, and hand;
  • the median and ulnar nerves; and
  • the ulnar and anterior interosseous arteries and veins.
— The posterior forearm compartment **(Table 14.10)** contains
  • muscles that extend joints of the elbow, wrist, and hand and supinate the radioulnar joint (one muscle, the brachioradialis, passes anterior to the elbow and therefore acts as a flexor, instead of an extensor of this joint);
  • the radial nerve; and
  • the radial and posterior interosseous arteries and veins.

CLINICAL CORRELATION

SUBLUXATION OF THE RADIAL HEAD (NURSEMAID'S ELBOW) In young children the immature radial head can be subluxated when the child's arm is jerked upward. The head of the radius can slip under the anular ligament, which can get trapped between the radius and capitulum. The injured arm is held in a flexed and pronated position. Supination of the flexed elbow returns the joint to the correct orientation **(Fig. 14.20)**.

CLINICAL CORRELATION

LATERAL EPICONDYLITIS Repetitive use of the forearm extensors can inflame the attachment of the common extensor tendon at the lateral epicondyle (lateral epicondylitis). Pain is focused over the tendon insertion but radiates along the extensor forearm and is exacerbated by stretching of the extensor tendons by pronation and wrist flexion.

A Superficial muscles of anterior compartment of forearm.

Humeral-ulnar head

Radial head

B Intermediate muscle of anterior compartment of forearm.

C Deep muscles of anterior compartment of forearm.

Table 14.9 **Forearm Muscles, Anterior Compartment**

Muscle	Origin	Insertion	Innervation	Action
Superficial muscles				
① Pronator teres	Humeral head: medial epicondyle of humerus Ulnar head: coronoid process	Lateral radius (distal to supinator insertion)	Median n. (C6, C7)	Elbow: weak flexion Forearm: pronation
② Flexor carpi radialis	Medial epicondyle of humerus	Base of 2nd metacarpal (variance: base of 3rd metacarpal)		Wrist: flexion and abduction (radial deviation) of hand
③ Palmaris longus		Palmar aponeurosis	Median n. (C7, C8)	Elbow: weak flexion Wrist: flexion tightens palmar aponeurosis
④ Flexor carpi ulnaris	Humeral head: medial epicondyle Ulnar head: olecranon	Pisiform; hook of hamate; base of 5th metacarpal	Ulnar n. (C7–T1)	Wrist: flexion and adduction (ulnar deviation) of hand
Intermediate muscles				
⑤ Flexor digitorum superficialis	Humeral-ulnar head: medial epicondyle of humerus and coronoid process of ulna Radial head: upper half of anterior border of radius	Sides of middle phalanges of 2nd to 5th digits	Median n. (C8, T1)	Elbow: weak flexion Wrist, MCP, and PIP joints of 2nd to 5th digits: flexion
Deep muscles				
⑥ Flexor digitorum profundus	Ulna (proximal two thirds of flexor surface) and interosseous membrane	Distal phalanges of 2nd to 5th digits (palmar surface)	Median n. (C8, T1, radial half of fingers 2 and 3) Ulnar n. (C8, T1, radial half of fingers 4 and 5)	Wrist, MCP, PIP, and DIP of 2nd to 5th digits: flexion
⑦ Flexor pollicis longus	Radius (midanterior surface) and adjacent interosseous membrane	Distal phalanx of thumb (palmar surface)	Median n. (C8, T1)	Wrist: flexion and abduction (radial deviation) of hand Carpometacarpal of thumb: flexion MCP and IP of thumb: flexion
⑧ Pronator quadratus	Distal quarter of ulna (anterior surface)	Distal quarter of radius (anterior surface)		Hand: pronation Distal radioulnar joint: stabilization

Abbreviations: DIP, distal interphalangeal; IP, interphalangeal; MCP, metacarpophalangeal; PIP, proximal interphalangeal.

A Superficial muscles of posterior compartment of forearm.

B Deep muscles of posterior compartment of forearm.

C Radialis muscle group of posterior compartment of forearm.

Table 14.10 **Forearm Muscles, Posterior Compartment**

Muscle	Origin	Insertion	Innervation	Action
Superficial muscles				
① Extensor digitorum	Common head (lateral epicondyle of humerus)	Dorsal digital expansion of 2nd to 5th digits	Radial n. (C7, C8)	Wrist: extension MCP, PIP, and DIP of 2nd to 5th digits: extension/abduction of fingers
② Extensor digiti minimi		Dorsal digital expansion of 5th digit		Wrist: extension, ulnar abduction of hand MCP, PIP, and DIP of 5th digit: extension and abduction of 5th digit
③ Extensor carpi ulnaris	Common head (lateral epicondyle of humerus) Ulnar head (dorsal surface)	Base of 5th metacarpal		Wrist: extension, adduction (ulnar deviation) of hand
Deep muscles				
④ Supinator	Olecranon, lateral epicondyle of humerus, radial collateral ligament, annular ligament of radius	Radius (between radial tuberosity and insertion of pronator teres)	Radial n. (C6, C7)	Radioulnar joints: supination
⑤ Abductor pollicis longus	Radius and ulna (dorsal surfaces, interosseous membrane)	Base of 1st metacarpal	Radial n. (C7, C8)	Radiocarpal joint: abduction of the hand Carpometacarpal joint of thumb: abduction
⑥ Extensor pollicis brevis	Radius (posterior surface) and interosseous membrane	Base of proximal phalanx of thumb		Radiocarpal joint: abduction (radial deviation) of hand Carpometacarpal and MCP of thumb: extension
⑦ Extensor pollicis longus	Ulna (posterior surface) and interosseous membrane	Base of distal phalanx of thumb		Wrist: extension and abduction (radial deviation) of hand Carpometacarpal of thumb: adduction MCP and IP of thumb: extension
⑧ Extensor indicis	Ulna (posterior surface) and interosseous membrane	Posterior digital extension of 2nd digit		Wrist: extension MCP, PIP, and DIP of 2nd digit: extension
Radialis muscles				
⑨ Brachioradialis	Distal humerus (distal surface), lateral intermuscular septum	Styloid process of the radius	Radial n. (C5, C6)	Elbow: flexion Forearm: semipronation
⑩ Extensor carpi radialis longus	Lateral supracondylar ridge of distal humerus, lateral intermuscular septum	2nd metacarpal (base)	Radial n. (C6, C7)	Elbow: weak flexion Wrist: extension and abduction
⑪ Extensor carpi radialis brevis	Lateral epicondyle of humerus	3rd metacarpal (base)	Radial n. (C7, C8)	

Abbreviations: DIP, distal interphalangeal; IP, interphalangeal; MCP, metacarpophalangeal; PIP, proximal interphalangeal.

14.5   The Wrist

The wrist, the narrow space between the forearm and hand, contains the carpal bones and the tendons of forearm muscles that move the wrist and fingers.

Joints of the Wrist

Joints of the wrist include the articulations between the distal radius and bones of the proximal row of carpals and the articulations between adjacent carpal bones **(Fig. 14.21)**. Movements at the wrist joints and the muscles that provide them are listed in **Table 14.11.**

- The **radiocarpal joint** is an articulation of the distal radius and articular disk of the distal radioulnar joint with the scaphoid and lunate.
  - Palmar and dorsal radiocarpal ligaments and radial and ulnar collateral ligaments strengthen the joint.
- **Intercarpal joints** are the articulations between the carpal bones within each row; the **midcarpal joint** is the articulation between the bones of the proximal and distal carpal rows.
  - Movements at these joints augment movements at the wrist joint.

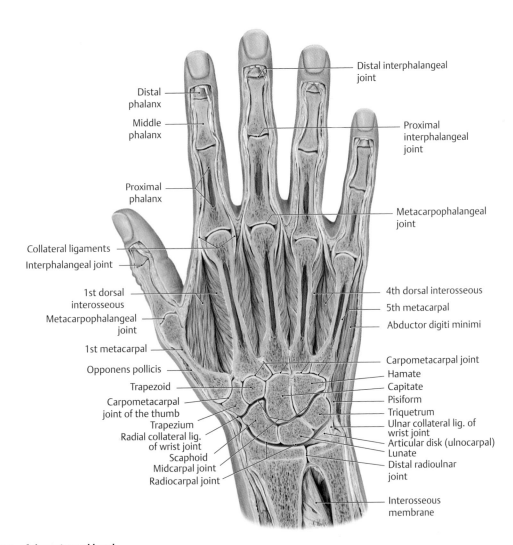

Fig. 14.21 Joints of the wrist and hand
Right hand, posterior (dorsal) view.

A Flexion

B Extension

C Abduction (radial deviation)   **D** Adduction (ulnar deviation)

Table 14.11 **Movements at the Wrist Joints**

Action	Primary Muscles
Flexion	Flexor carpi radialis
	Flexor carpi ulnaris
Extension	Extensor carpi radialis longus
	Extensor carpi radialis brevis
	Extensor carpi ulnaris
Abduction (radial deviation)	Flexor carpi radialis
	Extensor carpi radialis longus
	Extensor carpi radialis brevis
Adduction (ulnar deviation)	Flexor carpi ulnaris
	Extensor carpi ulnaris

Spaces of the Wrist

Neurovascular structures and the long tendons of the forearm muscles pass between the forearm and hand through narrow spaces that are usually defined by fascial thickenings.

— The **carpal tunnel** is a fascio-osseous space on the anterior wrist.
  • Carpal bones form the floor and sides; the flexor retinaculum forms the roof (**Fig. 14.22**).
  • The tendons of the flexor pollicis longus, flexor digitorum superficialis, and flexor digitorum profundus, and the median nerve pass through the tunnel (**Fig. 14.23**).
  • **A common flexor synovial tendon sheath** encloses the flexor tendons as they pass through the carpal tunnel.
  • The palmar carpal ligament and flexor retinaculum prevent bowing of the flexor tendons as they cross the wrist.
— The **ulnar tunnel** (Guyon's canal) is a narrow passageway on the medial side of the anterior wrist (**Figs. 14.24 and 14.25;** see **Fig. 14.23B**).

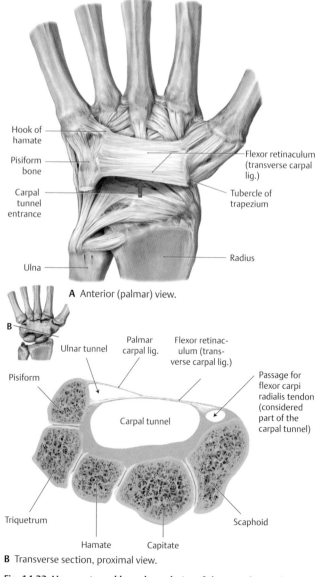

A Anterior (palmar) view.

B Transverse section, proximal view.

Fig. 14.22 **Ligaments and bony boundaries of the carpal tunnel**
Right hand.

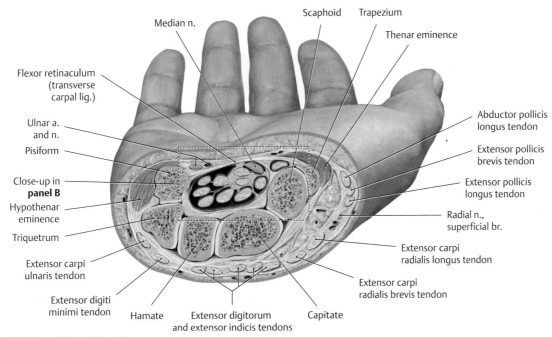

A Cross section through the right wrist.

B Blowup of area enclosed by *dashed lines* in **A**. Structures in the ulnar tunnel *(green)* and carpal tunnel *(blue)*.

Fig. 14.23 Contents within the carpal tunnel
Right hand, proximal view. The tight fit of sensitive neurovascular structures with closely apposed, frequently moving tendons in the carpal tunnel often causes problems (carpal tunnel syndrome) when any of the structures swell or degenerate.

CLINICAL CORRELATION

CARPAL TUNNEL SYNDROME The carpal tunnel, defined by inflexible fibrous and osseous boundaries, can be compromised by the swelling of its contents, infiltration of fluid from inflammation or infection, protrusion of a dislocated carpal bone, or pressure from an external source. The median nerve is most sensitive to the increased pressure, and signs of carpal tunnel syndrome reflect the nerve's distribution. These include tingling or numbness on the palmar surface of the lateral three and a half digits and weakness and eventual atrophy of the thenar muscles. The palmar cutaneous branch of the median nerve arises proximal to the canal and passes over the flexor retinaculum, so sensation of the palm remains intact.

- The flexor retinaculum forms the floor, and the **palmar carpal ligament** forms the roof. The pisiform and hamate form the medial and lateral borders.
- The ulnar artery and nerve pass through the tunnel into the palm of the hand.

CLINICAL CORRELATION

ULNAR NERVE COMPRESSION Compression of the ulnar nerve at the wrist affects the innervation of most intrinsic hand muscles. When the patient attempts to form a fist, it results in a deformity known as a "claw hand"—the metacarpophalangeal joints are hyperextended due to the loss of the interossei muscles, and the interphalangeal joints are flexed.

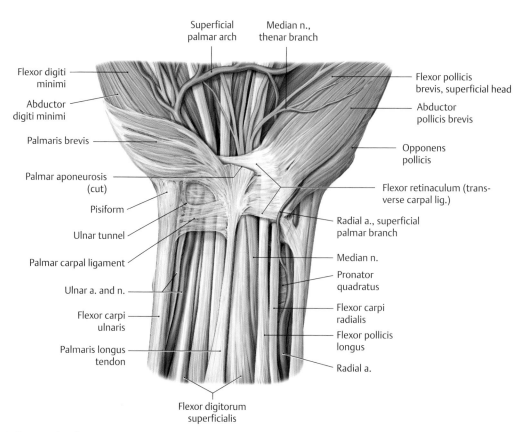

Fig. 14.24 Anterior carpal region
Right hand, anterior (palmar) view. Ulnar tunnel and deep palm. Carpal tunnel with flexor retinaculum transparent. *Removed:* Palmaris brevis, palmaris longus, palmar aponeurosis, and palmarcarpal ligament.

— The **anatomic snuffbox** is a small triangular depression on the radial side of the dorsum of the wrist (**Fig. 14.26**).
  • Tendons of the extensor pollicis longus, extensor pollicis brevis, and abductor pollicis longus form the borders. The scaphoid and trapezium form its floor.
  • The radial artery passes through the snuffbox.
  • The cephalic vein and superficial branch of the radial nerve cross the snuffbox superficially.
— Six small **dorsal compartments** (designated as 1st through 6th) form on the posterior surface of the wrist (**Table 14.12; Fig. I4.27**).
  • The extensor retinaculum forms their roof, and the dorsal surfaces of the distal radius and ulna form their floor.
  • Extensor tendons of forearm muscles pass through the compartments onto the dorsum of the hand.
  • **Dorsal carpal synovial tendon sheaths** enclose the extensor tendons as they pass through the dorsal compartments.

Fig. 14.25 Apertures and walls of the ulnar tunnel
Right hand, anterior (palmar) view.

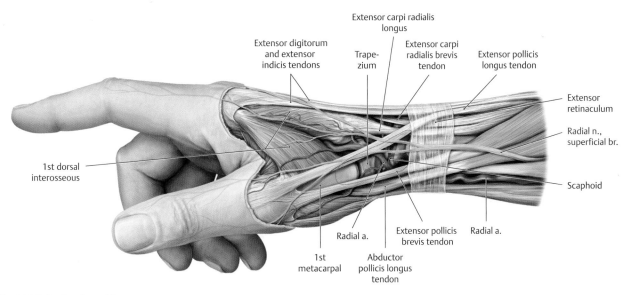

Fig. 14.26 Anatomic snuffbox
Right hand, radial view. The three-sided "anatomic snuffbox" *(shaded light yellow)* is bounded by the tendons of insertion of the abductor pollicis longus and the extensor pollicis brevis and extensor pollicis longus.

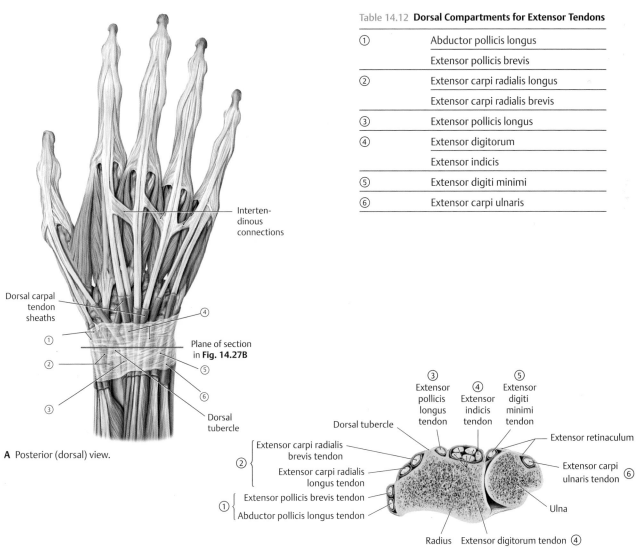

Table 14.12	**Dorsal Compartments for Extensor Tendons**
①	Abductor pollicis longus
	Extensor pollicis brevis
②	Extensor carpi radialis longus
	Extensor carpi radialis brevis
③	Extensor pollicis longus
④	Extensor digitorum
	Extensor indicis
⑤	Extensor digiti minimi
⑥	Extensor carpi ulnaris

A Posterior (dorsal) view.

B Proximal view of section indicated in **A**.

Fig. 14.27 Extensor retinaculum and dorsal compartments
Right hand.

14.6   The Hand

The muscles and joints of the hand create a flexible tool that is adept at fine motor movements. The ability to grasp objects by positioning the thumb in opposition to the other fingers is a feature that is unique to humans and apes.

Joints of the Hand and Fingers

Joints of the hand and fingers are the articulations between the distal carpal bones and proximal end of the metacarpal bones of the palms, the distal end of the metacarpal bones and the proximal phalanges, and between the proximal, middle, and distal phalanges of each digit (see **Fig. 14.20**). Movements at these joints and the muscles of the forearm and hand that provide them are listed in **Tables 14.13** and **14.14.**

— **Carpometacarpal joints** are the synovial articulations between the distal row of carpal bones and the metacarpals.
  • Little or no movement occurs at the plane-type joints of the 2nd, 3rd, and 4th digits.
  • The joint of the 5th digit between the metacarpus and the hamate is moderately mobile.
  • The saddle-type joint between the metacarpus of the thumb and the trapezium in the distal carpal row allows movement in all directions, which is essential for thumb opposition **(Fig. 14.28)**.
— **Metacarpophalangeal (MCP) joints** are condyloid synovial joints between the heads of the metacarpals and bases of the proximal phalanges.
  • Movement in two planes, flexion-extension and abduction-adduction, occurs in digits 2 through 5.
  • Only flexion and extension occur at the MCP joint of the thumb.
— **Interphalangeal (IP) joints** are hinge-type synovial joints between phalanges.
  • Digits 2 through 4 have proximal interphalangeal (PIP) and distal interphalangeal (DIP) joints.

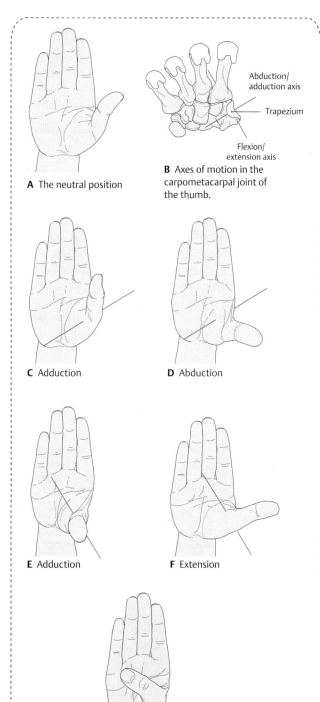

A The neutral position

B Axes of motion in the carpometacarpal joint of the thumb.

C Adduction   **D** Abduction

E Adduction   **F** Extension

G Opposition

Table 14.13 **Movements at the Joints of the Fingers (Digits 2 through 5)**

Action	Primary Muscles
Flexion at MCP	Lumbricals Palmer and dorsal interossei Flexor digiti minimi (only 5th digit)
Flexion at DIP	Flexor digitorum profundus
Flexion at PIP	Flexor digitorum profundus Flexor digitorum superficialis
Extension at MCP	Extensor digitorum Extensor indicis (only 2nd digit) Extensor digiti minimi (only 5th digit)
Extension at DIP and PIP	Lumbricals Palmer and dorsal interossei
Abduction at MCP	Dorsal interossei Abductor digiti minimi (only 5th digit)
Adduction	Palmer interossei (digits 2, 4, and 5 only)
Opposition	Opponens digiti minimi (only 5th digit)

Abbreviations: DIP, distal interphalangeal; MCP, metacarpophalangeal; PIP, proximal interphalangeal.

Table 14.14 **Movements at Joints of the Thumb**

Action	Primary Muscles
Flexion	Flexor pollicis longus Flexor pollicis brevis
Extension	Extensor pollicis longus Extensor pollicis brevis
Abduction	Abductor pollicis longus Abductor pollicis brevis
Adduction	Adductor pollicis
Opposition	Opponens pollicis

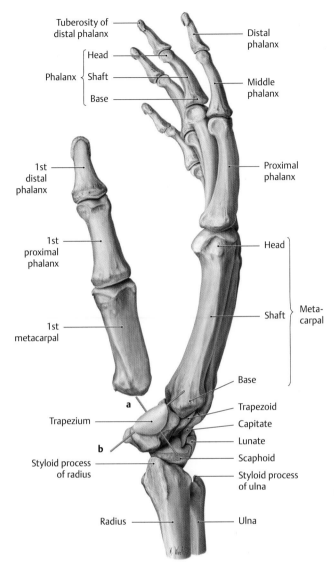

Fig. 14.28 **Carpometacarpal joint of the thumb**
Radial view. The 1st metacarpal bone has been moved slightly distally to expose the articular surface of the trapezium. Two cardinal axes of motion are shown here: *a*, abduction/adduction; and *b*, flexion/extension.

- The thumb has only a single IP joint.
- IP joints permit only flexion and extension.
— MCP and IP joints are surrounded by a fibrous capsule and supported by medial and lateral collateral ligaments.

The Dorsum of the Hand and Fingers

— The dorsum of the hand has the following surface anatomy (**Fig. 14.29**):
  - The skin is thin and loose.
  - A prominent superficial dorsal venous network gives rise to the cephalic and basilic veins.

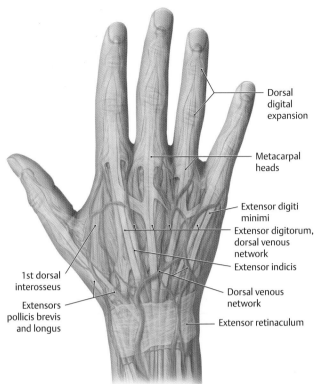

Fig. 14.29 **Surface anatomy of the dorsum of the hand**
Right hand.

- The heads of the metacarpals of the 2nd through 5th digits form distinct "knuckles" when the hand is flexed into a fist.
- The extensor tendons fan out from the wrist to the fingers.
— On the dorsum of the fingers, the long extensor tendons (of the posterior forearm compartment) flatten to form a **dorsal digital expansion** (extensor expansion, extensor hood), a triangular tendinous aponeurosis (**Fig. 14.30**). The dorsal digital expansion
  - forms a hood that wraps around the sides of the distal metacarpus and proximal phalanx and holds the extensor tendon in place;
  - inserts onto the middle and distal phalanges via a **central slip** and paired **lateral bands;** and
  - is reinforced by the lumbricals and interossei muscles of the palm, which connect to the lateral bands and assist in extension of the interphalangeal joints of the fingers.

CLINICAL CORRELATION

EXTENSOR TENDON RUPTURE Traumatic finger injuries can cause tendon ruptures that result in a variety of deformities. Rupture of the extensor tendon at the distal phalanx prohibits extension of the distal interphalangeal (DIP) joint. The unopposed action of the flexor digitorum profundus produces the characteristic "mallet finger" deformity in which the distal phalanx remains flexed.

A Posterior view.

Fig. 14.30 Dorsal digital expansion
Right hand, middle finger, posterior view. The dorsal digital expansion permits the long digital flexors and the short muscles of the hand to act on all three finger joints.

The Palm of the Hand and Fingers

— The palm of the hand has the following surface anatomy (**Fig. 14.31**):
  • The skin is thickened, firmly attached to the underlying fascia, and supplied with numerous sweat glands.
  • A central concavity separates a **thenar eminence** at the base of the thumb from a **hypothenar eminence** at the base of the 5th digit.
  • Longitudinal and transverse **flexion creases** form where the skin is tightly bound to the palmar fascia.
— Deep fascia over the central palm forms a tough, thickened palmar aponeurosis (**Fig. 14.32**), which
  • firmly adheres to the skin of the palm,
  • is continuous proximally with the flexor retinaculum and palmaris longus muscle, and
  • is continuous distally with a **transverse metacarpal ligament** and the four digital fibrous sheaths of the fingers that surround the long flexor tendons and their synovial digital tendon sheaths.
— The palmar aponeurosis and deep palmar fascia divide the palm into five muscular compartments (**Tables 14.15, 14.16, 14.17**):
  1. The **thenar compartment,** which contains thenar muscles that abduct, flex, and oppose the thumb.

  2. The **central compartment,** which contains forearm flexor tendons that flex the fingers and lumbricals that flex and extend joints of the fingers.
  3. The hypothenar **compartment,** which contains hypothenar muscles that flex, abduct, and oppose the 5th digit.
  4. The **adductor compartment,** which contains the adductor pollicis muscle that adducts the thumb.
  5. The interosseous **compartment,** which contains interossei muscles that abduct and adduct the fingers.
— **Thenar** and **midpalmar spaces** are potential spaces deep within the palm between the long flexor tendons and the fascia over the deep palmar muscles. The midpalmar space is continuous with the anterior forearm compartment through the carpal tunnel.

CLINICAL CORRELATION

DUPUYTREN'S DISEASE Dupuytren's disease is the progressive fibrosis and contracture of the longitudinal bands of the palmar fascia to the 4th and 5th digits, causing flexion of these fingers. It presents as painless nodular thickenings that progress to raised ridges on the palm. Surgical excision is usually required to release the bands.

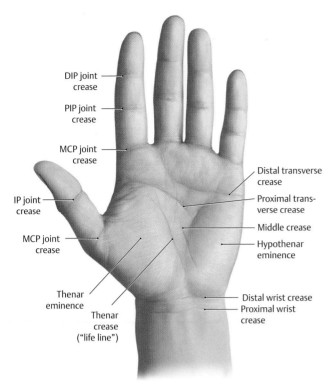

Fig. 14.31 Surface anatomy of the palm of the hand
Left hand. DIP, distal interphalangeal; IP, interphalangeal; MCP, meta-carpophalangeal; PIP, proximal interphalangeal.

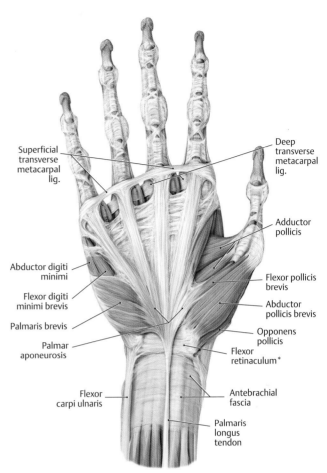

Fig. 14.32 Palmar aponeurosis
Right hand, palmar surface.
*Also known as transverse carpal ligament.

— On the palmar surface of the fingers
  • tendons of the flexor digitorum superficialis (FDS) split into two bands that insert on the middle phalanx,
  • tendons of the flexor digitorum profundus pass between the bands of the FDS to insert on the distal phalanx, and
  • **synovial tendon sheaths** surround the flexor tendons as they enter the **fibrous tendon sheaths** of the fingers.
    ◦ The digital synovial sheath of the 5th digit normally communicates with the common flexor sheath at the wrist.
    ◦ The synovial sheath of the thumb extends into the wrist and may communicate with the sheath of the 5th digit and with the common synovial sheath.
    ◦ The synovial sheaths of the 2nd, 3rd, and 4th digits usually remain independent from the common synovial sheath and other digital synovial sheaths.
— Muscles of the forearm and intrinsic muscles of the hand move the joints of the hand and fingers (see **Tables 14.13** and **14.14**).

CLINICAL CORRELATION

TENOSYNOVITIS A puncture wound of the finger can initiate an infection in the digital synovial sheaths (tenosynovitis). Swelling of the tissue is painful and inhibits movement. Although synovial sheath connections vary, sheaths of the 2nd, 3rd, and 4th digits are usually independent and can confine the infection to that digit (unless the sheath ruptures). The sheath of the 5th digit, however, normally communicates with the common synovial sheath in the palm and wrist. Infection can track via this route through the carpal tunnel and into the anterior compartment. Likewise, infection in the thumb can track into the wrist and palm.

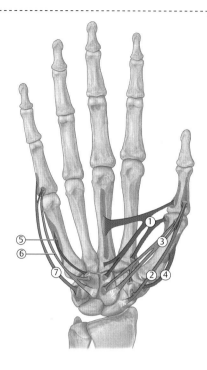

Thenar and hypothenar muscles, right hand, anterior (palmar) view.

Table 14.15 **Thenar Muscles**

Muscle	Origin	Insertion	Innervation	Action
① Adductor pollicis	Transverse head: 3rd metacarpal (palmar surface)	Thumb (base of proximal phalanx) via the ulnar sesamoid	Ulnar n. (C8, T1)	CMC joint of thumb: adduction
	Oblique head: capitate bone, 2nd and 3rd metacarpals (bases)			MCP joint of thumb: flexion
② Abductor pollicis brevis	Scaphoid bone and trapezium, flexor retinaculum	Thumb (base of proximal phalanx) via the radial sesamoid	Median n. (C8, T1)	CMC joint of thumb: abduction
③ Flexor pollicis brevis	Superficial head: flexor retinaculum		Superficial head: median n. (C8, T1)	CMC joint of thumb: flexion
	Deep head: capitate bone, trapezium		Deep head: ulnar n. (C8, T1)	
④ Opponens pollicis	Trapezium	1st metacarpal (radial border)	Median n. (C8, T1)	CMC joint of thumb: opposition

Abbreviations: CMC, carpometacarpal; MCP, metacarpophalangeal.

Table 14.16 **Hypothenar Muscles**

Muscle	Origin	Insertion	Innervation	Action
⑤ Opponens digiti minimi	Hook of hamate, flexor retinaculum	5th metacarpal (ulnar border)	Ulnar n. (C8, T1)	Draws metacarpal in palmar direction (opposition)
⑥ Flexor digiti minimi brevis		5th proximal phalanx (base)		MCP joint of little finger: flexion
⑦ Abductor digiti minimi	Pisiform bone	5th proximal phalanx (ulnar base) and dorsal digital expansion of 5th digit		MCP joint of little finger: flexion and abduction of little finger. PIP and DIP joints of little finger: extension
Palmaris brevis	Palmar aponeurosis (ulnar border)	Skin of hypothenar eminence		Tightens the palmar aponeurosis (protective function)

Abbreviations: DIP, distal inteiphalangeal; MCP, metacarpophalangeal; PIP, proximal inteiphalangeal.

A Lumbricals, right hand, palmar view.　　**B** Dorsal interossei, right hand, palmar view.　　**C** Palmar interossei, right hand, palmar view.

Table 14.17 **Metacarpal Muscles**

Muscle Group	Muscle	Origin	Insertion	Innervation	Action
Lumbricals	① 1st	Tendons of flexor digitorum profundus (radial sides)	2nd digit (dde)	Median n. (C8–T1)	2nd to 5th digits: • MCP joints: flexion • Proximal and distal IP joints: extension
	② 2nd		3rd digit (dde)		
	③ 3rd	Tendons of flexor digitorum profundus (bipennate from medial and lateral sides)	4th digit (dde)	Ulnar n. (C8–T1)	
	④ 4th		5th digit (dde)		
Dorsal interossei	⑤ 1st	1st and 2nd metacarpals (adjacent sides, two heads)	2nd digit (dde) 2nd proximal phalanx (radial side)		2nd to 4th digits: • MCP joints: flexion • Proximal and distal IP joints: extension and abduction from 3rd digit
	⑥ 2nd	2nd and 3rd metacarpals (adjacent sides, two heads)	3rd digit (dde) 3rd proximal phalanx (radial side)		
	⑦ 3rd	3rd and 4th metacarpals (adjacent sides, two heads)	3rd digit (dde) 3rd proximal phalanx (ulnar side)		
	⑧ 4th	4th and 5th metacarpals (adjacent sides, two heads)	4th digit (dde) 4th proximal phalanx (ulnar side)		
Palmar interossei	⑨ 1st	2nd metacarpal (ulnar side)	2nd digit (dde) 2nd proximal phalanx (base)		2nd to 4th, and 5th digits: • MCP joints: flexion • Proximal and distal IP joints: extension and abduction from 3rd digit
	⑩ 2nd	4th metacarpal (radial side)	4th digit (dde) 4th proximal phalanx (base)		
	⑪ 3rd	5th metacarpal (radial side)	5th digit (dde) 5th proximal phalanx (base)		

Abbreviations: dde, dorsal digital expansion; IP, inteiphalangeal; MCP, metacarpophalangeal.

14.7   Topographic Views of Upper Limb Musculature

Shoulder and Arm

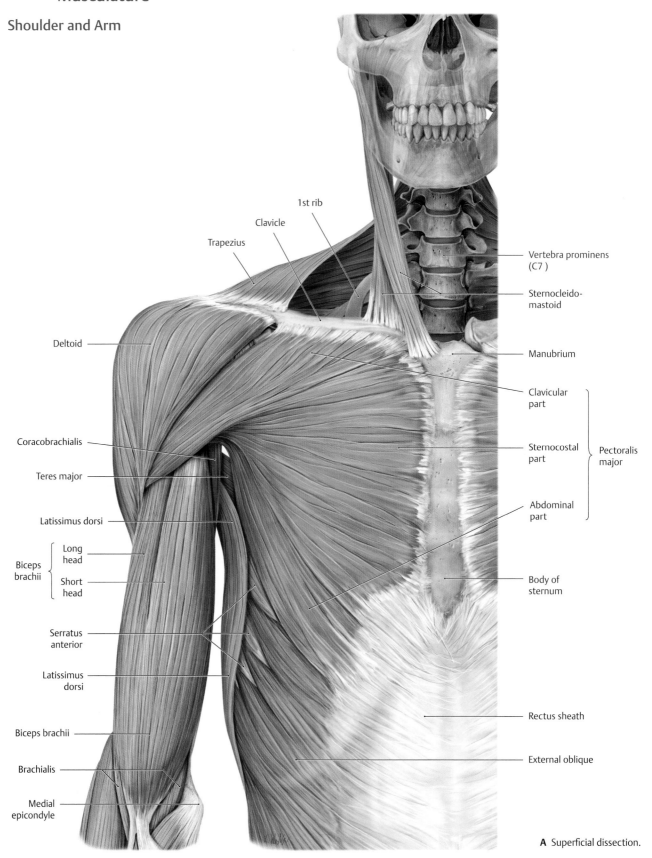

1st rib

Clavicle

Trapezius

Deltoid

Coracobrachialis

Teres major

Latissimus dorsi

Biceps brachii {
Long head

Short head

Serratus anterior

Latissimus dorsi

Biceps brachii

Brachialis

Medial epicondyle

Vertebra prominens (C7)

Sternocleido-mastoid

Manubrium

Clavicular part

Sternocostal part

Pectoralis major

Abdominal part

Body of sternum

Rectus sheath

External oblique

A Superficial dissection.

Fig. 14.33 Anterior shoulder muscles
Right side, anterior view. Muscle origins are shown in *red*, insertions in *gray*

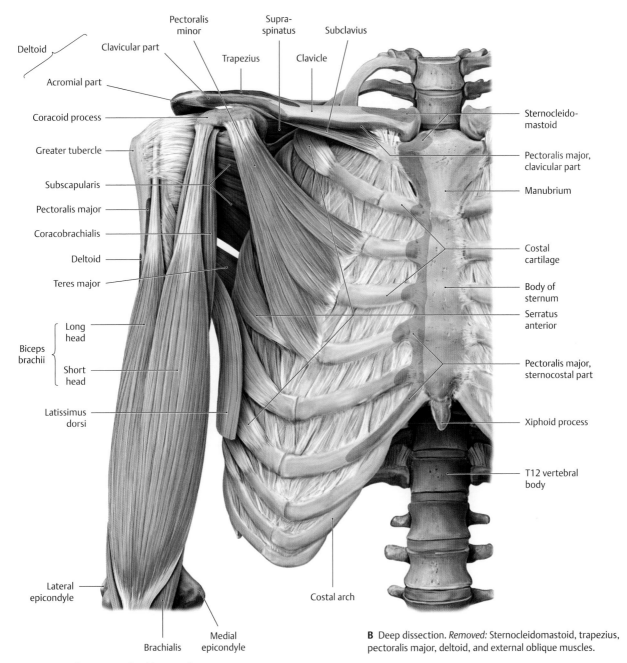

Fig. 14.33 (*continued*) **Anterior shoulder muscles**

B Deep dissection. *Removed:* Sternocleidomastoid, trapezius, pectoralis major, deltoid, and external oblique muscles.

Semispinalis
capitis

Sternocleidomastoid

Splenius
capitis

Descending
part

Trapezius

Transverse
part

Scapular spine

Deltoid

Ascending
part

Teres major

Long
head

Triceps
brachii

Lateral
head

Latissimus
dorsi

Extensor carpi
radialis brevis

Extensor carpi
radialis longus

Olecranon

Anconeus

External
oblique

Thoracolumbar
fascia

Flexor
carpi ulnaris

Extensor
carpi ulnaris

Extensor
digitorum

Iliac
crest

Internal
oblique

A Superficial dissection.

Fig. 14.34 Posterior shoulder muscles
Right side, posterior view.

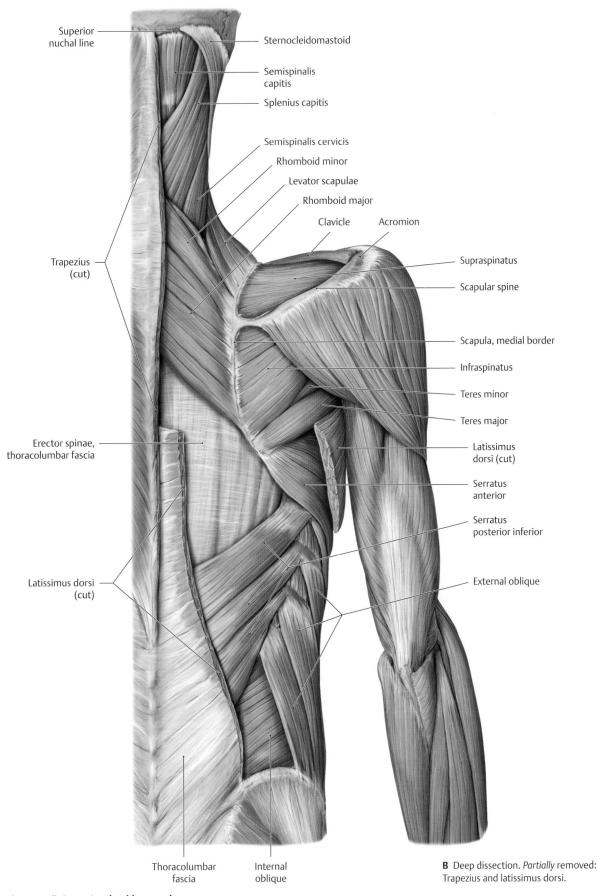

Fig. 14.34 (*continued*) **Posterior shoulder muscles**

B Deep dissection. *Partially* removed:
Trapezius and latissimus dorsi.

Forearm and Wrist

Biceps brachii

Biceps brachii tendon

Brachioradialis

Extensor carpi radialis longus

Extensor carpi radialis brevis

Flexor pollicis longus

Abductor pollicis longus

Flexor pollicis longus tendon

Triceps brachii

Brachialis

Medial epicondyle, common head of flexors

Bicipital aponeurosis

Pronator teres

Flexor carpi radialis

Palmaris longus

Flexor carpi ulnaris

Flexor digitorum superficialis

Palmaris longus

Flexor digitorum superficialis tendons

Flexor digitorum profundus tendons

Fig. 14.35 Anterior forearm muscles
Right forearm, anterior view. Muscle origins are shown in *red*, insertions in *gray*.
Superficial flexors and radialis group.

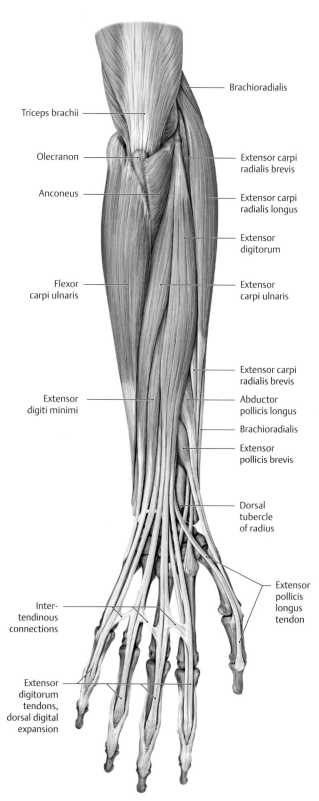

Triceps brachii

Olecranon

Anconeus

Flexor carpi ulnaris

Extensor digiti minimi

Inter-tendinous connections

Extensor digitorum tendons, dorsal digital expansion

Brachioradialis

Extensor carpi radialis brevis

Extensor carpi radialis longus

Extensor digitorum

Extensor carpi ulnaris

Extensor carpi radialis brevis

Abductor pollicis longus

Brachioradialis

Extensor pollicis brevis

Dorsal tubercle of radius

Extensor pollicis longus tendon

Fig. 14.36 Posterior forearm muscles
Right forearm, posterior view. Muscle origins are shown in *red*, insertions in *gray*.
Superficial extensors and radialis group.

Hand

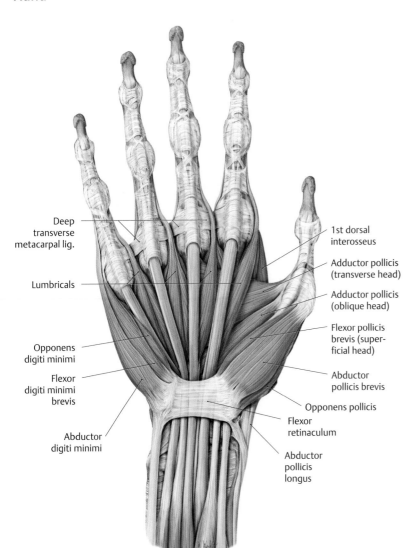

Deep transverse metacarpal lig.

Lumbricals

Opponens digiti minimi

Flexor digiti minimi brevis

Abductor digiti minimi

1st dorsal interosseus

Adductor pollicis (transverse head)

Adductor pollicis (oblique head)

Flexor pollicis brevis (superficial head)

Abductor pollicis brevis

Opponens pollicis

Flexor retinaculum

Abductor pollicis longus

Fig. 14.37 Intrinsic muscles of the hand: superficial and middle layers
Right hand, palmar surface.
Superficial layer, with carpal and digital tendon sheaths exposed. *Removed:* Palmar aponeurosis, palmaris longus, antebrachial fascia, and palmaris brevis.

Compartments in Arm and Forearm

Deltoid

Pectoralis major

Coraco-brachialis

Teres major

Biceps brachii, long head

Biceps brachii, short head

Humerus

Biceps brachii

Brachio-radialis

Brachialis

Medial epicondyle

A Dissection of the arm.

Biceps brachii

Brachialis

Medial epicondyle, common head of flexors

Bicipital aponeurosis

Biceps brachii tendon

Brachio-radialis

Pronator teres

Extensor carpi radialis longus

Flexor carpi radialis

Extensor carpi radialis brevis

Palmaris longus

Radius

Ulna

Brachio-radialis

Flexor carpi ulnaris

Flexor digitorum superficialis

Flexor pollicis longus

Abductor pollicis longus

Flexor carpi radialis tendon

Thenar muscles

Palmaris longus tendon

Flexor retinaculum (transverse carpal ligament)

Palmaris brevis

Palmar aponeurosis

B Dissection of the forearm.

Fig. 14.38 Windowed dissection
Right limb, anterior view.

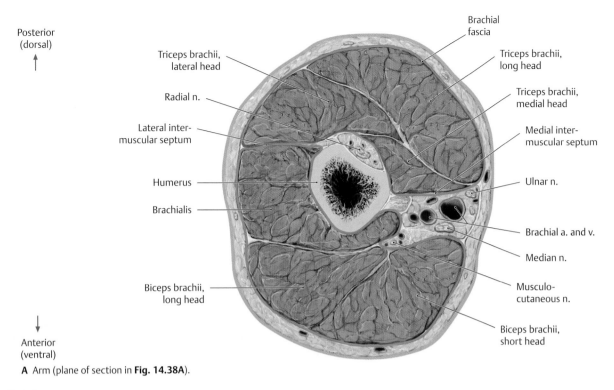

Posterior (dorsal)

Triceps brachii, lateral head

Radial n.

Lateral inter-muscular septum

Humerus

Brachialis

Biceps brachii, long head

Anterior (ventral)

Brachial fascia

Triceps brachii, long head

Triceps brachii, medial head

Medial inter-muscular septum

Ulnar n.

Brachial a. and v.

Median n.

Musculo-cutaneous n.

Biceps brachii, short head

A Arm (plane of section in **Fig. 14.38A**).

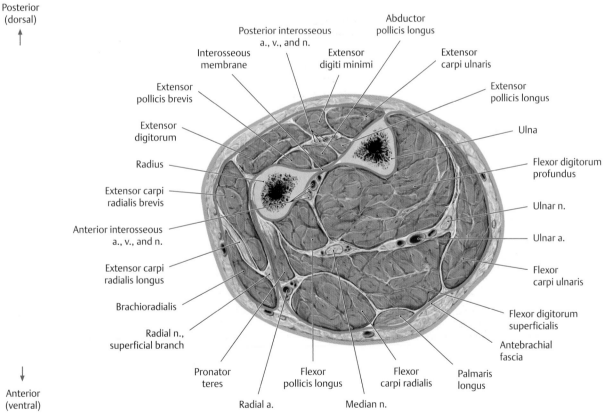

Posterior (dorsal)

Posterior interosseous a., v., and n.

Interosseous membrane

Extensor pollicis brevis

Extensor digitorum

Radius

Extensor carpi radialis brevis

Anterior interosseous a., v., and n.

Extensor carpi radialis longus

Brachioradialis

Radial n., superficial branch

Extensor digiti minimi

Abductor pollicis longus

Extensor carpi ulnaris

Extensor pollicis longus

Ulna

Flexor digitorum profundus

Ulnar n.

Ulnar a.

Flexor carpi ulnaris

Flexor digitorum superficialis

Antebrachial fascia

Pronator teres

Radial a.

Flexor pollicis longus

Flexor carpi radialis

Median n.

Palmaris longus

Anterior (ventral)

B Forearm (plane of section in **Fig. 14.38B**).

Fig. 14.39 Transverse sections
Right limb, proximal (superior) view.
The anterior compartment is outlined in *pink* and the posterior compartment in *green*.

Unit VI Clinical Imaging Basics of the Upper Limb

Radiographs are always the first imaging choice in evaluation of bones and joints in the setting of trauma or pain (**Table 14.18**). X-rays are highly sensitive for the detection of fractures and misalignment of joints.

Computed tomography (CT) provides significantly more detail of bone and is sometimes helpful for seeing subtle nondisplaced fractures, especially in older adults with decreased bone mass. The superior soft tissue contrast of magnetic resonance imaging (MRI) makes it the ideal imaging method for evaluation of the soft tissue components of joints.

Ultrasound has the benefit of real time imaging and is good for seeing superficial tissues, but its utility decreases with the size of the patient and the depth of the structure in question. However, in small children ultrasound is useful for the assessment of abnormal joint fluid and for anatomic evaluation of cartilaginous growth plates, especially in the growing elbow (see **Table 14.18**).

Since a radiograph is a summation shadow, all bones need to be evaluated in at least two projections (orthogonal) and all joints should be evaluated in at least three projections. The orthogonal view allows evaluation of the position of structures that may be overlapping in a single projection (**Fig. 14.40**). When viewing a bone X-ray, the cortical edge should be smooth along its entire length, and the trabecular pattern of the bone should be uniform throughout. Joints should be evaluated for even spacing, smoothness of the reticular surface, and alignment of the joint itself (**Fig. 14.41**).

While X-rays are best for evaluating bone, MRI is the choice for imaging soft tissues around the joints, since these are not visible on radiographs (**Figs. 14.42** and **14.43**).

Table 14.18 **Suitability of Imaging Modalities for the Upper Limb**

Modality	Clinical Uses
Radiographs (X-rays)	Primarily used to evaluate the bones and alignment of joints
CT (computed tomography)	Usually reserved as a troubleshooting tool to evaluate for subtle nondisplaced fractures
MRI (magnetic resonance imaging)	One of the most important imaging modalities for the evaluation of joints, specifically the non-osseous components of the joint—cartilage, ligaments, tendons, and muscles
Ultrasound	Limited role in evaluation of superficial soft tissue abnormalities, and for guidance of interventional procedures involving the joints. However, in children, due to their small size, ultrasound plays a larger role in diagnosis of joint disorders and for evaluation of cartilaginous growth plates.

B Coned down (magnified) view of the 5th digit *(arrow)* shows that the distal phalanx is dislocated and positioned dorsally. This is not seen on the frontal projection since there is no lateral displacement of the bone, and the ends of the bones at the DIP joint line up in the AP summation shadow.

A Anteroposterior (AP) view of the hand appears normal, even the 5th digit.

Fig. 14.40 **Radiograph of the hand demonstrating the importance of orthogonal views.** (Courtesy of Joseph Makris, MD, UMass Memorial Health Care.)

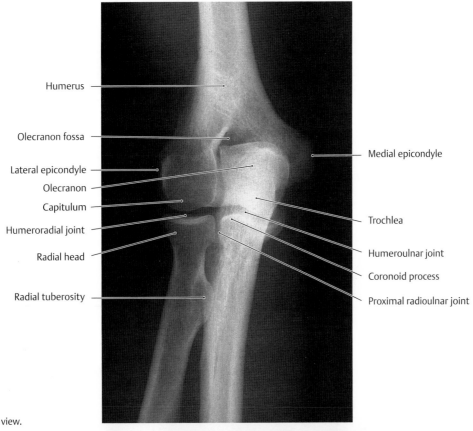

Humerus

Olecranon fossa

Lateral epicondyle

Olecranon

Capitulum

Humeroradial joint

Radial head

Radial tuberosity

Medial epicondyle

Trochlea

Humeroulnar joint

Coronoid process

Proximal radioulnar joint

A Anteroposterior view.

Humerus

Coronoid fossa

Coronoid process

Radial head

Radial tuberosity

Olecranon fossa

Lateral epicondyle

Humeroradial joint

Humeroulnar joint

Olecranon

Radius

Ulna

B Lateral view.

Fig. 14.41 **Radiograph of the elbow**

Brachioradialis

Extensor carpi radialis longus

Lateral epicondyle

Humeroradial joint

Radial head

Supinator

Radial tuberosity

Extensor digitorum

Brachialis

Medial epicondyle

Pronator teres

Medial collateral lig.

Humeroulnar joint

Ulna, coronoid process

Brachialis

Flexor carpi radialis

Fig. 14.42 MRI of the elbow
Coronal section.
In this sequence, fat is *white* (the fat in the bone marrow causes the bones to be a *very light gray/white* as well). Muscles are *dark gray* and ligaments and cortical bone are *black*.
The utility of MRI is the ability to see the ligaments, tendons, muscles, and cartilage. A muscle tear, tendon rupture, or ligamentous tear is invisible on an X-ray, but well demonstrated on MRI.

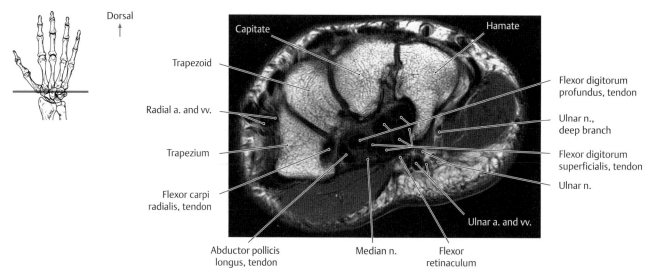

Dorsal

Capitate

Hamate

Trapezoid

Radial a. and vv.

Trapezium

Flexor carpi radialis, tendon

Flexor digitorum profundus, tendon

Ulnar n., deep branch

Flexor digitorum superficialis, tendon

Ulnar n.

Ulnar a. and vv.

Abductor pollicis longus, tendon

Median n.

Flexor retinaculum

Fig. 14.43 MRI of the right wrist
Transverse (axial) section, distal view.
In this sequence, fat is *white*, muscles are *dark gray*, and nerves and tendons are *black*. Note the detail of the tendons and nerves crossing the wrist through the carpal tunnel.

Unit VI   Review Questions: Upper Limb

1. A patient complains of tingling and pain in the upper arm. Upon further examination and additional tests, you determine that the axillary artery has been occluded by atherosclerosis. The patient, however, still has a radial pulse at the wrist. Which of the following arteries could provide a collateral circulation around the occlusion?
   A. Suprascapular and circumflex scapular arteries
   B. Suprascapular and lateral thoracic arteries
   C. Posterior circumflex humeral and anterior circumflex humeral arteries
   D. Superior thoracic and lateral thoracic arteries
   E. Posterior intercostals and lateral thoracic arteries

2. The deep palmar arch of the hand is formed mainly by the
   A. ulnar artery
   B. radial artery
   C. brachial artery
   D. palmar digital arteries
   E. palmar metacarpal arteries

3. Each cord of the brachial plexus
   A. contains nerve fibers from C5 to T1 levels of the spinal cord
   B. is formed from the junction of one anterior and one posterior division
   C. gives a branch to the median nerve
   D. lies within the axilla
   E. gives rise to a subscapular nerve (upper, middle, and lower)

4. Nerves often pair with arteries to travel as neurovascular bundles. Which of the following is *not* an accurate pairing?
   A. Axillary nerve and posterior circumflex humeral artery
   B. Median nerve and brachial artery
   C. Musculocutaneous nerve and circumflex scapular artery
   D. Radial nerve and deep brachial artery
   E. Long thoracic nerve and lateral thoracic artery

5. During a radical mastectomy on a 50-year-old woman, the surgeon does a careful but thorough axillary node dissection. What nerve lies along the medial wall of the axilla and is particularly vulnerable during this procedure?
   A. Lateral branch of posterior intercostal
   B. Musculocutaneous
   C. Lateral pectoral
   D. Long thoracic
   E. Dorsal scapular

6. One of your patients ruptured the tendon of the long head of the biceps brachii. Although he is bothered by the unattractive bulge that formed in his anterior arm, he is surprised to find that he has lost little flexor strength. You

confirm that the brachialis muscle has greater leverage at the joint and therefore is the more powerful flexor of the elbow. Where does the brachialis insert?
   A. Radial tuberosity
   B. Ulnar tuberosity
   C. Coronoid process
   D. Bicipital aponeurosis
   E. Olecranon

7. Which part(s) of the triceps brachii crosses/cross the glenohumeral joint?
   A. Medial head
   B. Lateral head
   C. Long head
   D. Lateral and medial heads
   E. Lateral and long heads

8. Structures that pass through the quadrangular space of the upper limb include the
   A. radial nerve
   B. suprascapular nerve
   C. posterior humeral circumflex artery
   D. anterior humeral circumflex artery
   E. deep brachial artery

9. Which of the following bones articulates with the radius at the wrist?
   A. Pisiform
   B. Hamate
   C. Capitate
   D. Trapezium
   E. Scaphoid

10. The flexor retinaculum
    A. forms the floor of the ulnar tunnel
    B. forms the roof of the carpal tunnel
    C. is continuous with the palmar aponeurosis
    D. is continuous with the palmaris longus
    E. All of the above

11. As a second-year resident doing a pediatric surgery rotation, you set up an arterial line on a 6-year-old girl prior to surgery. You choose the radial artery of her left (nondominant) hand. Because you know that the procedure can result in occlusion of the artery, you verify that the collateral circulation to the hand is patent. The radial artery
    A. forms the superficial arch of the hand
    B. passes superficial to the anatomic snuffbox
    C. supplies the muscles of the posterior compartment through its posterior interosseous branch
    D. supplies the princeps pollicis artery of the thumb
    E. lies medial to the tendon of the flexor carpi radialis in the wrist

12. During your first training session as a phlebotomist, you are relieved to find that your "patient" is a 24-year-old weight lifter whose superficial veins stand out dramatically against his overdeveloped muscles. Superficial veins of the upper limb
    A. include a basilic vein that runs in the deltopectoral groove
    B. include a cephalic vein that joins the brachial veins in the arm
    C. drain into the veins of the deep venous system via perforating veins
    D. course with the arteries as paired accompanying veins
    E. have bidirectional valves that allow flow in either direction

13. An injury to the lower brachial plexus (Klumpke's palsy) would affect
    A. sensation in the nail bed of the 5th digit
    B. abduction of the 2nd through 5th digits
    C. adduction of the thumb
    D. adduction of the wrist
    E. All of the above

14. While moonlighting in the emergency department one night, you treat a 14-year-old gang member who was stabbed in the supraclavicular region of the neck 2 cm above the middle third of the clavicle. A chest X-ray confirms that he has a pneumothorax. What other structure could be injured in this area?
    A. Axillary nerve
    B. Pectoralis minor
    C. Subscapular artery
    D. Posterior cord of the brachial plexus
    E. Cephalic vein

15. The serratus anterior muscle
    A. forms a scapulothoracic joint with the external intercostal muscles
    B. is innervated by a branch of the posterior cord
    C. elevates the scapula off the thoracic wall
    D. rotates the scapula laterally during abduction of the arm above the horizontal plane
    E. originates from the subscapular fossa

16. A professional rodeo cowboy fell off his horse and fractured his humerus at the anatomic neck and the lesser tubercle. Which of the following muscles inserts on this tubercle?
    A. Supraspinatus
    B. Infraspinatus
    C. Subscapularis
    D. Coracobrachialis
    E. Teres major

17. Damage to which nerve would most affect elbow flexion?
    A. Radial nerve
    B. Ulnar nerve
    C. Median nerve
    D. Musculocutaneous nerve
    E. Axillary nerve

18. At a neighborhood block party several children engage in a tug-of-war. Suddenly, Jason, a 5-year-old boy, hugs his right elbow and cries out in pain. The inconsolable child is eventually taken to the local clinic, where the pediatrician recognizes that Jason has subluxed (partially dislocated) his radial head. By gently supinating the flexed arm, the doctor restores it to its normal position. Which of the following is true regarding the proximal radioulnar joint?
    A. The radial head rotates within the annular ligament.
    B. It includes a hinge-type joint between the head of the radius and capitulum of the humerus.
    C. The biceps brachii pronates the joint.
    D. An articular disk separates the radius and ulna.
    E. The subluxation of the radial head results from a tear of the radial collateral ligament.

19. On your first day of shadowing in your preceptor's office, you are asked to get some baseline information on the patients. You start by taking their pulse. The radial artery is easiest to palpate in the wrist where it lies immediately lateral to the tendon of the
    A. flexor carpi radialis
    B. flexor digitorum
    C. flexor pollicis longus
    D. palmaris longus
    E. extensor carpi radialis

20. You examine a 14-year-old girl in the emergency department. She has a puncture wound from a dog bite in the flesh over the middle phalange of her 5th digit. The incident occurred 2 days ago, and the finger is inflamed and likely infected. What are your thoughts regarding possible spread of the infection via the synovial sheath?
    A. It will spread into the superficial space on the dorsum of the hand.
    B. It will spread to the common flexor sheath in the wrist.
    C. It will spread to the adjacent finger.
    D. It will remain confined to the sheath of the infected finger.
    E. A and B are correct.

21. The axillary artery
    A. begins at the lateral border of the 1st rib
    B. lies anterior to the axillary vein
    C. ends by dividing into brachial and deep brachial arteries
    D. passes through the axilla between the pectoralis major and pectoralis minor muscles
    E. branches include the thyrocervical trunk

22. Axillary lymph nodes that lie medial to the pectoralis minor include
    A. pectoral nodes
    B. humeral nodes
    C. apical nodes
    D. central nodes
    E. subscapular nodes

23. The C4 anterior ramus is a component of
    A. the pre-fixed plexus
    B. the upper trunk
    C. the posterior cord
    D. the axillary nerve
    E. All of the above

24. A young man suffered a crushing injury to his right arm, fracturing his humerus at midshaft and damaging the nerve that runs in the posterior compartment. What functional loss would you expect from this injury?
    A. Inability to extend the elbow
    B. Inability to supinate the hand
    C. Inability to abduct the thumb
    D. Inability to extend the wrist
    E. All of the above

25. One of your orthopedic colleagues introduces you, an anatomist, to his patient, a famous baseball pitcher, who suffers from chronic rotator cuff pain. He asks you to demonstrate the rotator cuff on a cadaver specimen and explain the anatomy of this type of injury. You tell him the following:
    A. Tendons of the rotator cuff muscles insert onto the capsule of the glenohumeral joint.
    B. The supraspinatus tendon passes through the subacromial space between the shoulder joint and the coracoacromial arch.
    C. An abnormal communication between the subacromial bursa and glenohumeral joint cavity can result from rupture of the supraspinatus tendon.
    D. Rupture of the supraspinatus tendon will impair the patient's ability to initiate abduction of the arm.
    E. All of the above

26. Which of the following muscles has no attachment on the humerus?
    A. Deltoid
    B. Coracobrachialis
    C. Flexor digitorum superficialis
    D. Pronator teres
    E. Biceps brachii

27. Which muscle provides strong adduction of the glenohumeral joint?
    A. Teres minor
    B. Pectoralis major
    C. Pectoralis minor
    D. Short head of the biceps brachii
    E. Subscapularis

28. A young woman riding a 10-speed bicycle accidentally engaged the front brake, was thrown over the handlebars, and landed on her outstretched hands. In the emergency department, imaging of the elbow revealed a subtle fracture of the radial neck that allowed proximal movement of the radius relative to the ulna, which also suggested a tear in the interosseous membrane. Which movements were most impaired by this injury?
    A. Flexion of the wrist
    B. Extension of the elbow
    C. Extension of the digits
    D. Abduction of the thumb
    E. Adduction of the thumb

29. An elderly man had injured his wrist in a fall and is now experiencing tingling in his fingers and a weakened grip. A lateral X-ray of the wrist shows that his lunate has dislocated and is pressing on the structures within the carpal tunnel. Which of the following structures pass through the carpal tunnel?
    A. Ulnar artery
    B. Radial artery
    C. Flexor carpi radialis
    D. Flexor pollicis longus
    E. Palmaris longus

30. In the anatomy lab you are fascinated by the deep dissection of the hand because as an amateur violinist you appreciate that the intrinsic muscles of the palm are important for the fine movements of the hand. Which of the following is true for both the lumbricals and the interossei muscles?
    A. All are innervated by the median nerve.
    B. All are innervated by the ulnar nerve.
    C. They flex the metacarpophalangeal joints.
    D. They arise from the tendons of the flexor digitorum profundus.
    E. They abduct or adduct the fingers.

Answers and Explanations

1. **A.** The suprascapular and transverse cervical branches of the subclavian artery and the thoracodorsal and circumflex scapular branches of the distal segment of the axillary artery participate in a scapular arcade that provides a collateral circulation that would circumvent the occlusion (Section 13.4).
   B. The lateral thoracic artery does not supply the scapula, nor does it anastomose with the suprascapular artery.
   C. The anterior and posterior humeral circumflex arteries anastomose around the neck of the humerus but do not anastomose with arteries proximal to the occlusion.
   D. Neither the superior thoracic artery nor the lateral thoracic artery supplies the scapular region.
   E. Posterior intercostal arteries supply the medial scapular region, but they do not anastomose with the lateral thoracic artery.

2. **B.** The deep palmar arch is formed mainly by the radial artery (Section 13.4).
   A. The ulnar artery forms the superficial palmar arch.
   C. The brachial artery begins at the lateral border of the axilla and terminates in the cubital fossa.
   D. The palmar digital arteries are branches of the superficial and deep palmar arches in the palm of the hand.
   E. The palmar metacarpal arteries arise from the superficial and deep palmar arches in the palm of the hand.

3. **D.** Each cord of the brachial plexus lies within the axilla (Section 13.4).
   A. The posterior cord contains fibers from C5 to T1; the medial cord contains fibers from C8 and T1; the lateral cord contains fibers from C5 to C7.
   B. The posterior divisions form the posterior cord; only anterior divisions form the medial and the lateral cords.
   C. The median nerve is formed from the medial and lateral cords.
   E. The subscapular nerves arise from the posterior cord.

4. **C.** The musculocutaneous nerve passes from the axilla to pierce the coracobrachialis of the anterior arm. The circumflex scapular artery passes through the triangular space into the scapular region (Section 14.2).
    A. The axillary artery and posterior circumflex humeral artery pass through the quadrangular space to the deltoid region.
    B. The median nerve and brachial artery descend on the medial side of the biceps brachii and enter the cubital fossa.
    D. The radial nerve and deep brachial artery wind around the posterior humerus through the triceps hiatus.
    E. The long thoracic nerve and lateral thoracic artery descend on the medial wall of the axilla to supply the serratus anterior muscle.

5. **D.** The long thoracic nerve runs superficial to, and innervates, the serratus anterior, which forms the medial wall of the axilla. Injury to this nerve can result in a "winged" scapula (Section 14.1).
    A. In the axilla the intercostal nerves run deep to the serratus anterior and external intercostal muscles and are not vulnerable to injury.
    B. The musculocutaneous nerve leaves the axilla just inferior to the glenohumeral joint where it enters the coracobrachialis muscle.
    C. The lateral pectoral nerve passes anteriorly to penetrate the pectoralis major muscle.
    E. The dorsal scapular nerve descends posteriorly from the upper roots of the plexus to innervate the levator scapulae and rhomboid muscles.

6. **B.** The brachialis muscle inserts on the ulnar tuberosity of the ulna (Section 14.3).
    A. The biceps brachii inserts on the radial tuberosity.
    C. The coronoid process forms the anterior lip of the trochlear notch of the ulna and is the origin of the ulnar head of the pronator teres.
    D. The bicipital aponeurosis is a fascial extension of the biceps brachii.
    E. The olecranon of the ulna forms the posterior prominence of the elbow and is the insertion for the triceps brachii and anconeus muscles.

7. **C.** The long head of the triceps brachii crosses the gleno-humeral joint to attach to the infraglenoid tubercle, where it contributes to extension of the joint (Section 14.2).
    A. The medial head arises from the medial aspect of the humeral shaft. It joins with the lateral and long heads to insert on the olecranon of the ulna.
    B. The lateral head arises from the lateral aspect of the humeral shaft. It joins with the medial and long heads to insert on the olecranon of the ulna.
    D. The medial and lateral heads arise from the humeral shaft and cross only the elbow joint.
    E. The lateral head arises from the shaft of the humerus and crosses the elbow joint. The long head originates on the infraglenoid tubercle of the scapula and crosses the glenohumeral and elbow joints.

8. **C.** The posterior humeral circumflex artery and the axillary nerve pass through the quadrangular space (Section 14.2).
    A. The radial nerve passes through the triceps hiatus.
    B. The suprascapular nerve passes through the scapular notch.

    D. The anterior humeral circumflex artery runs horizontally beneath the coracobrachialis and the short head of the biceps brachii to encircle the neck of the humerus.
    E. The deep brachial artery passes through the triceps hiatus with the radial nerve.

9. **E.** The radius articulates distally with the scaphoid and lunate bones of the wrist (Section 14.5).
    A. The pisiform on the medial side of the wrist articulates with the triquetrum.
    B. The hamate articulates with the capitate, lunate, triquetrum, and 4th and 5th metacarpal bones.
    C. The capitate articulates with the hamate, trapezoid, scaphoid, lunate, and 3rd metacarpal.
    D. The trapezium articulates with the trapezoid, scaphoid, and 1st metacarpal.

10. **E.** The flexor retinaculum forms the roof of the carpal tunnel and floor of the ulnar tunnel. As a thickening of the deep fascia of the palm, it is continuous with the palmar aponeurosis, palmaris longus, transverse metacarpal ligament, and fibrous digital sheaths (Sections 14.5 and 14.6).
    A. The flexor retinaculum forms the floor of the ulnar tunnel; the palmar carpal ligament form its roof. B through D are also correct (E).
    B. The carpal tunnel is a fascio-osseous tunnel. Carpal bones form the floor and sides; the flexor retinaculum forms the roof. A, C, and D are also correct (E).
    C. The flexor retinaculum is continuous with the tough palmar aponeurosis of the hand. A, B, and D are also correct (E).
    D. The palmaris longus passes over the carpal tunnel and inserts on the flexor retinaculum and palmar aponeurosis. A through C are also correct (E).

11. **D.** The princeps pollicis arises from the radial artery at the base of the 1st metacarpal and divides into two digital arteries of the thumb (Section 13.4).
    A. The ulnar artery forms the superficial palmar arch. The radial artery forms the deep palmar arch.
    B. The radial artery courses along the floor of the anatomic snuffbox.
    C. The posterior interosseous artery, which supplies muscles of the posterior forearm compartment, arises from the common interosseous artery, a branch of the ulnar artery in the cubital fossa.
    E. The radial artery lies lateral to the tendon of the flexor carpi radialis at the wrist.

12. **C.** The veins of the superficial venous system drain into the deep veins via perforating veins (Section 13.4).
    A. The cephalic vein courses along the deltopectoral groove before terminating in the axillary vein.
    B. The basilic vein joins with the paired brachial veins to form the axillary vein.
    D. Veins of the deep venous system travel with the arteries as paired accompanying veins. There is no superficial arterial system that accompanies the superficial veins.
    E. Veins of the limbs have unidirectional valves that prevent pooling of blood and facilitate flow back toward the heart.

13. **E.** The ulnar nerve arises from the lower part of the plexus. Its dorsal cutaneous branch in the hand supplies the palmar and dorsal surfaces of the 4th (half) and 5th digits, and its deep branch supplies the dorsal interossei muscles that abduct the fingers and the adductor pollicis that adducts the thumb. It also innervates the flexor carpi ulnaris that assists in adduction of the wrist (Section 13.4).

    A. The ulnar nerve's (C8–T1) dorsal cutaneous branch in the hand supplies the palmar and dorsal surfaces of 4th (half) and 5th digits. B through D are also correct (E).

    B. The ulnar nerve's (C8–T1) deep branch in the hand supplies the dorsal interossei muscles that abduct the fingers. A, C, and D are also correct (E).

    C. The ulnar nerve's (C8–T1) deep branch in the hand supplies the adductor pollicis muscle that adducts the thumb. A, B, and D are also correct (E).

    D. The ulnar nerve (C8–T1) innervates the flexor carpi ulnaris that assists the extensor carpi ulnaris (radial nerve) in adduction of the wrist. A through C are also correct (E).

14. **D.** The posterior cord is part of the supraclavicular brachial plexus and could be injured in the area (Section 13.4).

    A. The terminal nerves of the brachial plexus form below the clavicle. Although damage to the supraclavicular plexus could affect the axillary nerve, the stab wound would not directly damage the nerve itself.

    B. The pectoralis minor attaches to the coracoid process, which lies below the middle part of the clavicle.

    C. The subscapular artery is a branch of the distal part of the axillary artery, which is infraclavicular.

    E. The cephalic vein drains into the axillary vein below the clavicle and most likely would not be affected by this injury.

15. **D.** The serratus anterior pulls the inferior angle of the scapula laterally when the glenohumeral joint is abducted above the horizontal plane (Section 14.1).

    A. The scapulothoracic joint is a functional relationship between the serratus anterior and subscapularis muscles.

    B. The long thoracic nerve, which innervates the serratus anterior muscle, arises directly from the C5–C7 roots of the brachial plexus.

    C. The serratus anterior supports the scapula against the thoracic wall. Denervation of the muscle allows the scapula to lift away from the thoracic wall, a condition known as a "winged" scapula.

    E. The serratus anterior originates from the entire medial border of the scapula.

16. **C.** The subscapularis inserts on the lesser tubercle of the humerus and fibrous capsule of the glenohumeral joint (Section 14.2).

    A. The supraspinatus inserts on the greater tubercle of the humerus.

    B. The infraspinatus inserts on the greater tubercle of the humerus.

    D. The coracobrachialis inserts on the shaft of the middle part of the humerus.

    E. The teres major inserts on the crest that extends inferiorly from the lesser tuberosity.

17. **D.** The musculocutaneous nerve innervates the biceps brachii and brachialis muscles, the primary flexors of the elbow. There would also be loss of sensation to the skin of the lateral forearm (Sections 14.2 and 14.3).

    A. Damage to the radial nerve results in wrist drop and loss of sensation to the dorsum of the hand and the proximal segments of the 1st through 3rd digits and half of the 4th digit.

    B. Damage to the ulnar nerve may cause paresthesia (numbness and tingling) in the forearm, 4th and 5th fingers, or paralysis of the intrinsic muscles of the hand (so-called claw hand deformity).

    C. Damage to the median nerve above the cubital fossa will cause the inability to flex the proximal interphalangeal joint of the 1st to 3rd digits and the inability to flex the distal interphalangeal joints of the 2nd and 3rd digits. This results in "benediction hand" (2nd and 3rd finger are partially extended) when trying to form a fist. It also causes the inability to flex the terminal phalanx of the thumb (due to damage of flexor pollicis longus) and loss of sensation over the lateral aspect of the hand.

    E. Damage to the axillary nerve causes paralysis of the deltoid muscle, resulting in weakened flexion and extension of the shoulder and the inability to abduct the arm above the horizontal.

18. **A.** The annular ligament forms a circular cuff around the radial head that allows the bone to rotate in the joint (Section 14.4).

    B. The hinge-type joint between the radius and capitullum of the humerus is the humeroradial joint.

    C. The biceps brachii inserts on the tuberosity of the radius and therefore supinates the joint when contracted.

    D. In the proximal radioulnar joint the radius articulates at the radial notch of the ulna. An articular disk separates the radius and ulna in the distal radioulnar joint.

    E. Subluxation of the radial head results from a laxity of the annular ligament.

19. **A.** The radial artery descends on the lateral side of the forearm and at the wrist lies immediately lateral to the tendon of the flexor carpi radialis (Section 14.5).

    B. The tendons of the flexor digitorum lie in the middle of the wrist, medial to the radial artery.

    C. The tendon of the flexor pollicis longus lies lateral to the median nerve and medial to the tendon of the flexor carpi radialis and to the radial artery.

    D. The palmaris longus runs superficial to the flexor retinaculum and medial to the flexor pollicis longus.

    E. The radial artery lies medial (palmar) to the extensor carpi radialis tendon.

20. **B.** The synovial sheath of the 5th digit normally communicates with the common synovial sheath (Section 14.6).

    A. The synovial sheath of the 5th digit communicates with the common synovial sheath and with that of the thumb, but it does not normally communicate with the superficial space on the dorsum of the hand.

    C. The synovial sheaths of the 2nd, 3rd, and 4th digits do not normally communicate with any other tendon sheaths. It is unlikely the infection will spread to these fingers.

    D. Although the infection may remain confined to the infected finger, the synovial sheath of the 5th digit communicates with that of the thumb and with the common tendon sheath. Therefore, the concern is that it will spread via this route to the thumb, wrist, and forearm.

E. The synovial sheath of the 5th digit normally communicates with the common flexor sheath at the wrist but not with the superficial space on the dorsum of the hand.

21. **A.** The subclavian artery continues as the axillary artery at the lateral border of the 1st rib (Section 13.4).

    B. The axillary artery lies posterior to the axillary vein.

    C. The brachial artery is a continuation of the axillary artery in the axilla. The deep brachial artery is one of the branches of the brachial artery.

    D. The axillary artery passes through the axilla posterior to the pectoralis minor muscle.

    E. The thyrocervical trunk is a branch of the subclavian artery.

22. **C.** The apical nodes are the nodes of the upper infraclavicular group. These lie medial to the pectoralis minor muscle along the axillary vein and adjacent to the proximal part of the axillary artery (Section 13.4).

    A. Pectoral nodes are part of the lower axillary group that lies lateral to the pectoralis minor.

    B. Interpectoral nodes are part of the middle axillary group that lies between the pectoralis major and pectoralis minor muscles.

    D. Central nodes are part of the lower axillary group that lies lateral to the pectoralis minor.

    E. The subscapular nodes are part of the lower axillary group that lies lateral to the pectoralis minor.

23. **A.** The brachial plexus contains the anterior rami of C5 to T1. A prefixed plexus also contains the C4 anterior ramus (Section 13.4).

    B. The upper trunk contains C5 and C6 anterior rami.

    C. The posterior cord contains the anterior rami of C5 to T1.

    D. The axillary nerve contains the anterior rami of C5 and C6.

    E. B, C, and D are incorrect.

24. **D.** Damage to the radial nerve from a midhumeral fracture results in loss of innervation to the extensor carpi radialis and extensor carpi ulnaris (Sections 13.4 and 14.4).

    A. The branches of the radial nerve to the triceps brachii arise high in the arm, so a midhumeral lesion of the nerve would not affect the function of this muscle.

    B. The radial nerve innervates only one of the muscles that supinate the hand, the supinator. The biceps brachii, also a supinator, is innervated by the musculocutaneous nerve.

    C. Abduction of the thumb is weakened by damage to the radial nerve.

    E. A, B, and C are incorrect.

25. **E.** All of the rotator cuff muscles insert on the fibrous capsule of the glenohumeral joint. The supraspinatus muscle, the most frequently involved in rotator cuff tears, passes through the narrow subacromial space and, with repetitive use, becomes frayed. Rupture of the tendon allows the overlying bursa to communicate with the joint cavity and impairs the initial phase of abduction. Later phases of abduction remain intact through the action of the deltoid muscle (Section 14.2).

    A. The tendons of the rotator cuff muscles insert on, and reinforce, the fibrous capsule of the joint. B through D are also correct (E).

    B. The supraspinatus tendon and subacromial bursa pass through the narrow subacromial space between the capsule of the shoulder joint and the coracoacromial arch. A, C, and D are also correct (E).

    C. The supraspinatus tendon separates the subacromial and subdeltoid bursae from the joint cavity. With rupture of the tendon, a communication between the bursae and joint cavity may result. A, B, and D are also correct (E).

    D. The deltoid is the primary abductor of the glenohumeral joint, but the supraspinatus assists in the first 15 degrees of abduction. A through C are also correct (E).

26. **E.** The two heads of the biceps brachii originate on the supraglenoid tubercle and coracoid process of the scapula and insert on the radial tuberosity of the radius (Sections 14.2 and 14.3).

    A. The deltoid originates along the scapular spine and clavicle and inserts on the deltoid tuberosity of the humerus.

    B. The coracobrachialis originates on the coracoid process of the scapula and inserts on the shaft of the humerus.

    C. The flexor digitorum superficialis originates on the medial epicondyle of the humerus and upper part of the radius and inserts on the middle phalanx of the 2nd through 4th digits.

    D. The pronator teres originates on the medial epicondyle of the humerus and coronoid process of the ulna and inserts on the lateral radius.

27. **B.** The broad origin of the pectoralis major on the anterior trunk wall allows it to strongly adduct the arm (Section 14.2).

    A. As part of the rotator cuff, the teres minor supports the head of the humerus in the glenohumeral joint. It also weakly adducts and laterally rotates the arm.

    C. The pectoralis minor draws the scapula forward and down, causing the scapula to rotate medially.

    D. The short head of the biceps brachii provides some flexion, abduction, and internal rotation of the glenohumeral joint.

    E. The subscapularis supports the head of the humerus in the glenohumeral joint and medially rotates the arm.

28. **D.** The function of the abductor pollicis muscle, the primary abductor of the thumb, would be greatly impaired because it originates on the interosseous membrane (Section 14.4).

    A. The flexor carpi radialis and flexor carpi ulnaris originate from the medial epicondyle of the humerus and olecranon of the ulna and would be unaffected by this injury.

    B. The triceps brachii, which extends the elbow, inserts on the olecranon. It would not be impaired by this injury.

    C. The extensor digitorum originates from the humerus and ulna and would be unaffected by this injury.

    E. The adductor of the thumb, adductor pollicis, attaches to the 2nd and 3rd metacarpals and the capitate. It would not be affected by this injury.

29. **D.** The flexor pollicis longus passes through the carpal tunnel with the flexor digitorum superficialis, flexor digitorum profundus, and median nerve (Section 14.5).

   A. The ulnar artery and ulnar nerve pass through the ulnar canal at the wrist.

   B. At the wrist the radial artery turns dorsally to run through the floor of the anatomic snuffbox.

   C. The flexor carpi radialis crosses the wrist lateral to the carpal tunnel and inserts on the base of the 1st metacarpal.

   E. The palmaris longus passes superficial to the flexor retinaculum to insert into the palmar aponeurosis.

30. **C.** The interossei and lumbricals flex the metacarpophalangeal joints and extend the interphalangeal joints (Section 14.6).

   A. Only the lateral two lumbricals are innervated by the median nerve. The medial lumbricals and all of the interossei are innervated by the ulnar nerve.

   B. The ulnar nerve innervates all of the interossei and the medial two lumbricals. The lateral two lumbricals are innervated by the median nerve.

   D. Only the lumbricals arise from the flexor tendons. The interossei arise from the shafts of the metacarpal bones.

   E. The palmar interossei adduct the fingers, the dorsal interossei abduct the fingers. The lumbricals have no effect on these movements.

Unit VII   Lower Limb

15 Overview of the Lower Limb

The lower limb supports the weight of the entire body and therefore is designed for strength and stability. Bones, muscles, and tendons tend to be more robust and joints more stable than those found in the upper limb.

15.1 General Features

— In the anatomic position, the body is upright and supported by the lower limb. The feet are together and pointed forward.
— The regions of the lower limb (**Fig. 15.1**) include
  • the **gluteal region,** which includes the buttocks and lateral hip region and overlies the **pelvic girdle;**

A Anterior view.   **B** Posterior view.

Fig. 15.1 Regions of the lower limb
Right limb.

  • the **thigh,** between the hip and the knee;
  • the **popliteal** and **genual regions,** at the knee;
  • the **leg,** between the knee and ankle; and
  • the **foot,** which has dorsal and plantar surfaces. The plantar surface is also called the **sole** of the foot.
— Movements of the joints of the lower limb are similar to movements of the upper limb, with some variations. They include
  • flexion—**plantar flexion** indicates flexing the foot or toes downward;
  • extension—**dorsiflexion** indicates extension of the foot, as when lifting the foot or toes upward;
  • abduction and adduction—the axis for abduction and adduction of the toes is the 2nd digit;
  • external rotation and internal rotation—movement around a longitudinal axis;
  • **inversion,** or supination of the foot—lifting the medial edge of the sole; and
  • **eversion,** or pronation of the foot lifting the lateral edge of the sole.
— As in the upper limb, muscles of the lower limb can be described as intrinsic or extrinsic:
  • Intrinsic muscles of the foot originate and insert on bones of the foot and ankle.
  • Extrinsic flexor and extensor muscles of the foot originate in the leg.
    ○ Synovial tendon sheaths surround the long flexor and extensor tendons as they cross the ankle joint.

15.2 Bones of the Lower Limb

Bones of the lower limb include the hip (coxal) bone that articulates with the sacrum to form the pelvic girdle, the femur of the thigh, the tibia and fibula of the leg, the tarsal bones of the ankle and hindfoot, and the metatarsal bones and phalanges of the midfoot and forefoot (**Fig. 15.2**).
— The **hip (coxal) bone** forms the lateral part of the pelvic girdle. The features of the hip bone are discussed in Section 10.2 with the bony pelvis.
— The **femur** is the long bone of the thigh (**Fig. 15.3**).
  • Proximally, its large ball-shaped **head** articulates with the acetabulum of the hip bone.
  • The **neck,** angled inferolaterally, connects the head with the shaft.
  • **Greater** and **lesser trochanters,** sites for muscle attachments, are separated by an **intertrochanteric crest** posteriorly and an **intertrochanteric line** anteriorly.
  • The **shaft** is slightly bowed anteriorly and, in the anatomic position, is angled medially.
  • **Linea aspera,** paired ridges on the posterior surface of the shaft, diverge distally as the **medial** and **lateral supracondylar lines.**

Hip bone

Pelvic girdle (right side)

Femur

Thigh

Patella

Tibial plateau

Tibia

Leg

Fibula

Ankle mortise

Tarsals

Metatarsals

Foot

Phalanges

5th   1st

Digits

A Anterior view.

Hip bone

Hip joint

Femur

Medial condyle

Knee joint

Tibia

Fibula

Talocrural (ankle) joint

B Posterior view.

Fig. 15.2 Bones of the lower limb
Right limb. The skeleton of the lower limb consists of a limb girdle and an attached free limb. The free limb is divided into the thigh (femur), leg (tibia and fibula), and foot. It is connected to the pelvic girdle by the hip joint.

- Distally, the **medial** and **lateral epicondyles** are attachment sites for ligaments of the knee, and the **adductor tubercle** is an attachment site for muscle.
- The femur articulates with the tibia at the **medial** and **lateral condyles,** which are separated by the **intercondylar notch.**
- The femur articulates with the patella anteriorly at the **patellar surface.**
— The **patella,** a large sesamoid bone, forms the kneecap (**Figs. 15.4** and **15.5;** see also **Fig. 16.14**).
  - It articulates with the distal femur at the knee joint.
  - Superiorly, its **base** is attached to the **quadriceps tendon.**
  - Inferiorly, its **apex** is attached to the **patellar ligament.**
— The **tibia** is the large medial long bone of the leg (**Fig. 15.6**).
  - Proximally, it articulates with the femur at the **tibial plateau,** which has flat **medial** and **lateral condyles** separated by an **intercondylar eminence.**
  - It articulates with the fibula proximally at the **tibiofibular joint** and distally at the **tibiofibular syndesmosis.**
  - A triangular **anterolateral tubercle (Gerdy's tubercle)** separates the lateral condyle from the lateral surface of the tibial shaft.
  - A **tibial tuberosity** on the anterior surface below the tibial plateau is an attachment site for anterior thigh muscles via the patellar ligament.
  - Distally, the **medial malleolus** forms part of the mortise of the ankle joint.
  - The sharp anterior border of the **shaft** is palpable between the knee and ankle.
  - An **interosseous membrane** connects the shaft of the tibia and fibula.
— The **fibula** is the lateral bone of the leg (see **Fig. 15.6**).
  - Proximally, the **head** articulates with the lateral condyle of the tibia at the proximal tibiofibular joint.
  - A narrow **neck** connects the head to the shaft.
  - A distal tibiofibular syndesmosis binds the fibula to the distal tibia.
  - Distally, the **lateral malleolus** forms the lateral wall of the mortise of the ankle joint.
— The **tarsal bones** consist of seven short bones of the foot (**Fig. 15.7**).
  - The **talus** is the most superior tarsal bone.
    ○ The **body** articulates with the tibia and fibula at the ankle joint.
    ○ The **head,** which articulates with the navicular bone, is the highest part of the medial arch of the foot.
    ○ The inferior surface articulates with the calcaneus.
  - The **calcaneus** is the large tarsal bone of the heel.
    ○ It articulates superiorly with the talus and anteriorly with the cuboid.
    ○ The **sustentaculum tali,** a medial process, forms part of the medial arch of the foot.
  - The **navicular** lies anterior to the talus and forms part of the medial arch.
  - The **cuboid** lies anterior to the calcaneus on the lateral side of the foot.
  - The **medial, intermediate,** and **lateral cuneiform** bones lie anterior to the navicular and articulate distally with the metatarsal bones.

Head

Fovea

Trochanteric fossa

Greater trochanter

Intertrochan-teric crest

Greater trochanter

Neck

Intertrochan-teric line

Lesser trochanter

Shaft

Lateral lip

Medial lip

Linea aspera

Medial supracondylar line

Lateral supracondylar line

Adductor tubercle

Medial epicondyle

Lateral epicondyle

Lateral epicondyle

Lateral condyle

Lateral condyle

Medial condyle

Patellar surface

Intercondylar notch

A Anterior view.

B Posterior view.

Fig. 15.3 Right femur

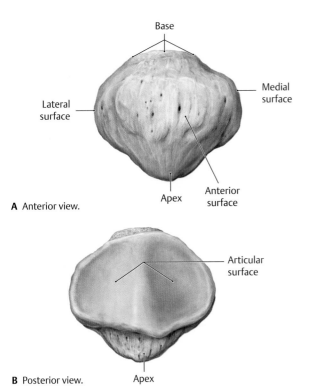

Base

Medial
surface

Lateral
surface

Apex

Anterior
surface

A Anterior view.

Articular
surface

B Posterior view.

Apex

Fig. 15.4 Patella
Right limb.

Fig. 15.5 Bipartite patella

— The **metatarsal bones** consist of five long bones that are designated 1st (medial) through 5th (lateral).
  • Proximally, their **bases** articulate with the tarsal bones.
  • Distally, their **heads** articulate with the proximal phalanges.
  • The **shaft** connects the heads and bases.
  • Paired **sesamoid bones** are associated with the head of the 1st metatarsal.
  • A prominent tuberosity at the base of the 5th metatarsal is a site of attachment for muscles of the leg.

DEVELOPMENT CORRELATION

BIPARTITE PATELLA Ossification of the patella occurs at ages 3 to 6 years, usually from several ossification centers. Occasionally, one center, most commonly the upper lateral segment, fails to fuse with the larger segment, resulting in a bipartite (two-part) patella. On imaging this may appear as a patellar fracture (**Fig. 15.5**).

— The **phalanges** are small long bones of the toes.
  • The 2nd through 5th digits have a proximal, middle, and distal phalanx.
  • The 1st digit, the **hallux,** or great toe, has only a proximal and a distal phalanx.

A Anterior view.

B Posterior view.

Fig. 15.6 Tibia and fibula
Right leg.

Phalanges

Metatarsal bones

Tarsal bones

1st distal phalanx

1st proximal phalanx
— Head
— Shaft
— Base

1st meta-tarsal
— Head
— Shaft
— Base

Medial cuneiform

Intermediate cuneiform

Navicular

Talus
— Head
— Neck
— Body

5th distal phalanx

5th middle phalanx

5th proximal phalanx

5th metatarsal

Lateral cuneiform

Tuberosity of 5th metatarsal

Cuboid

Calcaneus

Calcaneal tuberosity

A Dorsal (superior) view.

Talus

Neck

Body   Head

Posterior process

Calcaneus

Intermediate cuneiform

Navicular   Medial cuneiform

1st metatarsal

Cuboid   Tuberosity of 5th metatarsal

Lateral cuneiform

5th metatarsal

5th proximal phalanx

5th middle phalanx

5th distal phalanx

B Lateral view.

Fig. 15.7 Bones of the right foot (*continued on page 330*)

5th distal phalanx

5th middle phalanx

5th proximal phalanx

5th metatarsal

Tuberosity of 5th metatarsal

Groove for fibularis longus tendon

Tuberosity of cuboid

Cuboid

Calcaneus

1st distal phalanx

1st proximal phalanx

Sesamoids

1st metatarsal

Medial cuneiform

Intermediate cuneiform

Lateral cuneiform

Navicular

Head ⎫
Neck ⎬ Talus
Body ⎭

Posterior process ⎬ Talus

Sustentaculum tali

C Plantar (inferior) view.

15.3   Fascia and Compartments of the Lower Limb

— Similar to the upper limb, the lower limb musculature is enclosed within a snug sleeve of deep fascia, which is continuous from the iliac crest to the sole of the foot but has regional designations.
- **Fascia lata** surrounds muscles of the thigh. Laterally, longitudinal fibers of the fascia lata form a tough band, the **iliotibial tract,** which extends from the iliac crest to the anterolateral (Gerdy's) tubercle of the tibia (see **Fig. 16.46**).
- **Crural fascia** invests muscles of the leg, and at the ankle it forms the flexor and extensor retinacula.
- Fascia on the dorsum of the foot is thin, but on the sole it forms a thickened longitudinal band, the **plantar aponeurosis.**
- **Digital fibrous sheaths** are extensions of the plantar aponeurosis onto the toes, where they enclose the flexor tendons.
— The deep fascia creates compartments that separate the limb musculature. Muscles within each compartment are usually similar in function, innervation, and blood supply.

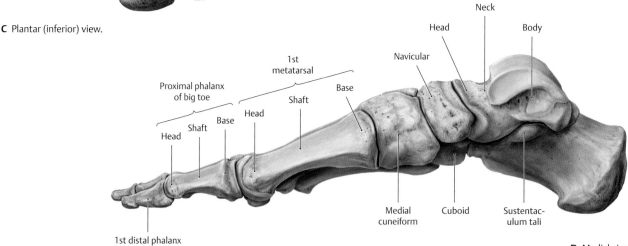

Talus

Neck

Head

Body

Navicular

Base

1st metatarsal

Shaft

Proximal phalanx of big toe

Head

Base

Shaft

Head

Shaft

Base

Medial cuneiform

Cuboid

Sustentaculum tali

1st distal phalanx

D Medial view.

Fig. 15.7 (*continued*) **Bones of the right foot**

Compartments of the lower limb (see **Fig. 16.53**) include the following:
- **Anterior, medial,** and **posterior compartments** of the thigh
- **Anterior, lateral, superficial posterior,** and **deep posterior** compartments of the leg (crural compartments)
- **Medial, lateral, central,** and **interosseous compartments** on the sole of the foot
- **Dorsal compartment** on the dorsum of the foot

15.4 Neurovasculature of the Lower Limb

Arteries of the Lower Limb

Branches of the internal iliac artery in the pelvis and the femoral artery (a continuation of the external iliac artery) supply blood to the lower limb (**Fig. 15.8**).
- The branches of the internal iliac artery that supply the lower limb include
  - the **superior gluteal** and **inferior gluteal arteries,** which exit the pelvis posteriorly through the greater sciatic foramen to supply the gluteal region; and
  - the **obturator artery,** which exits the pelvis anteriorly through the obturator foramen to supply the medial thigh.
- The **femoral artery** enters the anterior thigh deep to the inguinal ligament enclosed within a **femoral sheath** (formed by extensions of the deep fascia of the abdomen). The artery descends along the anteromedial thigh between the anterior and medial muscular compartments and ends at the **adductor hiatus,** a gap in the tendon of the **adductor magnus** muscle. Its branches include
  - the **superficial circumflex iliac** and **superficial epigastric arteries,** which supply the abdominal wall;
  - the **superficial** and **deep external pudendal arteries,** which supply the inguinal region;
  - the **descending genicular artery,** which contributes to the anastomosis around the knee; and
  - the **deep artery of the thigh,** which is the primary blood supply to the thigh.
- The deep artery of the thigh (deep femoral artery, profunda femoris), the largest branch of the femoral artery, arises in the proximal thigh. Its branches include
  - the **medial circumflex femoral artery,** which is the primary blood supply to the hip joint;
  - the **lateral circumflex femoral artery,** which supplies the hip joint and contributes to the anastomosis around the knee joint; and

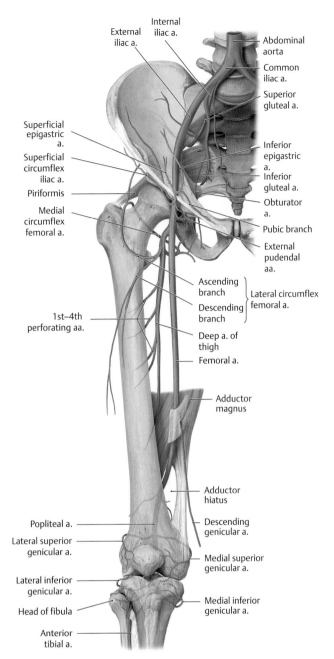

Fig. 15.8 **Course and branches of the femoral artery**

- the **1st through 3rd** (or 4th) **perforating arteries,** which supply muscles of the anterior, medial, and posterior muscles of the thigh.
- A **cruciate anastomosis** provides a collateral blood supply to structures around the hip. Contributions to the anastomosis include
  - the medial and lateral circumflex femoral arteries,
  - the 1st perforating artery, and
  - the inferior gluteal artery.
- The **popliteal artery** is the continuation of the femoral artery as it enters the **popliteal fossa,** a cavity posterior to the knee joint (**Fig. 15.9**).
  - Five **genicular branches** run medially and laterally around the knee.

CLINICAL CORRELATION

FEMORAL NECK FRACTURE Fractures of the femoral neck commonly occur following a low-energy impact in women over 60 years of age with osteoporosis. The distal fragment of bone is pulled upward by the quadriceps femoris, adductor, and hamstring muscles, causing shortening and lateral (external) rotation of the limb. Although an ample arterial anastomosis surrounds the hip joint, only the medial circumflex femoral artery supplies branches that enter the joint capsule and supply the femoral head. Tearing of those branches at the fracture site leads to avascular necrosis of the femoral head.

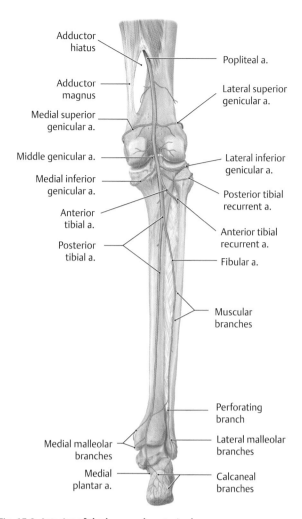

Fig. 15.9 Arteries of the knee and posterior leg
Right leg, posterior view.

- **Anterior tibial** and **posterior tibial arteries,** the terminal branches of the popliteal artery, arise in the proximal part of the posterior leg compartment.
— A **genicular anastomosis** that supplies the knee joint receives contributions from
  - the medial superior and inferior, lateral superior and inferior, and middle genicular arteries;
  - the descending genicular artery from the thigh;
  - the descending branch of the lateral circumflex artery; and

CLINICAL CORRELATION

POPLITEAL ANEURYSM Aneurysms of the popliteal artery are the most common peripheral arterial aneurysm. They can be distinguished by a thrill (palpable pulse) and bruits (abnormal arterial sounds) overlying the popliteal fossa. Because the artery lies deep to the tibial nerve, an aneurysm may stretch the nerve or occlude its blood supply. Pain from nerve compression is referred to the skin overlying the medial aspect of the calf, ankle, and foot. Half of all popliteal aneurysms remain asymptomatic, and ruptures are rare, but symptomatic patients present with distal leg ischemia from acute embolization or thrombosis. Fifty percent of patients with a popliteal aneurysm have an aneurysm in the contralateral artery, and 25% have an aortic aneurysm.

- the recurrent branches of anterior tibial and posterior tibial arteries.
— The posterior tibial artery descends into the deep posterior leg compartment to supply muscles in the deep and superficial posterior compartments (see **Fig. 15.9**). Its branches include
  - the **fibular artery,** which arises in the upper leg and descends within the posterior leg compartment; and
  - the **medial plantar** and **lateral plantar arteries,** which arise as the terminal branches posterior to the medial malleolus (**Fig. 15.10**).
— The fibular artery supplies muscles of the deep posterior compartment and, via small arteries that perforate the intermuscular septum, muscles of the lateral compartment. At the ankle it gives off
  - a **perforating branch** that arises at the ankle and anastomoses with the anterior tibial artery and
  - **malleolar branches** that contribute to an anastomosis around the ankle.
— Arteries of the sole (**Fig. 15.10**) arise from the posterior tibial artery and include
  - the medial plantar artery, a small branch of the posterior tibial artery that supplies the medial part of the sole;
  - the lateral plantar artery, the largest branch of the posterior tibial artery, which supplies the lateral side of the sole and curves medially to anastomose with the deep plantar artery;
  - a **deep plantar arch,** which forms through the anastomosis of the deep plantar artery and lateral plantar artery; and
  - four **plantar metatarsal arteries,** which arise from the deep plantar arch and their branches, the **common** and **proper plantar digital arteries,**
— The anterior tibial artery passes through an opening in the interosseous membrane to supply muscles of the anterior leg compartment (**Fig. 15.11**). Its branches are
  - proximally, a **recurrent branch** to the knee, and

Fig. 15.10 Arteries of the sole of the foot
Right foot, plantar view.

Fig. 15.11 Arteries of the anterior leg and foot
Right leg, anterior view.

Labels (top to bottom):
- Adductor magnus
- Adductor hiatus
- Popliteal a.
- Lateral superior genicular a.
- Medial superior genicular a.
- Lateral inferior genicular a.
- Medial inferior genicular a.
- Anterior tibial recurrent a.
- Interosseous membrane
- Anterior tibial a.
- Fibular a., perforating branch
- Anterior lateral malleolar a.
- Anterior medial malleolar a.
- Lateral tarsal a.
- Dorsal pedal a.
- Arcuate a.
- Deep plantar a.
- Dorsal metatarsal aa.
- Perforating branches
- Dorsal digital aa.

THE DORSAL PEDAL PULSE The dorsal pedal artery is readily palpable on the dorsum of the foot as it runs toward the first web space lateral to the extensor hallucis tendon. Absence of the dorsal pedal pulse suggests arterial occlusion in the peripheral vasculature.

LOWER LIMB ISCHEMIA Ischemia of the lower extremity is almost always related to atherosclerotic disease. Intermittent claudication is a symptom of chronic ischemic disease characterized by pain while walking, which intensifies over time and disappears at rest. Chronic disease has a benign course and, in the majority of patients, is treated conservatively. Acute ischemia has an abrupt onset from an embolitic or thrombolytic origin and usually requires aggressive treatment. The six signs (P signs) of acute ischemia are pain, pallor, pulselessness, paresthesia, paralysis, and poikilothermy.

Veins of the Lower Limb

The lower limb has both deep and superficial venous drainages, which anastomose through perforating veins. Veins of both systems have numerous valves along their length.

- Veins of the deep venous system travel with the major arteries and their branches and have similar names. As in the upper limb, these deep veins usually occur as paired accompanying veins in the distal part of the limb (**Fig. 15.12**).
  - The **femoral vein,** which drains the deep and superficial veins of the thigh and leg, passes under the inguinal ligament into the abdomen, where it becomes the external iliac vein.
  - **Superior** and **inferior gluteal veins,** which drain the gluteal region, pass through the greater sciatic foramen to empty into the internal iliac vein of the pelvis.
- Superficial veins are located in the subcutaneous tissue and normally drain, via perforating veins, to the deep venous system (**Fig. 15.13**).
  - The largest superficial veins, the **great saphenous** and **small saphenous veins,** originate at the **dorsal venous arch** on the dorsum of the foot.
  - The great saphenous vein arises from the medial side of the venous arch and passes superiorly, anterior to the medial malleolus and posteromedial to the knee. It drains into the femoral vein at the **saphenous opening,** an opening in the fascia lata in the upper thigh.
  - The small saphenous vein arises from the lateral side of the venous arch, passes posterior to the lateral malleolus, and ascends the posterior leg. It drains into the **popliteal vein** behind the knee.

- distally, the **dorsal pedal artery** as it emerges onto the dorsum of the foot.
- Arteries of the dorsum of the foot arise from the dorsal pedal artery and include
  - the **lateral tarsal** and **arcuate arteries,** which form a loop on the dorsum of the foot;
  - the **deep plantar artery,** which anastomoses with the lateral plantar artery on the sole; and
  - the **dorsal metatarsal arteries** and their branches, the **dorsal digital arteries,** which arise from the arcuate artery or the dorsal pedal artery.

DEEP VEIN THROMBOSES (DVT) Thromboses (blood clots) in the deep veins of the leg result from stasis, the slowing or pooling of blood. This can result from prolonged inactivity (extended airplane travel, immobilization following surgery) or anatomic abnormalities such as laxity of the crural fascia. Thrombi from the legs can break off and travel to the heart and lungs, lodging in the pulmonary arterial tree as pulmonary emboli. Large clots can severely impair lung function and even cause death. Thrombophlebitis is the inflammation of a vein caused by thrombosis.

Inguinal ligament
Piriformis
Lateral circumflex femoral vv.
Deep v. of thigh
Femoral v.
Adductor canal
Adductor hiatus
Popliteal v.
External iliac v.
Medial circumflex femoral vv.
Great saphenous v.
Accessory saphenous v.
Adductor magnus
Genicular vv.
Great saphenous v.
Anterior tibial vv.
Small saphenous v.
Dorsal venous network of the foot

A Anterior view.

Popliteal v.
Small saphenous v.
Anterior tibial v.
Fibular vv.
Small saphenous v.
Posterior tibial vv.
Lateral malleolus

B Posterior view.

Fig. 15.12 Deep veins of the lower limb
Right limb.

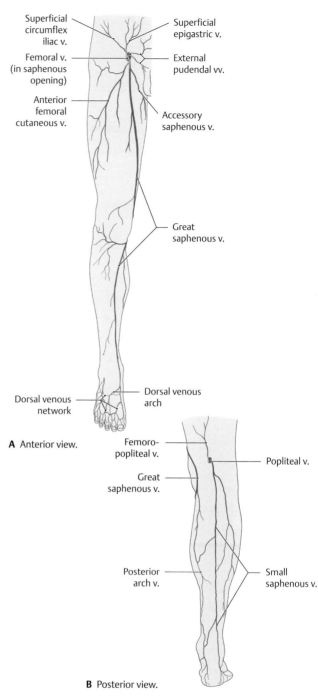

Superficial circumflex iliac v.
Femoral v. (in saphenous opening)
Anterior femoral cutaneous v.
Superficial epigastric v.
External pudendal vv.
Accessory saphenous v.
Great saphenous v.
Dorsal venous network
Dorsal venous arch

A Anterior view.

Femoro-popliteal v.
Great saphenous v.
Posterior arch v.
Popliteal v.
Small saphenous v.

B Posterior view.

Fig. 15.13 Superficial veins of the lower limb
Right limb.

CLINICAL CORRELATION

VARICOSE VEINS Varicose disease of the superficial veins of the lower limb is the most common chronic venous disease, affecting 15% of the adult population. Primary varices generally result from degeneration of the wall of the vein leading to dilated, tortuous vessels and incompetent venous valves. Secondary varices can develop from chronic occlusion of the deep veins with incompetence of the perforator veins. This causes a reversal of flow through the perforating veins. (Normal venous drainage flows from superficial to deep systems.) As the superficial veins dilate with increased volume, valve leaflets separate and become incompetent.

— The flow of blood from lower parts of the body must counter the downward force of gravity. In the lower limbs, venous return is assisted by
  • the presence of valves in the veins,
  • the pulsing of accompanying arteries, and
  • the contraction of surrounding muscles.

Lymphatics of the Lower Limb

Lymph from the lower limb drains superiorly from the foot following the deep and superficial veins. Upward flow is facilitated by the contraction of surrounding muscles (**Fig. 15.14**).
— Lymph from deep tissues of the
  • gluteal region drains along the gluteal vessels to internal iliac nodes.
  • thigh drains to deep inguinal nodes.
— Lymph from superficial tissues of the gluteal region and thigh drain to superficial inguinal nodes.
— Lymph from the dorsum and sole of the lateral foot and lateral leg drains along the short saphenous vein to the **deep popliteal nodes** at the knee. These drain directly to deep inguinal nodes.
— Lymph from the dorsum and sole of the medial foot and the medial leg drains along the long saphenous vein to superficial inguinal nodes.
— Lymph from the thigh drains first to superficial inguinal nodes, which in turn drain to deep inguinal nodes.
— Deep inguinal nodes drain sequentially to external iliac, common iliac, and lumbar nodes.

Fig. 15.14 Lymph nodes and drainage of the lower limbs
Right limb, anterior view.

Nerves of the Lower Limb: Lumbosacral Plexus

The lumbar and sacral plexuses, often combined as the **lumbosacral plexus,** innervate the lower limb (**Table 15.1; Figs. 15.15, 15.16, 15.17, 15.18**).

Nerves of the lumbar plexus enter the limb anteriorly to supply muscles of the anterior and medial thigh.

— The **iliohypogastric** (L1), **genital branch of the genitofemoral** (L1–L2), and **ilioinguinal** (L1) **nerves** are primarily nerves of the anterior abdominal wall and inguinal region. They also innervate small areas of skin over the upper lateral, anterior, and medial thigh, respectively.

— The **lateral cutaneous nerve of the thigh** (L2–L3), a sensory nerve that enters the lateral thigh anteromedial to the anterior superior iliac spine, innervates skin of the lateral thigh.

> **CLINICAL CORRELATION**
>
> **FEMORAL NERVE INJURY** Injuries of the femoral nerve can result in the following:
> — Weakened flexion of the hip
> — Loss of knee extension
> — Loss of sensation on the medial side of the leg and foot
> — Instability of the knee

— The **femoral nerve** enters the anterior thigh through the retroinguinal space (deep to the inguinal ligament), lateral to the femoral artery.
  • It innervates muscles of the anterior compartment.
  • Its **saphenous branch** is a sensory nerve that descends inferiorly to innervate the skin of the medial leg and foot.

Table 15.1 **Nerves of the Lower Limb**

Nerve	Level	Area of Innervation
Lumbar plexus		
Iliohypogastric n.	L1	Skin over upper lateral thigh and inguinal region
Ilioinguinal n.	L1	Skin over upper anterior thigh
Genitofemoral n.	L1–L2	Skin over upper thigh
Lateral cutaneous n. of the thigh	L2–L3	Skin of lateral thigh
Femoral n.	L2–L4	Iliopsoas, pectineus, sartorius, quadriceps femoris
—Anterior cutaneous n. of the thigh		Skin of anterior and medial thigh
—Saphenous n.		Skin of medial leg and foot
Obturator n.	L2–L4	Obturator externus, adductor longus, adductor brevis, adductor magnus, gracilis, pectineus; skin of medial thigh
Sacral plexus		
Superior gluteal n.	L4–S1	Gluteus medius, gluteus minimus, tensor fascia latae
Inferior gluteal n.	L5–S2	Gluteus maximus
Direct branches	L5–S2	Piriformis, obturator internus, gemelli, quadratus femoris
Posterior cutaneous n. of the thigh	S1–S3	Skin of posterior thigh and inferior gluteal region
Tibial n.	L4–S3	Biceps femoris (long head), semimembranosus, semitendinosus, adductor magnus (medial part), gastrocnemius, soleus, popliteus, tibialis posterior, flexor digitorum longus, flexor hallucis longus
—Medial plantar n.		Abductor hallucis, flexor digitorum brevis, flexor hallucis brevis (medial head), 1st lumbrical; skin of medial sole, 1st–3rd digits, and half of 4th digit
—Lateral plantar n.		Quadratus plantae, flexor hallucis brevis (lateral head), abductor digiti minimi, flexor digiti minimi brevis, interossei, 2nd–4th lumbricals, adductor hallucis; skin of lateral sole, 5th digit, and half of 4th digit
Common fibular n.	L4–S2	Biceps femoris (short head)
—Superficial fibular n.		Fibularis longus and brevis; skin of dorsum of foot
—Deep fibular n.		Anterior tibialis, extensor hallucis longus and brevis, extensor digitorum longus and brevis, fibularis tertius; skin of web space between 1st and 2nd digits
Pudendal n.	S2–S4	External anal sphincter, muscles of the deep and superficial perineal pouches, cutaneous brs. to scrotum and labia, sensory to penis and clitoris (see Section 10.6)
Sural n. (tibial and common fibular nn. contributions)	S1	Skin of posterior and lateral leg and lateral foot

Fig. 15.15 Lumbosacral plexus
Right side, lateral view.

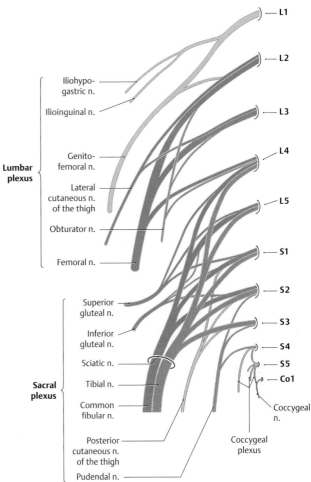

Fig. 15.16 Structure of the lumbosacral plexus
Right side, anterior view.

— The **obturator nerve** (L2–L4) enters the medial thigh through the obturator foramen and innervates muscles of the medial compartment.

The sacral plexus supplies muscles of the gluteal region, posterior thigh, and all muscular compartments of the leg and foot. Its branches enter the lower limb through the greater sciatic foramen in the gluteal region.

CLINICAL CORRELATION

OBTURATOR NERVE INJURY Injury to the obturator nerve is most commonly associated with pelvic surgery or pelvic fractures and results in the following:
— Weakened adduction of the hip (e.g., inability to move the leg from the gas pedal to the brake)
— Weakened external rotation of the hip
— Loss of sensation over a palm-size area on the medial side of the thigh
— Instability of the pelvis; lateral swing of the limb with locomotion

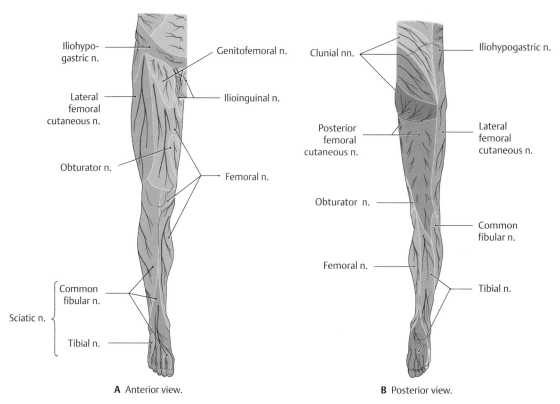

A Anterior view.

B Posterior view.

Fig. 15.17 Cutaneous innervation of the lower limb
Right limb.

A Anterior view.   **B** Posterior view.

Fig. 15.18 Dermatomes of the lower limb
Right limb.

CLINICAL CORRELATION

SUPERIOR GLUTEAL NERVE INJURY When one foot is lifted off the floor, as happens during the gait cycle, abduction of the hip by the contralateral gluteus medius and gluteus minimus muscles (the supported side) stabilizes the pelvis in the horizontal position. With injury to the superior gluteal nerve, the loss or weakness of abduction on that side allows the pelvis on the opposite (unsupported) side to sag. This results in a characteristic Duchenne's limp in which the weight of the trunk is shifted toward the nerve-damaged side to maintain the center of gravity **(Fig. 15.19)**.

— The **superior gluteal nerve** (L4–S1) enters the gluteal region above the piriformis muscle and runs laterally between the deep gluteal muscles. It supplies the abductors of the hip joint in the gluteal region.
— The **inferior gluteal nerve** (L5–S2) enters the gluteal region inferior to the piriformis muscle and innervates the large gluteus maximus muscle.
— The **posterior cutaneous nerve of the thigh** (L1–S3) is sensory to the thigh and posterior perineum. Its **inferior clunial branches** supply the inferior gluteal region.
— The **sciatic nerve** is made up of the **tibial** (L4–S3) and **common fibular** (L4–S2) **nerves,** which are bound together in a common sheath along their course in the posterior thigh. The two nerves diverge at the apex of the popliteal fossa.

Fig. 15.19 **Small gluteal muscle weakness**

Labels: Gluteus medius and minimus; Insufficient small gluteals; Shifted center of gravity; Pelvis sags; Stance leg; Swing leg

---

CLINICAL CORRELATION

SCIATIC NERVE INJURY The sciatic nerve can be injured by compression by the piriformis muscle, misplaced intramuscular injections in the gluteal region, pelvic fractures, or surgical procedures such as hip replacements. An injury in the gluteal region would affect muscles of the posterior thigh and all muscular compartments of the leg, the combined effects of damage to the tibial and common fibular nerves.

— The tibial nerve, the larger branch of the sciatic nerve, separates from the common fibular nerve and continues inferiorly through the popliteal fossa into the deep posterior leg compartment.
  • It innervates all of the muscles of the posterior thigh (except the short head of the biceps femoris) and the posterior leg.
  • At the ankle, it passes posterior to the medial malleolus, where it terminates as the **medial plantar** and **lateral plantar nerves.**

CLINICAL CORRELATION

TIBIAL NERVE INJURY Tibial nerve injury is unusual because the nerve is well protected in the thigh and posterior leg. Injury in the gluteal region results in the following:
— Impaired extension of the hip
— Loss of flexion of the knee
In the popliteal fossa, it can be affected by aneurysms of the popliteal artery and knee trauma. These can cause the following:
— Loss of plantar flexion at the ankle
— Loss of plantar flexion, abduction, and adduction of the digits
— Weakened inversion of the foot
— Loss of sensation on the posterolateral leg to the lateral malleolus, the sole and lateral side of the foot
— A shuffling gait with clawing of the toes

— The medial plantar nerve, comparable to the median nerve of the hand with small motor and large sensory components, is the largest branch of the tibial nerve.
  • It innervates plantar muscles on the medial side of the foot.
  • A superficial branch supplies a large area of skin on the medial side of the foot and the medial three and a half digits. It terminates as three **plantar digital nerves.**
— The lateral plantar nerve, the smaller branch of the tibial nerve, is comparable to the ulnar nerve of the hand.
  • It innervates the lateral plantar muscles and most deep muscles of the foot.
  • It innervates skin on the lateral sole and lateral one and a half digits and terminates as two **plantar digital nerves.**
— The common fibular nerve separates from the tibial nerve and, hugging the border of the biceps femoris muscle, passes laterally around the head of the fibula where it enters the lateral leg compartment.
  • In the thigh, it innervates the short head of the biceps femoris.
  • In the lateral leg compartment, it splits into its terminal branches, the **superficial fibular** and **deep fibular nerves.**

CLINICAL CORRELATION

COMMON FIBULAR NERVE INJURY The common fibular nerve is the most vulnerable of the peripheral nerves due to its exposed location around the neck of the fibula. Injuries result in the following:
— Loss of eversion of the foot
— Loss of dorsiflexion at the ankle and digits
— Weakened inversion of the foot
— Loss of sensation over the lateral leg and dorsum of the foot
— Footdrop compensated by a high-stepping gait; instability on uneven surfaces

---

— The superficial fibular nerve innervates the muscles in the lateral leg compartment. At the midleg, its sensory component pierces the crural fascia and runs onto the dorsum of the foot.
— From its division from the superficial fibular nerve, the deep fibular nerve circles anteriorly to enter the anterior leg compartment. It descends along the interosseous membrane, innervating all muscles of the compartment. It emerges onto the foot with the dorsal pedal artery to innervate the skin on adjacent surfaces of the 1st and 2nd digits.

CLINICAL CORRELATION

SUPERFICIAL AND DEEP FIBULAR NERVE INJURY Injury to the superficial fibular nerve only affects eversion of the foot and sensation over the lateral leg and most of the dorsum of the foot. Injury to the deep fibular has greater functional consequences, including the loss of all dorsiflexion. This results in footdrop and the compensating high-stepping gait.

— The **sural nerve** (S1), formed by communicating branches of the tibial and common fibular nerves on the surface of the posterior leg, runs posterior to the lateral malleolus at the ankle to innervate the skin of the lateral foot.

16 Functional Anatomy of the Lower Limb

The strong muscles and joints of the lower limb are adapted for bipedal locomotion and, in conjunction with the muscles of the trunk, maintain the body's center of gravity.

Schematics of lower limb muscles accompany the muscle tables (origin, attachment, innervation, and action) in the appropriate chapter sections. To see the muscles in situ, view the gallery of topographic images in Section 16.10 at the end of the chapter.

16.1 The Pelvic Girdle

The hip (coxal) bones and the sacrum form the pelvic girdle (bony pelvis), which is related anatomically and functionally to the pel-

vis and the lower limb (**Fig. 16.1**). (See Section 10.2 for a discussion of the pelvic girdle.)

— Articulations at the sacroiliac joint and pubic symphysis, supported by strong sacroiliac, sacrotuberous, and sacrospinous ligaments, create a stable framework that
  • supports and encloses the pelvic viscera,
  • transfers the weight of the trunk to the lower limb, and
  • forms part of the hip joint and provides attachment sites for lower limb muscles.

A Anterior view.

B Posterior view.

Fig. 16.1 The hip bones and their relation to bones of the trunk

16.2   The Gluteal Region

The gluteal region includes the buttock, which overlies the posterior part of the pelvic girdle, and the lateral hip region, which covers the hip joint and extends as far anteriorly as the anterior superior iliac spine.

– The muscular compartment of the gluteal region contains
  • muscles that laterally rotate, abduct, adduct, extend, and flex the hip joint (**Table 16.1**);
  • the superior gluteal, inferior gluteal, and sciatic nerves; and
  • the superior and inferior gluteal arteries and veins.

Iliotibial tract

A Vertically oriented gluteal muscles, right side, posterior view.

B Horizontally oriented gluteal muscles, right side, posterior view.

Table 16.1 **Gluteal Muscles**

Muscle	Origin	Insertion	Innervation	Action
① Gluteus maximus	Sacrum (dorsal surface, lateral part), ilium (gluteal surface, posterior part), thoracolumbar fascia, sacrotuberous ligament	• Upper fibers: iliotibial tract • Lower fibers: gluteal tuberosity	Inferior gluteal n. (L5–S2)	• Entire muscle: extends and externally rotates the hip in sagittal and coronal planes • Upper fibers: abduction • Lower fibers: adduction
② Gluteus medius	Ilium (gluteal surface below the iliac crest between the anterior and posterior gluteal line)	Greater trochanter of the femur (lateral surface)	Superior gluteal n. (L4–S1)	• Entire muscle: abducts the hip, stabilizes the pelvis in the coronal plane
③ Gluteus minimus	Ilium (gluteal surface below the origin of the gluteus medius)	Greater trochanter of the femur (anterolateral surface)		• Anterior part: flexion and internal rotation • Posterior part: extension and external rotation
④ Tensor fasciae latae	Anterior superior iliac spine	Iliotibial tract		• Tenses the fascia lata • Hip joint: abduction, flexion, and internal rotation
⑤ Piriformis	Pelvic surface of the sacrum	Apex of the greater trochanter of the femur	Direct branches from the sacral plexus (S1–S2)	• External rotation, abduction, and extension of the hip joint • Stabilizes the hip joint
⑥ Obturator internus	Inner surface of the obturator membrane and its bony boundaries	Medial surface of the greater trochanter	Direct branches from the sacral plexus (L5–S1)	External rotation, adduction, and extension of the hip joint (also active in abduction, depending on the joint's position)
⑦ Gemelli	• Gemellus superior: ischial spine • Gemellus inferior: ischial tuberosity	Jointly with obturator internus tendon (medial surface, greater trochanter)		
⑧ Quadratus femoris	Lateral border of the ischial tuberosity	Intertrochanteric crest of the femur		External rotation and adduction of the hip joint

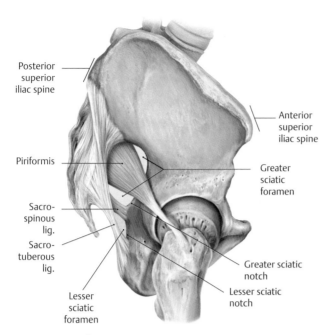

Fig. 16.2 **Sciatic foramina**
Right gluteal region.

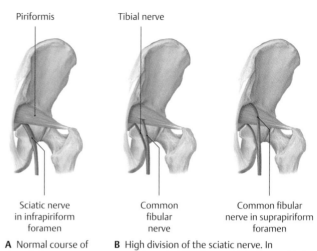

A Normal course of the sciatic nerve

B High division of the sciatic nerve. In approximately 15% of cases the common fibular n. passes through the piriformis where it may be compressed, causing a piriformis syndrome.

Fig. 16.3 **Variable course of the sciatic nerve in the gluteal region** (Rauber A, Kopsch F. Anatomie des Menschen. Bd. 1-4. Stuttgart: Thieme; Bd. 1. 2nd ed. 1997;Bde. 2 u. 3 1987: Bd. 4 1988)

— Posteriorly, structures pass between the pelvis and the gluteal region through the greater sciatic foramen (**Fig. 16.2**). These structures include
  • the piriformis muscle,
  • the superior gluteal and inferior gluteal vessels,
  • the superior gluteal and inferior gluteal nerves,
  • the sciatic nerve,
  • the pudendal nerve and internal pudendal vessels, and
  • the posterior femoral cutaneous nerve.

— The lesser sciatic foramen, a passageway between the gluteal region and perineum, transmits
  • the internal pudendal vessels,
  • the pudendal nerve, and
  • the tendon of the obturator internus muscle.

16.3   The Hip and Thigh

The Hip Joint

The **hip joint** is a highly mobile, yet stable, ball-and-socket joint between the proximal femur and the acetabulum of the hip bone (**Figs. 16.4** and **16.5**). Muscles crossing the joint, particularly in the gluteal region, provide additional stability as well as mobility.

— More than half of the large femoral head is seated in the bony acetabulum of the hip bone, which is oriented slightly anteriorly and inferiorly.

— The axis through the neck of the femur is laterally rotated with respect to the condylar axis of the distal femur; thus, when the femoral head is centered in the hip joint, the distal femur and knee joint are directed slightly inward (**Figs. 16.6** and **16.7**).

— A strong fibrous capsule surrounds the hip joint (**Fig. 16.8**).
  • **Iliofemoral, pubofemoral,** and **ischiofemoral ligaments** are extracapsular ligaments that strengthen the capsule. The iliofemoral ligament is the strongest and most supportive of these.

> **CLINICAL CORRELATION**
>
> **PIRIFORMIS SYNDROME** The sciatic nerve normally passes into the gluteal region inferior to the piriformis muscle. Tightening or shortening of the muscle can compress and irritate the sciatic nerve, causing pain and paresthesia (tingling and numbness) in the buttocks and posterior thigh. In some cases the sciatic nerve, or its common fibular component, is compressed as it passes through the muscle rather than inferior to it **(Fig. 16.3)**. Piriformis syndrome should be distinguished from sciatica in which the pain and paresthesia result from compression of lumbar nerve roots by a herniated intervertebral disk.

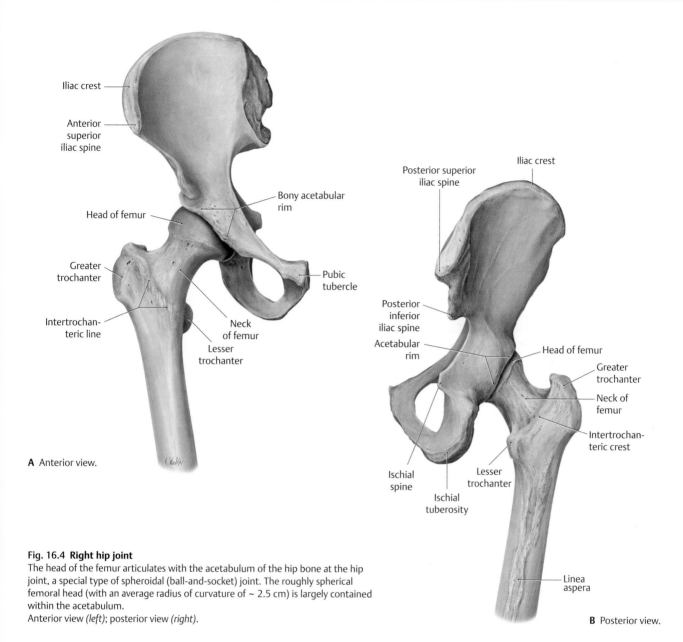

A Anterior view.

Iliac crest

Anterior superior iliac spine

Head of femur

Greater trochanter

Intertrochan-teric line

Bony acetabular rim

Pubic tubercle

Neck of femur

Lesser trochanter

Posterior superior iliac spine

Iliac crest

Posterior inferior iliac spine

Acetabular rim

Head of femur

Greater trochanter

Neck of femur

Intertrochan-teric crest

Ischial spine

Ischial tuberosity

Lesser trochanter

Linea aspera

B Posterior view.

Fig. 16.4 Right hip joint
The head of the femur articulates with the acetabulum of the hip bone at the hip joint, a special type of spheroidal (ball-and-socket) joint. The roughly spherical femoral head (with an average radius of curvature of ~ 2.5 cm) is largely contained within the acetabulum.
Anterior view (left); posterior view (right).

Anterior acetabular rim

Posterior acetabular rim

Femoral head

Greater trochanter

Femoral neck

Intertrochanteric crest

Lesser trochanter

Roof of the acetabulum

Fovea of the femoral head

Köhler's teardrop figure

Superior pubic ramus

Obturator foramen

Ischial tuberosity

Fig. 16.5 Radiograph of the right hip joint
Anteroposterior view.

— A fibrocartilaginous **acetabular labrum** attached to the acetabular rim deepens the joint (**Fig. 16.9**).

— A weak **ligament of the head of the femur** attaches to the acetabulum within the joint space but provides little support.

— Inferiorly, a **transverse ligament of the acetabulum** completes the circle of the C-shaped acetabular labrum.

— Muscles of the gluteal region and thigh move the hip joint (**Fig. 16.10, Table 16.2**).

CLINICAL CORRELATION

CONGENITAL HIP DISLOCATION Congenital hip dislocation (also known as hip dysplasia) is a common problem that occurs when the femoral head is not properly seated in the acetabulum. Hip abduction is impaired, and since the femoral head sits higher than normal, the affected limb is shorter than the contralateral limb. In routine neonatal screenings, a dislocated hip will "click" when it is adducted and pushed posteriorly.

CLINICAL CORRELATION

ACQUIRED HIP DISLOCATION Acquired hip dislocation usually occurs as a result of trauma that causes the femoral head to be displaced out of the acetabulum; anterior dislocations are rare, but posterior dislocations are common. Typically, in a head-on motor vehicle accident, the knees strike the dashboard, forcing the femoral head posteriorly through the joint capsule and onto the lateral surface of the ilium. The affected limb appears shortened and internally rotated. The sciatic nerve is particularly vulnerable to injury in these cases.

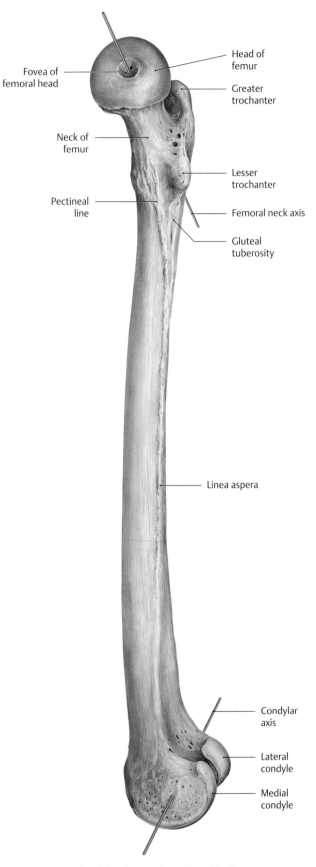

Fig. 16.6 Proximal and distal axes of rotation of the femur
Right femur.

B Hip joint in external rotation.

C Hip joint in medial rotation.

A Hip joint with femoral head centered in the acetabulum.

Fig. 16.7 Orientation of the hip joint relative to the knee joint

A Anterior view.

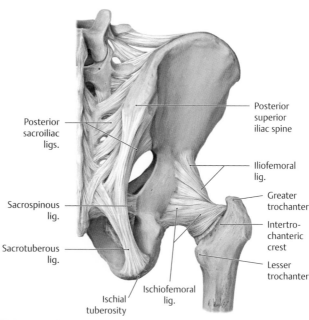

B Posterior view.

Fig. 16.8 Ligaments of the hip joint and pelvic girdle

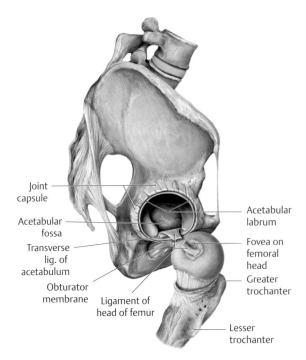

Fig. 16.9 Joint capsule of the hip joint
Lateral view. The capsule has been divided and the femoral head
dislocated to expose the cut ligament of the head of the femur.

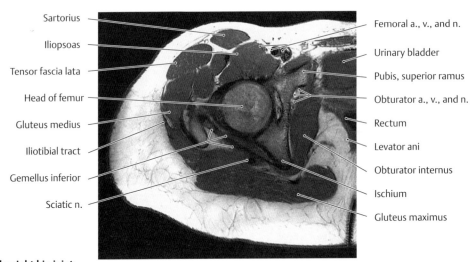

Fig. 16.10 MRI of the right hip joint
Transverse section, inferior view.

Table 16.2 **Movements of the Hip Joint**

Action	Primary Muscles
Flexion	Iliopsoas
	Tensor fascia latae
	Sartorius
	Rectus femoris
	Pectineus
Extension	Gluteus maximus
	Adductor magnus
	Biceps femoris, long head
	Semimembranosus
	Semitendinosus
Abduction	Gluteus medius
	Gluteus minimus
	Tensor fascia latae
Adduction	Gluteus maximus Adductor longus
	Adductor brevis
	Adductor magnus
	Pectineus
	Gracilis
Internal rotation	Gluteus medius
	Gluteus minimus
	Tensor fascia latae
External rotation	Gluteus maximus
	Quadratus femoris
	Piriformis
	Obturator externus
	Obturator internus

A Flexion

B Extension

C Abduction

D Adduction

E Internal rotation

F External rotation

Muscles of the Thigh

The powerful muscles of the thigh move the hip and knee joints and are separated into three compartments (see **Fig. 16.51A**).

— The anterior thigh compartment contains
  • muscles that primarily flex the hip joint and extend the knee joint (**Table 16.3**);
  • the femoral nerve; and
  • branches of the femoral artery, the deep artery of the thigh, and their accompanying veins.
— The medial thigh compartment contains
  • muscles that primarily adduct, flex, and extend the hip joint (**Table 16.4**);
  • the obturator and femoral nerves; and
  • the obturator artery and vein and deep artery and vein of the thigh.
— The posterior compartment contains
  • muscles that extend the hip joint and flex the knee joint (**Table 16.5**),

  • the sciatic nerve, and
  • branches of the deep artery and vein of the thigh.

HAMSTRING STRAINS Hamstring strains are tears of the hamstring (posterior thigh) muscles at their proximal attachment to the pelvic girdle. This is a common injury in individuals who participate in sports that involve sprinting with sudden starts and stops. Forced high kicks, especially with an extended knee, may avulse the muscle tendons from their origin at the ischial tuberosity. Symptoms include sudden, sharp pain in the back of the thigh during physical activity, a popping or tearing feeling in the muscle, swelling, muscle weakness, and an inability to bear weight on the affected leg.

— Three muscles of the thigh, the **sartorius, gracilis,** and **semitendinosus,** cross the knee medially and join to form the **pes anserinus,** a common tendon that overlies the **anserine bursa** inferomedial to the knee joint (see **Fig. 16.43**).

Thigh muscles, anterior compartment, right side.

Table 16.3 **Thigh Muscles, Anterior Compartment**

Muscle		Origin	Insertion	Innervation	Action
① Sartorius		Anterior superior iliac spine	Medial to the tibial tuberosity (together with gracilis and semitendinosus)	Femoral n. (L2–L3)	• Hip joint: flexion, abduction, and external rotation • Knee joint: flexion and internal rotation
	② Rectus femoris	Anterior inferior iliac spine, acetabular roof of hip joint	Tibial tuberosity (via patellar ligament)	Femoral n. (L2–L4)	• Hip joint: flexion • Knee joint: extension
	③ Vastus medialis	Linea aspera (medial lip), intertrochanteric line (distal part)	Both sides of tuberosity on the medial and lateral condyles (via the medial and longitudinal patellar retinacula)		Knee joint: extension
Quadriceps femoris*	④ Vastus lateralis	Linea aspera (lateral lip), greater trochanter (lateral surface)			
	⑤ Vastus intermedius	Femoral shaft (anterior side)	Tibial tuberosity (via patellar ligament)		
	Articularis genus (distal fibers of vastus intermedius)	Anterior side of femoral shaft at level of the suprapatellar recess	Suprapatellar recess of knee joint capsule		Knee joint: extension; prevents entrapment of capsule

*The entire muscle inserts on the tibial tuberosity via the patellar ligament.

A Thigh muscles, medial compartment, superficial layer, anterior view.

B Thigh muscles, medial compartment, deep layer, anterior view.

Table 16.4 **Thigh Muscles, Medial Compartment: Superficial and Deep Layers**

Muscle	Origin	Insertion	Innervation	Action
Superficial layer				
① Pectineus	Pecten pubis	Femur (pectineal line and the proximal linea aspera)	Femoral n., obturator n. (L2–L3)	• Hip joint: adduction, external rotation, and slight flexion • Stabilizes the pelvis in the coronal and sagittal planes
② Adductor longus	Superior pubic ramus and anterior side of the symphysis	Femur (linea aspera, medial lip in the middle third of the femur)	Obturator n. (L2–L4)	• Hip joint: adduction and flexion (up to 70 degrees); extension (past 80 degrees of flexion) • Stabilizes the pelvis in the coronal and sagittal planes
③ Adductor brevis	Inferior pubic ramus		Obturator n. (L2–L3)	
④ Gracilis	Inferior pubic ramus below the symphysis	Tibia (medial border of the tuberosity, along with the tendons of sartorius and semitendinosus)		• Hip joint: adduction and flexion • Knee joint: flexion and internal rotation
Deep layer				
⑤ Obturator externus	Outer surface of the obturator membrane and its bony boundaries	Trochanteric fossa of the femur	Obturator n. (L3–L4)	• Hip joint: adduction and external rotation • Stabilizes the pelvis in the sagittal plane
⑥ Adductor magnus	Inferior pubic ramus, ischial ramus, and ischial tuberosity	• Deep part ("fleshy insertion"): medial lip of the linea spine	• Deep part: obturator n. (L2–L4)	• Hip joint: adduction, extension, and slight flexion (the tendinous insertion is also active in internal rotation) • Stabilizes the pelvis in the coronal and sagittal planes
		• Superficial part ("tendinous insertion"): adductor tubercle of the femur	• Superficial part: tibial n. (L4)	

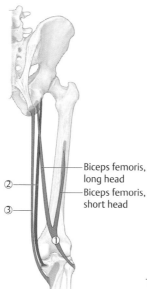

Biceps femoris, long head

Biceps femoris, short head

Thigh muscles, posterior compartment, right side.

Table 16.5 **Thigh Muscles, Posterior Compartment**

Muscle	Origin	Insertion	Innervation	Action
① Biceps femoris	Long head: ischial tuberosity, sacrotuberous ligament (common head with semitendinosus)	Head of fibula	Tibial n. (L5–S2)	• Hip joint (long head): extends the hip, stabilizes the pelvis in the sagittal plane • Knee joint: flexion and external rotation
	Short head: lateral lip of the linea aspera in the middle third of the femur		Common fibular n. (L5–S2)	Knee joint: flexion and external rotation
② Semimembranosus	Ischial tuberosity	Medial tibial condyle, oblique popliteal ligament, popliteus fascia	Tibial n. (L5–S2)	• Hip joint: extends the hip, stabilizes the pelvis in the sagittal plane • Knee joint: flexion and internal rotation
③ Semitendinosus	Ischial tuberosity and sacrotuberous ligament (common head with long head of biceps femoris)	Medial to the tibial tuberosity in the pes anserinus (along with the tendons of gracilis and sartorius)		

Spaces of the Thigh

The femoral nerve, artery, and vein descend through narrow passages in the thigh that are created by the inguinal ligament and anterior and medial thigh muscles.

— Anteriorly, structures pass from the abdomen into the thigh through the **retroinguinal space,** deep to the inguinal ligament. The retroinguinal space is divided into a lateral muscular compartment and a medial vascular compartment **(Fig. 16.11)**.

- The muscular compartment contains the femoral nerve and iliopsoas muscle.
- The vascular compartment contains the femoral vessels enclosed within the **femoral sheath.**
- The femoral sheath, formed by extensions of the transversalis and psoas fasciae, surrounds the femoral vessels as they pass under the inguinal ligament. Inferiorly, the sheath merges with the outer layer of the vessel walls (adventitia). Septa divide the sheath into compartments:

  ◦ Lateral and central compartments contain the femoral artery and femoral vein, respectively.
  ◦ A medial compartment within the sheath, the **femoral canal,** contains loose connective tissue, fat, and often a deep inguinal lymph node. The **femoral ring** defines the superior opening of the canal.

CLINICAL CORRELATION

FEMORAL HERNIAS Femoral hernias (usually of the small intestine) are always acquired and are more common in women. They pass inferior to the inguinal ligament, through the femoral ring and femoral canal, and appear in the femoral triangle inferior and lateral to the pubic tubercle **(Fig. 16.12)**. They should be distinguished from inguinal hernias, which occur superior and lateral to the pubic tubercle (above the inguinal ligament).

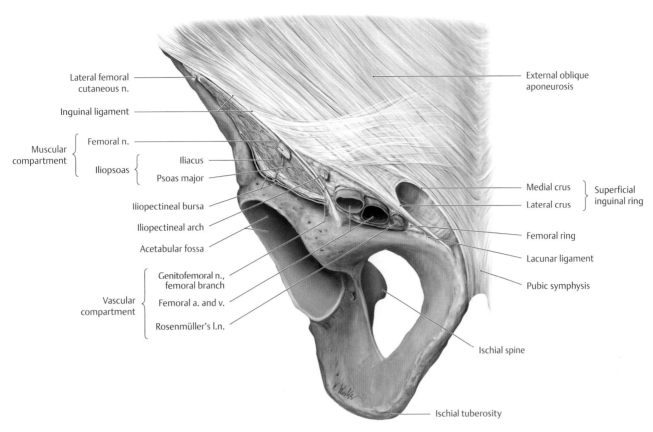

Fig. 16.11 Retroinguinal space: Muscular and vascular compartments
Right inguinal region, anterior view.

Lateral femoral cutaneous n.

Inguinal ligament

Muscular compartment { Femoral n.

Iliopsoas { Iliacus

Psoas major

Iliopectineal bursa

Iliopectineal arch

Acetabular fossa

Vascular compartment { Genitofemoral n., femoral branch

Femoral a. and v.

Rosenmüller's l.n.

External oblique aponeurosis

Medial crus } Superficial inguinal ring

Lateral crus

Femoral ring

Lacunar ligament

Pubic symphysis

Ischial spine

Ischial tuberosity

Fig. 16.12 Femoral hernia
Right female inguinal region, anterior view.

Rosenmüller lymph nodes (deep inguinal lymph nodes)

Femoral vessels in the saphenous opening

Peritoneum of hernial sac

Transversalis fascia

Fascia lata

Inferior epigastric vessels

Inguinal ligament

Superficial inguinal ring

Uterine round ligament

Lacunar ligament

Hernial sac

Great saphenous vein

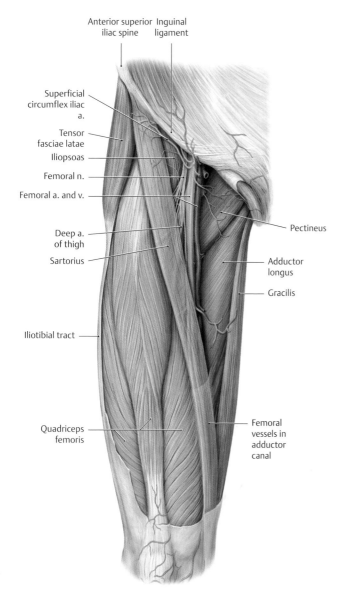

Fig. 16.13 Anterior thigh
Right thigh, anterior view. *Revealed:* Femoral triangle. *Removed:* Skin, subcutaneous tissue, and fascia lata. *Partially transparent:* Sartorius.

— The **femoral triangle** is an area of the anterior thigh (**Fig. 16.13**).
  • It contains the femoral artery and vein and their branches and the terminal branches of the femoral nerve.
  • Its boundaries are
    ◦ superiorly, the inguinal ligament;
    ◦ medially, the adductor longus muscle;
    ◦ laterally, the sartorius muscle;
    ◦ the floor, formed by the iliopsoas and pectineus muscles; and
    ◦ the apex, formed by the inferior junction of the medial and lateral borders.
— The **adductor canal** is an intermuscular passage between the anterior and medial thigh muscles.
  • It contains the femoral vessels and the saphenous branch of the femoral nerve.

• The canal begins at the inferior apex of the femoral triangle and ends at the **adductor hiatus,** an opening in the tendon of the adductor magnus muscle.

16.4 The Knee and Popliteal Region

The popliteal region connects the thigh and leg. It contains the knee joint and the popliteal fossa and its contents.

The Knee Joint

The knee joint is a modified hinge joint that includes the medial and lateral articulations between the condyles of the femur and tibia, and the articulation between the femur and patella (**Figs. 16.14** and **16.15**). Flexion and extension are the primary movements at the knee joint, but some rotation and sliding also occur.
— The patella articulates with the patellar surface of the femur between the medial and lateral condyles and protects the knee joint anteriorly. The patella is embedded in the tendon of the quadriceps femoris muscle, increasing the leverage of the muscle by holding the tendon away from the joint.
— Although the articular surfaces of the femur and tibia are extensive, there is little congruity between the bones, and stability depends chiefly on
  • ligaments that connect the tibia and femur; and
  • muscles that surround the joint, most importantly the quadriceps femoris.
— The fibrous capsule of the knee joint is thin and incomplete and derives additional support from **patellar retinacula** (capsular ligaments that attach anteriorly to the quadriceps tendon), the patella, and **extracapsular ligaments** around the joint (**Fig. 16.16**).
— Extracapsular (external) ligaments support the fibrous capsule (**Figs. 16.17** and **16.18**).
  • **The patellar ligament,** the distal part of the quadriceps tendon that supports the knee joint anteriorly, extends from the patella to the tibial tuberosity.
  • The two **collateral ligaments** limit rotation and prevent medial and lateral dislocation of the knee joint. They are tightest in extension and slacken during flexion.
    ◦ The **lateral (fibular) collateral ligament** is cordlike and remains unattached to the joint capsule. It extends from the lateral epicondyle of the femur to the head of the fibula.
    ◦ The **medial (tibial) collateral ligament** is flat and ribbonlike and is attached to the joint capsule and medial meniscus. It extends from the medial epicondyle of the femur to the medial condyle and anteromedial aspect of the tibia.

CLINICAL CORRELATION

PATELLAR TENDON REFLEX The patellar tendon reflex is initiated by tapping the patellar tendon to elicit contraction of the quadriceps femoris muscle (extension of the knee). It tests the integrity of the L2–L4 spinal cord segments carried by the femoral nerve.

• The **oblique popliteal ligament** is an expansion of the semimembranosus tendon, which supports the joint capsule posteriorly and laterally.

A Anterior view.

B Posterior view.

Fig. 16.14 Right knee joint

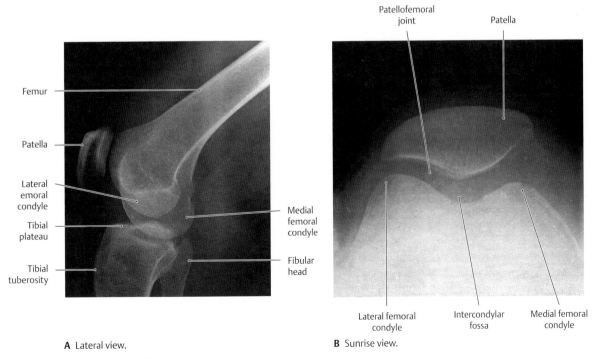

A Lateral view.

B Sunrise view.

Fig. 16.15 Radiograph of the knee in flexion

Fig. 16.16 Ligaments of the knee joint
Right knee, anterior view.

Femur

Vastus intermedius tendon of insertion

Vastus lateralis

Vastus medialis

Rectus femoris tendon of insertion

Lateral transverse patellar retinaculum

Medial collateral lig.

Lateral longitudinal patellar retinaculum

Medial transverse patellar retinaculum

Lateral collateral lig.

Medial longitudinal patellar retinaculum

Head of fibula

Patellar lig.

Tibial tuberosity

Fibula

Tibia

Interosseous membrane

A Medial view.

B Lateral view.

Fig. 16.17 Collateral and patellar ligaments of the knee joint
Right knee joint. Each knee joint has medial and lateral collateral
ligaments. The medial collateral ligament is attached to both the capsule
and the medial meniscus, whereas the lateral collateral ligament has no
direct contact with either the capsule or the lateral meniscus. Both
collateral ligaments are taut when the knee is in extension and stabilize
the joint in the coronal plane.

- The **arcuate popliteal ligament** extends from the fibular
  head to the posterior knee joint and reinforces the joint
  capsule posteriorly and laterally.
— In addition to the support provided by extracapsular
  ligaments, the capsule is strengthened by tendinous attachments of muscles that cross the joint. Bursae associated with
  these muscular attachments are numerous and include

- the **suprapatellar bursa** (pouch), which lies deep to the
  quadriceps femoris tendon and communicates with the
  cavity of the knee joint;
- the **prepatellar bursa,** which is subcutaneous over the
  patella;
- the **superficial infrapatellar bursa,** which is subcutaneous over the patellar ligament;

- • the **deep infrapatellar bursa,** which lies deep to the patellar ligament; and
- • the **anserine bursa,** which lies between the pes anserinus and tibial collateral ligament.
- — Additional bursae around the knee communicate with the joint cavity. They include the **subpopliteal recess**, the **semimembranosus bursa**, and the **medial subtendinous bursa** of the gastrocnemius (**Fig. 16.18**).
- — Intra-articular ligaments provide stability during movements of the joint (**Figs. 16.19** and **16.20**).
  - • Two **cruciate ligaments** are located within the joint capsule but lie external to the synovial layer. They provide stability in all positions, in addition to limiting rotation and preventing anterior and posterior dislocation of the joint.
    - ○ The **anterior cruciate ligament** arises from the anterior intercondylar part of the tibia and extends posterolaterally to the medial aspect of the lateral femoral condyle.
    - ○ The **posterior cruciate ligament** arises from the posterior intercondylar part of the tibia and extends anteromedially to the lateral aspect of the medial femoral condyle.
  - • A **transverse ligament** connects the menisci to each other along their anterior edges.
  - • A **posterior meniscofemoral ligament** joins the lateral meniscus to the posterior cruciate ligament and medial femoral condyle.

Fig. 16.18 Capsule, ligaments, and periarticular bursae of the knee joint
Right knee, posterior view.

Patellar surface of femur

Anterior cruciate lig.

Transverse lig. of knee

Lateral meniscus

Lateral collateral lig.

Anterior lig. of fibular head

Fibula

Medial femoral condyle

Posterior cruciate lig.

Medial meniscus

Medial collateral lig.

Patellar lig. (reflected inferiorly)

Patella

A Anterior view.

Intercondylar notch

Lateral femoral condyle

Anterior cruciate lig.

Posterior menisco-femoral lig.

Lateral meniscus

Lateral collateral lig.

Posterior lig. of fibular head

Head of fibula

Interosseous membrane

Tibia

B Posterior view.

Fig. 16.19 Cruciate and collateral ligaments of the knee joint
Right knee. The cruciate ligaments keep the articular surfaces of the femur and tibia in contact, while stabilizing the knee joint primarily in the sagittal plane. Portions of the cruciate ligaments are taut in every joint position.

Patella

Anterior cruciate ligament

Hoffa's fat pad

Patellar ligament

Femur

Posterior cruciate ligament

Tibia

Fig. 16.20 MRI of the knee joint
Sagittal section through the cruciate ligaments.

CLINICAL CORRELATION

LIGAMENTOUS INJURIES OF THE KNEE Most knee injuries occur during physical activity and involve rupture or strain of the knee ligaments. A forceful blow to the lateral side of the knee can strain the medial collateral ligament and, because of their intimate relationship, tear the medial meniscus as well. A similar injury can result from excessive lateral rotation of the knee and is often accompanied by rupture of the anterior cruciate ligament. The Lachman test is used to demonstrate instability of the knee joint resulting from rupture of the cruciate ligaments **(Fig. 16.21)**. Excessive anterior translation of the free-hanging tibia from under the stabilized femur is a positive anterior drawer sign, indicating anterior cruciate rupture. Posterior displacement of the tibia is a positive posterior drawer sign, indicating rupture of the posterior cruciate ligament.

A Right knee in flexion, rupture of anterior cruciate ligament, anterior view.

B Right knee in flexion, anterior "drawer sign," medial view. During examination the tibia can be pulled forward *(arrow)*.

Fig. 16.21 **Rupture of the anterior cruciate ligament**

— **Menisci,** crescent-shaped fibrocartilaginous pads, deepen the articular surfaces of the tibial plateau. Wedge-shaped in cross section, they are tallest at the outer rim, where they are attached to the joint capsule and the intercondylar ridge **(Figs. 16.22, 16.23, 16.24)**.
  • The **medial meniscus** is C-shaped and relatively immobile due to its additional attachment to the tibial collateral ligament.

  • The **lateral meniscus** is nearly circular and more mobile during flexion and extension of the joint than its medial counterpart.
— An extensive synovial layer lines the internal surface of the joint capsule. Its posterior aspect extends into the intercondylar space of the joint cavity and reflects around the intracapsular ligaments, dividing most of the joint space into medial and lateral parts **(Figs. 16.25 and 16.26)**.
— Muscles of the thigh and leg move the knee joint **(Table 16.6)**.

Anterior cruciate lig.

Patellar lig.

Medial meniscus

Transverse lig. of knee

Tibiofibular joint

Medial collateral lig.

Lateral collateral lig.

Posterior cruciate lig.

Posterior meniscofemoral lig.

Lateral meniscus

Head of fibula

Fig. 16.22 **Menisci in the knee joint**
Right tibial plateau with cruciate, patellar, and collateral ligaments divided, proximal view.

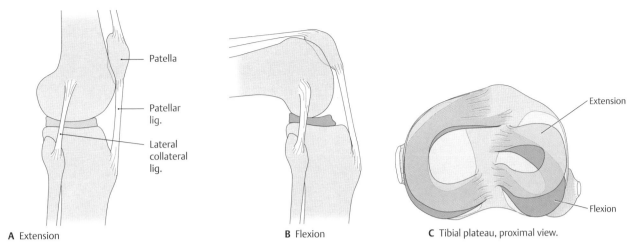

A Extension

B Flexion

C Tibial plateau, proximal view.

Patella

Patellar lig.

Lateral collateral lig.

Extension

Flexion

Fig. 16.23 Movements of the menisci

Quadriceps tendon

Suprapatellar bursa

Femur

Patella

Deep infrapatellar bursa

Lateral meniscus

Patellar lig.

Lateral collateral lig.

Subpopliteal recess

Infrapatellar bursa

Fibula

Tibia

Outer meniscus

Gastrocnemius, lateral head

Fig. 16.25 Joint cavity of the knee
Right knee, lateral view. The joint cavity was demonstrated by injecting liquid plastic into the knee joint and later removing the capsule.

Fig. 16.24 MRI of the knee joint
Sagittal section through the lateral meniscus.

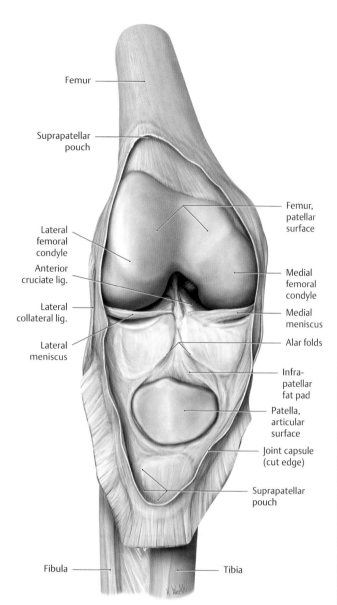

Fig. 16.26 Opened joint capsule of the knee
Right knee, anterior view, with patella reflected downward.

A Flexion

B Extension

C Internal rotation with the knee joint flexed

D External rotation with the knee joint flexed

Table 16.6 **Movements of the Knee Joint**

Action	Primary Muscles
Flexion	Biceps femoris—short and long heads
	Semimembranosus
	Semitendinosus
	Sartorius
	Gracilis
	Gastrocnemius
	Popliteus
Extension	Quadriceps femoris
Internal rotation	Semimembranosus
	Semitendinosus
	Sartorius
	Gracilis
	Popliteus (of nonbearing leg)
External rotation	Biceps femoris

Anatomic axis of the femur

Center of rotation of the femoral head (hip joint)

Mechanical axis (Mikulicz line)

Intercondylar eminence of the tibial plateau (knee joint)

Knee baseline

81°

174°

93°

Ankle mortise

Talocrural joint

A Normal mechanical axis, anterior view.

Gluteus maximus (superior part)

Iliotibial tract

Biceps femoris

B Axis in genu varum, posterior view.

Sartorius

Semi-tendinosus

Gracilis

Mechanical axis

C Axis in genu valgum, posterior view.

Fig. 16.27 The mechanical axis of the leg

CLINICAL CORRELATION

GENU VARUM AND GENU VALGUM Although the femur lies diagonally within the thigh, the tibia is nearly vertical in the leg. This creates a Q angle at the knee between the long axes of the two bones. The angle varies with developmental stage and sex, but it can also be altered by disease. Normally, the head of the femur sits over the center of the knee joint, distributing weight evenly on the tibial plateau. In genu varum (bowleg), the Q angle is smaller than normal because the femur is more vertical. This increases the weight on the medial side of the knee, putting additional stress on the medial meniscus and medial (tibial) collateral ligament. When a person is standing upright with feet and ankles together, the knees are wide apart. In genu valgum (knock knee), the Q angle is larger because the femur is more diagonal. Greater weight is put on the lateral side of the knee, stressing the lateral meniscus and lateral (fibular) collateral ligament. In the upright position, the knees touch, but the ankles do not **(Fig. 16.27)**.

The Popliteal Fossa

The popliteal fossa is a diamond-shaped space posterior to the knee joint **(Fig. 16.28** and **16.29)**.

— Its muscular boundaries are
  • superomedially, the semimembranosus muscle;
  • superolaterally, the biceps femoris muscle; and
  • inferiorly, the medial and lateral heads of the gastrocnemius muscle.

— The contents of the fossa, which are embedded within popliteal fat, include
  • the popliteal artery and vein and their genicular branches,
  • popliteal lymph nodes, and
  • tibial and common fibular nerves.

— At the superior apex of the popliteal fossa, the sciatic nerve splits into its two terminal branches.
  • The tibial nerve descends into the posterior leg compartment with the popliteal vessels.
  • The common fibular nerve courses laterally along the edge of the biceps femoris muscle to enter the lateral leg compartment.

A Superficial neurovascular structures.

Semitendinosus

Semimem-
branosus

Tibial n.

Gastrocnemius,
medial head

Gastrocnemius,
lateral head

Great
saphenous v.

Biceps
femoris

Plantaris

Common
fibular n.

Small
saphenous v.

Medial sural
cutaneous n.

Lateral sural
cutaneous n.

B Deep neurovascular structures.

Popliteal
a. and v.

Sciatic n.

Biceps femoris,
long head

Gracilis

Semi-
membranosus

Semi-
tendinosus

Gastrocnemius,
medial head

Medial
subtendinous
bursa of
gastrocnemius

Middle genicular a.

Semimembranosus
bursa

Oblique popliteal
lig.

Semimembranosus
tendon

Medial inferior
genicular a.

Tibial n.

Popliteus

Biceps
femoris,
short head

Common
fibular n.

Medial superior
genicular a.

Lateral superior
genicular a.

Plantaris

Gastroc-
nemius,
lateral head

Lateral inferior
genicular a.

Posterior tibial
recurrent a.

Plantaris
tendon

Soleus
Gastrocnemius

Triceps
surae

Fig. 16.28 Popliteal fossa
Right leg, posterior view.

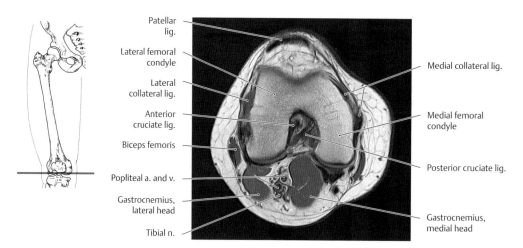

Patellar
lig.

Lateral femoral
condyle

Lateral
collateral lig.

Anterior
cruciate lig.

Biceps femoris

Popliteal a. and v.

Gastrocnemius,
lateral head

Tibial n.

Medial collateral lig.

Medial femoral
condyle

Posterior cruciate lig.

Gastrocnemius,
medial head

Fig. 16.29 MRI of the knee joint
Transverse section, inferior view.

Fig. 16.30 MRI of a Baker's cyst in the popliteal fossa
Transverse section, inferior view.

CLINICAL CORRELATION

POPLITEAL (BAKER'S) CYST Popliteal (Baker's) cysts, palpable fluid-filled synovial sacs that protrude into the popliteal fossa, are usually a consequence of chronic effusion of the knee joint. Often they result from a herniation of the bursae deep to the gastrocnemius or semimembranosus muscles. The sacs protrude through the fibrous layer of the joint capsule but maintain a communication with the synovial cavity. Some cysts may be asymptomatic, but others are painful and can impair flexion and extension of the knee joint **(Fig. 16.30)**.

16.5 The Leg

The leg extends from the knee to the ankle; it contains the tibia and fibula and the muscles of the leg (crural) compartments.

Tibiofibular Joints

The tibia and fibula are joined proximally at the knee and distally at the ankle. Unlike the extensive movement at the radioulnar joints in the forearm, only slight movement occurs at each tibiofibular joint, and no muscles are directly associated with them.

— The proximal **tibiofibular joint** is a plane-type synovial joint between the fibular head and an articular facet of the lateral condyle of the tibia. **Anterior** and **posterior ligaments of the fibular head** secure the joint (see **Fig. 16.19**).

— The distal **tibiofibular joint,** a compound fibrous joint, creates a mortise formed by the medial and lateral malleoli that cups the talus and stabilizes the ankle joint. Ligaments of the tibiofibular joint **(Fig. 16.31)** include

A Anterior view with talocrural joint in plantar flexion.

B Posterior view with foot in neutral (0-degree) position.

Fig. 16.31 Ligaments of the ankle and foot
Right foot.

• a deep **interosseous tibiofibular ligament,** the primary support of the joint, which is continuous with the interosseous membrane of the leg, and
• the external **anterior tibiofibular** and **posterior tibiofibular ligaments.**
— An interosseous membrane unites the shafts of the tibia and fibula and provides stability to the distal tibiofibular and ankle joints.

Muscles of the Leg

Muscles of the leg, which move the knee, ankle, and foot, are divided into four crural compartments (see **Fig. 16.51B**).
— The anterior compartment contains
• muscles that dorsiflex the foot and toes and invert the foot (**Table 16.7**),
• the deep fibular nerve, and
• the anterior tibial artery and veins.

CLINICAL CORRELATION

SHIN SPLINTS Shin splints result from chronic trauma of the tibialis anterior, usually incurred by overuse of the muscle during athletic activities. In what is considered a mild form of anterior compartment syndrome, small tears of the periosteum cause pain and swelling over the distal two thirds of the tibial shaft.

— The lateral compartment contains
• muscles that evert and plantar flex the foot (**Table 16.8**),
• the superficial fibular nerve, and
• the muscular branches of the fibular artery and veins from the posterior compartment.
— The superficial posterior compartment contains
• muscles that plantar flex the foot, two of which, the gastrocnemius and soleus, form the triceps surae and share a common tendon of insertion, the **calcaneal tendon (Table 16.9**);
• the tibial nerve; and
• the muscular branches of the posterior tibial artery and veins from the deep posterior compartment.

CLINICAL CORRELATION

RUPTURE OF THE CALCANEAL TENDON Rupture of the calcaneal tendon tends to occur following sudden forced plantar flexion of the foot, unexpected dorsiflexion of the foot, or violent dorsiflexion of a plantar-flexed foot in people unaccustomed to exercise or who exercise intermittently. The rupture disables the gastrocnemius, soleus, and plantaris muscles, rendering the patient unable to plantar flex the foot.

— The deep posterior compartment contains
• muscles that plantar flex the foot and toes and invert the foot (**Table 16.10**) (only one muscle, the popliteus, crosses the knee and laterally rotates the femur),
• the tibial nerve, and
• the posterior tibial and fibular artery and veins.

CLINICAL CORRELATION

COMPARTMENT SYNDROME Compartment syndrome is a condition that may follow burns, hemorrhage, complex fractures, or crush injuries. Swelling, infection, or bleeding into the compartment can increase intracompartmental pressure and, when high enough, compress the small vascular structures that supply the compartment contents. Nerves are particularly vulnerable to ischemia, and permanent loss of motor and sensory functions distal to the compartment can result. Symptoms include severe pain that is out of proportion to the injury, paresthesia (tingling and numbness), pallor of the skin, paralysis of muscles affected, and loss of distal pulses in the affected limb. Treatment is prompt surgery to decompress the compartment by making long cuts through the fascia (fasciotomy).

— Retinacula, thickened bands of the crural fascia, bind the tendons of the long extensor and flexor muscles as they cross the ankle (**Fig. 16.32**).
• **Superior extensor** and **inferior extensor retinacula** bind muscles of the anterior compartment.
• Medially, a **flexor retinaculum** binds muscles of the deep posterior compartment.
• **Superior fibular** and **inferior fibular retinacula** bind muscles of the lateral compartment.
— The **tarsal tunnel** is a passageway on the medial side of the ankle formed by the flexor retinaculum and its attachments to the medial malleolus and calcaneus. It transmits
• muscle tendons of the deep posterior compartment,
• posterior tibial artery and veins and their medial plantar and lateral plantar branches, and
• the tibial nerve and its medial plantar and lateral plantar branches.

CLINICAL CORRELATION

TARSAL TUNNEL SYNDROME Tarsal tunnel syndrome, similar to carpal tunnel syndrome of the hand, results from swelling of the synovial sheaths of the long flexor tendons within the tarsal tunnel. Compression of the tibial nerve can result in burning pain, numbness, and tingling that radiates to the heel.

Table 16.7 **Leg Muscles, Anterior Compartment**

Muscle	Origin	Insertion	Innervation	Action
① Tibialis anterior	Tibia (upper two thirds of the lateral surface), interosseous membrane, and superficial crural fascia (highest part)	Medial cuneiform (medial and plantar surface), first metatarsal (medial base)	Deep fibular n. (L4, L5)	• Talocrural joint: dorsiflexion • Subtalar joint: inversion (supination)
② Extensor hallucis longus	Fibula (middle third of the medial surface), interosseous membrane	1st toe (at the dorsal aponeurosis and the base of its distal phalanx)	Deep fibular n. (L4, L5)	• Talocrural joint: dorsiflexion • Subtalar joint: active in both eversion and inversion (pronation/supination), depending on the initial position of the foot • Extends the MTP and IP joints of the big toe
③ Extensor digitorum longus	Fibula (head and anterior border), tibia (lateral condyle), and interosseous membrane	2nd to 5th toes (at the dorsal aponeuroses at the bases of the distal phalanges)	Deep fibular n. (L4, L5)	• Talocrural joint: dorsiflexion • Subtalar joint: eversion (pronation) • Extends the MTP and IP joints of the 2nd to 5th toes
④ Fibularis tertius	Distal fibula (anterior border)	5th metatarsal (base)	Deep fibular n. (L4, L5)	• Talocrural joint: dorsiflexion • Subtalar joint: eversion (pronation)

Abbreviations: IP, interphalangeal; MTP, metatarsophalangeal.

Leg muscles, anterior compartment
Right leg, anterior view.

Table 16.8 **Leg Muscles, Lateral Compartment**

Muscle	Origin	Insertion	Innervation	Action
① Fibularis longus	Fibula (head and proximal two thirds of the lateral surface, arising partly from the intermuscular septa)	Medial cuneiform (plantar side), 1st metatarsal (base)	Superficial fibular n. (L5–S1)	• Talocrural joint: plantar flexion • Subtalar joint: eversion (pronation) • Supports the transverse arch of the foot
② Fibularis brevis	Fibula (distal half of the lateral surface), intermuscular septa	5th metatarsal (tuberosity at the base, with an occasional division to the dorsal aponeurosis of the 5th toe)		• Talocrural joint: plantar flexion • Subtalar joint: eversion (pronation)

Fibularis tertius

Leg muscles, lateral compartment
Right leg and foot, anterior view.

Table 16.9 **Leg Muscles, Posterior Compartment: Superficial Flexors**

Muscle		Origin	Insertion	Innervation	Action
Triceps surae	① Gastrocnemius	Femur (medial head: superior posterior part of the medial femoral condyle. lateral head: lateral surface of lateral femoral condyle)	Calcaneal tuberosity via the calcaneal (Achilles) tendon	Tibial n. (S1, S2)	• Talocrural joint: plantar flexion when knee is extended (gastrocnemius) • Knee joint: flexion (gastrocnemius) • Talocrural joint: plantar flexion (soleus)
	② Soleus	Fibula (head and neck, posterior surface), tibia (soleal line via a tendinous arch)	Calcaneal tuberosity		
③ Plantaris		Femur (lateral epicondyle, proximal to lateral head of gastrocnemius)			Negligible; may act with gastrocnemius in plantar flexion

Superficial flexors, posterior compartment of leg
Right leg with foot in plantar flexion, posterior view,

Table 16.10 **Leg Muscles, Posterior Compartment: Deep Flexors**

Muscle	Origin	Insertion	Innervation	Action
① Tibialis posterior	Interosseous membrane, adjacent borders of tibia and fibula	Navicular tuberosity; cuneiforms (medial, intermediate, and lateral); 2nd to 4th metatarsals (bases)	Tibial n. (L4, L5)	• Talocrural joint: plantar flexion • Subtalar joint: inversion (supination) • Supports the longitudinal and transverse arches
② Flexor digitorum longus	Tibia (middle third of posterior surface)	2nd to 5th distal phalanges (bases)	Tibial n. (L5–S2)	• Talocrural joint: plantar flexion • Subtalar joint: inversion (supination) • MTP and IP joints of the 2nd to 5th toes: plantar flexion
③ Flexor hallucis longus	Fibula (distal two thirds of posterior surface), adjacent interosseous membrane	1st distal phalanx (base)		• Talocrural joint: plantar flexion • Subtalar joint: inversion (supination) • MTP and IP joints of the 1st toe: plantar flexion • Supports the medial longitudinal arch
④ Popliteus	Lateral femoral condyle, posterior horn of the lateral meniscus	Posterior tibial surface (above the origin at the soleus)	Tibial n. (L4–S1)	Knee joint: flexes and unlocks the knee by internally rotating the femur on the fixed tibia 5 degrees

Abbreviations: IP, interphalangeal; MTP, metatarsophalangeal.

Deep flexors, posterior compartment of leg
Right leg with foot in plantar flexion, posterior view.

A Anterior view with talocrural joint in plantar flexion.

B Medial view.

C Lateral view.

Fig. 16.32 Tendon sheaths and retinacula of the ankle
Right foot. The superior and inferior extensor retinacula retain the long extensor tendons, the fibularis retinacula hold the fibular muscle tendons in place, and the flexor retinaculum retains the long flexor tendons through the tarsal tunnel.

16.6   The Ankle (Talocrural) Joint

The weight of the body is transferred along the tibia of the leg, through the talus at the ankle joint, and onto the heel and ball of the foot. Strong bony and ligamentous supports stabilize the ankle and facilitate this transfer of weight.

The **ankle joint** includes articulations between the distal tibia and fibula and the talus (**Figs. 16.33, 16.34, 16.35, 16.36**).

— At the ankle joint, the ankle mortise, which is formed by the distal tibiofibular joint, hugs the body of the talus. Tibiofibular ligaments that stabilize the ankle mortise also contribute to the stability of the ankle joint.

— The ankle joint is tighter and more stable with the foot in dorsiflexion, when the wider anterior part of the trochlea (of the talus) is wedged within the ankle mortise. Accordingly, the joint is looser and less stable in plantar flexion.

— Strong collateral talocrural ligaments connect the tibia and fibula to the tarsal bones and support the talocrural articulations (**Fig. 16.37**).

- The medial **deltoid ligament** of the ankle extends from the medial malleolus of the tibia to the talus, calcaneus, and navicular. Its components are
  - the **anterior tibiotalar part,**
  - the **posterior tibiotalar part,**
  - the **tibiocalcaneal part,** and
  - the **tibionavicular part.**
- The **lateral ligament of the ankle** extends from the lateral malleolus of the fibula to the talus and calcaneus. Its parts are
  - the **anterior talofibular ligament,**
  - the **posterior talofibular ligament,** and
  - the **calcaneofibular ligament.**

CLINICAL CORRELATION

ANKLE SPRAINS Ankle sprains (torn ligaments) are caused most often by forced inversion of the foot (e.g., walking on uneven ground). Damage to the lateral talocrural ligaments is correlated with the severity of the injury and proceeds from anterior to posterior: the anterior talofibular ligament is the most easily injured, followed by the calcaneofibular and the least frequently injured, the posterior talofibular ligament. Fracture of the lateral malleolus can also accompany inversion injuries.

- Movement at the ankle joint, provided by muscles of the leg, is limited primarily to dorsiflexion (extension) and plantar flexion (**Table 16.11**).

Subtalar (talocalcaneal) joint
Intercuneiform joints
Cuneocuboid joint
Tarsometatarsal joints
Proximal interphalangeal joints
Distal interphalangeal joints

Talocrural (ankle) joint
Talonavicular joint
Calcaneocuboid joint } Tranverse tarsal joint
Cuneonavicular joint
Intermetatarsal joints
Metatarsophalangeal joints
Interphalangeal joint of the hallux

Fig. 16.33 Joints of the foot
Right foot with talocrural joint in plantar flexion, anterior view.

Fig. 16.34 Talocrural and subtalar joints
Right foot with foot in neutral (0-degree) position, posterior view.

Tibia

Fibula

Ankle mortise

Medial malleolus

Lateral malleolus

Talocrural joint

Talus

Navicular

Subtalar (talocalcaneal) joint

Sustentaculum tali

1st metatarsal

Tuberosity of 5th metatarsal

Sesamoids

Calcaneal tuberosity

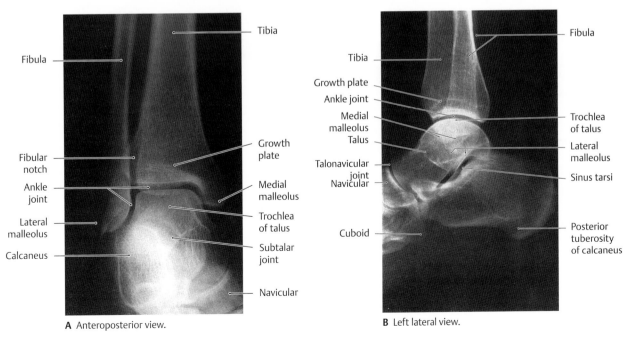

Tibia

Fibula

Fibula

Growth plate

Fibular notch

Medial malleolus

Ankle joint

Trochlea of talus

Lateral malleolus

Subtalar joint

Calcaneus

Navicular

Tibia

Fibula

Growth plate

Ankle joint

Trochlea of talus

Medial malleolus

Talus

Lateral malleolus

Talonavicular joint

Sinus tarsi

Navicular

Cuboid

Posterior tuberosity of calcaneus

A Anteroposterior view.

B Left lateral view.

Fig. 16.35 Radiograph of the ankle

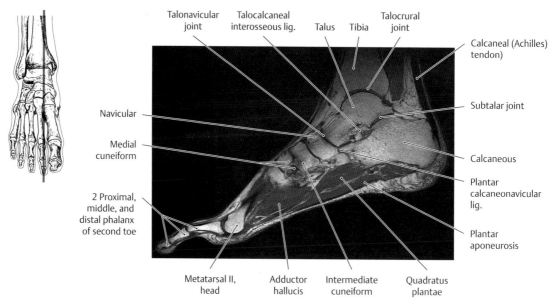

Fig. 16.36 MRI of the right ankle and foot
A Right foot and ankle, sagittal section.

A Medial view.

Fig. 16.37 Ligaments of the ankle and foot
Right foot.

B Lateral view.

Fig. 16.37 (*continued*) **Ligaments of the ankle and foot**

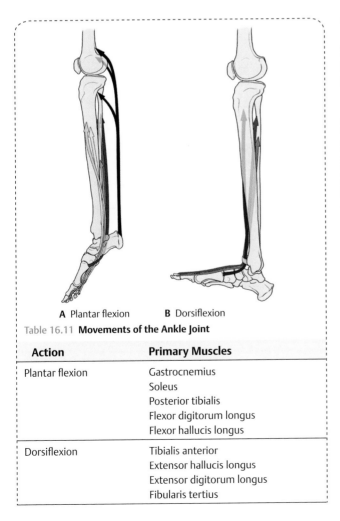

| **A** Plantar flexion | **B** Dorsiflexion |

Table 16.11 **Movements of the Ankle Joint**

Action	Primary Muscles
Plantar flexion	Gastrocnemius
	Soleus
	Posterior tibialis
	Flexor digitorum longus
	Flexor hallucis longus
Dorsiflexion	Tibialis anterior
	Extensor hallucis longus
	Extensor digitorum longus
	Fibularis tertius

16.7 The Foot

The numerous joints of the foot create a flexible unit that effectively absorbs shock, distributes the weight of vertical loads, and participates in locomotion.

Joints of the Foot and Toes

Movements at the joints of the foot, particularly the intertarsal (subtalar and transverse tarsal), metatarsophalangeal, and interphalangeal joints, contribute to smooth locomotion and maintenance of balance (see **Fig. 16.33**).

— The **subtalar joint** is an articulation between the inferior surface of the talus and underlying calcaneus (**Fig. 16.38;** see also **Figs. 16.35B** and **16.36**).

• It is a compound joint that has anterior and posterior compartments.

    ○ The anterior compartment contains the talocalcaneal component of the talocalcaneonavicular articulation.

    ○ The posterior compartment contains the posterior talocalcaneal articulation.

• A strong **interosseous talocalcaneal ligament** joins the bones and separates the anterior and posterior parts of the joint.

• This joint is the main articulation that allows inversion and eversion of the foot.

— The **transverse tarsal joint** is a compound joint that combines the talonavicular and calcaneocuboid articulations.

• Movement at this joint rotates the front of the foot relative to the heel, augmenting the inversion and eversion at the subtalar joint.

• This joint is a common site for surgical amputation of the foot.

Fig. 16.38 Subtalar joint and ligaments
Right foot with opened subtalar joint, dorsal view. The subtalar joint consists of two distinct articulations separated by the interosseous talocalcaneal ligament: the posterior compartment (talocalcaneal joint) and the anterior compartment (talocalcaneonavicular joint).

A Inversion and supination (lifting the medial border of the foot)

B Eversion and pronation (lifting the lateral border of the foot)

Table 16.12 **Movements of the Subtalor and Transverse Tarsal Joints**

Action	Primary Muscles
Inversion and supination	Tibialis anterior
	Tibialis posterior
	Flexor hallucis longus
	Flexor digitorum longus
Eversion and pronation	Fibularis longus
	Fibularis brevis
	Fibularis tertius

— **The tarsometatarsal** and **intermetatarsal joints** are small and relatively immobile.
— **Metatarsophalangeal joints** are condyloid synovial joints between the heads of the metatarsals and base of the phalanges.
  • Flexion, extension, and some abduction and adduction occur at this joint.
— **Interphalangeal joints** are hinge–type synovial joints that primarily allow flexion and extension of the toes, with some inversion and eversion of the foot.
  • Digits 2 through 4 have **proximal interphalangeal (PIP)** and **distal interphalangeal (DIP) joints.**
  • The great toe has only a single interphalangeal joint.
— Muscles of the leg and foot move the joints of the foot (**Tables 16.12** and **16.13**).

Table 16.13 **Movements of the Metatarsophalangeal and Interphalangeal Joints**

Action	Primary Muscles
Flexion	Flexor hallucis longus
	Flexor hallucis brevis
	Flexor digitorum longus
	Flexor digitorum brevis
	Lumbricals
	Dorsal and palmar interossei
Extension	Extensor hallucis longus
	Extensor hallucis brevis
	Extensor digitorum longus
	Extensor digitorum brevis
Abduction	Abductor hallucis
	Abductor digiti minimi
	Dorsal interossei
Adduction	Adductor hallucis
	Plantar interossei

Arches of the Foot

The tarsal and metatarsal bones form flexible longitudinal and transverse arches on the sole of the foot.

— The arches function as a unit to
  - distribute weight onto the heel and ball of the foot,
  - act as shock absorbers during locomotion, and
  - enhance the flexibility of the foot when planted on uneven surfaces.
— The longitudinal arch has medial and lateral parts (**Fig. 16.39**).
  - The medial arch is the highest part of the longitudinal arch, formed by the talus, navicular, three cuneiforms, and medial metatarsals. The head of the talus is the keystone of the arch.
  - The lateral arch is flatter than the medial arch and is formed by the calcaneus, cuboid, and lateral metatarsals.
— The transverse arch, formed by the cuboid, cuneiforms, and bases of the metatarsals, crosses the midfoot.
— The arches are supported by active and passive stabilizers (**Figs. 16.40** and **16.41**).
  - The primary active stabilizers of the arches are muscles of the leg and foot:
    ○ The tibialis posterior and fibularis longus of the leg
    ○ The short flexors, abductors, and adductors of the foot
  - The primary passive stabilizers of the arches are ligaments of the foot:
    ○ The plantar aponeurosis
    ○ The **plantar calcaneonavicular ligament** (spring ligament)
    ○ The **long plantar ligament**
    ○ The **plantar calcaneocuboid ligament** (short plantar ligament)

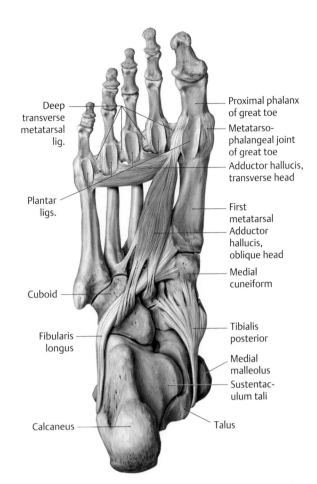

Fig. 16.40 Stabilizers of the transverse arch
Right foot, plantar view. The transverse pedal arch is supported by both active and passive stabilizing structures (muscles and ligaments, respectively). *Note:* The arch of the forefoot has only passive stabilizers, whereas the arches of the metatarsus and tarsus have only active stabilizers.

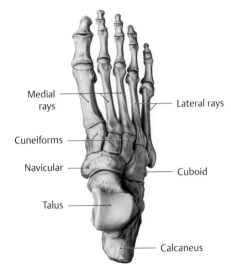

Fig. 16.39 Plantar vault
Right foot. The forces of the foot are distributed between two lateral and three medial rays. The arrangement of these rays creates a longitudinal and transverse arch in the sole of the foot, helping the foot absorb vertical loads.

CLINICAL CORRELATION

PES PLANUS Pes planus, or flatfoot, is a condition in which both the active and the passive stabilizers of the medial longitudinal arch are lax or absent. Because the head of the talus is not supported, it can displace inferomedially, and the forefoot everts and abducts, putting increased stress on the plantar calcaneonavicular (spring) ligament. Pes planus commonly occurs in older individuals who stand for long periods. Flatfoot is normal in children younger than 3 years, but this resolves with maturity.

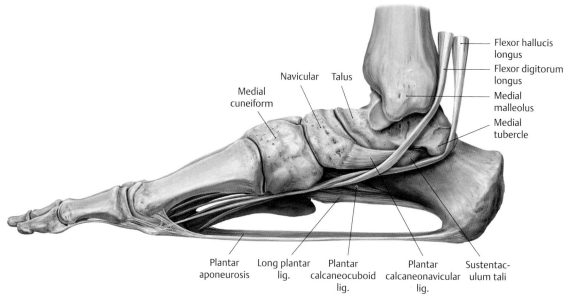

A Passive stabilizers (ligaments) of the longitudinal arch.

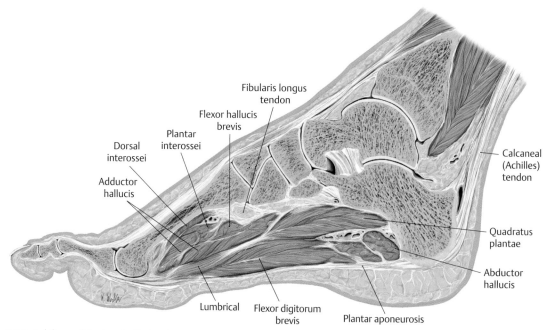

B Active stabilizers of the longitudinal arch.

Fig. 16.41 Stabilizers of the longitudinal arch
Right foot, medial view.

Dorsum of the Foot

— Surface anatomy on the dorsum of the foot reveals
- skin that is thin and loose,
- a superficial dorsal venous arch that is the origin of the great saphenous and small saphenous veins, and
- tendons of extensor muscles of the anterior leg compartment.
— A **dorsal muscular compartment** of the foot contains two intrinsic muscles, the **extensor digitorum brevis** and the **extensor hallucis brevis,** which extend the toes (**Table 16.14**).

Table 16.14 Intrinsic Muscles of the Dorsum of the Foot

Muscle	Origin	Insertion	Innervation	Action
① Extensor digitorum brevis	Calcaneus (dorsal surface)	2nd to 4th toes (at dorsal aponeuroses and bases of the middle phalanges)	Deep fibular n. (L5–S1)	Extension of the MTP and PIP joints of the 2nd to 4th toes
② Extensor hallucis brevis		1st toe (at dorsal aponeurosis and proximal phalanx)		Extension of the MTP joints of the 1st toe

Abbreviations: MTP, metatarsophalangeal; PIP, proximal interphalangeal.

Intrinsic muscles of the dorsum of the foot, right foot, dorsal view.

Sole of the Foot

— Surface anatomy on the sole of the foot reveals
  • tough, thickened skin, particularly on the heel, lateral side, and ball of the foot;
  • skin that is firmly attached to the underlying plantar aponeurosis; and
  • subcutaneous tissue divided by fibrous septa into fat-filled areas that act as shock absorbers, especially in the heel.
— The tough, longitudinal plantar aponeurosis (see **Fig. 16.48**)
  • attaches tightly to the skin of the sole,
  • originates at the calcaneus and is continuous distally with the fibrous digital sheaths that contain the flexor tendons of the toes,

  • protects the sole of the foot from injury, and
  • acts as a tie rod that supports the arches of the foot.
— The musculature of the sole is usually described as having four layers (**Tables 16.15** and **16.16**). However, as in the palm of the hand, the deep fascia separates the muscles of the sole into four fascial compartments:
  • The **medial compartment,** which contains the abductor and flexors of the 1st digit (hallux)
  • The **central compartment,** which contains the short and long flexors of the 2nd through 4th digits, the adductor hallucis, the lumbricals, and the quadratus plantae
  • The **lateral compartment,** which contains the abductor and flexor of the 5th digit
  • The **interosseous compartment,** which contains the interossei muscles

Table 16.15 Superficial Intrinsic Muscles of the Sole of the Foot

Muscle	Origin	Insertion	Innervation	Action
① Abductor hallucis	Calcaneal tuberosity (medial process); flexor retinaculum, plantar aponeurosis	1st toe (base of proximal phalanx via the medial sesamoid)	Medial plantar n. (S1, S2)	• 1st MTP joint: flexion and abduction of the 1st toe • Supports the longitudinal arch
② Flexor digitorum brevis	Calcaneal tuberosity (medial tubercle), plantar aponeurosis	2nd to 5th toes (sides of middle phalanges)		• Flexes the MTP and PIP joints of the 2nd to 5th toes • Supports the longitudinal arch
③ Abductor digiti minimi		5th toe (base of proximal phalanx), 5th metatarsal (at tuberosity)	Lateral plantar n. (S1–S3)	• Flexes the MTP joint of the 5th toe • Abducts the 5th toe • Supports the longitudinal arch

Superficial intrinsic muscles of the sole of the foot, right foot, first layer, plantar view.

Abbreviations: MTP, metatarsophalangeal; PIP, proximal interphalangeal.

Deep intrinsic muscles of the sole of the foot, right foot, plantar view.

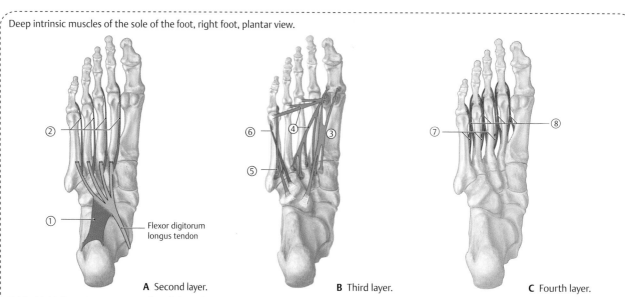

A Second layer.   **B** Third layer.   **C** Fourth layer.

Table 16.16 **Deep Intrinsic Muscles of the Sole**

Muscle	Origin	Insertion	Innervation	Action
① Quadratus plantae	Calcaneal tuberosity (medial and plantar borders on plantar side)	Flexor digitorum longus tendon (lateral border)	Lateral plantar n. (S1–S3)	Redirects and augments the pull of flexor digitorum longus
② Lumbricals (four muscles)	Flexor digitorum longus tendons (medial borders)	2nd to 5th toes (at dorsal aponeuroses)	1st lumbrical: medial plantar n. (S2, S3) 2nd and 4th lumbrical: lateral plantar n. (S2, S3)	• Flexes the MTP joints of 2nd to 5th toes • Extension of IP joints of 2nd to 5th toes • Adducts 2nd to 5th toes toward the big toe
③ Flexor hallucis brevis	Cuboid, lateral cuneiforms, and plantar calcaneocuboid lig.	1st toe (at base of proximal phalanx via medial and lateral sesamoids)	Medial head: medial plantar n. (S1, S2) Lateral head: lateral plantar n. (S1, S2)	• Flexes the first MTP joint • Supports the longitudinal arch
④ Adductor hallucis	Oblique head: 2nd to 4th metatarsals (at bases) cuboid and lateral cuneiforms Transverse head: MTPs of 3rd to 5th toes, deep transverse metatarsal lig.	1st proximal phalanx (at base, by a common tendon via the lateral sesamoid)	Lateral plantar n., deep branch (S2, S3)	• Flexes the first MTP joint • Adducts big toe • Transverse head: supports transverse arch • Oblique head: supports longitudinal arch
⑤ Flexor digiti minimi brevis	5th metatarsal (base), long plantar lig.	5th toe (base of proximal phalanx)	Lateral plantar n., superficial branch (S2, S3)	Flexes the MTP joint of the little toe
⑥ Opponens digiti minimi*	Long plantar lig.; fibularis longus (at plantar tendon sheath)	5th metatarsal		Pulls 5th metatarsal in plantar and medial direction
⑦ Plantar interossei (three muscles)	3rd to 5th metatarsals (medial border)	3rd to 5th toes (medial base of proximal phalanx)	Lateral plantar n. (S2, S3)	• Flexes the MTP joints of 3rd to 5th toes • Extension of IP joints of 3rd to 5th toes • Adducts 3rd to 5th toes toward 2nd toe
⑧ Dorsal interossei (four muscles)	1st to 5th metatarsals (by two heads on opposing sides)	1st interosseus: 2nd proximal phalanx (medial base) 2nd to 4th interossei: 2nd to 4th proximal phalanges (lateral base), 2nd to 4th toes (at dorsal aponeuroses)		• Flexes the MTP joints of 2nd to 4th toes • Extension of IP joints of 2nd to 4th toes • Abducts 3rd and 4th toes from 2nd toe

Abbreviations: IP, interphalangeal; MTP, metatarsophalangeal.
*May be absent.

16.8 The Gait Cycle

Gait is a complex activity that requires the coordinated action of muscles of the hip, thigh, and leg. **Table 16.17** is a summary of muscle action during the gait cycle.

— Gait is described in two phases: in normal walking, the stance phase makes up ~ 60%, and the swing phase makes up ~ 40%.

— One cycle of gait consists of the action of one leg through each of the two phases.

Table 16.17 **Muscle Action Sequence During the Gait Cycle**

Activity	Active Muscle Groups
Stance phase	
This phase begins with the heel strike.	Hip extensors Dorsiflexors
The foot begins to accept the weight of the body, and the pelvis is stabilized.	Hip adductors Knee extensors Plantar flexors
At midstance, the pelvis, knee, and ankle are stabilized.	Hip abductors Knee extensors Plantar flexors
This phase ends with the push off that includes "heel lift" and "toe off." Pelvis is stabilized.	Hip abductors Plantar flexors
Throughout the stance phase, the arches of the foot are preserved.	Long tendons of the foot Intrinsic muscles of the foot
Swing phase	
This phase begins with forward acceleration of the thigh.	Hip flexors
The foot needs to clear the ground as it swings forward.	Dorsiflexors
The thigh decelerates in preparation for landing.	Hip extensors
As the foot prepares for heel strike, the knee extends and positions the foot.	Knee extensor Dorsiflexors

16.9　Topographic Anatomy of Lower Limb Musculature

Thigh, Hip, and Gluteal Region

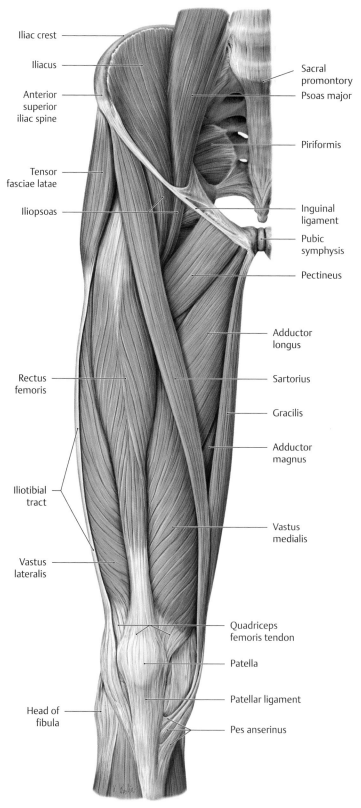

Iliac crest

Iliacus

Anterior superior iliac spine

Tensor fasciae latae

Iliopsoas

Rectus femoris

Iliotibial tract

Vastus lateralis

Head of fibula

Sacral promontory

Psoas major

Piriformis

Inguinal ligament

Pubic symphysis

Pectineus

Adductor longus

Sartorius

Gracilis

Adductor magnus

Vastus medialis

Quadriceps femoris tendon

Patella

Patellar ligament

Pes anserinus

Fig. 16.42　Muscles of the hip and thigh
Right limb, anterior view. Muscle origins are shown in *red*, insertions in *gray*.
Removed: Fascia lata of the thigh (to the lateral iliotibial tract).

Fig. 16.43 Muscles of the hip, thigh, and gluteal region
Midsagittal section, medial view.

Fig. 16.44 Muscles of the hip, thigh, and gluteal region
Right limb, posterior view.
Removed: Fascia lata (to iliotibial tract).

The Leg (Figs. 16.45, 16.46 and 16.47)

Fig. 16.45 Muscles of the leg
Right leg, anterior view.

Fig. 16.46 Muscles of the leg
Right leg, lateral view.

Fig. 16.47 Muscles of the leg

Right leg, posterior view. Muscle origins shown in *red*, insertions in *gray*.
Note: The bulge of the calf is produced mainly by the triceps surae (soleus
and the two heads of the gastrocnemius).

The Foot (Figs. 16.48 and 16.49)

Fig. 16.48 Plantar aponeurosis
Right foot, plantar view. The plantar aponeurosis is a tough aponeurotic sheet, thickest at the center, that blends with the dorsal fascia (not shown) at the borders of the foot.

Fig. 16.49 Intrinsic muscles of the sole of the foot
Right foot, plantar view.
Superficial (first) layer. *Removed:* Plantar aponeurosis, including the superficial transverse metacarpal ligament.

Compartments (Figs. 16.50 and 16.51)

Fig. 16.50 Windowed dissection
Right limb, posterior view.

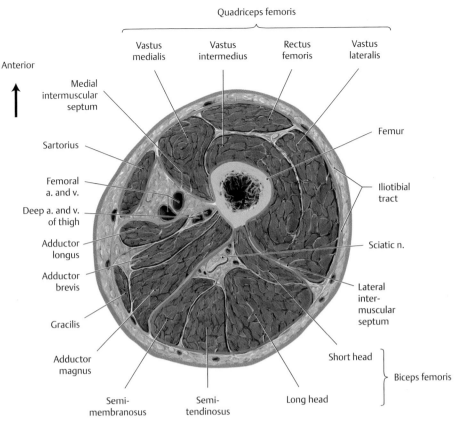

Anterior

Quadriceps femoris

Vastus medialis

Vastus intermedius

Rectus femoris

Vastus lateralis

Medial intermuscular septum

Sartorius

Femoral a. and v.

Deep a. and v. of thigh

Adductor longus

Adductor brevis

Gracilis

Adductor magnus

Semi- membranosus

Semi- tendinosus

Long head

Femur

Iliotibial tract

Sciatic n.

Lateral inter- muscular septum

Short head

Biceps femoris

A Thigh (plane of upper section in **Fig. 16.50).** The anterior compartment is outlined in *pink*, the posterior compartment in *green*, and the medial compart- ment in *orange*.

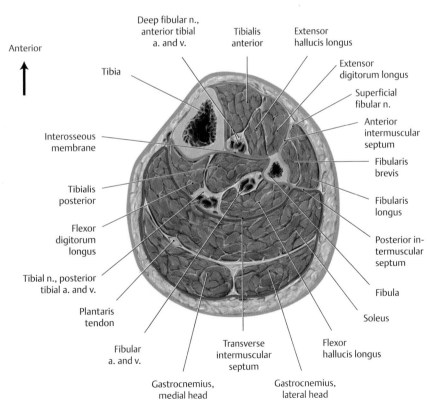

Anterior

Deep fibular n., anterior tibial a. and v.

Tibialis anterior

Extensor hallucis longus

Extensor digitorum longus

Superficial fibular n.

Anterior intermuscular septum

Fibularis brevis

Fibularis longus

Posterior in- termuscular septum

Fibula

Soleus

Flexor hallucis longus

Transverse intermuscular septum

Gastrocnemius, lateral head

Gastrocnemius, medial head

Fibular a. and v.

Plantaris tendon

Tibial n., posterior tibial a. and v.

Flexor digitorum longus

Tibialis posterior

Interosseous membrane

Tibia

B Leg (plane of lower section in **Fig. 16.50).** The anterior compartment is outlined in *pink*, the lateral compartment in *orange*, the deep posterior compartment in *green*, and the superficial posterior compartment in *blue*.

Fig. 16.51 Transverse sections}
Right limb, proximal (superior) view.

Unit VII   Clinical Imaging Basics of the Lower Limb

As in the upper extremity, radiographs are always the first imaging choice in evaluation of bones and joints in the setting of trauma or pain, and magnetic resonance imaging (MRI) is the primary method for evaluating the soft tissue components of the joints. In infants, ultrasound is used to diagnose developmental hip dysplasia and to assess for abnormal joint fluid (**Table 16.18**).

The principles and practices used in evaluating images of bones, joints, and soft tissues in the lower limb are similar to those used in the upper limb, except lower limb radiographs are often obtained with the patient standing or in a weight-bearing position. This distinction is important especially in the evaluation of weight-bearing joints (hips, knees, and ankles) because the joint is evaluated under the stress of everyday use (**Fig. 16.52**). MRIs cannot be taken with the patient in a weight-bearing position; nonetheless, they provide excellent detail of the internal soft tissue structures of the joint (**Fig. 16.53**).

Table 16.18 **Suitability of Imaging Modalities for the Lower Limb**

Modality	Clinical Uses
Radiographs (X-rays)	First-line imaging evaluation tool for the extremities; used primarily to evaluate for fractures, bone lesions, and alignment of joints
CT (computed tomography)	Reserved as a troubleshooting tool to evaluate for subtle nondisplaced fractures
MRI (magnetic resonance imaging)	One of the most important imaging modalities for the evaluation of joints, specifically the non-osseous components of the joint, e.g., cartilage, ligaments, tendons, and muscles
Ultrasound	In children, due to their small size, it plays a larger role in diagnosis of hip disorders (developmental dysplasia, toxic synovitis, or joint effusion) and in evaluation of cartilaginous growth plates. Ultrasound has a limited role in evaluation of superficial soft tissue abnormalities and for guidance of interventional procedures involving the joints.

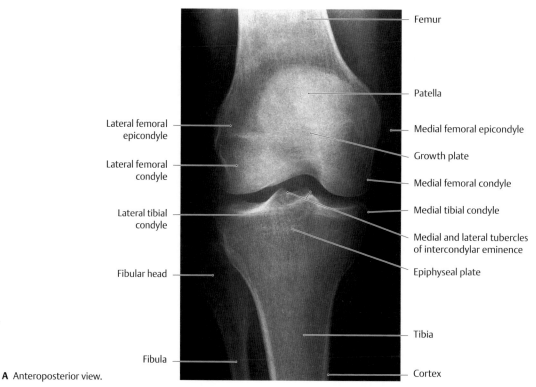

A Anteroposterior view.

Fig. 16.52 Radiograph of the right knee

Knee radiographs are usually performed with the patient upright in order to assess the knee joint in a weight-bearing stance. The articular surfaces of the bones should be smooth and the medial and lateral joint compartments should be equally spaced. There should be no bone fragments in the joint spaces. The cortical edge of each bone should be traced around the entire bone and should be smooth. Note how the patella overlaps the femur in the frontal projection (A) and is difficult to see clearly. The lateral view (B) affords a non-overlapping view of the patella.

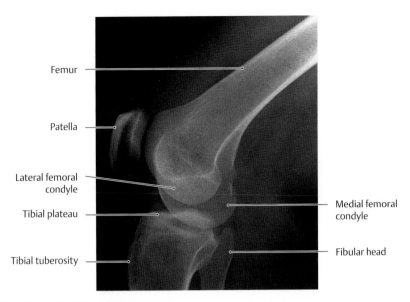

B Lateral view.

Fig. 16.52 (*continued*) **Radiograph of the right knee**

A Coronal section

B Midsagittal section

Fig. 16.53 MRI of the knee

In this sequence fat is *dark gray,* muscle is *light gray,* and fluid is *white.* Note how the cartilage lining the joint spaces (hyaline cartilage) is very bright because of its high fluid content. Conversely, the bone marrow is dark because of its fat content. Cortical bone is *black.* The tissue characteristics of this sequence allow for very sensitive assessment of pathology, as fluid from edema will stand out as bright white.

Unit VII Review Questions: Lower Limb

1. A young girl has recovered well from the severe injuries she sustained in a motor vehicle accident 9 months ago, but because of some lingering nerve problems, she still has difficulty walking. She is balanced during the midstance phase but has difficulty bringing her limb forward to initiate movement. What nerve seems to be affected?
   A. Superior gluteal
   B. Inferior gluteal
   C. Femoral
   D. Obturator
   E. Tibial

2. A young woman searching for driftwood walked several miles on the soft sandy beach of a Caribbean island. While walking on this uneven surface, the balance between inversion and eversion at her subtalar joint was maintained by the opposing actions of the fibularis longus and the
   A. fibularis brevis
   B. fibularis tertius
   C. soleus
   D. tibialis anterior
   E. extensor digitorum longus

3. Structures at the knee that are *not* attached to the joint capsule include the
   A. medial meniscus
   B. medial collateral ligament
   C. lateral collateral ligament
   D. patellar retinacula
   E. All of the above (A–D) are attached to the joint cavity.

4. A woman in her early 40s discovered a small lump at the top of her thigh that was later diagnosed as a femoral hernia. Where would this hernia be located?
   A. Retroinguinal space
   B. Femoral canal
   C. Femoral sheath
   D. Femoral ring
   E. All of the above

5. An elderly woman shopping with her daughter fell in the mall parking lot. After examining the woman, the paramedics who responded to the call noted that the limb was pulled upward, and the hip was rotated laterally. They confided to the daughter that it appeared that the woman had fractured her femoral neck. Which of the following muscles would be responsible for the lateral (external) rotation?
   A. Gluteus medius
   B. Tensor of the fascia lata
   C. Pectineus
   D. Vastus lateralis
   E. All of the above

6. The strongest and most supportive ligament of the hip joint is the
   A. transverse ligament of the acetabulum
   B. ligament of the head of the femur
   C. pubofemoral ligament
   D. ischiofemoral ligament
   E. iliofemoral ligament

7. A young man running on the beach severely lacerated his foot when he accidentally stepped into a pit with broken glass left by late-night partygoers. Surgery was required to remove the glass fragments and treat the lacerations. You opt to use regional anesthesia, injecting anesthetic near each of the nerves that cross the ankle. Where would you anesthetize the sural nerve?
   A. Anterior to the medial malleolus
   B. Posterior to the medial malleolus
   C. Posterior to the lateral malleolus
   D. Anterior to the lateral malleolus
   E. First web space

8. Sensation along the lateral side of the first toe is transmitted by branches of the
   A. saphenous nerve
   B. medial plantar nerve
   C. deep fibular nerve
   D. superficial fibular nerve
   E. lateral plantar nerve

9. Superficial veins of the lower limb
   A. lie deep to the fascia lata
   B. include the great saphenous vein that terminates at the popliteal vein
   C. include the small saphenous vein whose course runs anterior to the lateral malleolus
   D. drain to deep veins via perforating veins
   E. originate from the plantar venous arch on the sole

10. The dorsal pedal artery is a continuation of the
    A. posterior tibial artery
    B. fibular artery
    C. anterior tibial artery
    D. popliteal artery
    E. inferior medial genicular artery

11. The deep plantar arch of the foot is an anastomosis between the dorsal pedal artery and which structure on the sole of the foot?
    A. Fibular artery
    B. Lateral plantar artery
    C. Plantar metatarsal arteries
    D. Plantar digital arteries
    E. Arcuate artery

12. An obese woman suffers from peripheral edema (swelling of the legs) and large varicose veins in her leg. Which of the following might be coexisting symptoms related to her condition?
    A. Incompetent valves in the great saphenous vein
    B. Reversed flow in the perforating veins
    C. Deep vein thrombosis
    D. Thrombophlebitis
    E. All of the above

13. "Footdrop" occurs when the plantar flexor muscles are unopposed. This condition may be caused by damage to which of the following nerves?
    A. Superficial fibular
    B. Deep fibular
    C. Sural
    D. Tibial
    E. Medial plantar

14. As she was riding her bike home from her job as a camp counselor, Kristin was sideswiped by a large pickup trunk. She suffered multiple bruises, a fractured tibia, and a fractured pelvis. Several months later she still had an area of numbness on the medial side of her thigh and walked with a lateral swing to her gait. Which muscle was affected by her injury?
    A. Gluteus medius
    B. Gluteus maximus
    C. Semimembranosus
    D. Adductor longus
    E. Rectus femoris

15. In the anatomy laboratory you have just dissected the gluteal region of your cadaver. You are surprised to discover that in your cadaver the lateral component of the sciatic nerve passes *through* the piriformis muscle instead of *inferior* to it. Being a dedicated student, you investigate this further and find this anomaly can cause a piriformis syndrome in which the nerve is compressed by contraction of the muscle. What symptom might this particular patient have experienced?
    A. Paresthesia (tingling) on the sole of the foot
    B. Loss of knee flexion
    C. Loss of knee extension
    D. Footdrop
    E. Sagging of the unsupported hip when walking

16. The adductor magnus muscle
    A. extends and adducts the hip joint
    B. is innervated by the femoral and obturator nerves
    C. inserts on the linea aspera of the femur and adductor tubercle of the tibia
    D. forms the anterior wall of the adductor canal
    E. originates from the superior pubic ramus

17. Which muscle(s) of the lower limb is/are capable of producing flexion at one joint and extension at a second joint?
    A. Semimembranosus
    B. Rectus femoris
    C. Lumbricals of foot
    D. Long head of biceps femoris
    E. All of the above

18. During a street fight between two local gangs, one boy received a violent blow to the anterior knee that knocked him to the ground. In the emergency department, the physical exam of his knee revealed a positive posterior drawer sign. What structure appears to be injured?
    A. Anterior cruciate ligament
    B. Posterior cruciate ligament
    C. Patellar ligament
    D. Medial collateral ligament
    E. Lateral collateral ligament

19. A single woman looking for adventure signed up for a walking tour of the Scottish highlands. She was unprepared for the effort that it required but kept up with the more experienced walkers. After a few days she began to experience extreme tenderness in her anterior leg deep to the ridge of the tibia. The tour guide had seen this in previous clients and suggested that her pain was due to shin splints. Her pain originated from overuse of the
    A. extensor digitorum longus
    B. extensor digitorum brevis
    C. extensor hallucis longus
    D. fibularis tertius
    E. tibialis anterior

20. Which fibrous structure on the sole of the foot originates at the calcaneus and continues distally as digital fibrous sheaths?
    A. Plantar aponeurosis
    B. Plantar calcaneonavicular ligament
    C. Long plantar ligament
    D. Short plantar ligament
    E. Deltoid ligament

21. A man was on a hunting trip with friends when he was accidentally shot in the midthigh. He bled profusely from his femoral artery until his friends applied constant pressure over the wound and drove him to a local emergency clinic. Although examination of the wound site in surgery revealed a badly torn femoral artery, the man continued to have distal pulses in his leg. What vessel arises proximal to the injury site and can provide collateral blood supply to the distal limb?
    A. Medial circumflex femoral artery
    B. Lateral circumflex femoral artery
    C. Obturator artery
    D. Descending genicular artery
    E. Popliteal artery

22. An elderly woman slipped on a patch of ice in her driveway when she went to pick up the morning newspaper. Her neighbor witnessed the accident and called an ambulance. In the emergency department, X-rays revealed that she had fractured the neck of her femur. Her physician explained to her that avascular necrosis was a common complication of this injury in elderly women and convinced her to agree to a hip replacement. What vessel contributes most significantly to the blood supply of the hip joint?
    A. Obturator
    B. Superior gluteal
    C. Inferior gluteal
    D. Medial circumflex femoral
    E. Lateral circumflex femoral

23. Which of the following spaces contain the femoral nerve?
    A. Femoral sheath
    B. Adductor hiatus
    C. Popliteal fossa
    D. Femoral canal
    E. Retroinguinal space

24. The inferior gluteal nerve innervates the
    A. gluteus maximus
    B. gluteus medius
    C. gluteus minimus
    D. piriformis
    E. All of the above

25. Which of the following muscles insert on the iliotibial tract?
- A. Gluteus maximus
- B. Gluteus medius
- C. Gluteus minimus
- D. Quadratus femoris
- E. None of the above

26. Your 13-year-old son who studies martial arts is particularly flexible and is praised for his high kicks. After several weeks of training in preparation for an upcoming tournament, he complains of tenderness in his lower buttocks during practice and even when he sits on the hard stadium benches. As his pediatrician, how do you explain his problem?
- A. Inflammation of the ischial tuberosity
- B. Rupture of the obturator internus tendon from its insertion
- C. Compression of the sciatic nerve in the gluteal region
- D. Irritation of the tibial nerve in the thigh
- E. Irritation of the inferior gluteal nerve

27. Which of the following muscles are involved in knee flexion?
- A. Flexor hallucis longus
- B. Soleus
- C. Tibialis posterior
- D. Biceps femoris
- E. Rectus femoris

28. The lateral border of the femoral triangle is formed by the
- A. tensor fasciae latae
- B. femoral nerve
- C. sartorius
- D. adductor longus
- E. rectus femoris

29. An 18-year-old marathon runner finished fourth in the Detroit marathon but limped away from the finish line. He had been suffering from excruciating pain on the sole of his foot and immediately sought advice from the medical volunteers. Following a thorough exam, the EMTs explained that the muscle tendons running through his tarsal tunnel had swollen and were compressing the nerve that accompanies them. What bones form the wall of this tunnel?
- A. Navicular and talus
- B. Cuboid and calcaneus
- C. Talus and calcaneus
- D. Medial malleolus of the tibia and calcaneus
- E. Talus and base of the 1st metatarsal

30. An experienced 24-year-old backpacker has spent the last 4 months hiking the entire Appalachian trail. Although he has sturdy hiking boots, he often changes to the lightweight sneakers he brought as a backup. For the last few miles of the trek, he has been experiencing shooting pain along the side of his foot at the apex of his medial arch. What structure is probably the cause of the pain?
- A. Plantar calcaneonavicular (spring) ligament
- B. Deltoid ligament
- C. Posterior talofibular ligament
- D. Superior extensor retinaculum
- E. Tendon of fibularis longus

Answers and Explanations

1. **C.** Forward movement at the beginning of the swing phase depends on the action of her hip flexors, particularly the rectus femoris, which is innervated by the femoral nerve (Sections 16.2, 16.3, and 16.8).

A. The superior gluteal nerve innervates the abductors of the hip. Damage to this nerve would cause a sagging of the hip on the contralateral side just before the midstance.

B. The inferior gluteal nerve innervates the gluteus maximus. Injury to this nerve would affect the deceleration of the swing phase.

D. Injury to the obturator nerve, which innervates the adductors of the hip, would cause an outward swing of the limb but would not inhibit acceleration of the thigh.

E. The tibial nerve innervates the hamstring muscles of the posterior thigh, which are responsible for the deceleration at the end of the swing phase.

2. **D.** The tibialis anterior and tibialis posterior are the strong inverters of the foot that counter the action of the fibularis longus and fibularis brevis (Section 16.7).

A. The fibularis brevis, in the lateral crural compartment, inserts on the base of the 5th metatarsal, which allows it to evert the foot.

B. The fibularis tertius, a muscle of the anterior crural compartment, inserts on the base of the 5th metatarsal and everts the foot.

C. The soleus, in the posterior crural compartment, plantar flexes the foot.

E. The extensor digitorum, in the anterior crural compartment, everts the foot.

3. **C.** The lateral (fibular) collateral ligament is an extracapsular ligament that extends from the lateral epicondyle of the femur to the head of the fibula and remains separate from the joint capsule of the knee (Section 16.4).

A. The medial and lateral menisci attach along their outer rims to the joint capsule.

B. The medial (tibial) collateral ligament is a capsular ligament that extends from the medial epicondyle of the femur to the medial condyle and superior part of the medial tibia. It attaches to the joint capsule and to the medial meniscus.

D. The patellar retinacula are fibrous expansions of the tendons of the quadriceps femoris muscle. They form the joint capsule on either side of the patella.

E. Only the lateral (fibular) collateral ligament (C) is correct.

4. **E.** A vascular compartment of the retroinguinal space contains the femoral sheath and the femoral canal. The femoral ring defines the upper edge of the femoral canal. A femoral hernia protrudes into the femoral canal (Section 16.3).

A. The retroinguinal space contains the femoral canal, the site of the femoral hernia. B through D are also correct (E).

B. The femoral canal is a space within the femoral sheath that normally contains loose connective tissue, fat, and often a deep inguinal lymph node. A, C, and D are also correct (E).

C. The femoral sheath contains the femoral vessels and the femoral canal. A, B, and D are also correct (E).

D. The femoral ring defines the superior opening of the femoral canal. A, B, and C are also correct (E).

5. **C.** The pectineus in the medial thigh compartment adducts and laterally rotates the hip (Section 16.3).

  A. The gluteus medius is an abductor of the hip.

  B. The tensor fascia lata abducts, flexes, and internally rotates the hip.

  D. The vastus lateralis extends the knee and has no influence over the hip joint.

  E. A, B, and D are incorrect.

6. **E.** The iliofemoral ligament attaches proximally to the anterior inferior iliac spine and rim of the acetabulum and distally to the intertrochanteric line of the femur. It supports the hip joint during standing (Section 16.3).

  A. The transverse ligament completes the rim of the C-shaped acetabulum inferiorly.

  B. The ligament of the head of the femur attaches to the acetabulum within the joint but provides little support. A small artery runs within the ligament to the femoral head.

  C. The pubofemoral ligament runs laterally from the inferior aspect of the acetabular rim to merge with the iliofemoral ligament. It assists the iliofemoral ligament and limits abduction of the joint.

  D. The ischiofemoral ligament is the weakest of the three ligaments of the capsule. It arises from the ischial part of the acetabular rim and spirals anteriorly to insert on the femoral neck.

7. **C.** The sural nerve innervates the lateral side of the foot and runs posterior to the lateral malleolus (Section 15.4).

  A. The saphenous nerve runs anterior to the medial malleolus.

  B. The tibial nerve courses through the tarsal tunnel posterior to the medial malleolus.

  D. The superficial fibular nerve runs onto the dorsum of the foot anterior to the lateral malleolus.

  E. The deep fibular nerve accompanies the dorsal pedal artery onto the dorsum of the foot. It innervates the skin of the first web space.

8. **C.** The deep fibular nerve, a branch of the common fibular nerve, supplies cutaneous innervation to the first web space, including the skin adjacent to the first and second digits. It also supplies motor innervation to the muscles of the anterior compartment of the leg (Section 15.4).

  A. The saphenous nerve transmits sensation from the medial side of the foot.

  B. The medial plantar branch of the tibial nerve supplies cutaneous innervation to a large area of skin on the medial side of the foot and the medial three and a half digits.

  D. The superficial fibular nerve supplies cutaneous innervation to the dorsum of the foot.

  E. The lateral plantar branch supplies cutaneous innervation to the lateral foot and the lateral one and a half digits.

9. **D.** Similar to superficial veins of the upper limb, superficial veins of the lower limb drain to deep veins via perforating veins (Section 15.4).

  A. Superficial veins lie in the subcutaneous tissue, superficial to the deep fascia (fascia lata).

  B. The great saphenous vein pierces the fascia lata at the saphenous hiatus in the proximal thigh and terminates in the femoral vein.

  C. The small saphenous vein runs posterior to the lateral malleolus and superiorly to the popliteal fossa.

  E. The large superficial veins, the great and small saphenous veins, originate from the venous arch on the dorsum of the foot.

10. **C.** The anterior tibial artery descends within the anterior crural compartment and emerges onto the dorsum of the foot as the dorsal pedal artery (Section 15.4).

  A. The posterior tibial artery descends within posterior crural compartment and branches into the medial plantar and lateral plantar arteries that supply the sole of the foot.

  B. The fibular artery arises in the lateral part of the posterior leg and anastomoses with the anterior tibial artery to supply the ankle.

  D. The popliteal artery lies posterior to the knee. It gives rise to the genicular and tibial arteries.

  E. The inferior medial genicular artery is a branch of the popliteal artery and supplies blood to the patella and insertions of the sartorius, gracilis, and semitendinosus.

11. **B.** The lateral plantar artery, similar to the ulnar artery in the hand, is the largest branch of the posterior tibial artery. It supplies the lateral side of the foot and forms the deep plantar arch with the dorsal pedal artery (Section 15.4).

  A. The fibular artery supplies muscles in the posterior and lateral compartments of the leg and forms an anastomosis with the anterior tibial artery at the ankle, but it has no branches on the sole of the foot.

  C. The plantar metatarsal arteries arise from the deep plantar arch.

  D. Proper digital arteries arise from the plantar metatarsal arteries, which are branches of the deep plantar arch.

  E. The arcuate artery, a branch of the dorsal pedal artery, forms a loop on the dorsum of the foot and supplies the 2nd, 3rd, and 4th dorsal metatarsal arteries.

12. **E.** Varicose, or dilated, veins can occur in conjunction with deep vein thromboses. When the deep veins are obstructed, the normal superficial-to-deep flow in the perforating veins reverses. With the increased volume, the superficial veins dilate, and their valves become incompetent. Thrombophlebitis, or venous inflammation, often occurs with thrombus formation (Section 15.4).

  A. When venous valves are incompetent, upward flow is impeded, and blood pools in the veins. The resulting dilated veins are known as varicose veins. B through D are also correct (E).

  B. Superficial veins normally drain into the deep venous system through the perforating veins. If the deep veins are obstructed by thrombus, blood flows outward through the perforating veins into the superficial system, dilating the superficial veins. A, C, and D are also correct (E).

  C. When thrombus obstructs the deep veins of the leg, blood flows outward into the superficial veins, causing them to dilate. A, B, and D are also correct (E).

  D. Inflammation of veins can occur with thrombus formation. A through C are also correct (E).

13. **B.** Footdrop is caused by an injury to the deep (or common) fibular nerve causing paralysis of the dorsiflexor muscles in the foot, leaving the plantar flexor muscles unopposed (Section 15.4).

A. Injury to the superficial fibular nerve results in an inability to evert the foot and therefore an overall loss of balance and loss of sensation on the dorsum of the foot.

C. Injury to the sural nerve causes loss of sensation over the skin on the lateral side of the foot.

D. Injury to the tibial nerve causes paralysis of all of the muscles of the posterior thigh (except the short head of the biceps femoris) and posterior leg.

E. Injury to the medial plantar nerve causes paralysis of the muscles on the medial side of the foot and loss of sensation over a large area of skin on the medial side of the foot and the medial three and a half digits.

14. **D.** A lateral swinging gait is caused by unopposed hip abduction, which occurs when the adductors are paralyzed. The obturator nerve innervates the adductor muscles of the thigh and can be injured by pelvic fractures. The area of numbness on the medial thigh also suggests an obturator nerve injury (Section 15.4).

A. The gluteus medius is an abductor of the hip. Injury to this muscle results in a gluteal, or waddling, gait.

B. The injury to the inferior gluteal nerve, which innervates the gluteus maximus, impairs extension of the hip but does not cause any sensory loss.

C. Injury to the semimembranosus or its nerve, the tibial nerve, impairs hip extension, knee flexion, and sensation on the sole of the foot.

E. Injury to the femoral nerve, which innervates the rectus femoris, weakens flexion of the hip and extension of the knee. There is a sensory loss from the anterior thigh and the medial side of the leg and foot.

15. **D.** The common fibular nerve is the lateral component of the sciatic nerve. Compression will affect the dorsiflexors of the anterior leg compartment (through its deep fibular branch), resulting in footdrop (Sections 15.4 and 16.2).

A. Paresthesia on the sole of the foot would be a consequence of compression of the tibial nerve.

B. The tibial nerve, the medial component of the sciatic nerve, innervates the hamstring muscles, which flex the knee. This action would remain intact.

C. The knee extensors on the anterior thigh extend the knee and would not be affected by this anomaly.

E. Sagging of the unsupported hip is characteristic of an injury to the superior gluteal nerve.

16. **A.** The adductor magnus is the largest adductor of the hip but also works with the gluteus maximus to provide powerful extension of the hip joint (Section 16.3).

B. The adductor magnus has a dual innervation, the obturator and tibial nerves.

C. The adductor magnus inserts entirely on the femur; the adductor tubercle is a feature on the distal femur.

D. The adductor canal passes between the anterior and medial thigh compartments. The vastus medialis forms the anterior wall, and the adductor muscles form the posterior wall.

E. The adductor magnus originates on the ischiopubic ramus, which includes the inferior pubic ramus and ischial ramus.

17. **E.** Semimembranosus (A) produces flexion at the knee joint and extension at the hip joint. Rectus femoris (B) produces flexion at the hip joint and extension at the knee joint. The lumbricals of the foot (C) produce flexion of the metatarsophalangeal (MTP) joints of the 2nd to 5th toes and extension of the interphalangeal (IP) joints of the 2nd to 5th toes. The long head of the biceps femoris (D) produces extension of the hip joint and flexion of the knee joint (Sections 16.3 and 16.7).

A. Semimembranosus produces flexion at the knee joint and extension at the hip joint. B through D are also correct (E).

B. Rectus femoris produces flexion at the hip joint and extension at the knee joint. A, C, and D are also correct (E).

C. The lumbricals of the foot produce flexion of the MTP joints of the 2nd to 5th toes and extension of the IP joints of the 2nd to 5th toes. A, B, and D are also correct (E).

D. The long head of the biceps femoris produces extension of the hip joint and flexion of the knee joint. A through C are also correct (E).

18. **B.** The posterior displacement of the tibia is a positive posterior drawer sign that indicates an injury to the posterior cruciate ligament (Section 16.4).

A. Injury to the anterior cruciate ligament is recognized by the positive anterior drawer sign in which the tibia can be pulled anteriorly from under the femur.

C. A positive drawer sign suggests anterior or posterior displacement of the tibia relative to the femur. Rupture of the patellar ligament destabilizes the knee joint but does not disrupt the alignment of the tibia and femur.

D. Although the medial collateral ligament may be damaged by a forceful blow, it is not diagnosed by a posterior drawer sign.

E. The lateral collateral ligament is unlikely to be damaged by a blow to the anterior knee and is not diagnosed by either anterior or posterior drawer signs.

19. **E.** Shin splints are a result of inflammation of the tibialis anterior and small tears of the periosteum where the muscle attaches to the bone (Section 16.5).

A. The extensor digitorum originates from the head of the fibula, lateral condyle of the tibia, and interosseous membrane.

B. The extensor digitorum brevis is an intrinsic muscle of the foot. It arises from the calcaneus.

C. The extensor hallucis longus arises from the middle of the fibular shaft and the interosseous membrane.

D. Fibularis tertius is a lateral muscle that arises from the distal fibula.

20. **A.** The plantar aponeurosis is a thick fibrous band on the sole that is continuous with the deep fascia of the leg (Section 16.7).

B. The plantar calcaneonavicular ligament, or spring ligament, supports the head of the talus and maintains the medial side of the longitudinal arch of the foot.

C. The long plantar ligament supports the lateral side of the longitudinal arch of the foot and extends from the calcaneus to the bases of the 1st, 2nd, and 3rd metatarsals.

D. The short plantar ligament, or plantar calcaneocuboid ligament, supports the lateral arch of the foot.

E. The deltoid ligament is a four-part ligament that supports the medial side of the ankle joint.

21. **B.** The lateral circumflex femoral artery a rises from the deep artery of the thigh in the proximal thigh. It supplies structures around the hip as well as a descending branch that anastomoses with the genicular arteries at the knee. Reverse flow in these branches could supply the popliteal artery and its branches in the leg (Section 15.4).

A. The medial circumflex femoral artery arises from the deep artery of the thigh and supplies the hip joint. It does not anastomose with the popliteal artery or other branches of the knee and leg.

C. The obturator artery supplies the medial compartment of the thigh and does not anastomose with vessels of the leg.

D. The descending genicular artery is a branch of the femoral artery, but it arises distal to the site of injury and therefore cannot provide collateral circulation.

E. The popliteal artery anastomoses with the proximal femoral artery only through the lateral circumflex femoral artery.

22. **D.** Although the medial and lateral circumflex femoral arteries and inferior gluteal artery anastomose around the hip, branches that supply the hip joint arise primarily from the medial circumflex femoral artery (Section 15.4).

A. The obturator artery supplies the medial thigh muscles and a small artery to the head of the femur. It is not a significant blood supply to the joint.

B. The superior gluteal artery supplies muscles of the gluteal region but does not supply the hip joint.

C. The inferior gluteal artery contributes to an anastomosis around the hip and primarily supplies muscles of the gluteal region.

E. The lateral circumflex femoral artery anastomoses with the medial circumflex artery around the femoral neck, but it contributes less to the hip joint and more to the muscles of the lateral thigh.

23. **E.** The femoral nerve enters the anterior thigh through the muscular compartment of the retroinguinal space. It branches immediately to innervate the muscles of the anterior thigh (Section 15.4).

A. The femoral sheath encloses only the femoral artery and vein.

B. The femoral artery and vein pass through the adductor hiatus into the popliteal fossa.

C. The popliteal fossa contains the tibial and common fibular nerves.

D. The femoral canal lies medially within the femoral sheath and contains only loose connective tissue, fat, and lymph nodes.

24. **A.** The inferior gluteal nerve innervates only the gluteus maximus muscle (Section 15.4).

B. The superior gluteal nerve innervates the gluteus medius and minimus and tensor of the fascia lata.

C. The superior gluteal nerve innervates the gluteus medius and minimus and tensor of the fascia lata.

D. The piriformis is innervated by the S1 and S2 branches of the sacral plexus.

E. B, C, and D are incorrect

25. **A.** The upper fibers of the gluteus maximus insert onto the iliotibial tract (Section 16.2).

B. Gluteus medius inserts onto the lateral surface of the greater trochanter of the femur.

C. Gluteus minimus inserts onto the anterolateral surface of the greater trochanter of the femur.

D. Quadratus femoris inserts onto the intertrochanteric crest of the femur.

E. Not applicable.

26. **A.** The hamstring muscles originate at the ischial tuberosity and insert on the tibia and fibula. Repetitive stretching of these muscles over two joints (the flexed hip and extended knee) can irritate the site of origin (Section 16.3).

B. Pain from a tear at the insertion site of the obturator internus tendon would be focused over the greater trochanter of the femur.

C. The sciatic nerve emerges from behind the piriformis muscle and can be compressed at this location. However, pain would reflect the sensory areas of the tibial and common fibular nerves, which include the anterolateral and posterior leg and the dorsum and lateral edge of the foot.

D. Irritation of the tibial nerve would manifest as pain in the sole of the foot.

E. The inferior gluteal nerve does not have a sensory component. Injury to the nerve would affect the gluteus maximus muscle and manifest as weakened extension and lateral rotation.

27. **D.** The biceps femoris is one of the hamstring muscles (biceps femoris, semitendinosus, semimembranosus), which are the primary flexors of the knee (Section 16.3).

A. The flexor hallucis longus flexes the 1st digit and plantar flexes the foot.

B. The soleus does not cross the knee joint and only plantar flexes the foot at the ankle.

C. The tibialis posterior plantar flexes and inverts the foot.

E. The rectus femoris extends the leg at the knee.

28. **C.** The borders of the femoral triangle are the sartorius, adductor longus, and inguinal ligament (Section 16.3).

A. The tensor fasciae latae is the lateral boundary of the anterior thigh. The femoral triangle lies between the anterior and medial thigh compartments.

B. The femoral nerve is one of the contents (lateral) of the femoral triangle but not a boundary.

D. The adductor longus is the medial border of the triangle.

E. The rectus femoris is lateral to the femoral triangle and lies inside the anterior compartment of the thigh.

29. **D.** The tarsal tunnel is formed by the flexor retinaculum and its attachments to the calcaneus and medial malleolus of the tibia (Section 16.5).

A. The navicular and talus lie distal to the tarsal tunnel, and neither provide attachment for the flexor retinaculum, which forms the roof of the tunnel.

B. The cuboid lies on the lateral side of the foot; the tarsal tunnel lies on the medial side of the ankle.

C. The talus is not part of the tarsal tunnel.

E. Neither the talus nor the 1st metatarsal is part of the tarsal tunnel.

30.   **A.** The plantar calcaneonavicular ligament supports the head of the talus, which forms the apex of the medial longitudinal arch (Section 16.7).

B. The deltoid ligament is the collateral ligament on the medial side of the ankle. It is not associated with the medial arch.

C. The posterior talofibular ligament is part of the lateral ligament of the ankle and is not associated with the medial arch.

D. The superior extensor retinaculum restrains the tendons on the dorsum of the foot (dorsiflexors).

E. The tendon of the fibularis longus supports the transverse arch on the lateral side of the sole of the foot.

Unit VIII   Head and Neck

17 Overview of the Head and Neck

The head and neck region contains the brain, cranial meninges, cranial nerves, and sensory organs, as well as components of the respiratory, gastrointestinal, and endocrine systems. The skull encloses the brain, provides the bony framework for soft tissues of the head, and contains the nasal and oral cavities and bony orbits. The head and neck communicate with the thorax through the superior thoracic aperture and with the upper limb through the cervicoaxillary canal.

17.1 Bones of the Head: The Skull

The skull is made up of two parts: the large **neurocranium** and the smaller **viscerocranium (Fig. 17.1** and **Table 17.1).**
- The neurocranium, which makes up the largest part of the skull, houses and protects the brain.
- The viscerocranium includes the lower jaw and the thin-walled bones of the facial skeleton.

Neurocranium

Viscerocranium

Fig. 17.1 Bones of the neurocranium and viscerocranium
Left lateral view.

Table 17.1 **Bones of the Neurocranium and Viscerocranium (see Fig. 17.1)**

Neurocranium	Viscerocranium
• Frontal bone	• Nasal bone
• Sphenoid bone (excluding the pterygoid process)	• Lacrimal bone
	• Ethmoid bone (excluding the cribriform plate)
• Temporal bone (squamous part, petrous part)	• Sphenoid bone (pterygoid process) maxilla
• Parietal bone	
• Occipital bone	• Zygomatic bone
• Ethmoid bone (cribriform plate)	• Temporal bone (tympanic part, styloid process)
• Auditory ossicles	• Mandible
	• Vomer
	• Inferior nasal concha
	• Palatine bone
	• Hyoid bone

The Neurocranium

The neurocranium is formed by eight bones: the frontal, occipital, sphenoid, and ethmoid bones, and paired parietal and temporal bones. Four of these, the frontal, occipital, and two parietal bones, form the **calvaria**, or skullcap. These bones are composed of three layers: a dense **outer table**, a thin **inner table**, and a middle **diploë layer (Fig. 17.2)**.

— The **frontal bone (Figs. 17.3**, **17.4**, and **17.5**) forms the forehead, the roof, and the superior rim of the orbit (eye socket), and the floor of the anterior cranial fossa.
— The paired **parietal bones** (see **Figs. 17.2** and **17.3**) are flat bones that form the superolateral parts of the calvaria. Their internal surface has grooves for the middle meningeal arteries and the superior sagittal sinus.

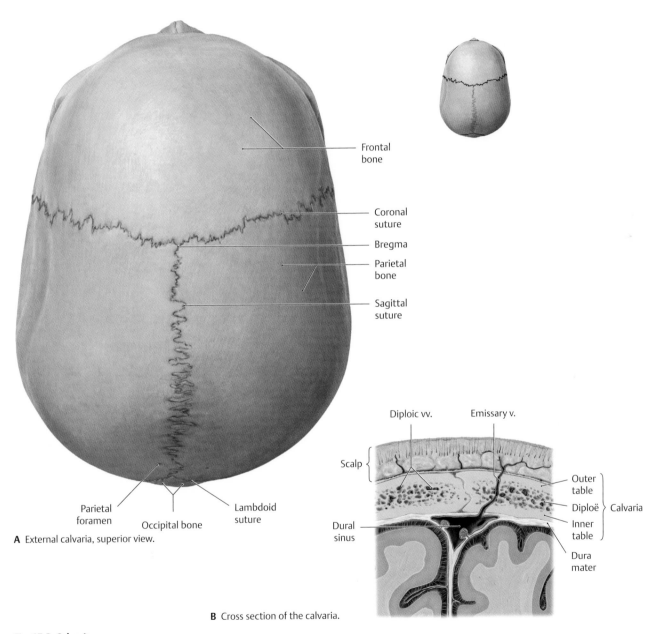

A External calvaria, superior view.

B Cross section of the calvaria.

Fig. 17.2 **Calvaria**

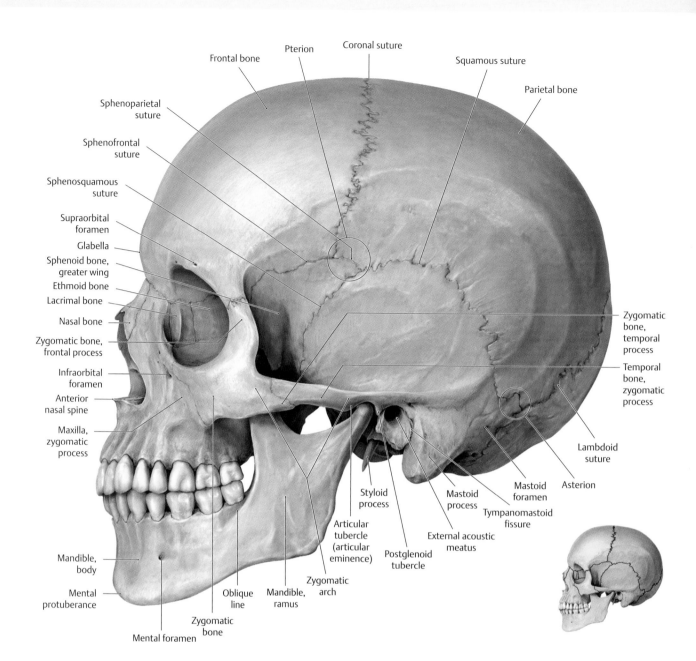

Fig. 17.3 Lateral skull
Left lateral view.

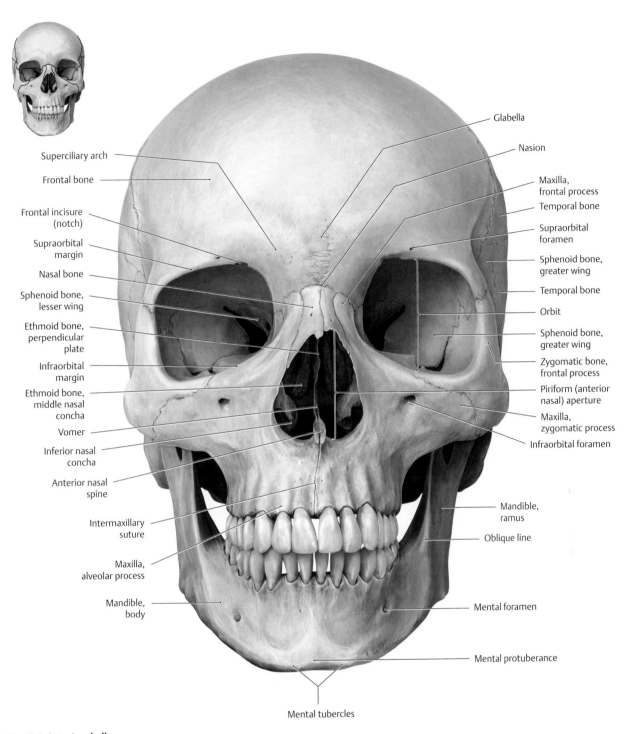

Superciliary arch

Frontal bone

Frontal incisure (notch)

Supraorbital margin

Nasal bone

Sphenoid bone, lesser wing

Ethmoid bone, perpendicular plate

Infraorbital margin

Ethmoid bone, middle nasal concha

Vomer

Inferior nasal concha

Anterior nasal spine

Intermaxillary suture

Maxilla, alveolar process

Mandible, body

Glabella

Nasion

Maxilla, frontal process

Temporal bone

Supraorbital foramen

Sphenoid bone, greater wing

Temporal bone

Orbit

Sphenoid bone, greater wing

Zygomatic bone, frontal process

Piriform (anterior nasal) aperture

Maxilla, zygomatic process

Infraorbital foramen

Mandible, ramus

Oblique line

Mental foramen

Mental protuberance

Mental tubercles

Fig. 17.4 Anterior skull
Anterior view.

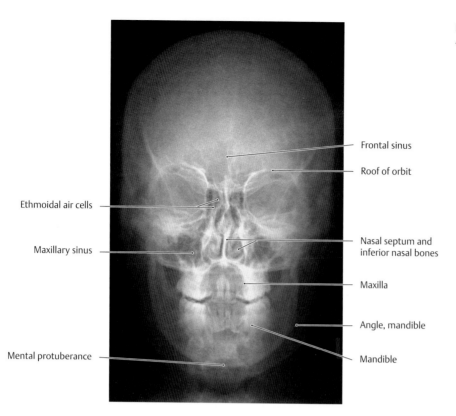

Fig. 17.5 Radiograph of the skull
Anteroposterior view.

Frontal sinus

Roof of orbit

Ethmoidal air cells

Nasal septum and
inferior nasal bones

Maxillary sinus

Maxilla

Angle, mandible

Mental protuberance

Mandible

- The **occipital bone (Figs. 17.6**, **17.7**, and **17.8)** forms the
  posterior cranial fossa of the skull base.
  A small anterior portion is called the **clivus.**
  - Foramina (openings) include the large **foramen magnum,**
    the **jugular foramina,** and the **condylar canals.**
  - Inferiorly, **occipital condyles** articulate with the first
    cervical vertebra.
  - The internal surface has grooves for the sigmoid and
    transverse dural sinuses.
  - The external surface is marked with **superior** and
    inferior nuchal lines and an **external occipital
    protuberance.**
- The paired **temporal bones (Figs. 17.9** and **17.10)** form part
  of the middle and posterior cranial fossae.
  - An outer **squamous part** forms the lateral skull, an
    inner **petrous part** encloses the middle and inner ear
    (neurocranium), and a **tympanic part** encloses the
    external auditory canal and tympanic membrane
    (viscerocranium).
  - Processes include a **mastoid process** composed of a mesh
    of **mastoid air cells,** the posterior part of the **zygomatic
    arch,** and a long, pointed **styloid process.**

- Foramina (openings) include an **internal acoustic meatus,
  external acoustic meatus, carotid canal,** and **stylomastoid foramen.**
- A **mandibular fossa** and **articular tubercle** articulate
  with the mandible.
- The **sphenoid bone (Figs. 17.11** and **17.12)** forms the posterior
  part of the orbit and the floor and the lateral wall of the
  middle cranial fossa between the frontal and temporal bones.
  - It has two **greater wings** that form parts of the middle
    cranial fossa and lateral walls of the skull.
  - Two **lesser wings** form the posterior part of the anterior
    cranial fossa and end in **anterior clinoid processes.**
  - The **sphenoid body** encloses the **sphenoid sinus.**
  - A midline saddle-shaped formation, the **sella turcica,**
    contains the **hypophyseal fossa** and is limited anteriorly
    by the **tuberculum sellae** and posteriorly by the **dorsum
    sellae** and its **posterior clinoid processes.**
  - Paired **pterygoid processes,** each with a **medial** and a
    lateral pterygoid plate, project inferiorly (viscerocranium).
  - Paired openings include the **optic canal, superior orbital
    fissure, foramen rotundum, foramen ovale,** and **foramen
    spinosum.**

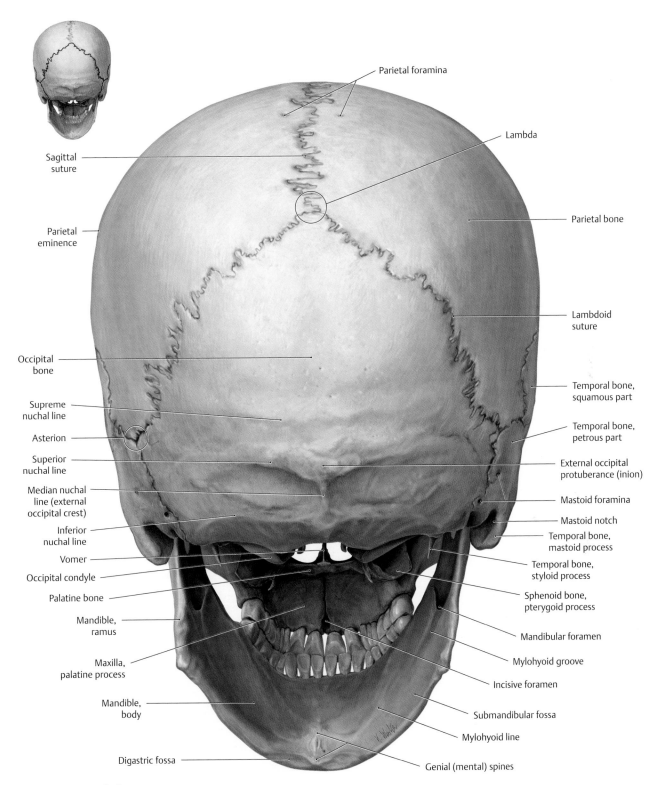

Parietal foramina

Lambda

Sagittal suture

Parietal bone

Parietal eminence

Lambdoid suture

Occipital bone

Temporal bone, squamous part

Supreme nuchal line

Temporal bone, petrous part

Asterion

External occipital protuberance (inion)

Superior nuchal line

Mastoid foramina

Median nuchal line (external occipital crest)

Mastoid notch

Inferior nuchal line

Temporal bone, mastoid process

Vomer

Temporal bone, styloid process

Occipital condyle

Sphenoid bone, pterygoid process

Palatine bone

Mandibular foramen

Mandible, ramus

Mylohyoid groove

Maxilla, palatine process

Incisive foramen

Mandible, body

Submandibular fossa

Mylohyoid line

Digastric fossa

Genial (mental) spines

Fig. 17.6 Posterior skull
Posterior view.

Median palatine suture

Incisive foramen

Maxillary dental arch with maxillary teeth in alveoli

Transverse palatine suture

Palatine process

Zygomatic process

Maxilla

Palatine bone, horizontal plate

Choana

Greater palatine foramen

Zygomatic bone, temporal surface

Lesser palatine foramen

Inferior orbital fissure

Vomer

Hamulus (of medial pterygoid plate)

Pterygoid process { Medial plate / Lateral plate }

Zygomatic arch

Palatovaginal (pharyngeal) canal

Temporal bone, articular tubercle

Foramen ovale

Pharyngeal tubercle

Foramen spinosum

Foramen lacerum

Mandibular fossa

Petrotympanic fissure

Carotid canal

Styloid process

Jugular foramen

Occipital condyle

Stylomastoid foramen

Mastoid process

Hypoglossal canal

Mastoid notch (for digastric belly)

Foramen magnum

Condylar canal

Mastoid foramen

Inferior nuchal line

Parietal bone

External occipital crest

Superior nuchal line

Supreme nuchal line

External occipital protuberance

Fig. 17.7 Base of the skull: exterior
Inferior view.

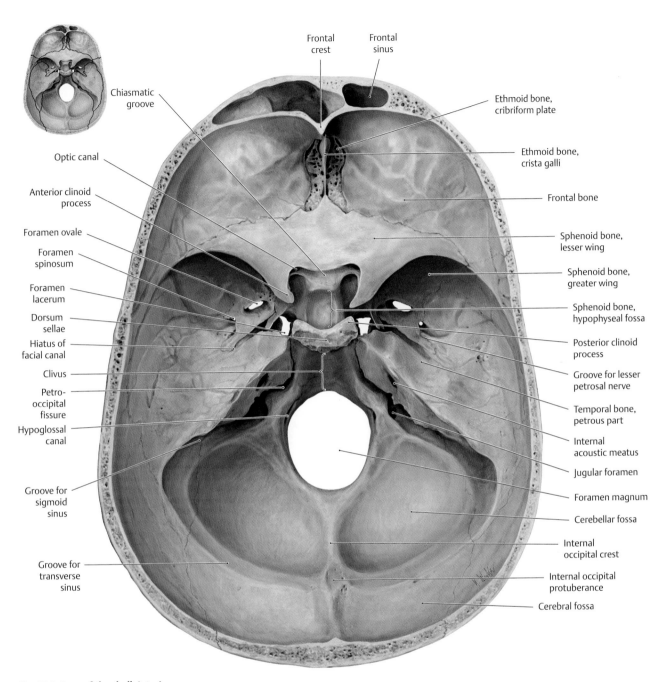

Fig. 17.8 **Base of the skull: Interior**
Superior view.

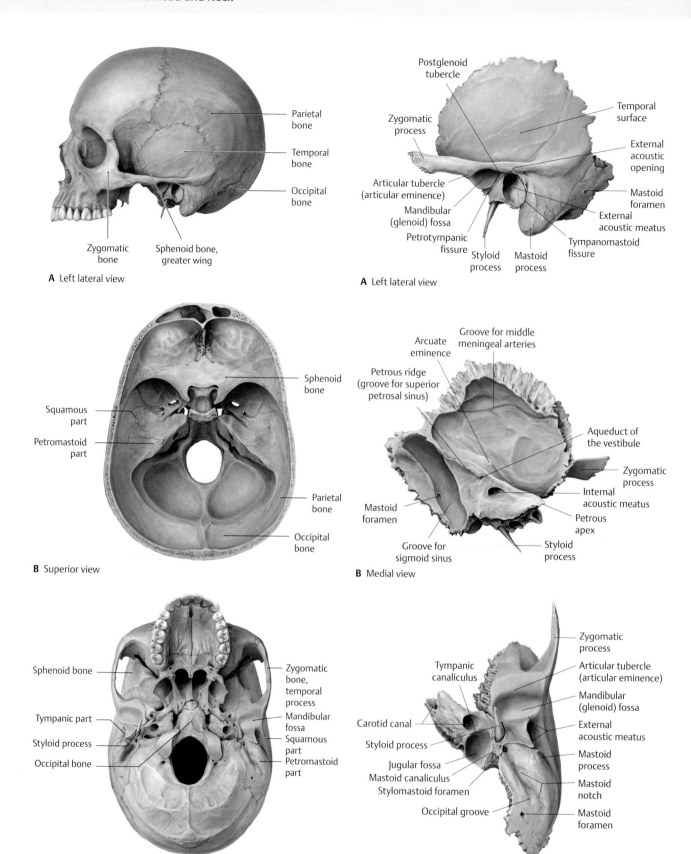

A Left lateral view

B Superior view

C Inferior view

Fig. 17.9 Temporal bone in situ
Squamous part *(light green)*, petromastoid part *(pale green)*, tympanic part *(dark green)*.

A Left lateral view

B Medial view

C Inferior view

Fig. 17.10 Temporal bone

A Left lateral view.

B Superior view.

C Inferior view.

D Anterior view.

Fig. 17.11 **Sphenoid bone in situ**

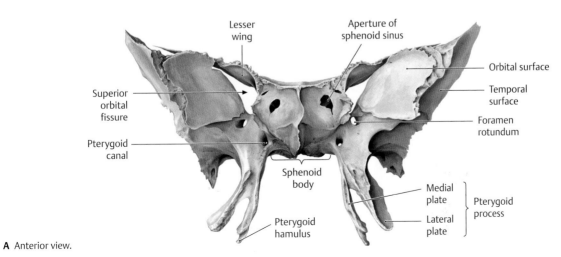

A Anterior view.

Fig. 17.12 **Sphenoid bone** (*continued on page 404*)

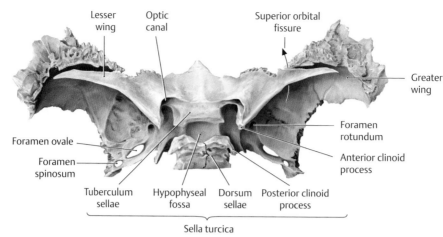

B Superior view.

Fig. 17.12 (*continued*) **Sphenoid bone**

The Viscerocranium

The **viscerocraniun**, or facial skeleton, is composed of 15 bones: the ethmoid, mandible, and vomer, and the paired inferior nasal concha, maxillary, nasal, lacrimal, zygomatic, and palatine bones (see **Figs. 17.3** and **17.4**).

— The **ethmoid bone (Figs. 17.13** and **17.14)** forms part of the anterior cranial fossa, the medial walls of the orbits, and parts of the nasal septum and lateral nasal walls.

• The **cribriform plate** (neurocranium) sits in the anterior cranial fossa above the nasal cavity.

• The **perpendicular plate** forms part of the nasal septum.

• Ethmoid processes include the **crista galli** superiorly and **superior** and **middle nasal concha** inferiorly on the lateral wall of the nasal cavity.

• Numerous thin-walled **ethmoid air cells** form the **ethmoid sinuses**.

— Paired **maxillary bones** (maxilla) **(Fig. 17.15;** see **Figs. 17.4** and **17.7)** form the upper jaw, floors of the orbits, and parts of the nose and palate.

• The **maxillary dental arch** contains **alveoli** (sockets) for the upper teeth.

• **Palatine processes** form the anterior part of the palate, and **frontal processes** form part of the external nose.

A Superior view.

A Superior view.

B Anterior view.

Fig. 17.13 Ethmoid bone in situ

B Anterior view.

Fig. 17.14 Ethmoid bone

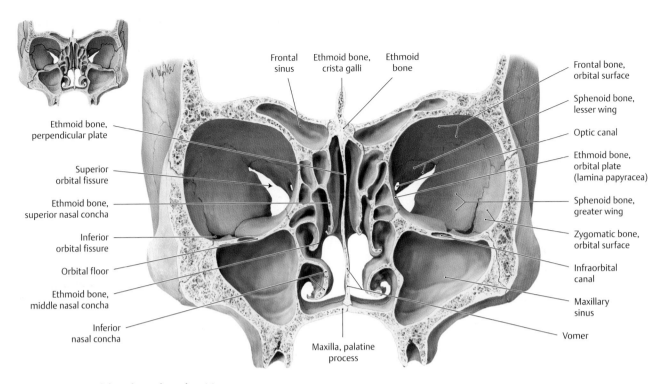

Frontal sinus

Ethmoid bone, crista galli

Ethmoid bone

Ethmoid bone, perpendicular plate

Superior orbital fissure

Ethmoid bone, superior nasal concha

Inferior orbital fissure

Orbital floor

Ethmoid bone, middle nasal concha

Inferior nasal concha

Maxilla, palatine process

Frontal bone, orbital surface

Sphenoid bone, lesser wing

Optic canal

Ethmoid bone, orbital plate (lamina papyracea)

Sphenoid bone, greater wing

Zygomatic bone, orbital surface

Infraorbital canal

Maxillary sinus

Vomer

Fig. 17.15 Bones of the orbit and nasal cavities
Coronal section, anterior view.

- An **infraorbital foramen** opens onto the face.
- A large **maxillary sinus** within the maxilla sits below each orbit.
— The **mandible (Fig. 17.16**; see also **Fig. 17.3**) forms the lower jaw.
  - A horizontal **body** connects posteriorly with a vertical **ramus** on each side.
  - An **angle** forms on each side at the junction between the body and the ramus.
  - The superior end of each ramus has an anterior **coronoid process** that is separated from the posterior **condylar process** by a **mandibular notch**.

- The **head** of the condylar process articulates with the mandibular fossa of the temporal bone.
- Foramina include a **mental foramen** externally and a **mandibular foramen** internally.
- The **mandibular dental arch** contains alveoli that house the lower teeth.
— Paired **nasal bones** (see **Fig. 17.4**) form the bridge of the nose.
— Paired **lacrimal bones** (see **Fig. 17.3**) form the anterior medial walls of the orbits and contain **fossae for the lacrimal sacs**.
— Paired **zygomatic bones** (see **Fig. 17.3**) form the bony prominences of the cheeks, anterior parts of the zygomatic arches, and lateral walls of the orbits.
— Paired **palatine bones** (see **Fig. 17.7**) have vertical parts that form the posterior lateral walls of the nasal cavity and **horizontal processes** that form the posterior parts of the palate.
— The **vomer** (see **Fig. 17.15**) forms the inferior and posterior part of nasal septum.
— Paired **inferior nasal conchae** (see **Fig. 17.15**) form the lowest scroll-like processes on the lateral walls of the nasal cavity.

Sutures of the Skull

— During development, the bones of the calvaria grow outward from their center toward adjacent bones; the bones eventually fuse to form fibrous joints called **sutures**.
— Although there are many smaller sutures, the major sutures of the calvaria (see **Figs. 17.2, 17.3, 17.5**) are
  - the **sagittal suture** between the right and left parietal bones,
  - the **coronal suture** between the frontal and parietal bones,
  - the **lambdoid suture** between the occipital and parietal bones, and

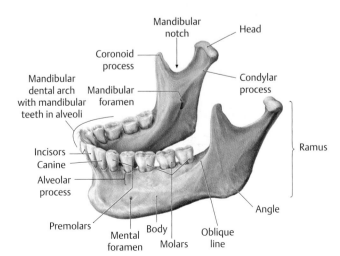

Mandibular notch

Head

Coronoid process

Condylar process

Mandibular dental arch with mandibular teeth in alveoli

Mandibular foramen

Incisors

Canine

Alveolar process

Ramus

Premolars

Mental foramen

Body

Molars

Oblique line

Angle

Fig. 17.16 Mandible
Oblique, left lateral view.

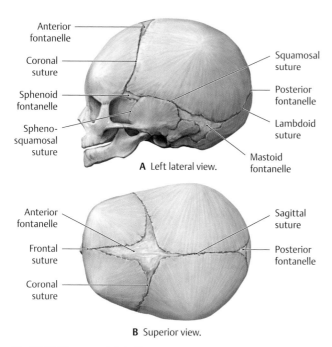

Fig. 17.17 **The neonatal skull**

A Left lateral view.

B Superior view.

Table 17.2 **Landmarks of the Skull (see Figs. 17.2, 17.3, 17.4, 17.6)**

Landmark	Location of Point or Area
Nasion	Junction of frontonasal and internasal sutures
Glabella	Most anterior prominence of frontal bone at the top of the nose
Bregma	Junction of coronal and sagittal sutures
Pterion	Area encompassing junction of frontal, parietal, sphenoid, and temporal bones along the spheno-parietal suture
Vertex	Most superior point of the skull along the sagittal suture
Lambda	Junction of lambdoid and sagittal sutures
Asterion	Junction of sutures joining occipital, temporal, and parietal bones

• the **squamous sutures** between the parietal and temporal bones.

— At birth, growth of the skull bones and formation of the sutures are incomplete. Large fibrous areas, known as **fontanelles**, remain between the bones and allow for continued growth of the brain. The largest of these, the **anterior fontanelle** at the junction of the frontal and parietal bones, closes between 18 and 24 months of age (**Fig. 17.17**).

— Junctions of the sutures and other prominent points of the skull are useful for measuring growth of the skull and brain; determining race, gender, and age; and locating deep cranial structures (**Table 17.2**).

Cranial Fossae

— The floor of the cranial cavity is divided into three fossae, or spaces (**Fig. 17.18**; see also **Fig. 17.8**).
  • The **anterior cranial fossa,** formed by the frontal and ethmoid bones and lesser wing of the sphenoid bone,

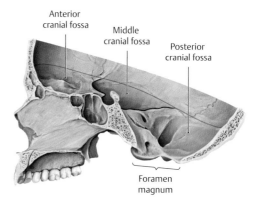

A Midsagittal section, left lateral view.

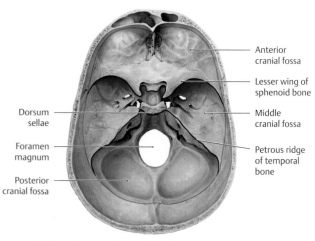

B Superior view of opened skull.

Fig. 17.18 **Cranial fossae**
The interior of the skull base consists of three successive fossae that become progressively deeper in the frontal-to-occipital direction.

contains the frontal lobe of the brain and the olfactory bulbs (see Section 18.2 for a description of the brain).

- The **middle cranial fossa,** formed by the greater and lesser wings of the sphenoid bone and squamous and petrous parts of the temporal bones, contains the temporal lobes of the brain, the optic chiasm, and the pituitary gland. The hypophyseal fossa separates the right and left halves of the middle cranial fossa.

- The **posterior cranial fossa,** formed primarily by the occipital bone and petrous parts of the temporal bones,

contains the pons, medulla oblongata, and cerebellum of the brain. The medulla oblongata exits the skull through the foramen magnum located on the floor of the fossa, and grooves on the posterior and lateral walls accommodate the transverse and sigmoid dural venous sinuses.

— Foramina within the anterior, middle, and posterior fossae allow blood vessels and nerves to pass through the skull (**Fig. 17.19**).

(See Sections 17.3, 17.4, and 18.3 for arteries of the head, veins of the head, and cranial nerves, respectively.)

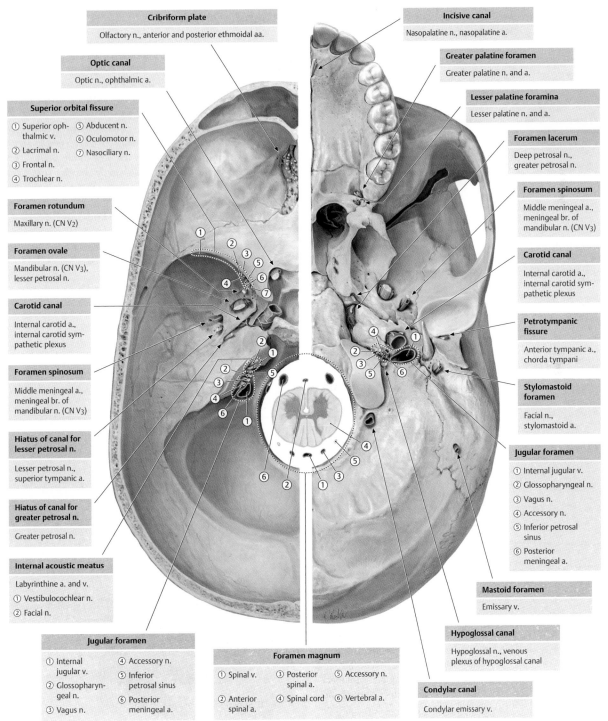

Cribriform plate
Olfactory n., anterior and posterior ethmoidal aa.

Optic canal
Optic n., ophthalmic a.

Superior orbital fissure
① Superior ophthalmic v. ⑤ Abducent n.
② Lacrimal n. ⑥ Oculomotor n.
③ Frontal n. ⑦ Nasociliary n.
④ Trochlear n.

Foramen rotundum
Maxillary n. (CN V₂)

Foramen ovale
Mandibular n. (CN V₃), lesser petrosal n.

Carotid canal
Internal carotid a., internal carotid sympathetic plexus

Foramen spinosum
Middle meningeal a., meningeal br. of mandibular n. (CN V₃)

Hiatus of canal for lesser petrosal n.
Lesser petrosal n., superior tympanic a.

Hiatus of canal for greater petrosal n.
Greater petrosal n.

Internal acoustic meatus
Labyrinthine a. and v.
① Vestibulocochlear n.
② Facial n.

Jugular foramen
① Internal jugular v.   ④ Accessory n.
② Glossopharyngeal n.   ⑤ Inferior petrosal sinus
③ Vagus n.   ⑥ Posterior meningeal a.

Foramen magnum
① Spinal v.   ③ Posterior spinal a.   ⑤ Accessory n.
② Anterior spinal a.   ④ Spinal cord   ⑥ Vertebral a.

Incisive canal
Nasopalatine n., nasopalatine a.

Greater palatine foramen
Greater palatine n. and a.

Lesser palatine foramina
Lesser palatine n. and a.

Foramen lacerum
Deep petrosal n., greater petrosal n.

Foramen spinosum
Middle meningeal a., meningeal br. of mandibular n. (CN V₃)

Carotid canal
Internal carotid a., internal carotid sympathetic plexus

Petrotympanic fissure
Anterior tympanic a., chorda tympani

Stylomastoid foramen
Facial n., stylomastoid a.

Jugular foramen
① Internal jugular v.
② Glossopharyngeal n.
③ Vagus n.
④ Accessory n.
⑤ Inferior petrosal sinus
⑥ Posterior meningeal a.

Mastoid foramen
Emissary v.

Hypoglossal canal
Hypoglossal n., venous plexus of hypoglossal canal

Condylar canal
Condylar emissary v.

A Cranial cavity (interior of skull base). Left side, superior view.

B Exterior of skull base. Left side, inferior view.

Fig. 17.19 **Neurovascular structures entering or exiting the cranial cavity**

17.2 Bones of the Neck

Most bones of the neck are parts of the vertebral column, thoracic skeleton, or pectoral girdle (see **Fig. 1.5A**).

— The seven cervical vertebrae support the head on the vertebral column and provide attachment for neck muscles.
— The manubrium of the sternum forms the inferior midline boundary of the anterior neck.
— The clavicles form the lateral boundaries of the neck.
— The **hyoid bone,** a small U-shaped bone, lies anterior to the C3 vertebra in the neck (**Fig. 17.20**).
  • It has a **body** and paired **lesser** and **greater horns.**
  • The hyoid does not articulate directly with any other bones of the skeleton, but muscles and ligaments attach it to the mandible, styloid processes of the temporal bones, larynx, clavicles, sternum, and scapulae.

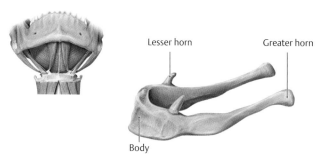

Lesser horn   Greater horn

Body

Fig. 17.20 Hyoid bone
The hyoid bone is suspended in the neck by muscles between the floor of the mouth and the larynx.

17.3 Arteries of the Head and Neck

Arteries of the head and neck are branches of the right and left **subclavian** and **common carotid arteries** (see **Fig. 3.6**).

— The brachiocephalic trunk arises from the aortic arch and divides behind the right sternoclavicular joint to form the right subclavian and right common carotid arteries.
— The left subclavian and left common carotid arteries are direct branches of the aortic arch in the superior mediastinum of the thorax.

The Subclavian Artery

The subclavian arteries enter the neck through the superior thoracic aperture and pass laterally between the anterior and middle scalene muscles. Two branches, the vertebral artery and the thyrocervical trunk, arise medial to the anterior scalene muscles on each side and supply structures in the head and neck (**Fig. 17.21**).

— The **vertebral artery** passes posteriorly in the neck to ascend through the transverse foramina of C1–C6 vertebrae and enters the foramen magnum at the base of the skull.
  • In the neck, it contributes the single anterior spinal artery and paired posterior spinal arteries that supply the upper spinal cord.
  • In the skull, it gives off the **posteroinferior cerebellar arteries.**
  • It terminates by joining the contralateral vertebral artery to form a single **basilar artery,** which supplies the posterior circulation of the brain.

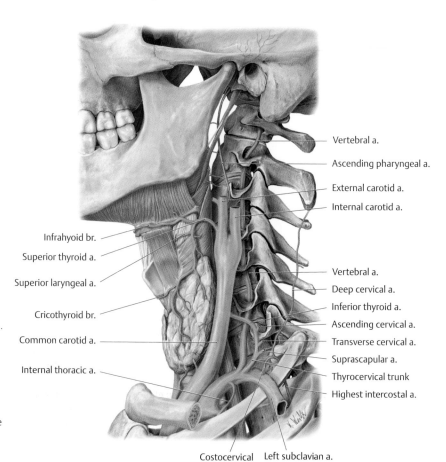

Vertebral a.
Ascending pharyngeal a.
External carotid a.
Internal carotid a.

Infrahyoid br.
Superior thyroid a.
Superior laryngeal a.

Vertebral a.
Deep cervical a.
Inferior thyroid a.
Ascending cervical a.

Cricothyroid br.

Common carotid a.

Transverse cervical a.
Suprascapular a.
Thyrocervical trunk

Internal thoracic a.

Highest intercostal a.

Costocervical   Left subclavian a.
trunk

A Left lateral view. The structures of the neck are primarily supplied by the external carotid artery and subclavian artery.

Fig. 17.21 Arteries of the neck

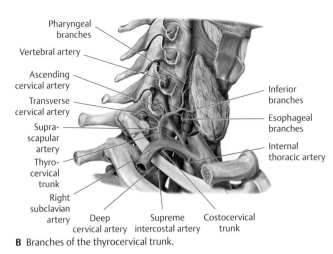

B Branches of the thyrocervical trunk.

Fig. 17.21 (*continued*) **Arteries of the neck**

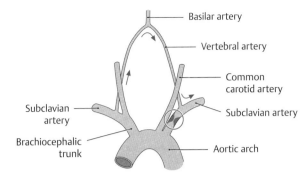

Fig. 17.22 Subclavian steal syndrome
Red circle indicates area of stenosis; *arrows* indicate direction of blood flow.

CLINICAL CORRELATION

SUBCLAVIAN STEAL SYNDROME "Subclavian steal" usually results from a stenosis of the left subclavian artery located proximal to the origin of the vertebral artery. When the left arm is exercised, there may be insufficient blood flow to the arm. As a result, blood is "stolen" from the vertebral artery circulation, causing a reversal of flow in the vertebral artery on the *affected* side. This leads to a deficient blood flow in the basilar artery and may deprive the brain of blood, producing a feeling of lightheadedness **(Fig. 17.22)**.

— The **thyrocervical trunk** is a short trunk that branches into four arteries:
  - The **inferior thyroid artery,** the largest branch, which turns medially to supply the larynx, trachea, esophagus, and thyroid and parathyroid glands
  - The **suprascapular** and **transverse cervical arteries,** which supply muscles of the back and scapular region
  - The **ascending cervical artery,** a small branch that supplies muscles in the neck

The Carotid Artery System

The carotid artery system supplies structures of the neck, face, skull, and brain and consists of paired common carotid, external carotid, and internal carotid arteries and their branches.

— The **common carotid artery** enters the neck from the thorax and ascends, with the internal jugular vein and vagus nerve, within a fascial sleeve, the **carotid sheath.**
  - Its only branches, the **external carotid** and **internal carotid arteries,** arise from its bifurcation at the C4 vertebral level **(Fig. 17.23)**.
— The **external carotid artery** supplies most structures of the face and head except the brain and the orbits. Six branches arise from the external carotid artery in the neck before it passes behind the mandible and finally bifurcates into two terminal branches, the **maxillary** and **superficial temporal arteries (Table 17.3)**.
  1. The **superior thyroid artery** supplies the thyroid gland and, through its **superior laryngeal artery,** the larynx.
  2. The **lingual artery** supplies the posterior tongue and floor of the mouth.
  3. The **facial artery** ascends deep to the submandibular gland, which it supplies, and crosses the mandible from

below to enter the face. It passes lateral to the corners of the mouth and terminates near the medial angle of the eye as the **angular artery.** The branches of the facial artery include
  - the **submental** and **tonsillar branches** in the neck, and
  - the **superior** and **inferior labial arteries** and a **lateral nasal artery** on the face.
  4. The **occipital artery** supplies branches to the posterior scalp.
  5. The **ascending pharyngeal artery** sends branches to the pharynx, ear, and deep neck muscles.
  6. The **posterior auricular artery** passes posteriorly to supply the scalp behind the ear.
— The maxillary artery arises posterior to the mandible and passes medially through the **infratemporal** and **pterygopalatine fossae** (see Sections 19.5 and 19.6). Branches from its three parts, the **mandibular, pterygoid,** and **pterygopalatine parts,** supply most structures of the face **(Table 17.4; Figs. 17.24** and **17.25)**.
— The superficial temporal artery passes superiorly through the temporal region anterior to the ear and terminates as **frontal** and **parietal arteries** on the scalp. Its branches on the face **(Fig. 17.26;** see **Table 17.4)** include the following:
  - The **transverse facial artery,** which supplies the parotid gland and duct and crosses anteriorly to supply the skin of the face
  - The **zygomatico-orbital artery,** which supplies the lateral orbit
  - The **middle temporal artery,** which supplies the temporal region
— The **internal carotid artery** is the continuation of the common carotid artery **(Fig. 17.27)**.
  - It is described in four parts:
    - A cervical part in the neck that has no branches
    - A petrous part that courses within the carotid canal of the temporal bone
    - A cavernous part that passes through the **cavernous sinus** (a venous sinus lateral to the sella turcica; see **Figs. 18.5** and **18.6)**
    - A cerebral part that emerges into the middle cranial fossa posterior to the orbit
  - Two receptors are located within the internal carotid artery near its origin.
    - The **carotid sinus,** a baroreceptor that responds to changes in arterial pressure, is noticeable as a small dilation near the origin of the internal carotid artery.

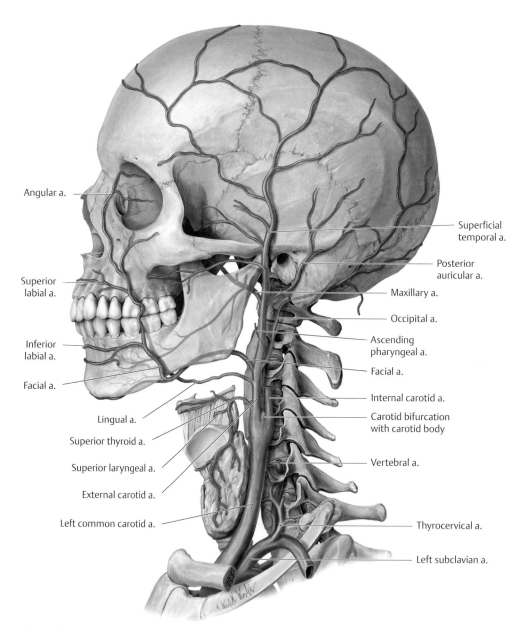

Fig. 17.23 External carotid artery
Left lateral view.

Angular a.

Superficial temporal a.

Posterior auricular a.

Superior labial a.

Maxillary a.

Occipital a.

Inferior labial a.

Ascending pharyngeal a.

Facial a.

Facial a.

Internal carotid a.

Lingual a.

Carotid bifurcation with carotid body

Superior thyroid a.

Superior laryngeal a.

Vertebral a.

External carotid a.

Left common carotid a.

Thyrocervical a.

Left subclavian a.

Table 17.3 **Anterior, Medial, and Posterior Branches of the External Carotid Artery**

Branch	Artery	Divisions and Distributions
Anterior brs.	Superior thyroid a.	Glandular br. (to thyroid gland); superior laryngeal a.; sternocleidomastoid br.
	Lingual a.	Dorsal lingual brs. (to base of tongue, epiglottis); sublingual a. (to sublingual gland, tongue, oral floor, oral cavity)
	Facial a.	Ascending palatine a. (to pharyngeal wall, soft palate, pharyngotympanic tube); tonsillar branch (to palatine tonsils); submental a. (to oral floor, submandibular gland); labial aa.; angular a. (to nasal root)
Medial br.	Ascending pharyngeal a.	Pharyngeal brs.; interior tympanic a. (to mucosa of inner ear); posterior meningeal a.
Posterior brs.	Occipital a.	Occipital brs.; descending br. (to posterior neck muscles)
	Posterior auricular a.	Stylomastoid a. (to facial n. in facial canal); posterior tympanic a.; auricular br.; occipital br.; parotid br.

Note: For terminal brs, see **Table 17.4.**

Table 17.4 Terminal Branches of the External Carotid Artery

Artery		Divisions and Distribution
Superficial temporal a.		Transverse facial a. (to soft tissues below the zygomatic arch); frontal branches; parietal branches; zygomaticoorbital a. (to lateral orbital wall)
Maxillary a.	Mandibular part	Inferior alveolar a. (to mandible, teeth, gingiva); middle meningeal a.; deep auricular a. (to temporomandibular joint, external auditory canal); anterior tympanic a.
	Pterygoid part	Masseteric a.; deep temporal branches; pterygoid branches; buccal a.
	Pterygopalatine part	Posterior superior alveolar a. (to maxillary molars, maxillary sinus, gingiva); infraorbital a. (to maxillary alveoli)
	Descending palatine a.	Greater palatine a. (to hard palate)
		Lesser palatine a. (to soft palate, palatine tonsil, pharyngeal wall)
	Sphenopalatine a.	Lateral posterior nasal aa. (to lateral wall of nasal cavity, conchae)
		Posterior septal branches (to nasal septum)

A Divisions of the maxillary artery: mandibular *(blue)*, pterygoid *(green)*, pterygopalatine *(yellow)*.

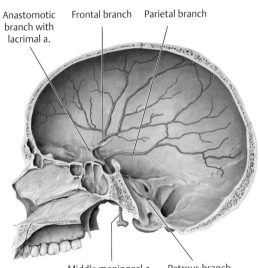

B Course of the maxillary artery.

Fig. 17.24 Maxillary artery
Left lateral view.

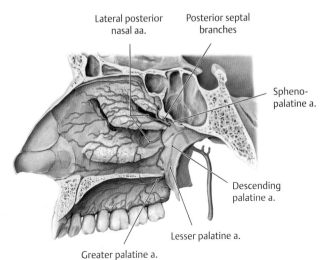

A Right middle meningeal artery. Opened skull, medial view.

B Lateral wall of right nasal cavity and palate, medial view.

Fig. 17.25 Deep branches of the maxillary artery

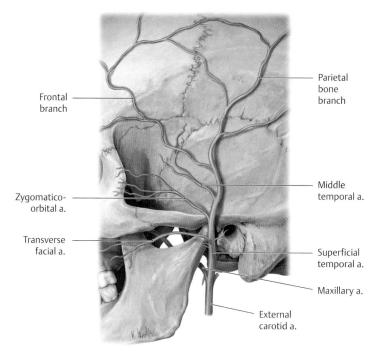

Fig. 17.26 Superficial temporal artery
Left lateral view.

Frontal branch

Parietal bone branch

Zygomatico-orbital a.

Middle temporal a.

Transverse facial a.

Superficial temporal a.

Maxillary a.

External carotid a.

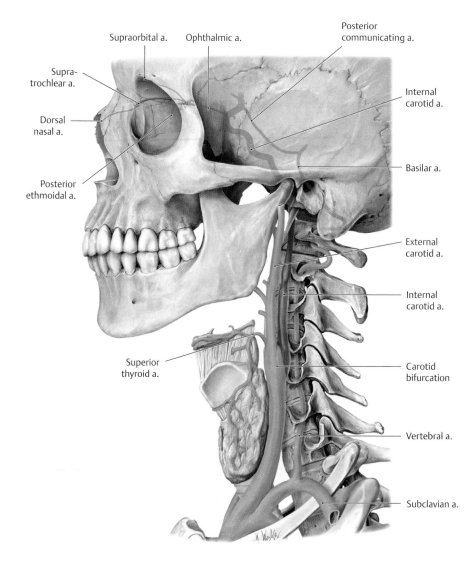

Supraorbital a.

Ophthalmic a.

Posterior communicating a.

Supra-trochlear a.

Internal carotid a.

Dorsal nasal a.

Basilar a.

Posterior ethmoidal a.

External carotid a.

Internal carotid a.

Carotid bifurcation

Superior thyroid a.

Vertebral a.

Subclavian a.

Fig. 17.27 Internal carotid artery
Left lateral view.

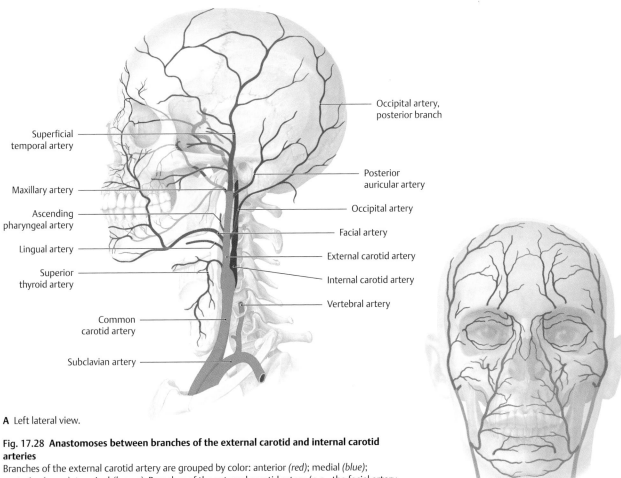

A Left lateral view.

Fig. 17.28 Anastomoses between branches of the external carotid and internal carotid arteries
Branches of the external carotid artery are grouped by color: anterior *(red)*; medial *(blue)*; posterior *(green)*; terminal *(brown)*. Branches of the external carotid artery (e.g., the facial artery *[red]*) communicate with terminal branches of the internal carotid artery (e.g., the ophthalmic artery *[purple]*).

B Anterior view.

- ○ The **carotid body,** a small mass of tissue located near the carotid sinus, is a chemoreceptor that monitors blood oxygen levels. Stimulation of the carotid body initiates an increase in heart rate, respiration rate, and blood pressure.
- • The **ophthalmic artery,** which arises within the skull as the first major branch of the internal carotid artery, passes through the optic canal to supply the orbital contents, including the retina of the eye through its **central retinal artery.**
  - ○ Branches of the ophthalmic artery, the **supraorbital** and **supratrochlear arteries** to the anterior scalp and **ethmoidal arteries** to the nasal cavity, anastomose with branches of the external carotid artery (**Fig. 17.28**).
- • The **anterior** and **middle cerebral arteries** arise from the internal carotid artery to supply the anterior circulation of the brain (see Section 18.2).

17.4   Veins of the Head and Neck

— Superficial and deep veins of the head and neck drain almost exclusively to the external and internal jugular veins, although some also communicate with the vertebral venous plexus of the vertebral column (**Figs. 17.29** and **17.30**).

— Superficial veins generally follow the course of the arteries, but the veins are usually more numerous, more variable, and more interconnected than the arteries.

— The most prominent superficial veins on each side of the head include
  - • the **supratrochlear** and **supraorbital veins,** which drain to the angular vein;
  - • the **angular vein,** which joins with the deep facial vein and continues inferiorly as the facial vein;
  - • the **pterygoid venous plexus,** which drains areas supplied by the maxillary artery, including the orbit, nasal cavity, and oral cavity (it drains to the maxillary and deep facial veins);
  - • the **deep facial vein,** which arises from the pterygoid venous plexus and drains to the facial vein;
  - • the **facial vein,** which drains to the **internal jugular vein;**
  - • the **superficial temporal** and **maxillary veins,** which join to form the retromandibular vein;
  - • the **retromandibular vein,** which joins the **posterior auricular vein** to form the **external jugular vein;** and
  - • the **occipital vein,** which drains to the external jugular vein.

— When present, right and left external jugular veins form posterior to the angle of the mandible by the union of the posterior auricular veins and the posterior division of the retromandibular veins.

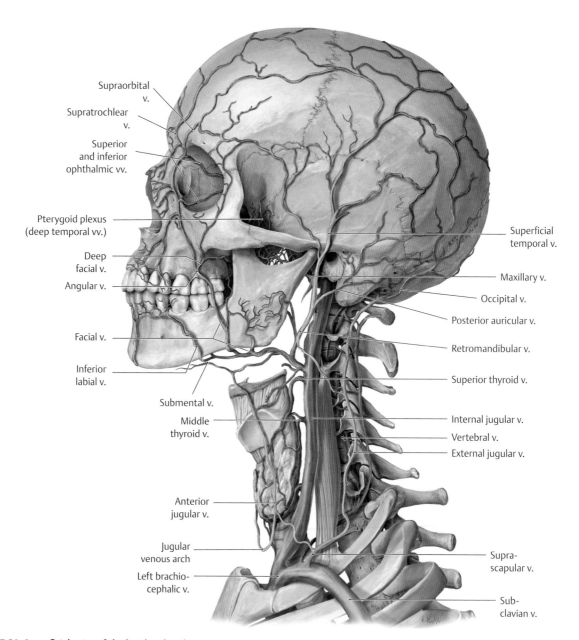

Fig. 17.29 Superficial veins of the head and neck
Left lateral view.

- They cross the sternocleidomastoid muscle in the neck and drain into the subclavian vein.
- They drain the scalp and side of the face.
- Their tributaries include the retromandibular, posterior auricular, occipital, transverse cervical, suprascapular, and anterior jugular veins.
- A right and left **internal jugular vein** forms at the jugular foramen at the skull base and descends within the carotid sheath with the common carotid artery and vagus nerve.
  - It joins the subclavian vein in the root of the neck to form the brachiocephalic vein. The junction of the internal jugular and subclavian veins is called the **jugulosubclavian**

CLINICAL CORRELATION

VENOUS ANASTOMOSES AS PORTALS OF INFECTION The extensive anastomoses between superficial veins of the face and the deep veins of the head (e.g., pterygoid plexus) and dural sinuses (e.g., cavernous sinus) is clinically very important. Veins in the triangular danger zone of the face are, in general, valveless. Thus, bacterial infections from the face are easily disseminated into the cranial cavity. An infection on the lip, for example, may travel via the facial vein to the cavernous sinus, resulting in a cavernous sinus thrombosis (infection leading to clot formation that may occlude the sinus) or even meningitis **(Fig. 17.31)**.

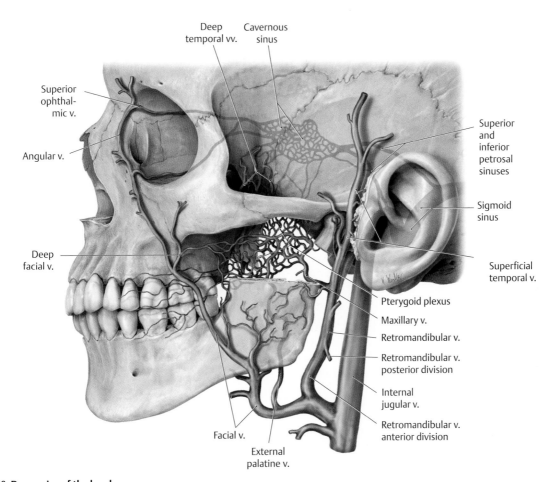

Fig. 17.30 **Deep veins of the head**

Left lateral view. The pterygoid plexus is a venous network situated between the mandibular ramus and the muscles of mastication. The cavernous sinus connects branches of the facial vein to the sigmoid sinuses.

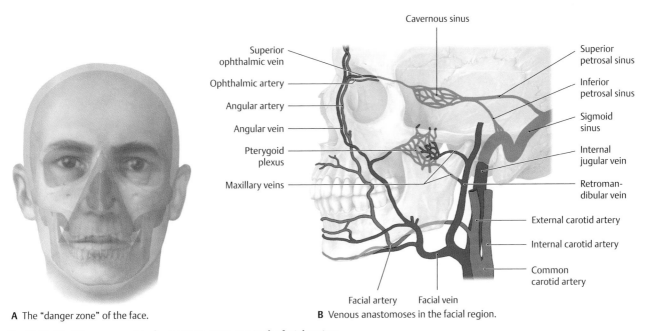

A The "danger zone" of the face.

B Venous anastomoses in the facial region.

Fig. 17.31 **The "danger zone" and venous anastomoses in the facial region**

junction, or **venous angle.** The thoracic duct and right lymphatic duct terminate at this junction.

- It drains the brain, the anterior face and scalp, and the viscera and deep muscles of the neck.
- Its tributaries include the dural venous sinuses, facial vein, lingual vein, pharyngeal veins, and superior and middle thyroid veins.

— A small **anterior jugular vein** originates from superficial veins on each side near the hyoid bone.

- It descends to the base of the neck and terminates in the external jugular or subclavian vein.
- A **jugular venous arch** may connect the right and left anterior jugular veins at the base of the neck, above the sternum.

— Deep veins of the orbit and brain drain to **dural venous sinuses,** venous channels formed within the outer covering of the brain that have no arterial counterpart (see Section 18.1). Dural venous sinuses drain eventually to the internal jugular vein.

17.5   Lymphatic Drainage of the Head and Neck

— Superficial lymph nodes of the head and neck extend along the external jugular vein.

- They receive lymph from local areas and drain to the deep cervical nodes.

- Superficial node groups include occipital, retroauricular, mastoid, parotid, anterior cervical, and lateral cervical nodes (**Fig. 17.32; Table 17.5**).

— Lymph from structures in the head and neck ultimately drains into **deep cervical lymph nodes** that lie along the internal jugular vein deep to the sternocleidomastoid muscle (**Fig. 17.33; Table 17.6**). There are two groups of deep cervical nodes:

- **Superior deep cervical nodes**, known as the jugulodigastric group, lie near the facial and internal jugular veins and posterior belly of the digastric muscle. Submandibular and submental nodes also drain to this group. Superior deep cervical nodes drain either to the inferior deep cervical nodes or directly to the jugular lymphatic trunks.

Table 17.5 **Superficial Cervical Lymph Nodes**

Lymph Node (LN)	Drainage Region
Retroauricular LN	Occiput
Occipital LN	
Mastoid LN	
Superficial parotid LN	Parotid-auricular region
Deep parotid LN	
Anterior superficial cervical LN	Sternocleidomastoid region
Lateral superficial cervical LN	

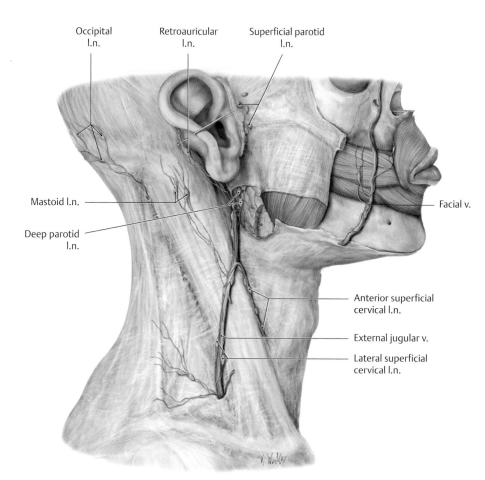

Occipital l.n. Retroauricular l.n. Superficial parotid l.n.

Mastoid l.n.

Deep parotid l.n.

Facial v.

Anterior superficial cervical l.n.

External jugular v.

Lateral superficial cervical l.n.

Fig. 17.32 Superficial cervical lymph nodes
Right lateral view.

Fig. 17.33 Deep cervical lymph nodes
Right lateral view.

Submandibular l.n.

Submental l.n.

Internal jugular v.

Table 17.6 **Deep Cervical Lymph Nodes**

Level	Lymph Node (l.N)		Drainage Region
I	Submental LN		Face
	Submandibular LN		
II	Lateral jugular LN group	Upper lateral group	Nuchal region, laryngo-tracheo-thyroidal region
III		Middle lateral group	
IV		Lower lateral group	
V	LN in posterior cervical triangle		Nuchal region
VI	Anterior cervical LN		Laryngo-tracheo-thyroidal region

- **Inferior deep cervical nodes** are usually associated with the lower internal jugular vein, but some nodes also reside in the area around the subclavian vein and brachial plexus. Inferior deep cervical nodes drain directly to the jugular lymphatic trunks.
— Lymphatic vessels from the deep cervical nodes join to form **jugular lymphatic trunks**.
  - On the right, these trunks drain directly or indirectly (via the right lymphatic duct) into the right jugulosubclavian junction (right venous angle).
  - On the left, these trunks join the thoracic duct, which drains into the left jugulosubclavian junction (left venous angle).

17.6 Nerves of the Head and Neck

Innervation of head and neck structures is a complex combination of somatic and autonomic nerves arising from the cervical spinal cord, cranial nerves, and the sympathetic trunk. A brief overview

is provided here. For more detailed discussions see Section 18.3 (cranial nerves), Section 18.4 (autonomic innervation), and Section 21.4 (nerves of the neck).
— Somatic nerves of the head and neck include the following:
  - spinal nerves C1 through C4, which innervate structures in the head and neck
    ○ The **cervical plexus** is derived from anterior rami of cervical spinal nerves C1–C4.
    ○ The **suboccipital**, **greater occipital**, and **third occipital nerves** are derived from posterior rami of cervical spinal nerves.
  - spinal nerves C5 through T1, whose anterior rami form the brachial plexus that innervates the upper limb (see Section 13.4)
  - Cranial nerves (CN I to CN XII), which arise from the brain.
— Autonomic nerves of the head and neck include
  - parasympathetic nerves, which arise in association with four of the cranial nerves (CN III, VII, XI, and X), and
  - sympathetic nerves, which arise from the cervical sympathetic trunk.

18 Meninges, Brain, and Cranial Nerves

The cranial meninges continuous with the meninges of the spinal cord, as well as the 12 cranial nerves that arise from the brain, are essential parts of the gross anatomy of the head and neck region and are discussed in detail in this unit. The study of the brain, however, is generally confined to the neuroanatomy curriculum, and only a brief overview is provided here.

18.1 The Meninges

The cranial meninges, coverings that protect the brain, consist of the external fibrous **dura mater,** the thin intermediate **arachnoid mater,** and the delicate inner **pia mater (Fig. 18.1).**

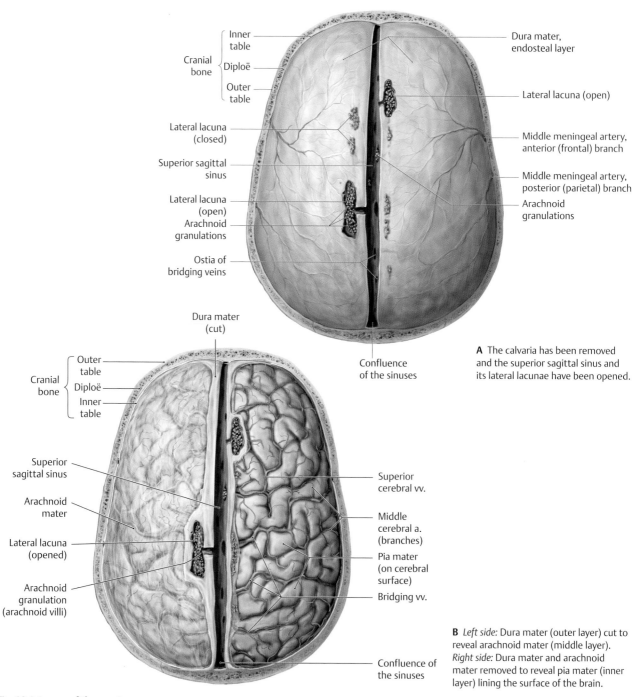

A The calvaria has been removed and the superior sagittal sinus and its lateral lacunae have been opened.

B *Left side:* Dura mater (outer layer) cut to reveal arachnoid mater (middle layer). *Right side:* Dura mater and arachnoid mater removed to reveal pia mater (inner layer) lining the surface of the brain.

Fig. 18.1 Layers of the meninges
Opened cranium, superior view. Arachnoid granulations, sites for loss of cerebral spinal fluid into the venous blood, are protrusions of the arachnoid layer of the meninges into the venous sinus system.

Dura mater

- The dura mater, or dura, a tough outer membrane surrounding the brain, is composed of a **periosteal (endosteal) layer** and a **meningeal layer.** The two layers are inseparable except where they enclose the venous sinuses that drain the brain (e.g., the superior sagittal sinus; see **Fig. 18.5**).
  - The outer periosteal layer, formed by the periosteum of the skull, adheres tightly to the inner surface of the skull, particularly at the sutures. This layer ends at the foramen magnum and is not continuous with the dura around the spinal cord.
  - The inner meningeal layer, a strong membranous sheet that adheres to the inner surface of the periosteal layer, provides sheaths for the cranial nerves as they pass through the skull foramina. It is closely applied, although not attached, to the underlying **arachnoid mater.** It continues into the vertebral canal as dura of the spinal cord (**Fig. 18.2**).
- The middle meningeal arteries, branches of the maxillary arteries, supply most of the dura, with contributions from the ophthalmic, occipital, and vertebral arteries. Veins accompany the arteries and drain into the pterygoid venous plexus.
- Branches of the trigeminal nerve (cranial nerve [CN] V) transmit sensation from the dura of the anterior and middle cranial fossa. Spinal nerves C1, C2, and C3 and small branches of the vagus nerve (CN X) innervate the dura of the posterior cranial fossa.

Dural Partitions

Infoldings of the meningeal layer of the dura form incomplete membranous partitions that separate and support parts of the brain (**Fig. 18.3**).

- The **falx cerebri,** a vertical sickle-shaped partition separating the right and left cerebral hemispheres, is attached anteriorly to the crista galli and the inner crest of the frontal bone and is continuous posteriorly with the tentorium cerebelli. The inferior, free edge of the falx cerebri is unattached.
- The **tentorium cerebelli,** a horizontal continuation of the falx cerebri, separates the occipital lobes of the cerebrum

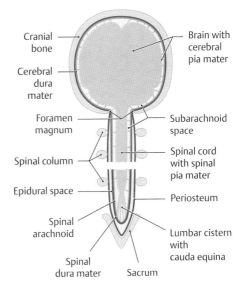

Fig. 18.2 Meninges in the cranial cavity and spinal cord
The two layers of the dura mater (periosteal and meningeal) form a single structural unit in the cranial cavity. In the spinal canal, however, the dura is separated from the periosteum of the vertebrae by the epidural space.

from the cerebellar hemispheres in the posterior cranial fossae.

- It is attached to the posterior clinoid processes and the petrous part of the temporal bones anteriorly and to the parietal and occipital bones posterolaterally.
- A U-shaped **tentorial notch** separates the attachments to the petrous ridge on each side and connects the middle and posterior cranial fossae.
- The **falx cerebelli,** a vertical partition separating the cerebellar hemispheres, is continuous superiorly with the tentorium cerebelli and is attached posteriorly to the occipital crest.
- The **diaphragma sellae,** a small dural fold attached to the anterior and posterior clinoid processes, forms a roof over the sella turcica, which encloses the hypophysis (pituitary gland).

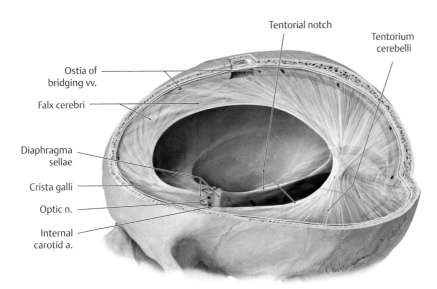

Fig. 18.3 Dural septa (folds)
Left anterior oblique view.

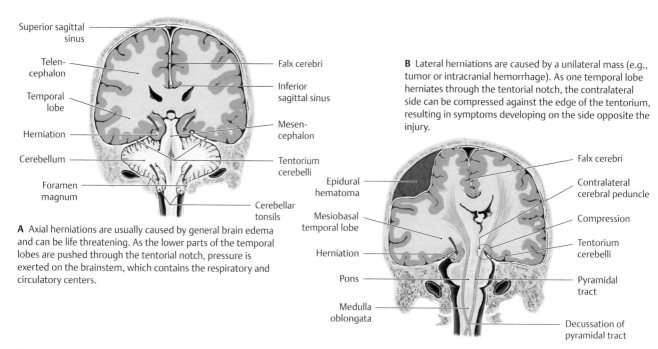

B Lateral herniations are caused by a unilateral mass (e.g., tumor or intracranial hemorrhage). As one temporal lobe herniates through the tentorial notch, the contralateral side can be compressed against the edge of the tentorium, resulting in symptoms developing on the side opposite the injury.

A Axial herniations are usually caused by general brain edema and can be life threatening. As the lower parts of the temporal lobes are pushed through the tentorial notch, pressure is exerted on the brainstem, which contains the respiratory and circulatory centers.

Fig. 18.4 Potential sites of herniation beneath the free edges of the meninges
Coronal section, anterior view.

CLINICAL CORRELATION

TENTORIAL HERNIATION Increased pressure within the middle cranial fossa created by edema or a space-occupying lesion such as a tumor can squeeze the brain tissue and force part of the temporal lobe to herniate through the tentorial notch **(Fig. 18.4)**. Pressure on the adjacent brainstem can be fatal in this situation. The oculomotor nerve (CN III) can also be stretched or damaged, leading to fixed pupil dilation (loss of parasympathetic function) and a "down and out" gaze due to paralysis of most of the extraocular muscles.

Dural Venous Sinuses

Dural venous sinuses are valveless venous spaces that form as a result of the separation of the periosteal and meningeal layers of the dura. Most of the large veins of the brain, skull, orbit, and inner ear drain through the dural sinuses and into the internal jugular veins in the neck **(Figs. 18.5 and 18.6; Table 18.1)**.

— The **confluence of sinuses** at the posterior edge of the tentorium cerebelli is a junction of the superior sagittal, straight, occipital, and transverse sinuses.

— The **superior sagittal sinus** runs in the attached superior border of the falx cerebri and ends in the confluence of sinuses.

— The **inferior sagittal sinus** runs in the free inferior edge of the falx cerebri and ends in the straight sinus.

— The **straight sinus** runs in the space formed by the union of the falx cerebri and tentorium cerebelli. It receives the inferior sagittal sinus and **great cerebral vein** and drains into the confluence of sinuses.

— The paired **transverse sinuses** run along the attached posterolateral margins of the tentorium cerebelli. Posteriorly, they join at the confluence of sinuses, and anteriorly they drain into the sigmoid sinuses, forming grooves in the occipital and parietal bones along their course.

— The paired **sigmoid sinuses** run in deep grooves of the occipital and temporal bones and drain into the internal jugular veins at the jugular foramen.

— The **occipital sinus** runs in the free edge of the falx cerebelli and ends in the confluence of sinuses.

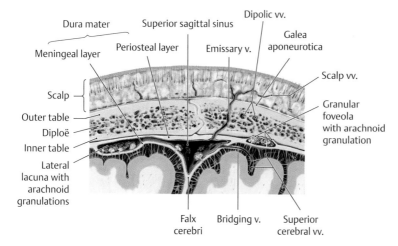

Fig. 18.5 Structure of a dural sinus
Superior sagittal sinus, coronal section, anterior view.

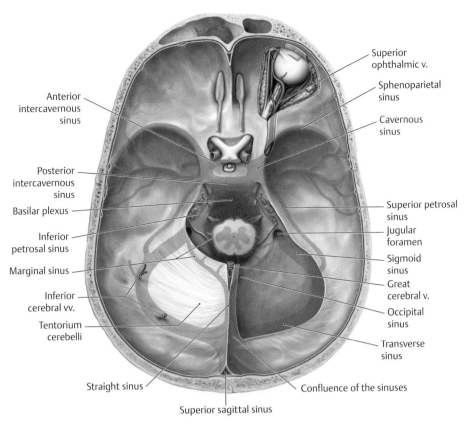

Fig. 18.6 Dural sinuses in the cranial cavity
Opened cranial cavity with dural sinus system ghosted in *blue*, superior view. *Removed:* Tentorium cerebelli.

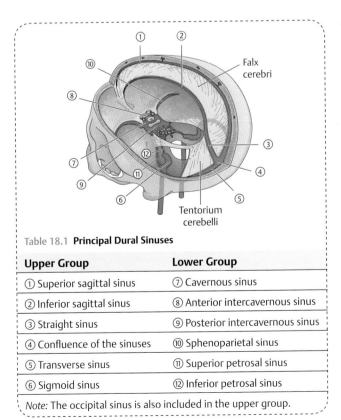

Table 18.1 **Principal Dural Sinuses**

Upper Group	Lower Group
① Superior sagittal sinus	⑦ Cavernous sinus
② Inferior sagittal sinus	⑧ Anterior intercavernous sinus
③ Straight sinus	⑨ Posterior intercavernous sinus
④ Confluence of the sinuses	⑩ Sphenoparietal sinus
⑤ Transverse sinus	⑪ Superior petrosal sinus
⑥ Sigmoid sinus	⑫ Inferior petrosal sinus

Note: The occipital sinus is also included in the upper group.

— The paired **cavernous sinuses,** located on either side of the sella turcica, have characteristics that distinguish them from other dural sinuses (**Figs. 18.7** and **18.8**).
• Each cavernous sinus contains a large plexus of thin-walled veins.
• Several important structures are associated with each cavernous sinus:
   ○ Internal carotid artery, which is surrounded by the sympathetic internal carotid nerve plexus
   ○ Oculomotor nerve (CN III)
   ○ Trochlear nerve (CN IV)
   ○ Ophthalmic and maxillary divisions (CN V_1, V_2) of the trigeminal nerve
   ○ Abducent nerve (CN VI)

CLINICAL CORRELATION

CAVERNOUS SINUS THROMBOPHLEBITIS Cavernous sinus thrombophlebitis can occur secondary to thrombophlebitis of the facial vein. Although blood from the angle of the eye, lips, nose, and face usually drains inferiorly, it can also drain through the veins of the orbit to the cavernous sinus. Infections from the face, particularly from the *danger zone of the face* (which extends from the bridge of the nose to the angles of the mouth) can spread infected thrombi to the cavernous sinus. This can affect the nerves that traverse the sinus (CN III, CN IV, CN V_1 and V_2, and CN VI) and result in acute meningitis.

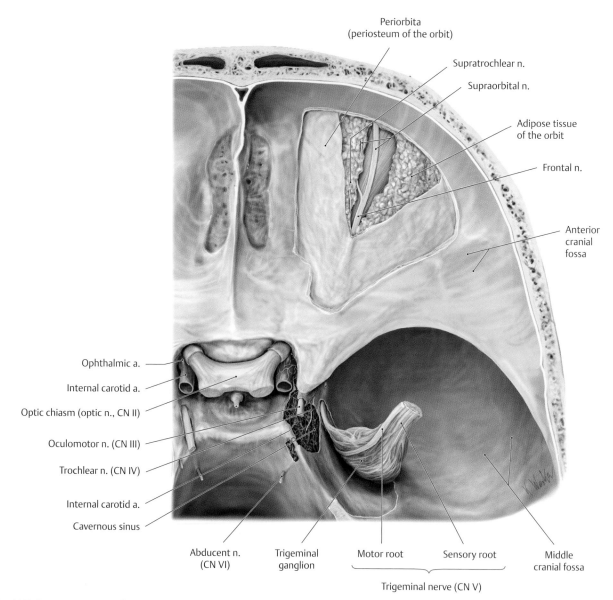

Fig. 18.7 Cavernous sinus and cranial nerves
Left anterior and middle cranial fossae, superior view. *Removed:* Lateral dural wall and roof of the cavernous sinus. The trigeminal ganglion is cut and retracted laterally following removal of its dural covering.

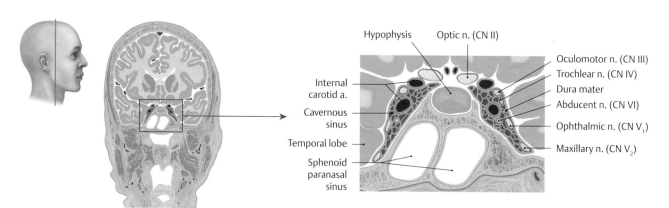

Fig. 18.8 Cavernous sinus
Middle cranial fossa, coronal section, anterior view.

- The cavernous sinuses receive the superior and inferior ophthalmic veins, the sphenoparietal sinuses, the superficial middle cerebral veins, and the central veins of the retina.
- The cavernous sinuses drain into the superior and inferior petrosal sinuses posteriorly and the pterygoid venous plexus inferiorly.
- Anterior and posterior **intercavernous sinuses** (see **Fig. 18.6**) connect the right and left cavernous sinuses.
- Paired **superior petrosal sinuses,** which drain the cavernous sinuses, travel within the attached margins of the tentorium cerebelli along the top of the petrous part of the temporal bones and empty into the sigmoid sinuses.
- Paired **inferior petrosal sinuses** drain the cavernous sinuses, passing through a groove between the petrous part of the temporal bones and the basilar part of the occipital bone and emptying into the sigmoid sinuses at the origin of the internal jugular veins. The inferior petrosal sinuses communicate, through a **basilar plexus,** with the vertebral venous plexus.

Arachnoid and Pia Mater (see Figs. 18.1 and 18.5)

- **Arachnoid** is a thin, avascular, fibrous layer underlying the meningeal layer of the dura.
  - Cerebrospinal fluid in the subarachnoid space presses the arachnoid against the overlying dura, but the two layers are not attached. Weblike **arachnoid trabeculae** attach the arachnoid to the underlying **pia mater.**
  - Delicate fingers of the arachnoid layer, the **arachnoid villi,** pierce the dura to allow the reabsorption of cerebrospinal fluid into the venous circulation and are especially numerous in the superior sagittal sinus. They form aggregations called **arachnoid granulations** that protrude into the largest dural venous sinuses and can push the dura ahead of them into the parietal bone, forming "pits."
  - Congregations of arachnoid granulations also occur in **lateral lacunae,** lateral expansions of the superior sagittal sinus.
- **Pia mater,** or pia, is a thin, highly vascular layer that adheres to the surface of the brain and closely follows its contours.

Meningeal Spaces

- The **epidural space** between the cranium and dura is not a natural space because the dura adheres to the skull. Meningeal vessels that supply the skull and dura travel in this space **(Fig. 18.9).**

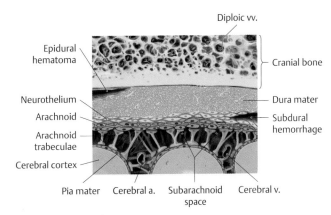

Fig. 18.9 Meningeal spaces
Meninges, coronal section, anterior view.

- The **subdural space** between the dura and arachnoid is a potential space, open only in pathologic conditions such as a subdural hematoma. Superficial cerebral veins ("bridging veins") cross this space, connecting the venous circulation of the brain with the dural venous sinuses (see **Fig. 18.9**).

EXTRACEREBRAL HEMORRHAGE Bleeding from vessels between the bony skull and the brain (extracerebral hemorrhage) increases intracranial pressure and can damage brain tissue. Three types of cerebral hemorrhages are distinguished based on their relationship to the meningeal layers **(Fig. 18.10).**

Epidural hemorrhages commonly originate from a torn middle meningeal artery following a skull fracture at the pterion and result in bleeding into the epidural space. The hemorrhagic spread is usually limited by suture lines because the dura is attached to the skull at these points. As a result, the local accumulation of blood causes compression of the brain in that area.

Subdural hematomas result from tearing of the bridging veins as they traverse the gap between the dural sinus and cerebral cortex. The elderly are more susceptible to this type of hemorrhage because with brain shrinkage these veins bridge a larger gap and are more vulnerable to injury from head trauma. This condition may mimic a slowly evolving stroke with a fluctuating level of consciousness and localizing neurologic signs.

Most subarachnoid hemorrhages occur due to the rupture of aneurysms associated with vessels of the circle of Willis and most frequently with vessels of the anterior cerebral circulation. These hemorrhages into the subarachnoid space begin with a sudden, severe headache, neck stiffness, and drowsiness but can progress to severe consequences such as hemiplegia and coma.

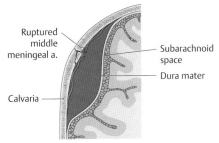

A Epidural hematoma (above the dura).

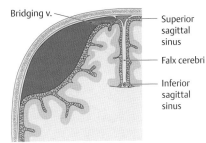

B Subdural hematoma (below the dura).

C Subarachnoid hemorrhage

Fig. 18.10 Extracerebral hemorrhages

— The **subarachnoid space,** between the arachnoid and pia layers, contains cerebrospinal fluid, arteries, and veins (see **Fig. 18.9**).

- • **Subarachnoid cisterns** are spaces that form where the subarachnoid space enlarges around large infoldings of the brain. The largest of these include the **cerebellomedullary, pontomedullary, interpeduncular, chiasmatic, quadrigeminal,** and **ambient cisterns** (see Section 18.2; see **Fig. 18.13**).

18.2 The Brain

The brain, enclosed within the bony skull, is the largest part of the central nervous system. It communicates with the peripheral nervous system through the spinal cord and spinal nerves and through the 12 pairs of cranial nerves.

Regions of the Brain

The major regions of the brain are the cerebrum, diencephalon, brainstem (mesencephalon, pons, medulla oblongata), and cerebellum (**Fig. 18.11**).

— The **cerebrum** is the largest part of the brain and the center for integration within the central nervous system.

- • The falx cerebri lies in a **longitudinal fissure** between the **right** and **left cerebral hemispheres.**
- • Each cerebral hemisphere is further divided into **frontal, parietal, occipital,** and **temporal lobes** that occupy the anterior and middle cranial fossae.
- • Posteriorly, the cerebrum rests on the tentorium cerebelli.
- • The surface layer of the cerebrum (cortex) forms **gyri** (folds) separated by **sulci** (grooves).

— The **diencephalon** forms the central core of the brain and consists of the **thalamus, hypophysis,** and **hypothalamus.**

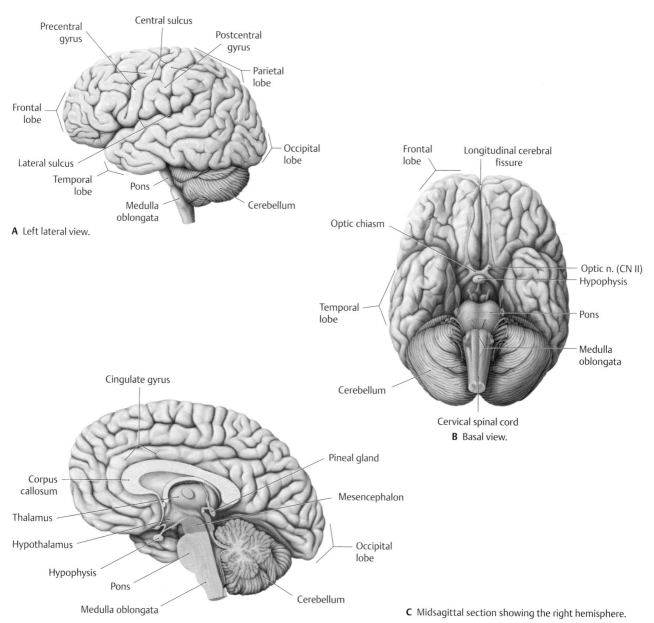

A Left lateral view.

B Basal view.

C Midsagittal section showing the right hemisphere.

Fig. 18.11 Adult brain
CN, cranial nerve.

— The **mesencephalon** (midbrain), the most anterior part of the brainstem, passes through the tentorial notch between the middle and posterior cranial fossae.
  • It is associated with the oculomotor (CN III) and trochlear (CN IV) nerves.
— The **pons,** the middle part of the brainstem, lies in the anterior part of the posterior cranial fossa below the mesencephalon.
  • Several ascending and descending fiber tracts connect the pons to the cerebellum.
  • The pons is associated with the trigeminal (CN V), abducent (CN VI), and facial (CN VII) nerves.
— The **medulla oblongata,** the most posterior part of the brainstem, connects the brain and spinal cord.
  • It contains nuclei for the vestibulocochlear (CN VIII), glossopharyngeal (CN IX), vagus (CN X), and hypoglossal (XII) nerves.
— The **cerebellum,** which occupies most of the posterior cranial fossa, lies inferior to the cerebrum and is separated from it by the tentorium cerebelli.
  • It consists of paired hemispheres and a small middle section, the vermis.

Ventricular System and Cerebrospinal Fluid

The brain and spinal cord are suspended in cerebrospinal fluid (CSF). The buoyant environment created by the CSF reduces the pressure of the brain on the nerves and vessels on its inferior surface.
— CSF is produced in the **choroid plexuses,** vascular networks within four ventricles (spaces) of the brain. The first two of these ventricles are large and paired; the third and fourth are smaller and lie in the midline (**Fig. 18.12**).

• The **1st** and **2nd (lateral) ventricles,** paired cavities that occupy a large portion of each cerebral hemisphere, communicate with the 3rd ventricle through the **interventricular foramina.**
• The **3rd ventricle,** a slitlike space between the two halves of the diencephalon, communicates posteriorly with the 4th ventricle through a narrow passage, the **cerebral aqueduct,** which passes through the mesencephalon.
• The **4th ventricle,** a pyramidally shaped space that extends from the pons to the medulla oblongata, is continuous with the spinal canal inferiorly and with the subarachnoid space through the **median** and **lateral apertures** in its roof.
— CSF circulates through the ventricles and passes into the subarachnoid space and subarachnoid cisterns through the median and lateral apertures of the 4th ventricle. It flows superiorly through the fissures and sulci of the cerebrum and is reabsorbed into the venous circulation through the arachnoid granulations that protrude into the superior sagittal sinus (**Fig. 18.13**).

CLINICAL CORRELATION

HYDROCEPHALUS Hydrocephalus, an excessive accumulation of cerebrospinal fluid (CSF) in the ventricles of the brain, can occur as a result of partial obstruction of the flow of CSF within the ventricular system, interference of CSF reabsorption into the venous circulation, or, in rare cases, overproduction of CSF. Excess CSF in the ventricles causes them to dilate and exert pressure on the surrounding cortex, causing the bones of the calvaria to separate, thus creating the characteristic increase in head size. Treatment involves the placement of a shunt between the ventricles and the abdomen, which allows CSF to drain to the peritoneal cavity, where it can be easily absorbed.

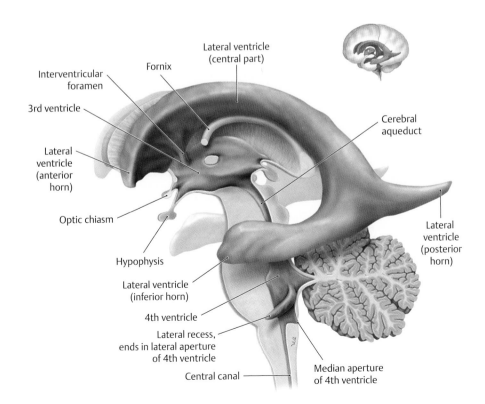

Fig. 18.12 Ventricular system in situ
Ventricular system with neighboring structures, left lateral view.

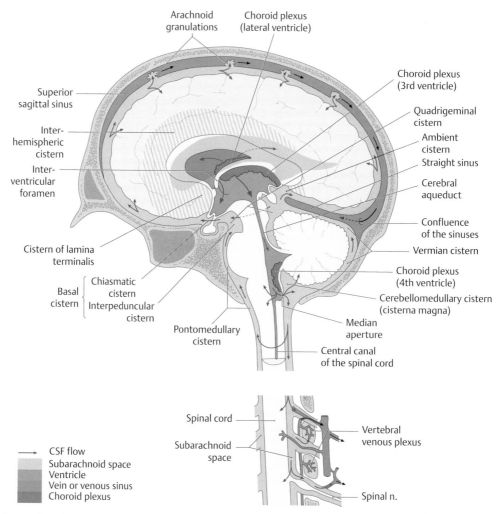

Fig. 18.13 **Circulation of cerebrospinal fluid (CSF)**

Arteries of the Brain

As a result of its high metabolic demand, the brain receives one sixth of the cardiac output and one fifth of the oxygen consumed by the body at rest. This blood supply, derived from the internal carotid and vertebral arteries, is divided into **anterior** and **posterior cerebral circulations (Fig. 18.14)**, which unite on the ventral surface of the brain to form a **cerebral arterial circle** (of Willis).

— The internal carotid artery supplies the anterior cerebral circulation.

- Its **petrous part** has a tortuous course as it enters the skull and follows the carotid canal horizontally and medially within the temporal bone. Small branches pass into the middle ear and pterygoid canal.
- The **cavernous part** crosses over the foramen lacerum and runs anteriorly within the cavernous sinus **(Fig. 18.15)**. Small branches supply the meninges, hypophysis, and cranial nerves within the cavernous sinus.
- The **cerebral part** in the middle cranial fossa gives off the ophthalmic artery (see **Fig. 20.8**) and immediately makes a U-turn to run posteriorly, where it divides into the anterior cerebral and middle cerebral arteries.

— The vertebral and basilar arteries supply the posterior cerebral circulation.

- The vertebral artery enters the skull through the foramen magnum and supplies branches to the spinal cord and cerebellum before merging with the opposite vertebral artery to form a single basilar artery.
  - Intracranial branches of the vertebral artery include the posterior inferior cerebellar artery and the anterior and posterior spinal arteries.

CLINICAL CORRELATION

STROKE A stroke is the manifestation of a neurologic deficiency resulting from a cerebral vascular impairment. Ischemic strokes are usually caused by an embolus obstructing one of the major cerebral arteries. Although the vessels of the circle of Willis can provide collateral circulation to circumvent the obstruction, anastomoses between the vessels are often incomplete or of insufficient size to provide adequate flow. Hemorrhagic strokes are usually due to rupture of an aneurysm, most often a saccular, or berry, aneurysm that bleeds into the subarachnoid space. Symptoms occur shortly after the cerebral event and relate to the area of brain affected. They may include difficulty speaking, understanding language, or walking; vision problems; contralateral paralysis or numbness; and headache.

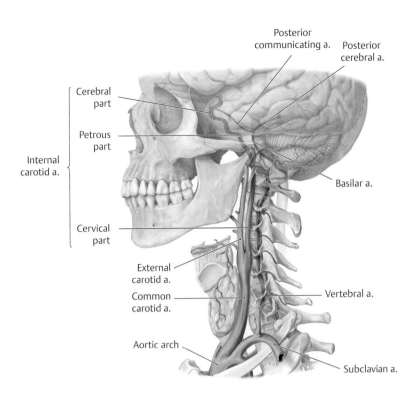

Fig. 18.14 Internal carotid artery
Left lateral view.

Posterior communicating a.
Posterior cerebral a.
Cerebral part
Petrous part
Internal carotid a.
Cervical part
Basilar a.
External carotid a.
Common carotid a.
Vertebral a.
Aortic arch
Subclavian a.

- The **basilar artery** ascends on the ventral surface of the brainstem, distributing branches to the brainstem, cerebellum, and cerebrum. It terminates as the right and left **posterior cerebral arteries.**
  ○ Major branches of the basilar artery are the **anterior inferior cerebellar artery** and the **superior cerebellar artery.**
- The cerebral arterial circle (of Willis), an important arterial anastomosis on the ventral surface of the brain, supplies the brain and connects the circulations of the internal carotid and vertebral arteries (**Figs. 18.16** and **18.17**).
  - A small **anterior communicating artery** connects the two anterior cerebral arteries, linking the right and left anterior cerebral circulations.
  - A pair of **posterior communicating arteries** connects the internal carotid and posterior cerebral arteries on each side, completing the communication between the anterior and posterior cerebral circulations.
  - The branches of the circle are
    ○ the anterior communicating arteries,
    ○ the anterior cerebral arteries,
    ○ the internal carotid arteries,
    ○ the posterior communicating arteries, and
    ○ the posterior cerebral arteries.
  - The cerebral arteries that arise from the cerebral arterial circle provide the blood supply to the cerebral hemispheres (**Table 18.2**).

Cavernous sinus
Middle cranial fossa
Carotid canal
Fibro-cartilage
Temporal bone, petrous part
Sphenoid sinus
Internal carotid artery
Foramen lacerum

Fig. 18.15 The foramen lacerum and the internal carotid artery in the carotid canal
Left lateral view. The foramen lacerum is not a true aperture, being occluded in life by a layer of fibrocartilage; it appears as an opening only in the dried skull. It is closely related to the internal carotid artery that traverses the canal.

Table 18.2 **Distribution of the Cerebral Arteries**

Artery	Origin	Distribution
Anterior cerebral	Internal carotid artery	Frontal pole and medial and superior surfaces of the cerebral hemispheres
Middle cerebral	Internal carotid artery	Most of the lateral surface of the cerebral hemispheres
Posterior cerebral	Basilar artery	Occipital pole and inferior part of temporal lobe

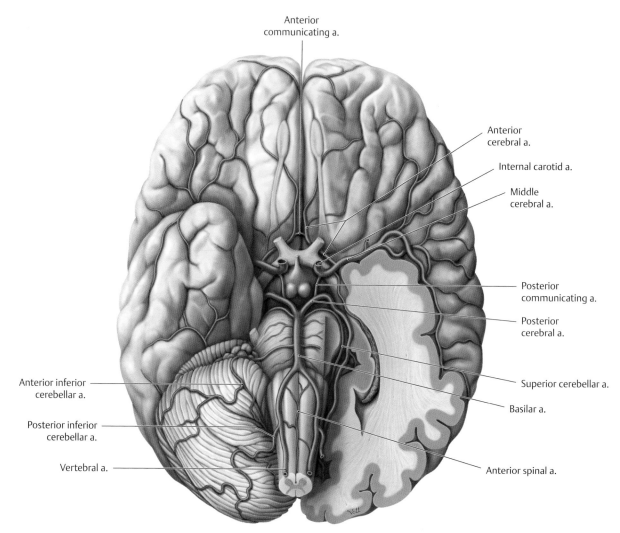

Anterior communicating a.

Anterior cerebral a.

Internal carotid a.

Middle cerebral a.

Posterior communicating a.

Posterior cerebral a.

Superior cerebellar a.

Basilar a.

Anterior spinal a.

Anterior inferior cerebellar a.

Posterior inferior cerebellar a.

Vertebral a.

Fig. 18.16 Arteries of the brain
Inferior (basal) view.

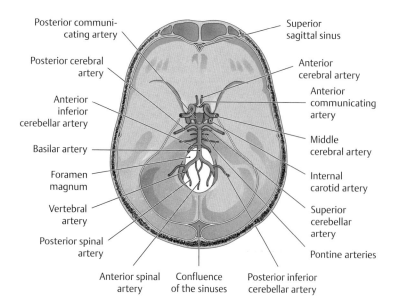

Posterior communicating artery

Posterior cerebral artery

Anterior inferior cerebellar artery

Basilar artery

Foramen magnum

Vertebral artery

Posterior spinal artery

Superior sagittal sinus

Anterior cerebral artery

Anterior communicating artery

Middle cerebral artery

Internal carotid artery

Superior cerebellar artery

Pontine arteries

Anterior spinal artery   Confluence of the sinuses   Posterior inferior cerebellar artery

Fig. 18.17 Projection of the circle of Willis onto the base of the skull
Superior view.

Veins of the Brain

Veins that drain the brain are thin-walled and valveless and usually drain into one of the dural venous sinuses (**Fig. 18.18**).

- Superficial (external) veins that drain the cerebral hemispheres include
  - the **superior cerebral veins,** which drain the supralateral and medial aspects. These "bridging veins" traverse the subdural space and drain into the superior sagittal sinus (**Fig. 18.19**);
  - the **middle cerebral veins,** which drain the lateral hemispheres and empty into the cavernous sinus and from there into the petrosal and transverse sinuses; and

- the **inferior cerebral veins,** which drain inferior aspects of the brain and join either the superior cerebral or the **basilar veins.**
- Basilar veins drain the small anterior cerebral veins and deep middle cerebral veins.
- **Internal cerebral veins** drain the 3rd and 4th ventricles and deep parts of the cerebrum. These unite to form the **great cerebral vein.**
- The great cerebral vein receives the basilar veins and merges with the inferior sagittal sinus to form the straight sinus.
- **Superior** and **inferior cerebellar veins** drain the cerebellum into adjacent dural sinuses or superficially into the great cerebral vein.

A Lateral view of the left hemisphere.

B Medial view of the right hemisphere.

Fig. 18.18 Cerebral veins

Fig. 18.19 Bridging veins

Viewed from upper left; the dura has been opened and reflected upward. Before superficial cerebral veins terminate in the dural sinus, they leave the subarachnoid space for a short distance and course between the arachnoid and meningeal layers of the dura to the superior sagittal sinus. Injury to these segments of cerebral veins, called "bridging veins," leads to subdural hemorrhage.

18.3   Cranial Nerves

The 12 cranial nerves arise from the base of the brain (**Figs. 18.20** and **18.21; Tables 18.3** and **18.4**). Like spinal nerves, cranial nerves can stimulate muscles or transmit sensation from a peripheral structure to the central nervous system. Some cranial nerves also carry fibers from the cranial portion of the parasympathetic nervous system. Seven types of nerve fibers are found (alone or in combination) in cranial nerves.

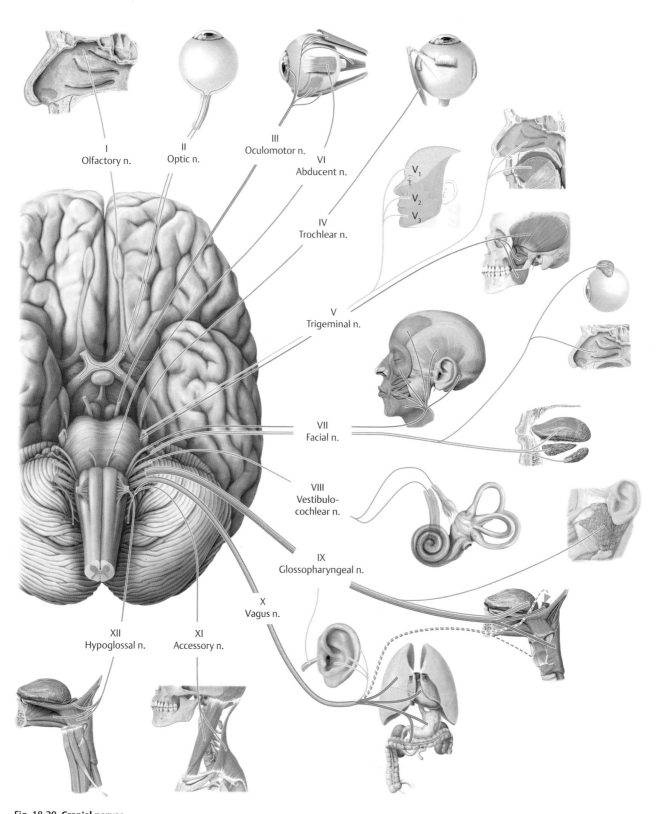

Fig. 18.20 Cranial nerves
Inferior (basal) view. The 12 pairs of cranial nerves (CN) are numbered according to their emergence from the brainstem. *(See Table 18.3 for explanation of color coding.)*

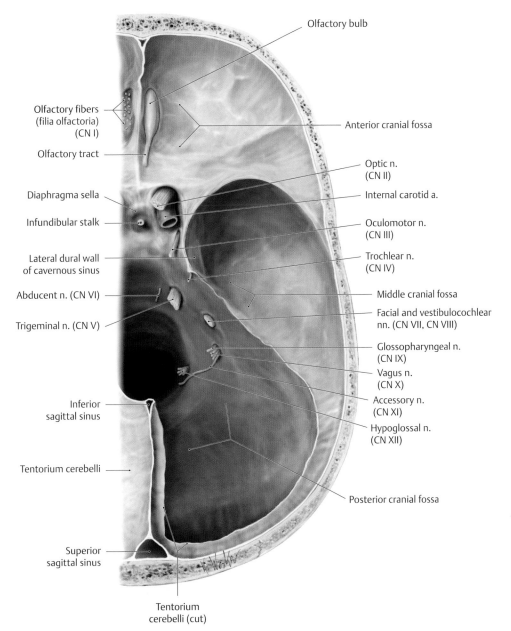

Fig. 18.21 Cranial nerves exiting the cranial cavity
Cranial cavity (superior view of interior skull base), right side. *Removed:* Brain and tentorium cerebelli. The ends of the cranial nerves have been cut to reveal the fissures, fossa, or dural cave where they pass through the cranial fossa.

Table 18.3 **Classification of Cranial Nerve Fibers**

Fiber Type	Function
General somatomotor	● Innervate voluntary muscle
General visceromotor (parasympathetic)	● Constitute the cranial component of the parasympathetic system, innervate involuntary muscles and glands
Special visceromotor (branchiomotor)	● Innervate muscles that developed from the primitive pharynx (pharyngeal arches)
General somatosensory	● Carry sensations such as touch, temperature, pain, and pressure
Special somatosensory	● Carry impulses from the eye for sight and from the ear for hearing and balance
General viscerosensory	● Transmit information from viscera such as carotid bodies, the heart, esophagus, trachea, and gastrointestinal tract
Special viscerosensory	● Transmit information regarding smell and taste

See **Fig. 18.20** for explanation of color coding.

Table 18.4 **Cranial Nerves: Function Overview**

Cranial Nerve		Passage Through Skull	Sensory Territory (Afferent)/Target Organ (Efferent)
CN I: Olfactory n.		Ethmoid bone (cribriform plate)	Smell: special viscerosensory fibers from olfactory mucosa of nasal cavity
CN II: Optic n.		Optic canal	Sight: special somatosensory fibers from retina
CN III: Oculomotor n.		Superior orbital fissure	Somatomotor innervation: to levator palpebrae superioris and four extraocular mm. (superior, medial, and inferior rectus, and inferior oblique)
			Parasympathetic innervation: preganglionic fibers to ciliary ganglion; postganglionic fibers to intraocular mm. (ciliary mm. and pupillary sphincter)
CN IV: Trochlear n.		Superior orbital fissure	Somatomotor innervation: to one extraocular m. (superior oblique)
CN V: Trigeminal n.	CN V$_1$	Superior orbital fissure	General somatic sensation: from orbit, nasal cavity, paranasal sinuses, and face
	CN V$_2$	Foramen rotundum	General somatic sensation: from nasal cavity, paranasal sinuses, superior nasopharynx, upper oral cavity, internal skull, and face
	CN V$_3$	Foramen ovale	General somatic sensation: from lower oral cavity, ear, internal skull, and face
			Branchiomotor innervation: to the eight mm. derived from the 1st pharyngeal (branchial) arch (including mm. of mastication)
CN VI: Abducent n.		Superior orbital fissure	Somatomotor innervation: to one extraocular m. (lateral rectus)
CN VII: Facial n.		Internal acoustic meatus	General somatic sensation: from external ear
			Taste: special viscerosensory fibers from tongue (anterior two thirds) and soft palate
			Parasympathetic innervation: preganglionic fibers to submandibular and pterygopalatine ganglia; postganglionic fibers to glands (e.g., lacrimal, submandibular, sublingual, palatine) and mucosa of nasal cavity, palate, and paranasal sinuses
			Branchiomotor innervation: to mm. derived from the 2nd pharyngeal arch (including mm. of facial expression, stylohyoid, and stapedius)
CN VIII: Vestibulocochlear n.		Internal acoustic meatus	Hearing and balance: special somatosensory fibers from cochlea (hearing) and vestibular apparatus (balance)
CN IX: Glossopharyngeal n.		Jugular foramen	General somatic sensation: from oral cavity, pharynx, tongue (posterior third), and middle ear
			Taste: special visceral sensation from tongue (posterior third)
			General visceral sensation: from carotid body and sinus
			Parasympathetic innervation: preganglionic fibers to otic ganglion; postganglionic fibers to parotid gland and inferior labial glands
			Branchiomotor innervation: to the one m. derived from the 3rd pharyngeal arch (stylopharyngeus)
CN X: Vagus n.		Jugular foramen	General somatic sensation: from ear and internal skull
			Taste: special visceral sensation from epiglottis and root of tongue
			General visceral sensation: from aortic body, laryngopharynx and larynx, respiratory tract, and thoracoabdominal viscera
			Parasympathetic innervation: preganglionic fibers to small, unnamed ganglia near target organs or embedded in smooth muscle walls; postganglionic fibers to glands, mucosa, and smooth muscle of pharynx, larynx, and thoracic and abdominal viscera
			Branchiomotor innervation: to pharyngeal and laryngeal mm. derived from the 4th and 6th pharyngeal arches; also distributes branchiomotor fibers from CN XI
CN XI: Accessory n.		Jugular foramen	Somatomotor innervation: to trapezius and sternocleidomastoid
			Branchiomotor innervation: to laryngeal mm. (except cricothyroid) via pharyngeal plexus and CN X (*Note:* The branchiomotor fibers from the cranial root of CN XI are distributed by CN X [vagus n.].)
CN XII: Hypoglossal n.		Hypoglossal canal	Somatomotor innervation: to all intrinsic and extrinsic lingual mm. (except palatoglossus)

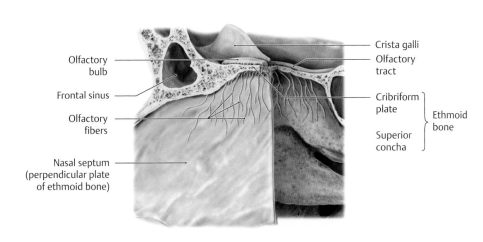

Fig. 18.22 Olfactory nerve (CN I)
Olfactory fibers, bulb, and tract. Portion of left nasal septum and lateral wall of right nasal cavity, left lateral view.

CN I, the **olfactory nerve,** carries special sensory fibers that transmit sensation of smell from the superior aspect of the lateral and septal walls of the nasal cavity (**Fig. 18.22**).
— Olfactory neurons pass through the cribriform plate of the ethmoid bone and synapse with secondary neurons in the **olfactory bulbs.**
  • The axons of these secondary neurons form the **olfactory tracts.**
  • The olfactory bulbs and tracts are extensions of the cerebral cortex.

CN II, the **optic nerve,** is a collection of special sensory nerve fibers that originate on the **retina** of the eye and converge at the **optic disk** at the back of the eyeball (**Fig. 18.23;** see also Section 20.1).
— The nerve exits the orbit through the optic canal and joins the contralateral optic nerve to form the **optic chiasm.**
— The optic chiasm is a redistribution center where nerve fibers from the medial half of each optic nerve cross to the opposite side.
— Two **optic tracts** diverge from the chiasm. Each tract contains nerve fibers from the medial half of one eye and the lateral half of the other eye.

CN III, the **oculomotor nerve; CN IV,** the **trochlear nerve;** and **CN VI,** the **abducent nerve** innervate structures of the orbit (**Fig. 18.24;** see also Section 20.1). They pass through the cavernous sinus before entering the orbit through the superior orbital fissure.
— The oculomotor nerve has somatic and visceral components.
  • General somatic motor fibers innervate four of the extraocular muscles (superior rectus, medial rectus, inferior rectus, and inferior oblique), which move the eyeball, and the levator palpebrae superioris muscle, which elevates the eyelid.
  • General visceral motor fibers carry preganglionic parasympathetic fibers that synapse in the **ciliary ganglion** and innervate the **pupillary sphincter muscle** (which constricts the pupil) and **ciliary body** (which changes the curvature of the lens of the eye) (see **Fig. 20.6**).
— The trochlear nerve carries general somatic motor fibers and innervates the superior oblique muscle, which depresses and medially rotates the eye.
— The abducent nerve carries general somatic motor fibers and innervates the lateral rectus muscle, which abducts the eye.

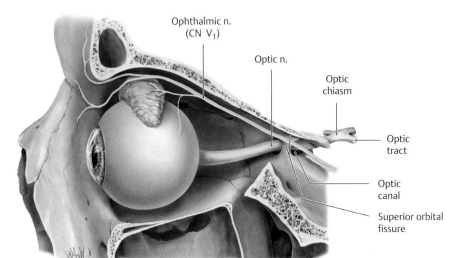

Fig. 18.23 Optic nerve (CN II)
Optic nerve in the left orbit, left lateral view.

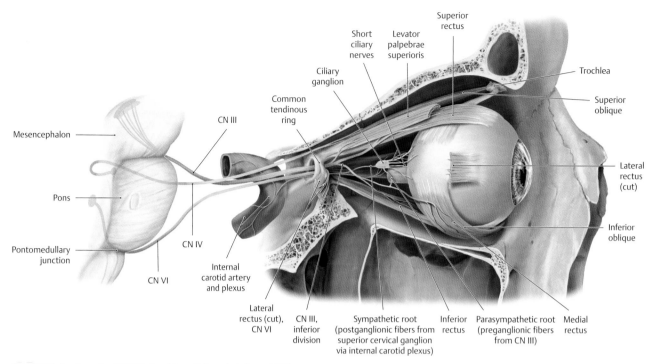

Fig. 18.24 Oculomotor (CN III), trochlear (IV), and abducent (VI) nerves
Course of the nerves innervating the extraocular muscles, right orbit, lateral view.

CN V, the **trigeminal nerve,** is the primary sensory nerve of the face (**Figs. 18.25** and **18.26**). Its small motor component innervates the muscles of mastication (chewing).

– The general somatic sensory neurons, which form the sensory root, synapse in the trigeminal ganglion located in a dural space on the petrous part of the temporal bone.
– A small motor root in the mandibular division (CN V$_3$) contains branchial motor fibers.
– Branches of the trigeminal nerve are associated with the parasympathetic ganglia of the head and distribute postganglionic parasympathetic fibers to their target organs.

– The trigeminal nerve has three divisions:
   1. The **ophthalmic division (CN V$_1$)** (see Section 20.1)
      ○ contains only somatic sensory fibers;
      ○ passes through the cavernous sinus and superior orbital fissure into the orbit;
      ○ is associated with the **ciliary ganglion** (see Section 18.4);
      ○ distributes visceral motor fibers from the facial nerve (CN VII) to the lacrimal gland via the lacrimal nerve;
      ○ innervates the orbit, the cornea, and the skin on the top of the nose, forehead, and scalp;
      ○ functions as the sensory component of the corneal reflex via the **nasociliary branch;** and
      ○ has **lacrimal, frontal,** and **nasociliary** branches.

Fig. 18.25 Divisions of the trigeminal nerve
Right lateral view.

CLINICAL CORRELATION

TRIGEMINAL NEURALGIA Trigeminal neuralgia, a pathology of the sensory root of the trigeminal nerve (CN V), most commonly affects the maxillary division (CN V$_2$) and least frequently affects the ophthalmic division (CN V$_1$). The disorder is characterized by unilateral electric shock-like pain in the area supplied by the nerve. It usually lasts several seconds to several minutes. As the condition progresses, the pain may last longer, and there may be a shorter period between attacks. The pain may be initiated by touching a trigger point in the face by eating, talking, brushing teeth, or shaving. It is believed that trigeminal neuralgia is caused by the loss of myelin on the sensory root due to the pressure from an abnormal blood vessel. Surgery to destroy the nerve root or ganglion may be effective but may lead to permanent facial numbness.

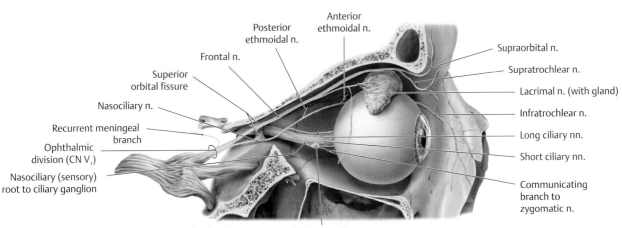

A Ophthalmic division (CN V1), partially opened right orbit.

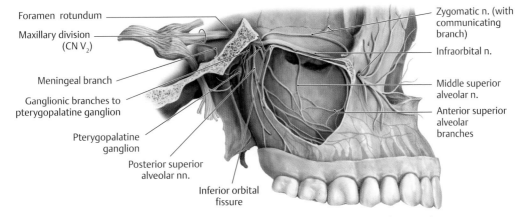

B Maxillary division (CN V2), partially opened right maxillary sinus with the zygomatic arch removed.

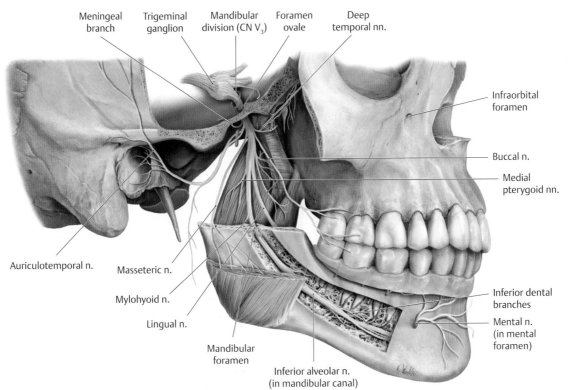

C Mandibular division (CN V3), partially opened mandible with the zygomatic arch removed. *Note*: The mylohyoid nerve branches from the inferior alveolar nerve just before the mandibular foramen.

Fig. 18.26 Trigeminal nerve (CN V)
Course of the trigeminal nerve divisions.

2. The **maxillary division (CN V₂)** (see Section 19.6)
    ○ contains only somatic sensory fibers;
    ○ travels through the cavernous sinus and the foramen rotundum to enter the **pterygopalatine fossa;**
    ○ is associated with the **pterygopalatine ganglion** (see Section 18.4);
    ○ distributes visceral motor fibers to the palatal and nasal glands via the nasopalatine and greater and lesser palatine nerves;
    ○ distributes visceral motor fibers to the lacrimal gland via the zygomatic branch which joins the lacrimal nerve of CN V₁;
    ○ innervates the skin of the midface (from the lower eyelid to the upper lip) and structures associated with the maxilla, such as the maxillary sinus, hard palate, nasal cavity, and maxillary teeth; and
    ○ has **infraorbital, zygomatic, greater** and **lesser palatine, superior alveolar,** and **nasopalatine** branches (see also **Fig. 19.25**).
3. The **mandibular division (CN V₃)** (see Sections 19.4 and 19.5)
    ○ contains somatic sensory and branchial motor fibers;
    ○ passes through the foramen ovale into the **infra-temporal fossa;**

○ is associated with the **otic** and **submandibular ganglia** (see Section 18.4);
○ distributes visceral motor fibers of the facial nerve (CN VII) to the submandibular and sublingual glands via the lingual nerve;
○ distributes visceral motor fibers of the glossopharyngeal nerve (CN IX) to the parotid gland via the auriculotemporal nerve;
○ has a sensory component that innervates skin over the lower jaw and lateral face and structures associated with the mandible, such as the lower teeth, **temporomandibular joint,** floor of the mouth, and anterior tongue;
○ has a motor component that innervates the **digastric** (anterior belly), **mylohyoid, tensor veli palatini,** and **tensor tympani muscles** and the **muscles of mastication** (see Sections 19.2 and 19.8); and
○ has **meningeal, buccal, auriculotemporal, lingual, inferior alveolar,** and **muscular branches** (to muscles noted above).

CN VII, the **facial nerve,** is the primary motor nerve of the face but also has sensory and visceral components (**Figs. 18.27, 18.28, 18.29**). It contains a motor root that innervates the muscles of facial

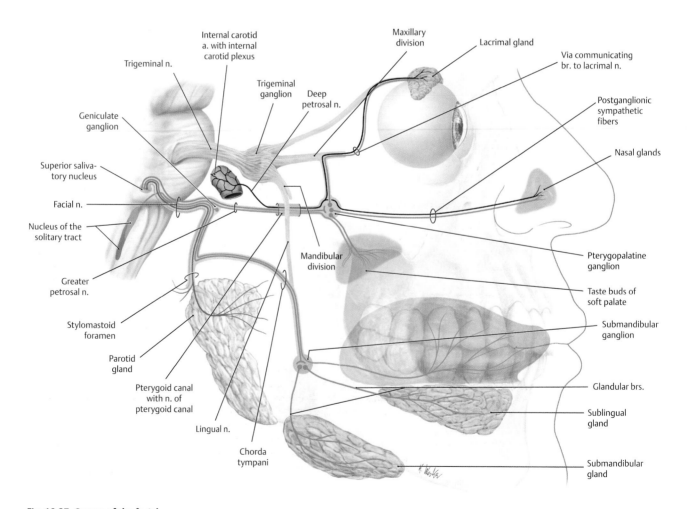

Fig. 18.27 Course of the facial nerve
Visceral motor (parasympathetic) and special visceral sensory (taste) fibers shown in black, right lateral view.

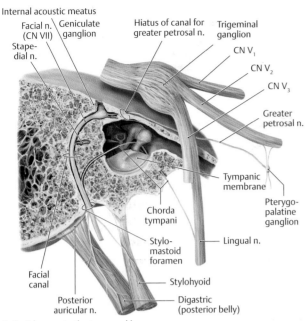

A Facial nerve in the temporal bone.

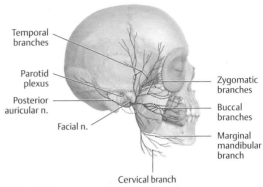

B Parotid plexus.

Fig. 18.28 Facial nerve (CN VII)
Branches of the facial nerve, right lateral view.

expression, and an intermediate nerve that carries special sensory (for taste) and visceral motor fibers (parasympathetic) and somatic sensory fibers. Both the motor root and the intermediate nerve pass through the internal acoustic meatus into the **facial canal** of the temporal bone, where three branches arise: the greater petrosal nerve, stapedial nerve, and chorda tympani.

— The motor root
  • exits the skull through the stylomastoid foramen and
  • contains branchial motor fibers, which
    ○ innervate the **stylohyoid, stapedius,** and **digastric (posterior belly) muscles** (see **Table 19.7, Figs. 19.29** and **20.17,** and Section 19.2) and
    ○ form the **parotid plexus within the parotid gland,** which innervates the **muscles of facial expression** (see Section 19.1). Branches of the parotid plexus include the posterior auricular, **temporal, zygomatic, buccal, marginal mandibular,** and **cervical branches.**
— The intermediate nerve (**nervus intermedius**) contains the following:
  • The **greater petrosal nerve** (parasympathetic), which passes through the middle cranial fossa and combines with the **deep petrosal nerve** (sympathetic) to form the **nerve of the pterygoid canal** (see Section 19.6). The visceral motor (parasympathetic) fibers synapse in the pterygopalatine ganglion and are distributed to glands of the nasal mucosa and palate and to the lacrimal gland.

• The **chorda tympani,** which passes through the middle ear cavity, exits through the petrotympanic fissure to the infratemporal fossa and travels with the lingual nerve of CN V$_3$. It carries
  ○ visceral motor fibers that synapse in the submandibular ganglion and supply the submandibular and sublingual salivary glands, and
  ○ special sensory fibers for taste from the anterior part of the tongue and palate.
• General somatic sensory fibers, which transmit sensations from the external ear to the **geniculate ganglion,** the sensory ganglion of the facial nerve, located in the temporal bone.

CLINICAL CORRELATION

BELL'S PALSY Bell's palsy is paralysis of the facial muscles due to a lesion of the facial nerve (CN VII). Symptoms usually begin suddenly and affect one side of the face only. They include drooping of the corner of the mouth, eyebrow, and lower eyelid, and the inability to smile, whistle, blow out cheeks, wrinkle the forehead, blink, or close the eyes forcefully. Taste is impaired on the anterior two thirds of the tongue (due to involvement of the chorda tympani), decreased tear production leads to dry eyes (due to involvement of the greater petrosal nerve), sensitivity to sounds is increased (due to paralysis of the stapedius), and the lower jaw and tongue deviate to the opposite side (due to paralysis of the posterior belly of the digastric muscle).

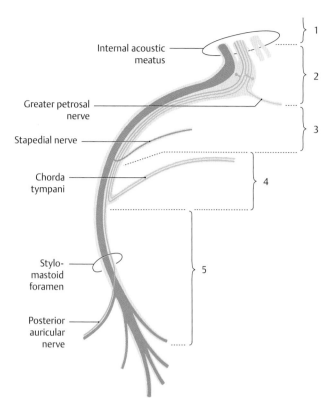

Internal acoustic meatus

Greater petrosal nerve

Stapedial nerve

Chorda tympani

Stylo-mastoid foramen

Posterior auricular nerve

Fig. 18.29 Branching pattern of the facial nerve: diagnostic significance in temporal bone fractures

The principal signs and symptoms are different depending upon the exact site of the lesion in the course of the facial nerve through the petrous bone.

Note: Only the principal signs and symptoms associated with a particular lesion site are described here. The more peripheral the site of the nerve injury, the less diverse the signs and symptoms become.

1 A lesion at this level affects the facial nerve in addition to the vestibulochochlear nerve. As a result, peripheral motor facial paralysis is accompanied by hearing loss (deafness) and vestibular dysfunction (dizziness).

2 Peripheral motor facial paralysis is accompanied by disturbances of taste sensation (chorda tympani), lacrimation, and salivation.

3 Motor paralysis is accompanied by disturbances of salivation and taste. Hyperacusis due to paralysis of the stapedius muscle has little clinical importance.

4 Peripheral motor paralysis is accompanied by disturbances of taste and salivation.

5 Peripheral motor (facial) paralysis is the only manifestation of a lesion at this level.

CN VIII, the **vestibulocochlear nerve,** is the sensory nerve of hearing and balance. The nerve enters the temporal bone with the facial nerve through the internal acoustic meatus.

— The two branches of the vestibulocochlear nerve carry special sensory fibers (**Fig. 18.30;** see Section 20.2):
  • The **cochlear root** supplies the **cochlea** and its **spiral organ,** the organ of hearing.
  • The **vestibular root,** which contains the **vestibular ganglia,** supplies the **utricle, saccule,** and **semicircular ducts,** the organs of balance.

CN IX, the **glossopharyngeal nerve,** leaves the skull through the jugular foramen and contains special sensory (taste), visceral sensory, somatic motor, and visceral motor components (**Figs. 18.31** and **18.32; Table 18.5**).

— Somatic motor fibers innervate the **stylopharyngeus muscle.**
— Visceral motor fibers arise with the **tympanic nerve,** a branch of the glossopharyngeal nerve. Carrying sensory and visceral motor fibers, it runs through the **tympanic cavity** of the **middle ear** (see Section 20.2), where it contributes to the **tympanic plexus.** It gives rise to the lesser petrosal nerve.

PETROSAL NERVES OF THE HEAD Three petrosal nerves are associated with autonomic innervation of the head. Two nerves carry preganglionic parasympathetic nerves:

— The greater petrosal nerve, a branch of CN VII, forms the parasympathetic part of the nerve of the pterygoid canal, which synapses in the pterygopalatine ganglion. Postganglionic fibers travel via the zygomatic n. (CN V$_2$) to the lacrimal n. (CN V$_1$) in the orbit where they innervate the lacrimal gland. They also innervate glands in the nasal cavity via branches of the maxillary nerve (CN V$_2$).

— The lesser petrosal nerve, a branch of CN IX, arises from the tympanic plexus in the middle ear and synapses in the otic ganglion. Postganglionic fibers travel briefly with the auriculotemporal n. (CN V$_3$) before innervating the parotid gland.

One nerve carries postganglionic sympathetic fibers:

— The deep petrosal nerve arises from the internal carotid plexus and forms the sympathetic component of the nerve of the pterygoid canal. These fibers pass through the pterygopalatine fossa without synapsing in the ganglion, and are distributed to the lacrimal gland and nasal glands along the same routes as the greater petrosal nerve.

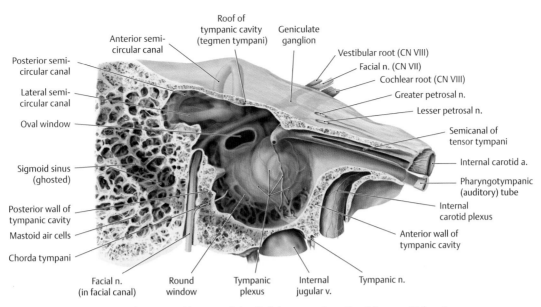

A Vestibulocochlear nerve in the temporal bone, medial wall of the tympanic cavity, oblique sagittal section.

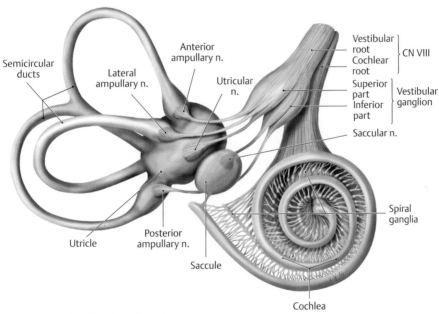

B Vestibular and cochlear (spiral) ganglia.

Fig. 18.30 Vestibulocochlear nerve (CN VIII)

- The **lesser petrosal nerve** passes through the middle cranial fossa and foramen ovale carrying visceral motor fibers that synapse in the otic ganglion. Postganglionic fibers travel with the auriculotemporal nerve (CN V$_3$) to innervate the parotid gland.
- Sensory fibers of the tympanic plexus supply the tympanic cavity and **pharyngotympanic** (auditory) **tube.**

- Special sensory fibers transmit taste from the posterior third of the tongue.
- Visceral sensory fibers transmit information from the **tonsils, soft palate,** posterior third of the tongue, **pharynx,** and, via the **branch to the carotid sinus,** from receptors in the carotid body and carotid sinus at the bifurcation of the common carotid artery.

Table 18.5 **Glossopharyngeal Nerve Branches**

①	Tympanic n.
②	Br. to carotid sinus
③	Br. to stylopharyngeus muscle
④	Tonsillar brs.
⑤	Lingual brs.
⑥	Pharyngeal brs.

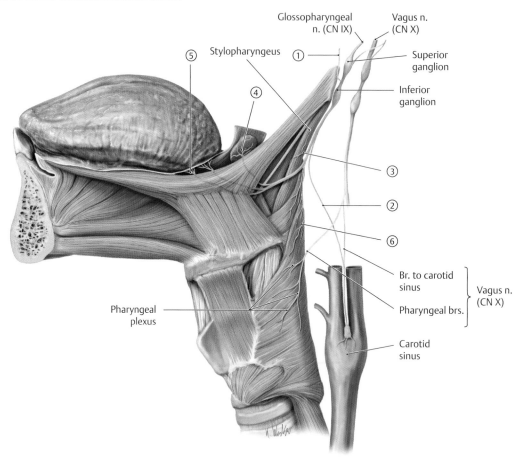

Fig. 18.31 Glossopharyngeal nerve (CN IX)
Course of the glossopharyngeal nerve, left lateral view. The numbers are explained in Table 18.5.

CN X, the **vagus nerve,** has the most extensive distribution of the cranial nerves **(Fig. 18.33; Table 18.6)**.
— Branchial motor fibers innervate the muscles of the soft palate (except tensor veli palatini), pharynx (except stylopharyngeus), and larynx, and the palatoglossus muscle of the tongue.
— Visceral motor fibers innervate smooth muscle and glands of the pharynx, larynx, thoracic organs, and abdominal foregut and midgut.

— General somatic sensory fibers transmit sensation from the dura in the posterior cranial fossa, the skin of the external ear, and the external auditory canal.
— Visceral sensory fibers transmit sensation from mucosa of the lower pharynx, the larynx, lungs and airway, the heart, the abdominal foregut and midgut, and the chemoreceptors of the aortic body and baroreceptors of the aortic arch.
— Special sensory fibers carry taste from the epiglottis.

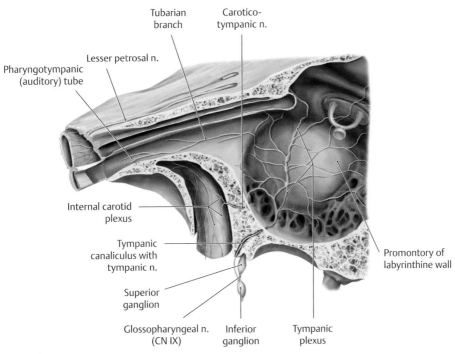

A Glossopharyngeal nerve in the tympanic cavity, left anterolateral view.

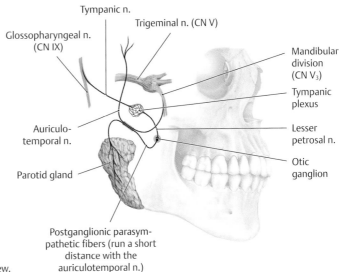

B Visceral motor fibers of the glossopharyngeal nerve, right lateral view.

Fig. 18.32 Branches of the glossopharyngeal nerve

— The vagus nerve has cervical, thoracic, and abdominal segments.
- In the neck
  - each vagus nerve leaves the skull through the jugular foramen and descends within the carotid sheath of the neck, and
  - its branches are **pharyngeal branches, the superior laryngeal nerve, cervical cardiac** (parasympathetic) **branches,** and the **right recurrent laryngeal nerve** (which arises from the right vagus and recurs around the right subclavian artery).
- In the thorax
  - the right and left vagus nerves enter the thorax posterior to the sternoclavicular joints and merge on the surface of the esophagus as the esophageal plexus (see Section 3.2), and
  - their branches are the left recurrent laryngeal nerve (which arises from the left vagus and recurs around the arch of the aorta) and the thoracic cardiac and pulmonary branches (parasympathetic).
- In the abdomen
  - right and left vagal trunks arise from the esophageal plexus and pass through the esophageal hiatus of the

Vagus n.
(CN X)

① Pharyngeal brs.

② Superior laryngeal n.

Internal br.
(internal laryngeal n.)

External br.
(external laryngeal n.)

Cricothyroid

Right inferior
laryngeal n.

Left inferior
laryngeal n.

Subclavian a.

③R

Brachio-
cephalic
trunk

③L

④

Table 18.6 **Vagus Nerve Branches in the Neck**	
①	Pharyngeal brs.
②	Superior laryngeal n.
③R	Right recurrent laryngeal n.
③L	Left recurrent laryngeal n.
④	Cervical cardiac brs.

Vagus n.
(CN X)

①

②

Internal br. (sensory)

Cricothyroid

External br. (motor)

A Branches of the vagus nerve in the neck. Anterior view. The numbers are explained in Table 18.6.

B Innervation of the pharyngeal and laryngeal muscles. Left lateral view.

Fig. 18.33 Vagus nerve (CN X)

diaphragm as the anterior and posterior vagal trunks; and

  ○ their parasympathetic branches are distributed to organs of the foregut, midgut, and retroperitoneum.

CN XI, the **accessory nerve**, contains general somatic motor fibers, which originate in a nucleus of the upper segments of the spinal cord (**Fig. 18.34**).

— The nerve emerges with the upper five or six cervical spinal nerves and ascends within the vertebral canal. It enters the skull through the foramen magnum and exits through the jugular foramen with the vagus and glossopharyngeal nerves.

— It innervates the sternocleidomastoid muscle in the neck and then crosses the lateral region of the neck to innervate the trapezius muscle.

CN XII, the **hypoglossal nerve**, contains only general somatic motor fibers (**Fig. 18.35**).

— The hypoglossal nerve leaves the skull through the hypoglossal canal and runs forward, medial to the angle of the mandible, to enter the oral cavity.

— It innervates all of the muscles of the tongue except the palatoglossus.

CLINICAL CORRELATION

INJURY TO THE HYPOGLOSSAL NERVE Injury to the hypoglossal nerve causes ipsilateral paralysis of half of the tongue. When the tongue is protruded, the tip deviates toward the paralyzed side because the action of the genioglossus muscle on the unaffected side is unopposed (**Fig. 18.36**). Symptoms mainly manifest as slurring of speech. Over time, the tongue becomes weak and atrophies.

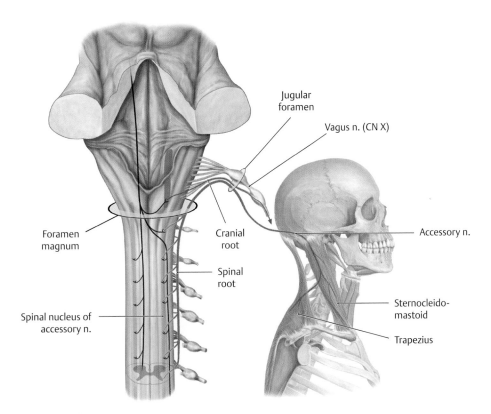

Fig. 18.34 Accessory nerve (CN XI)
Brainstem with the cerebellum removed, posterior view.

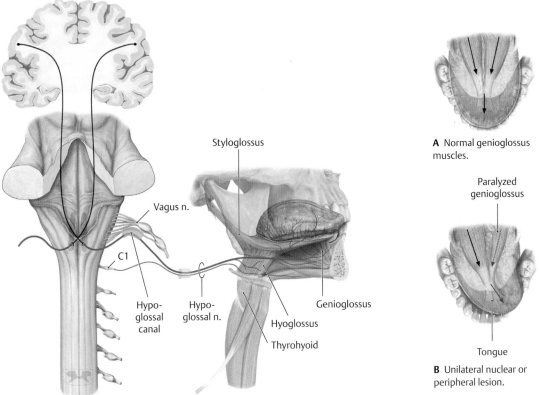

Fig. 18.35 Hypoglossal nerve (CN XII)
Brainstem with the cerebellum removed, posterior view. *Note*: C1, which innervates the thyrohyoid and geniohyoid, runs briefly with the hypoglossal nerve.

A Normal genioglossus muscles.

B Unilateral nuclear or peripheral lesion.

Fig. 18.36 Hypoglossal nerve lesions

18.4 Autonomic Nerves of the Head

— Sympathetic nerves of the head arise as postganglionic fibers from the superior cervical ganglia (**Fig. 18.37; Table 18.7;** see Section 21.3).
   • The **internal carotid plexus** of sympathetic fibers surrounds the internal carotid artery and its branches within the skull. A similar **external carotid plexus** follows the branches of the external carotid artery on the face.
   • Sympathetic fibers often travel with the parasympathetic nerves, but they do not synapse in the parasympathetic ganglia.
— The cranial portion of the parasympathetic (visceral motor) system is associated with the oculomotor (CN III), facial

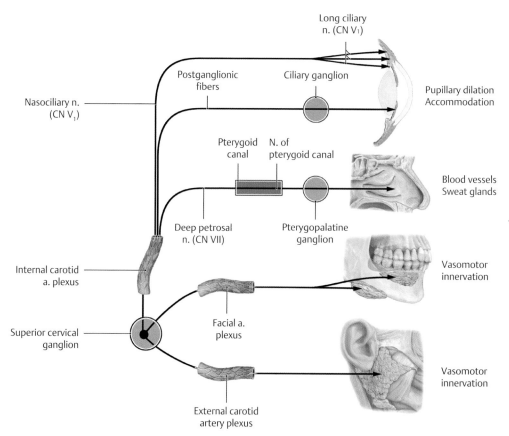

Fig. 18.37 Sympathetic innervation of the head
Sympathetic preganglionic fibers of the head originate in the lateral horn of the spinal cord (T1–L2). They exit into the sympathetic trunk and ascend to synapse in the superior cervical ganglion. Postganglionic fibers then travel with arterial plexuses (internal carotid a., facial a., and external carotid a.). Although these fibers often travel with parasympathetic fibers through the parasympathetic ganglia, they do not synapse in these ganglia. Similar to parasympathetic fibers, sympathetic nerves may "piggyback" on branches of the trigeminal nerve (CN V) to reach their target organ.

Table 18.7 **Sympathetic Fibers in the Head**

Nucleus	Path of Presynaptic Fibers	Ganglion	Postsynaptic Fibers	Target Organs
Lateral horn of spinal cord (T1–L2)	Enter sympathetic trunk and ascend to superior cervical ganglion	Superior cervical ganglion	ICA plexus → nasociliary nn. (CN V_1) → long ciliary nn. (CN V_1)	Dilator pupillae muscle (mydriasis)
			Postganglionic fibers → ciliary ganglion* → short ciliary nn.	Ciliary muscle (accommodation)
			ICA plexus → deep petrosal n. → n. of pterygoid canal → pterygopalatine ganglion* → branches of maxillary n. (CN V_2)	Glands of nasal cavity Sweat glands Blood vessels
			Facial a. plexus → submandibular ganglion*	Submandibular gland Sublingual gland
			External carotid a. plexus	Parotid gland

*Passes through without synapsing.
→, is continuous with.
ICA, internal carotid a.

(CN VII), glossopharyngeal (CN IX), and vagus (CN X) nerves **(Fig. 18.38; Table 18.8)**.

- Preganglionic parasympathetic fibers traveling with the oculomotor (CN III), facial (CN VII), and glossopharyngeal (CN IX) nerves synapse in the four parasympathetic ganglia of the head: the ciliary, pterygopalatine, submandibular, and otic ganglia.
- Parasympathetic nerves traveling with the vagus nerve (CN X) extend into the thorax and abdomen and synapse in ganglia of nerve plexuses in those regions.
- Parasympathetic ganglia of the head are usually attached to, or in close association with, a branch of the trigeminal nerve (CN V). The postganglionic parasympathetic fibers travel to their target organ by "piggybacking" on these trigeminal branches.

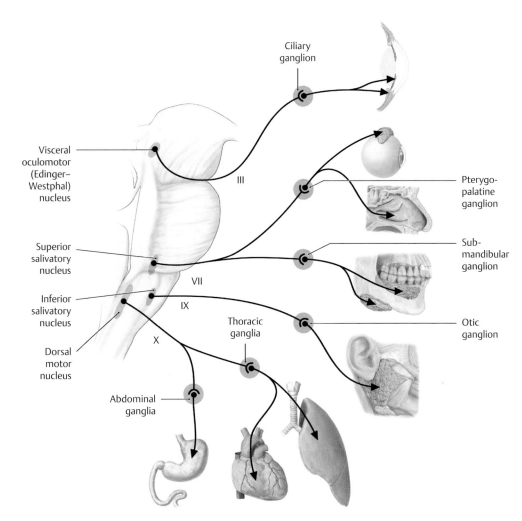

Fig. 18.38 Parasympathetic nervous system (cranial part): Overview
There are four parasympathetic nuclei in the brainstem. The visceral motor fibers of these nuclei travel along specific cranial nerves as shown. The postganglionic fibers often travel with branches of the trigeminal nerve (CN V) to reach their target organs.

Table 18.8 **Parasympathetic Ganglia in the Head**

Nucleus	Path of Presynaptic Fibers	Ganglion	Postsynaptic Fibers	Target Organs
Edinger-Westphal nucleus	Oculomotor n. (CN III)	Ciliary ganglion	Short ciliary nn. (CN V$_1$)	Ciliary muscle (accommodation) Pupillary sphincter (miosis)
Superior salivary nucleus	Nervus intermedius (CN VII root) → greater petrosal n. → n. of pterygoid canal	Pterygopalatine ganglion	• Maxillary n. (CN V$_2$) → zygomatic n. → anastomosis → lacrimal n. (CN V$_1$) • Orbital branches • Posterior superior nasal brs. • Nasopalatine nn. • Greater and lesser palatine nn.	• Lacrimal gland • Glands of nasal cavity and paranasal sinuses • Glands of gingiva • Glands of hard and soft palate • Glands of pharynx
	Nervus intermedius (CN VII root) → chorda tympani → lingual n. (CN V$_3$)	Submandibular ganglion	Glandular branches	Submandibular gland Sublingual gland
Inferior salivatory nucleus	Glossopharyngeal n. (CN IX) → tympanic n. → lesser petrosal n.	Otic ganglion	Auriculotemporal n. (CN V$_3$)	Parotid gland
Dorsal motor (vagal) nucleus	Vagus n. (X)	Ganglia near organs	Fine fibers in organs, not individually named	Thoracic and abdominal viscera

→, is continuous with.

19 Anterior, Lateral, and Deep Regions of the Head

The anatomy of the head can be divided into smaller regions that lie anterior and lateral to the neurocranium and form the superficial and deep structures of the face. They include the scalp; the parotid region; the temporal, infratemporal, and pterygopalatine fossae; and the nasal and oral cavities.

19.1 The Scalp and Face

The **scalp** covers the neurocranium and extends from the superior nuchal lines of the occipital bone, which mark the superior limit of the neck, to the supraorbital ridge of the frontal bone. The face extends from the forehead to the chin and to the ears on either side.

— The scalp is composed of five layers (**Fig. 19.1**):
  • Skin
  • Connective tissue containing the vessels of the scalp
  • Aponeurosis of the **occipitofrontalis, temporoparietalis,** and **superior auricular** muscles (gala aponeurotica)
  • Loose areolar tissue
  • Periosteum of the skull (pericranium)

Note that the first letter of each layer spells **"SCALP"**—a handy mnemonic.

— Muscles of facial expression lie in the loose connective tissue layer of the face and scalp. Their origin on bones of the face and insertion into the overlying skin allows them to create facial movements (**Fig. 19.2; Tables 19.1** and **19.2**).
— Most arteries that supply the face and scalp are branches of the external carotid artery (see **Fig. 17.23**) and include the following:
  • The superior and inferior labial arteries, the lateral nasal artery, and the angular branches of the facial artery, which supply the face between the eye and lower lip
  • The mental branch of the inferior alveolar artery, which supplies the chin
  • The superficial temporal, posterior auricular, and occipital arteries, which supply the lateral and posterior parts of the scalp
  • The supratrochlear and supraorbital branches of the ophthalmic artery (a branch of the internal carotid artery), which supply the anterior scalp. These arteries anastomose

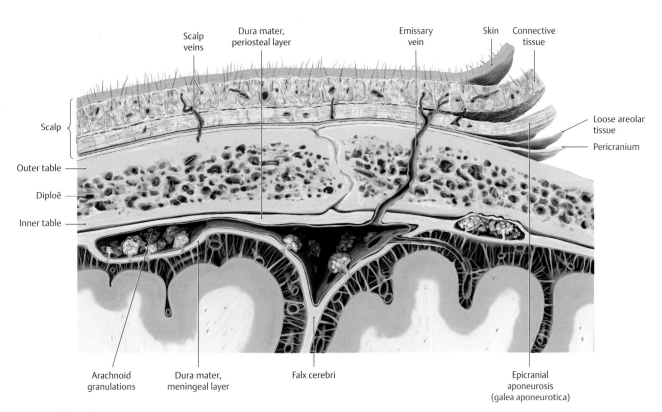

Fig. 19.1 **The scalp**

with the angular artery on the face and form a connection between internal carotid and external carotid circulations (see **Fig. 17.28**).

— Superficial veins of the head drain the face and scalp. Most of these veins follow the arteries of similar name and territory but drain to the facial and retromandibular veins, which terminate in the internal and external jugular veins.

— Veins of the scalp have deep connections to
  - **diploic veins,** which run within the diploë layer of the skull, and
  - **emissary veins,** which drain through the skull from the dural venous sinuses.

A Anterior view. Muscle origins (0) and insertion (I) indicated on left side of face.

Fig. 19.2 Muscles of facial expression

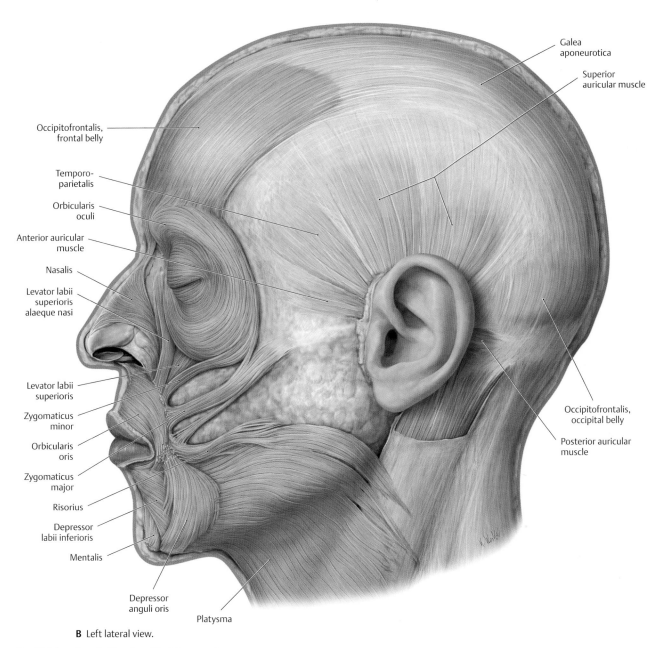

B Left lateral view.

Fig. 19.2 (*continued*) **Muscles of facial expression**

Table 19.1 **Muscles of Facial Expression: Forehead, Nose, and Ear**

Muscle	Origin	Insertion*	Main Action(s)**
Calvaria			
Occipitofrontalis (frontal belly)	Epicranial aponeurosis	Skin and subcutaneous tissue of eyebrows and forehead	Elevates eyebrows, wrinkles skin of forehead
Palpebral fissure and nose			
Procerus	Nasal bone, lateral nasal cartilage (upper part)	Skin of lower forehead between eyebrows	Pulls medial angle of eyebrows inferiorly, producing transverse wrinkles over bridge of nose
Orbicularis oculi	Medial orbital margin, medial palpebral ligament; lacrimal bone	Skin around margin of orbit, superior and inferior tarsal plates	Acts as orbital sphincter (closes eyelids) • Palpebral portion gently closes • Orbital portion tightly closes (as in winking)
Nasalis	Maxilla (superior region of canine ridge)	Nasal cartilages	Flares nostrils by drawing ala (side) of nose toward nasal septum

(continued on page 450)

Table 19.1 (*continued*) **Muscles of Facial Expression: Forehead, Nose, and Ear**

Muscle	Origin	Insertion*	Main Action(s)**
Levator labii superioris alaeque nasi	Maxilla (frontal process)	Alar cartilage of nose and upper lip	Elevates upper lip, opens nostril
Ear			
Anterior auricular muscles	Temporal fascia (anterior portion)	Helix of the ear	Pull ear superiorly and anteriorly
Superior auricular muscles	Epicranial aponeurosis on side of head	Upper portion of auricle	Elevate ear
Posterior auricular muscles	Mastoid process	Convexity of concha of ear	Pull ear superiorly and posteriorly

* There are no bony insertions for the muscles of facial expression.
** All muscles of facial expression are innervated by the facial nerve (CN VII) via temporal, zygomatic, buccal, mandibular, or cervical branches arising from the parotid plexus.

Table 19.2 **Muscles of Facial Expression: Mouth and Neck**

Muscle	Origin	Insertion*	Main Action(s)**
Mouth			
Zygomaticus major	Zygomatic bone (lateral surface, posterior part)	Skin at corner of the mouth	Pulls corner of mouth superiorly and laterally
Zygomaticus minor		Upper lip just medial to corner of the mouth	Pulls upper lip superiorly
Levator labii superioris alaeque nasi	Maxilla (frontal process)	Alar cartilage of nose and upper lip	Elevates upper lip, opens nostril
Levator labii superioris	Maxilla (frontal process) and infraorbital region	Skin of upper lip, alar cartilages of nose	Elevates upper lip, dilates nostril, raises angle of the mouth
Depressor labii inferioris	Mandible (anterior portion of oblique line)	Lower lip at midline; blends with muscle from opposite side	Pulls lower lip inferiorly and laterally
Levator anguli oris	Maxilla (below infraorbital foramen)	Skin at corner of the mouth	Raises angle of mouth, helps form nasolabial furrow
Depressor anguli oris	Mandible (oblique line below canine, premolar, and first molar teeth)	Skin at corner of the mouth; blends with orbicularis oris	Pulls angle of mouth inferiorly and laterally
Buccinator	Mandible, alveolar processes of maxilla and mandible, pterygo-mandibular raphe	Angle of mouth, orbicularis oris	Presses cheek against molar teeth, working with tongue to keep food between occlusal surfaces and out of oral vestibule; expels air from oral cavity/resists distension when blowing. *Unilateral:* Draws mouth to one side
Orbicularis oris	Deep surface of skin Superiorly: maxilla (median plane) Inferiorly: mandible	Mucous membrane of lips	Acts as oral sphincter • Compresses and protrudes lips (e.g., when whistling, sucking, and kissing) • Resists distension (when blowing)
Risorius	Fascia over masseter	Skin of corner of the mouth	Retracts corner of mouth as in grimacing
Mentalis	Mandible (incisive fossa)	Skin of chin	Elevates and protrudes lower lip
Neck			
Platysma	Skin over lower neck and upper lateral thorax	Mandible (inferior border), skin over lower face, angle of mouth	Depresses and wrinkles skin of lower face and mouth; tenses skin of neck; aids in forced depression of the mandible

* There are no bony insertions for the muscles of facial expression.
** All muscles of facial expression are innervated by the facial nerve (CN VII) via temporal, zygomatic, buccal, mandibular, or cervical branches arising from its parotid plexus.

— Primary sensory nerves of the face and scalp **(Fig. 19.3)** include
  - the **supraorbital** and **supratrochlear nerves** (cranial nerve [CN] V_1);
  - the infraorbital nerve and **zygomaticotemporal** and **zygomaticofacial nerves** (V_2);
  - the auriculotemporal, buccal, and **mental** (a branch of the inferior alveolar nerve) nerves (V_3);
  - the **great auricular** and **lesser occipital nerve,** which are anterior rami of C2 and C3 via the cervical plexus; and
  - the **greater occipital** and **third occipital nerves,** which are posterior rami of C2 and C3, respectively.

— Motor nerves of the face and scalp (see **Figs. 19.3B** and **18.28B**) include
  - the temporal, zygomatic, buccal, and marginal mandibular branches of the facial nerve (CN VII), which innervate muscles of the face;
  - the temporal and posterior auricular branches of the facial nerve, which innervate muscles of the scalp; and
  - the muscular branches of the mandibular division of the trigeminal nerve (CN V_3), which innervate the muscles of mastication.

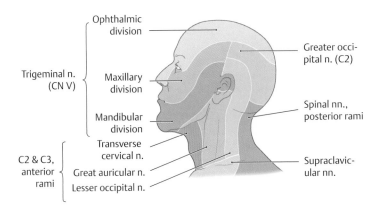

A Cutaneous innervation of the head and neck, left lateral view. The occiput and nuchal regions are supplied by the dorsal rami *(blue)* of the spinal nerves (the greater occipital nerve is the dorsal ramus of C2).

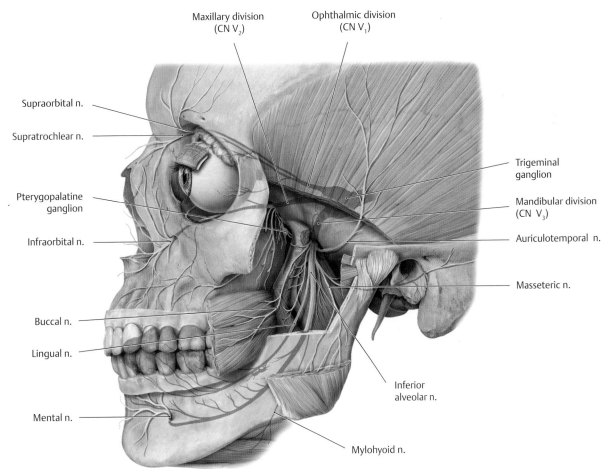

B Divisions of the trigeminal nerve, left lateral view.

Fig. 19.3 **Cutaneous innervation of the face**

19.2   The Temporomandibular Joint and Muscles of Mastication

— The **temporomandibular joint** (TMJ), which joins the mandible to the skull, is a synovial articulation between the head of the mandible and the mandibular fossa and articular tubercle of the temporal bone (**Figs. 19.4** and **19.5**).
  • An articular disk divides the joint cavity into a separate upper part for gliding movement and a lower part for hinge movement.

• The **lateral ligament** strengthens the fibrous capsule that surrounds the joint.
• **Sphenomandibular** and **stylomandibular ligaments** support the joint during chewing.
— Muscles of mastication, which include the **masseter, temporalis, lateral pterygoid, and medial pterygoid muscles,** act at the temporomandibular joint to move the mandible during chewing (**Figs. 19.6, 19.7, 19.8; Table 19.3**). They reside in the parotid region and in the temporal and infratemporal fossae.

CLINICAL CORRELATION

DISLOCATION OF THE TEMPOROMANDIBULAR JOINT During yawning (or other activities in which the mouth opens very widely), the head of the mandible moves forward from the mandibular fossa onto the articular tubercle. In some individuals this may cause the condyle of the mandible to slide in front of the anterior tubercle, where it locks the mandible in the protruded position. The ligaments supporting the joint become stretched, which causes severe spasm (trismus) of the masseter, medial pterygoid, and temporalis muscles.

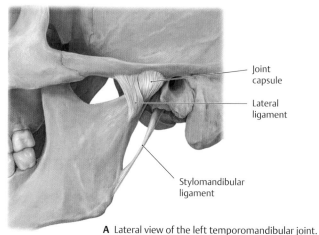

A Lateral view of the left temporomandibular joint.

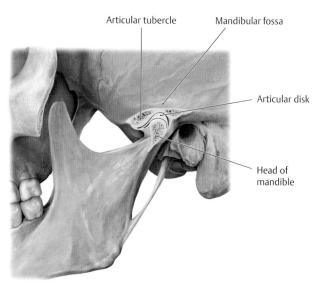

Fig. 19.4 Temporomandibular joint
The head of the mandible articulates with the mandibular fossa in the temporomandibular joint. Temporomandibularjoint, sagittal section, left lateral view.

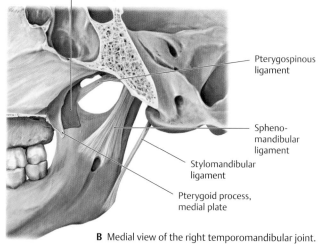

B Medial view of the right temporomandibular joint.

Fig. 19.5 Ligaments of the temporomandibular joint

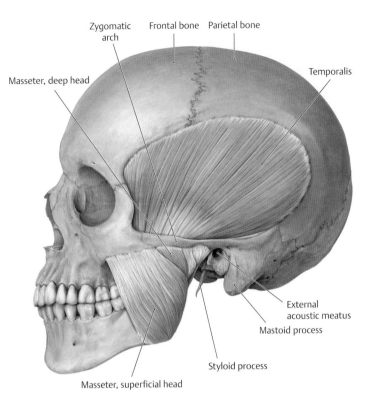

Fig. 19.6 Masseter and temporalis muscles
Left lateral view.

Labels (clockwise): Zygomatic arch; Frontal bone; Parietal bone; Temporalis; Masseter, deep head; External acoustic meatus; Mastoid process; Styloid process; Masseter, superficial head.

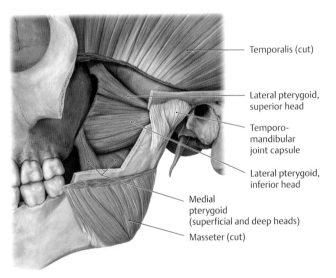

A Lateral pterygoid m. *Removed:* Coronoid process of mandible.

Labels: Temporalis (cut); Lateral pterygoid, superior head; Temporomandibular joint capsule; Lateral pterygoid, inferior head; Medial pterygoid (superficial and deep heads); Masseter (cut).

Fig. 19.7 Lateral and medial pterygoid muscles
Left lateral view.

B Medial pterygoid m. *Removed:* Temporalis, masseter; *Cut:* Lateral pterygoid.

Labels: Lateral pterygoid, superior head (cut); Articular disk; Lateral pterygoid, inferior head (cut); Medial pterygoid, deep (internal) head; Pterygoid process, lateral plate; Medial pterygoid, superficial (external) head.

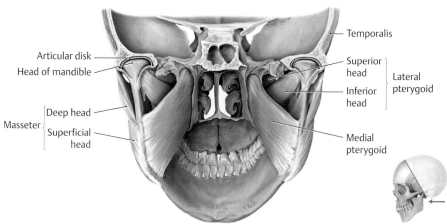

Fig. 19.8 Masticatory muscular sling
Oblique posterior view. *Revealed:* Muscular sling formed by the masseter and medial pterygoid muscles that embed the mandible.

Table 19.3 **Muscles of Mastication**

Muscle		Origin	Insertion	Innervation	Action
Masseter		Superficial head: zygomatic arch (anterior two thirds)	Mandibular angle (masseteric tuberosity)	Mandibular n. (CN V₃) via masseteric n.	Elevates (adducts) and protrudes mandible
		Deep part: zygomatic arch (posterior one third)			
Temporalis		Temporal fossa (inferior temporal line)	Coronoid process of mandible (apex and medial surface)	Mandibular n. (CN V₃) via deep temporal nn.	*Vertical fibers:* elevate (adduct) mandible *Horizontal fibers:* retract (retrude) mandible *Unilateral:* lateral movement of mandible (chewing)
Lateral pterygoid	Superior head	Greater wing of sphenoid bone (infratemporal crest)	Temporomandibular joint (articular disk)	Mandibular n. (CN V₃) via lateral pterygoid n.	*Bilateral:* protrudes mandible (pulls articular disk forward) *Unilateral:* lateral movements of mandible (chewing)
	Inferior head	Lateral pterygoid plate (lateral surface)	Mandible (condylar process)		
Medial pterygoid	Superficial head	Maxilla (tuberosity)	Pterygoid tuberosity on medial surface of the mandibular angle	Mandibular n. (CN V₃) via medial pterygoid n.	*Bilateral:* elevates (adducts) mandible with massater; contributes to protrusion *Unilateral:* small grinding movements
	Deep head	Medial surface of lateral pterygoid plate and pterygoid fossa			

19.3 Parotid Region

The parotid region lies superficial to the ramus of the mandible and includes the parotid gland and its surrounding structures (**Figs. 19.9** and **19.10**).

— The **parotid gland,** the largest of the three salivary glands, lies anterior to the ear on the lateral side of the face.
  • A superficial part of the gland lies on the masseter muscle.
  • A deep part of the gland curves around the posterior edge of the ramus of the mandible.
  • A tough parotid fascia derived from the deep cervical fascia encloses the gland.
  • Secretomotor (parasympathetic) fibers to the parotid gland arise with the glossopharyngeal nerve (CN IX) and synapse in the otic ganglion. Postganglionic fibers hitchhike on the auriculotemporal nerve of CN V₃.

— The **parotid duct** crosses the masseter muscle superficially to pierce the buccinator muscle and enter the mouth, where it opens opposite the second upper molar tooth.

— The parotid plexus, formed by the facial nerve (CN VII), is embedded within the parotid gland and gives rise to five branches that supply muscles of the face: the temporal, zygomatic, buccal, marginal mandibular, and cervical branches (see **Fig. 18.28B**).

— Structures traversing, or embedded within, the parotid gland include
  • the parotid plexus of the facial nerve (CN VII);
  • the retromandibular vein, formed by the superficial temporal and maxillary veins;

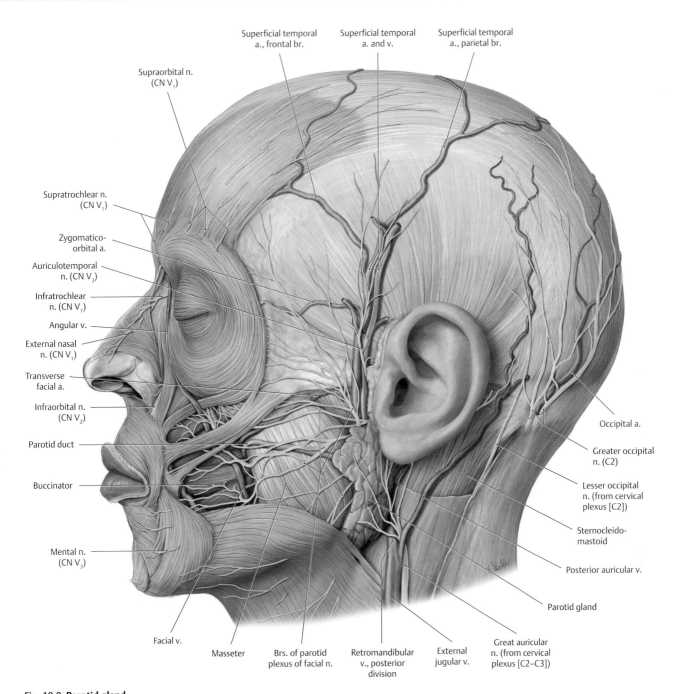

Fig. 19.9 Parotid gland
Left lateral view. *Note:* The parotid duct penetrates the buccinator muscle to open opposite the second upper molar.

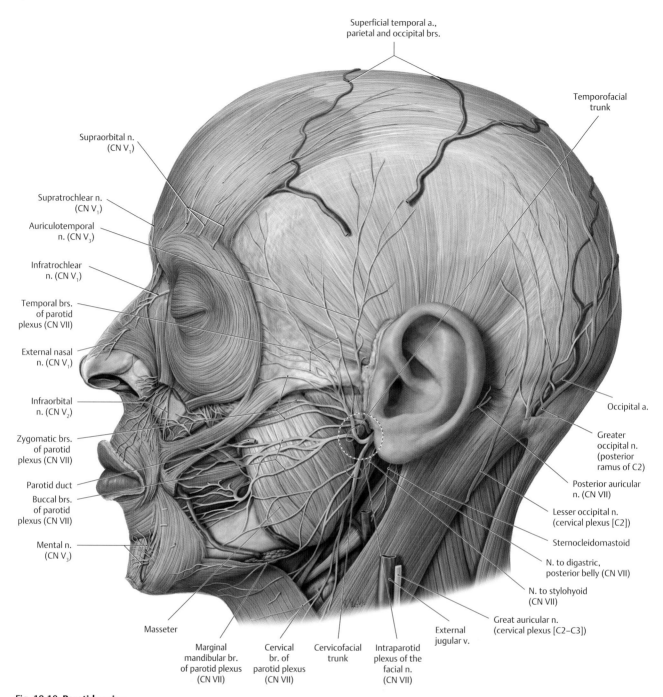

Fig. 19.10 Parotid region
Left lateral view. *Removed:* Parotid gland, sternocleidomastoid, and veins of the head. *Revealed:* Parotid bed and carotid triangle.

- the external carotid artery and the origin of its terminal branches, the superficial temporal and maxillary arteries; and
- the parotid lymph nodes, which drain the parotid gland, the external ear, the forehead, and the temporal region.

19.4   Temporal Fossa

The temporal fossa lies superior and medial to the parotid region and covers the lateral aspect of the head (**Figs. 19.11** and **19.12**).
— The boundaries of the temporal fossa are
  - anteriorly, the frontal process of the zygomatic bone and zygomatic process of the frontal bone;

- laterally, the zygomatic arch;
- medially, the frontal bone, parietal bone, greater wing of the sphenoid bone, and squamous part of the temporal bone; and
- inferiorly, the infratemporal fossa.
— The temporal fossa contains
  - the temporalis muscle and **temporal fascia,**
  - the superficial temporal artery and vein,
  - the **deep temporal branches** of the maxillary artery, and
  - the **deep temporal nerves** and auriculotemporal nerve of the mandibular division of the trigeminal nerve (CN V$_3$).

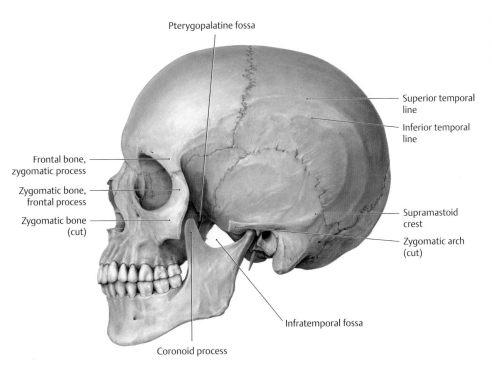

Pterygopalatine fossa

Superior temporal line

Inferior temporal line

Frontal bone, zygomatic process

Zygomatic bone, frontal process

Zygomatic bone (cut)

Supramastoid crest

Zygomatic arch (cut)

Infratemporal fossa

Coronoid process

Fig. 19.11 Temporal fossa
Left lateral view. The temporal fossa lies on the lateral surface of the skull, medial and superior to the zygomatic arch.

Occipitofrontalis, frontal belly (frontalis)

Temporal branches (CN VII)

Zygomatic branch (CN VII)

Zygomatic arch

Temporalis tendon

Coronoid process

Parotid duct

Masseter (cut)

Auriculotemporal nerve (CN V₃)

Deep temporal artery

Lateral pterygoid

Lateral (temporo-mandibular) ligament

Facial nerve

Fig. 19.12 Topography of the temporal fossa
Left lateral view. *Cut:* Masseter. *Revealed:* Temporal fossa and temporomandibular joint.

19.5   Infratemporal Fossa

The infratemporal fossa lies deep to the ramus of the mandible and is continuous superiorly with the temporal fossa (**Fig. 19.13**; see also **Fig. 17.6**).

—   The bony boundaries of the infratemporal region are
   •   anteriorly, the posterior wall of the maxilla;
   •   posteriorly, the mandibular fossa of the temporal bone;
   •   medially, the lateral pterygoid plate of the sphenoid bone;
   •   laterally the ramus of the mandible; and
   •   superiorly, the temporal bone and greater wing of the sphenoid bone.
—   The infratemporal fossa communicates with the orbit anteriorly, the pterygopalatine fossa medially, and the middle cranial fossa superiorly.

—   The contents of the infratemporal fossa (**Figs. 19.14** and **19.15**) include
   •   the temporomandibular joint,
   •   the medial and lateral pterygoid muscles and the inferior part of the temporalis muscle,
   •   the maxillary artery and its branches (**Table 19.4**),
   •   the pterygoid venous plexus,
   •   the mandibular division of the trigeminal nerve (CN V_3) and its branches,
   •   the otic ganglion, and
   •   the chorda tympani of the facial nerve (CN VII).
—   The mandibular nerve (CN V_3), the nerve of the infratemporal fossa and the only division of the trigeminal nerve that carries general sensory and somatic motor fibers, distributes post-ganglionic parasympathetic (visceral motor) fibers that arise from the otic and submandibular ganglia (**Fig. 19.16, Table 19.5**; see **Fig. 18.26C**).

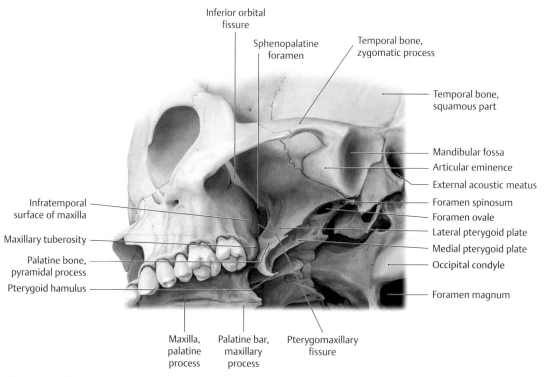

Fig. 19.13 Infratemporal fossa
Oblique external view of the base of the skull.

Temporalis (cut)

Deep temporal
nn. (CN V₃)

Superior alveolar nn.,
posterior superior
alveolar br. (CN V₂)

Maxillary a.

Buccal a. and n.
(CN V₃)

Medial pterygoid,
superficial and
deep heads

Lingual n. (CN V₃)

Facial a. and v.

Masseter (cut)

Superficial temporal
a. and v.

Deep temporal aa.

Auriculotemporal
n. (CN V₃)

Lateral pterygoid,
superior and
inferior heads

Facial n. (CN VII)

Ramus of mandible
(cut)

Inferior alveolar
a. and n. (CN V₃)

Sternocleidomastoid

Retromandibular v.,
posterior division

Fig. 19.14 Infratemporal fossa: Superficial layer
Left lateral view. *Removed:* Ramus of the mandible.

Temporalis (cut)

Deep temporal
nn. (CN V₃)

Infraorbital a.

Sphenopalatine a.

Posterior superior
alveolar a.

Buccal a. and n.
(CN V₃)

Buccinator

Medial pterygoid,
superficial head

Lingual n. (CN V₃)

Facial a. and v.

Masseter (cut)

Superficial temporal
a. and v.

Lateral pterygoid
(cut)

Auriculotemporal n.

Trigeminal n.,
mandibular division
(CN V₃)

Middle meningeal a.

Maxillary a.

Medial pterygoid,
deep head

Facial n. (CN VII)

Inferior alveolar
a. and n. (CN V₃)

Fig. 19.15 Infratemporal fossa: Deep dissection
Left lateral view. *Removed:* Lateral pterygoid muscle (both heads).
Revealed: Deep infratemporal fossa and mandibular nerve as it enters the mandibular canal via the foramen ovale in the roof of the fossa.

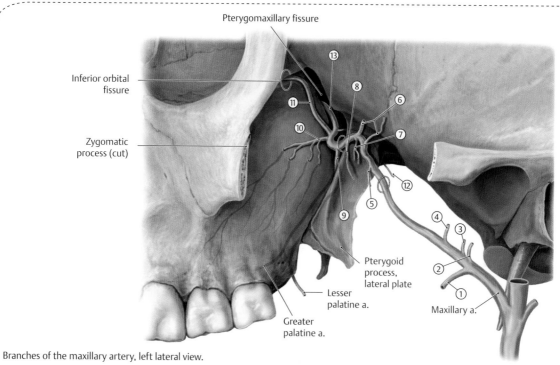

Branches of the maxillary artery, left lateral view.

Table 19.4 **Branches of the Maxillary Artery, Left Lateral View**

Part	Artery		Distribution
Mandibular part (between the origin and the first circle around artery)	① Inferior alveolar a.		Mandible, teeth, gingiva
	② Anterior tympanic a.		Tympanic cavity
	③ Deep auricular a.		Temporomandibular joint, external auditory canal
	④ Middle meningeal a.		Calvaria, dura, anterior and middle cranial fossae
Pterygoid part (between circles around the artery)	⑤ Masseteric a.		Masseter muscle
	⑥ Deep temporal aa.		Temporalis muscle
	⑦ Pterygoid branches		Pterygoid muscles
	⑧ Buccal a.		Buccal mucosa
Pterygopalatine part (from second circle through the pterygomaxillary fissure)	⑨ Descending palatine a.	Greater palatine a.	Hard palate
		Lesser palatine a.	Soft palate, palatine tonsil, pharyngeal wall
	⑩ Posterior superior alveolar a.		Maxillary molars, maxillary sinus, gingiva
	⑪ Infraorbital a.		Maxillary alveoli
	⑫ A. of pterygoid canal		
	⑬ Sphenopalatine a.	Lateral posterior nasal aa.	Lateral wall of nasal cavity, choanae
		Posterior septal branches	Nasal septum

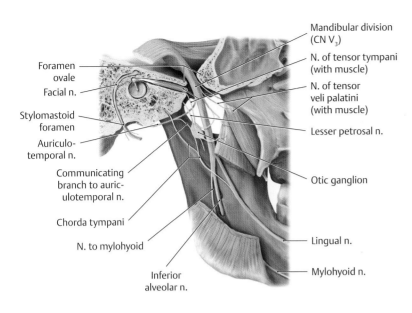

Fig. 19.16 **Mandibular nerve (CN V₃) in the infratemporal fossa**
Left medial view.

Labels: Mandibular division (CN V₃); N. of tensor tympani (with muscle); N. of tensor veli palatini (with muscle); Lesser petrosal n.; Otic ganglion; Lingual n.; Mylohyoid n.; Foramen ovale; Facial n.; Stylomastoid foramen; Auriculotemporal n.; Communicating branch to auriculotemporal n.; Chorda tympani; N. to mylohyoid; Inferior alveolar n.

Table 19.5 **Nerves of the Infratemporal Fossa**

Nerve	Nerve Fibers	Distribution
Muscular branches (CN V₃)	Branchial motor	Muscles of mastication; mylohyoid; tensor tympani; tensor veli palatini; anterior belly of digastric
Auriculotemporal (CN V₃)	General sensory	Auricle, temporal region, and temporomandibular joint
	Visceral motor from glossopharyngeal n. (CN IX)	Parotid gland
Inferior alveolar (CN V₃)	General sensory	Mandibular teeth; mental branch supplies skin of lower lip and chin
Lingual (CN V₃)	General sensory	Anterior two thirds of tongue, floor of mouth
Buccal (CN V₃)	General sensory	Skin and mucous membrane of cheek
Meningeal (CN V₃)	General sensory	Dura of middle cranial fossa
Chorda tympani (CN VII)	Special sensory taste	Anterior two thirds of tongue
	Visceral motor	Submandibular and sublingual glands via submandibular ganglion and lingual n. (CN V₃).

19.6 Pterygopalatine Fossa

The **pterygopalatine fossa,** a narrow space located medial to the infratemporal fossa, is an important distribution center for branches of the maxillary division of the trigeminal nerve (CN V₂) and the accompanying branches of the maxillary artery.

— The bony boundaries of the pterygopalatine fossa (**Fig. 19.17**) are
  • superiorly, the apex of the orbit;
  • anteriorly, the maxillary sinus;
  • posteriorly, the lateral pterygoid plate of the sphenoid bone;
  • laterally, the pterygomaxillary fissure; and
  • medially, the vertical plate of the palatine bone.
— Contents of the pterygopalatine fossa include
  • the pterygopalatine part of the maxillary artery, its branches, and its accompanying veins;
  • the nerve of the pterygoid canal;
  • the pterygopalatine ganglion; and

  • the maxillary division of the trigeminal nerve (CN V₂) and its branches.
— The pterygopalatine fossa communicates anteriorly with the orbit, medially with the nasal cavity and palate, and posteriorly with the middle cranial fossa and base of the skull (**Table 19.6**).
— The maxillary artery passes from the infratemporal fossa to the pterygopalatine fossa through the **pterygomaxillary fissure** (see **Table 19.4**). Its branches accompany the branches of the maxillary nerve (CN V₂) to supply the nose, palate, and pharynx.
— The **nerve of the pterygoid canal,** which enters the pterygopalatine fossa from the middle cranial fossa, is an autonomic nerve that carries
  • preganglionic parasympathetic fibers from the **greater petrosal nerve,** a branch of the facial nerve (CN VII); and
  • postganglionic sympathetic fibers from the **deep petrosal nerve,** which arises from the internal carotid plexus.

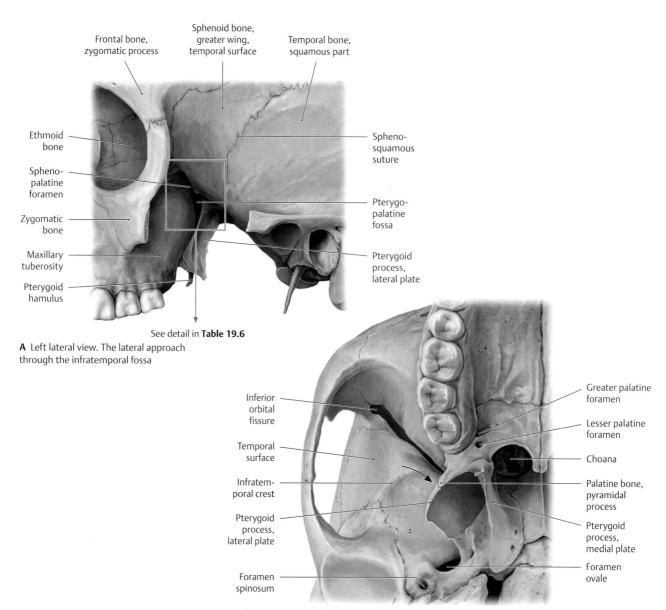

Frontal bone,
zygomatic process

Sphenoid bone,
greater wing,
temporal surface

Temporal bone,
squamous part

Ethmoid
bone

Spheno-
squamous
suture

Spheno-
palatine
foramen

Pterygo-
palatine
fossa

Zygomatic
bone

Maxillary
tuberosity

Pterygoid
process,
lateral plate

Pterygoid
hamulus

See detail in **Table 19.6**

A Left lateral view. The lateral approach
through the infratemporal fossa

Inferior
orbital
fissure

Greater palatine
foramen

Lesser palatine
foramen

Temporal
surface

Choana

Infratem-
poral crest

Palatine bone,
pyramidal
process

Pterygoid
process,
lateral plate

Pterygoid
process,
medial plate

Foramen
ovale

Foramen
spinosum

Fig. 19.17 **Pterygopalatine fossa**

B Inferior view, right side. The lateral approach through the infratemporal fossa viewed from the skull
base. The sphenoid is shown in *green*.

— The pterygopalatine ganglion receives general sensory fibers
from the maxillary nerve (CN V$_2$) and parasympathetic and
sympathetic fibers from the nerve of the pterygoid canal. Only
the parasympathetic fibers synapse in the ganglion; general
sensory and sympathetic fibers pass through the ganglion but
do not synapse there (**Table 19.7**).

— The maxillary division of the trigeminal nerve (CN V$_2$)
  • passes from the middle cranial fossa to the pterygopalatine
    fossa through the **foramen rotundum;**

• suspends the pterygopalatine ganglion by two small
  ganglionic nerves, which transmit general sensory fibers
  of the maxillary nerve;
• distributes postganglionic parasympathetic (secretomotor)
  and sympathetic (vasoconstrictive) fibers to the lacrimal,
  nasal, palatal, and pharyngeal glands; and
• distributes general sensory fibers to the midface, maxillary
  sinus, maxillary teeth, nasal cavity, palate, and superior
  pharynx.

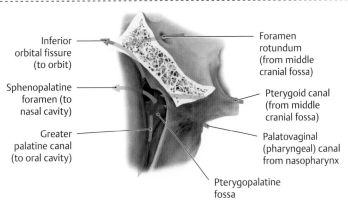

Inferior orbital fissure (to orbit)

Sphenopalatine foramen (to nasal cavity)

Greater palatine canal (to oral cavity)

Foramen rotundum (from middle cranial fossa)

Pterygoid canal (from middle cranial fossa)

Palatovaginal (pharyngeal) canal from nasopharynx

Pterygopalatine fossa

Table 19.6 **Communications of the Pterygopalatine Fossa**

Communication	Direction	Via	Transmitted structures
Middle cranial fossa	Posterosuperiorly	Foramen rotundum	• Maxillary n. (CN V$_2$)

Middle cranial fossa	Posteriorly in anterior wall of foramen lacerum	Pterygoid (vidian) canal	• N. of pterygoid canal, formed from:
			  ◦ Greater petrosal n. (preganglionic parasympathetic fibers from CN VII)
			  ◦ Deep petrosal n. (postganglionic sympathetic fibers from internal carotid plexus)
			• A. of pterygoid canal
			• Vv. of pterygoid canal

Orbit	Anterosuperiorly	Inferior orbital fissure	• Branches of maxillary n. (CN V$_2$):
			  ◦ Infraorbital n.
			  ◦ Zygomatic n.
			• Infraorbital a. and vv.
			• Communicating vv. between inferior ophthalmic v. and pterygoid plexus of vv.

Nasal cavity	Medially	Sphenopalatine foramen	• Nasopalatine n. (CN V$_2$), lateral and medial superior posterior nasal branches • Sphenopalatine a. and vv.
Oral cavity	Inferiorly	Greater palatine canal (foramen)	• Greater (descending) palatine n. (CN V$_2$) and a. • Branches that emerge through lesser palatine canals: ◦ Lesser palatine nn. (CN V2) and aa.
Nasopharynx	Inferoposteriorly	Palatovaginal (pharyngeal) canal	• CN V2, pharyngeal branches, and pharyngeal a.
Infratemporal fossa	Laterally	Pterygomaxillary fissure	• Maxillary a., pterygopalatine (third) part • Posterior superior alveolar n., a., and v.

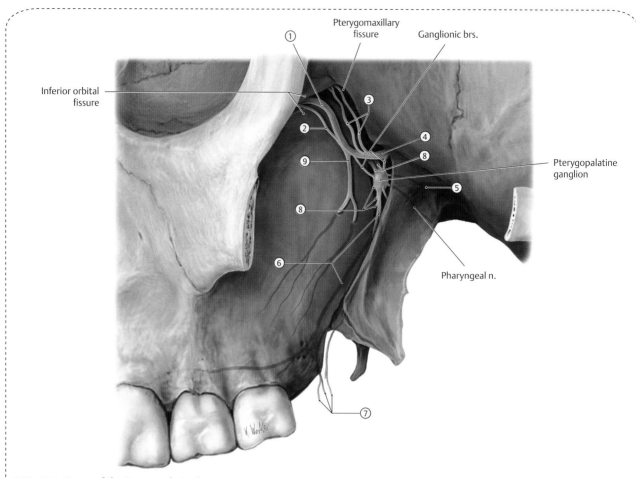

Table 19.7 **Nerves of the Pterygopalatine Fossa**

Nerve	Motor Innervation	Sensory Distribution
① Infraorbital n. (CN V$_2$)		Skin of the midface, maxillary sinus, teeth, and gingiva
② Zygomatic n. (CN V$_2$)–communicating branch from zygomaticotemporal n.	Visceral motor (postganglionic parasympathetic and postganglionic sympathetic) to lacrimal gland	Skin of lateral cheek, temple
③ Orbital branches (CN V$_2$)		Orbit, ethmoid and sphenoid sinuses
④ Maxillary (CN V$_2$)		
⑤ N. of the pterygoid canal (CN VII)	Visceral motor (preganglionic parasympathetic and postganglionic sympathetic) to glands of the nasal mucosa, and palate; lacrimal gland	
⑥ Greater palatine n. (CN V$_2$)		Hard palate
⑦ Lesser palatine n. (CN V$_2$)		Soft palate, palatine tonsil
⑧ Medial and lateral posterior superior and posterior inferior nasal nn. (CN V$_2$)		Nasal septum, upper lateral nasal wall, ethmoid sinuses
⑨ Posterior superior alveolar n. (CN V$_2$)		Maxillary sinus, cheeks, gingiva, maxillary molars

19.7 Nasal Cavity

The **nasal cavity** is located in the middle of the face between the orbits and maxillary sinuses and above the oral cavity.

Structure of the Nasal Cavity

The nose has an external portion and paired internal nasal cavities that are separated by a nasal septum (**Figs. 19.18** and **19.19**).
— The external nose consists of
  • anteriorly, the **alar** and **lateral nasal cartilages,** which form the nasal **ala** and **crura** surrounding the nostrils and the **apex,** or tip of the nose; and
  • posteriorly, the frontal, maxillary, and nasal bones, which form the **root,** or bridge, of the nose.
— The nasal cavities are pyramidally shaped spaces that communicate anteriorly with the outside through the **nares** (nostrils) and posteriorly with the nasopharynx through the **choanae.**
— The lateral walls of the nasal cavities are formed by the superior and middle nasal conchae of the ethmoid bone; the inferior nasal conchae; and the maxillary, palatine, lacrimal, and nasal bones.
  • The superior, middle, and inferior nasal conchae are scrolllike bony processes that project into the nasal cavity.
  • The **superior, middle,** and **inferior nasal meatuses** are recesses below the respective nasal conchae.
— The nasal septum forms the medial wall of each nasal cavity and consists of the vomer, the perpendicular plate of the ethmoid bone, and the septal cartilage.
— The **hard palate,** consisting of the maxilla and palatine bones, forms the floor of the nasal cavities and separates them from the oral cavity (see Section 19.8).
— **Paranasal sinuses** are air-filled cavities within bones of the skull that communicate with the nasal cavities (**Figs. 19.20, 19.21, 19.22; Table 19.8**).
  • Paired **frontal sinuses,** which are usually asymmetrical, lie above the root of the nose and drain into the middle meatus through a **frontonasal duct** into the **hiatus semilunaris.**
  • **Sphenoid sinuses,** which form within the body of the sphenoid bone, lie between the right and left cavernous sinuses and drain into the **sphenoethmoidal recess** in the posterosuperior part of the nasal cavities above the superior concha.
  • **Ethmoid sinuses** compose the medial wall of the orbit and are formed by numerous thin-walled ethmoid air cells. They lie between the orbits above the nasal cavities and drain into the superior and middle meatuses.
  • Paired **maxillary sinuses,** the largest of the paranasal sinuses, lie on either side of the nasal cavities, inferior to the orbits, and drain into the middle meatuses.
— A **nasolacrimal duct** drains tears from the medial corner of each eye and empties into the inferior meatus on each side.

A Left lateral view.

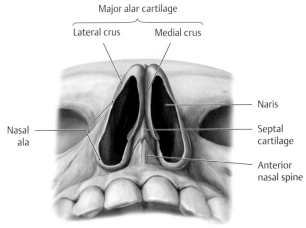

B Inferior view.

Fig. 19.18 Skeleton of the nose
The skeleton of the nose is composed of an upper bony portion and a lower cartilaginous portion. The proximal portions of the nostrils (alae) are composed of connective tissue with small embedded pieces of cartilage.

CLINICAL CORRELATION

INFECTION OF THE MAXILLARY SINUSES Infections arising in the nasal cavity may spread to any of the paranasal sinuses, but the maxillary sinuses are the most commonly affected. Mucus builds up within the maxillary sinuses and is unable to drain because their ostia are located high on the superomedial walls. The ostia are also commonly obstructed by inflammation of the mucous membranes of the sinuses (maxillary sinusitis). Maxillary sinusitis usually follows the common cold or influenza virus but may also arise from the spread of infections from posterior maxillary teeth.

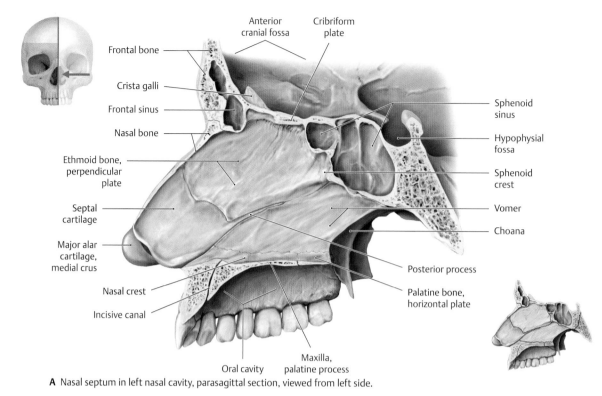

A Nasal septum in left nasal cavity, parasagittal section, viewed from left side.

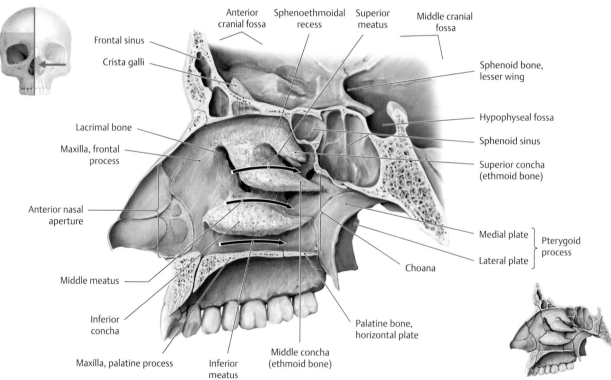

B Lateral wall of the right nasal cavity, sagittal section, medial view. *Removed:* Nasal septum. *Note:* The superior and middle conchae are parts of the ethmoid bone, whereas the inferior nasal conchae is a separate bone. *Arrows* indicate the direction of airflow through the nasal conchae.

Fig. 19.19 Bones of the nasal cavity

The left and right nasal cavities are flanked by lateral walls and separated by the nasal septum. Air enters the nasal cavity through the anterior nasal aperture and travels through three passages: the superior, middle, and inferior meatuses (**B**, *arrows*). These passages are separated by the superior, middle, and inferior conchae. Air leaves the nose through the choanae, entering the nasopharynx.

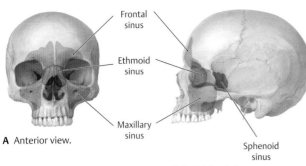

A Anterior view.

B Left lateral view.

Fig. 19.20 Location of the paranasal sinuses
The paranasal sinuses (frontal, ethmoid, maxillary, and sphenoid) are air-filled cavities that reduce the weight of the skull.

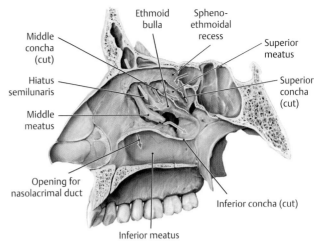

Fig. 19.22 Openings of the paranasal sinuses and nasolacrimal duct
Right nasal cavity, sagittal section, medial view. Mucosal secretions from the sinuses and nasolacrimal duct drain into the nose. *(See Table 19.8 for color coding.)*

Table 19.8 **Nasal Passages into which Sinuses Empty (Colors Refer to Fig. 19.22)**

Sinuses/duct		Nasal Passage	Via
Sphenoid sinus *(blue)*		Sphenoethmoidal recess	Direct
Ethmoid sinus *(green)*	Posterior cells	Superior meatus	Direct
	Anterior and middle cells	Middle meatus	Ethmoid bulla
Frontal sinus *(yellow)*		Middle meatus	Frontonasal duct into hiatus semilunaris
Maxillary sinus *(orange)*		Middle meatus	Hiatus semilunaris
Nasolacrimal duct *(red)*		Inferior meatus	Direct

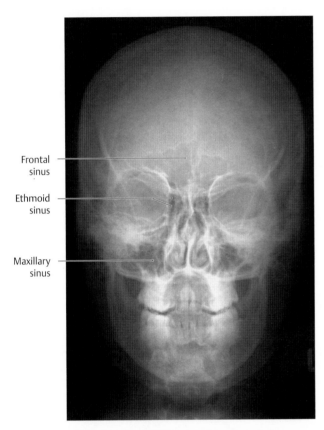

Fig. 19.21 Radiograph of the skull showing the paranasal sinuses
(From Moeller T. Color Atlas of Radiographic Anatomy, 3rd ed. Stuttgart: Thieme; 2010.)

Neurovasculature of the Nasal Cavity

— The external carotid artery, via its maxillary and facial branches, and the internal carotid artery, via its ophthalmic branch, supply the nasal cavity. The area of overlap between the external and internal circulations is referred to as Kiesselbach's area **(Fig. 19.23)**.
  • Branches of the maxillary artery include
    ○ the lateral posterior nasal and posterior septal arteries, branches of the sphenopalatine artery; and

CLINICAL CORRELATION

EPISTAXIS Bleeding, or epistaxis, of the highly vascular nasal mucosa is a common consequence of nasal trauma, and even minor trauma can disrupt the veins in the vestibule. Most bleeding originates from the arteries of Kiesselbach's area, where branches of the internal carotid and external carotid arteries anastomose in the anterior third of the nasal cavity. These include the sphenopalatine, greater palatine, anterior ethmoidal, and superior labial arteries.

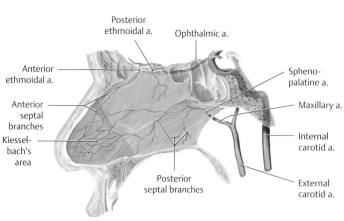

A Arteries of the nasal septum, left lateral view.

B Arteries of the right lateral nasal wall, medial view.

Fig. 19.23 Arteries of the nasal cavity

- the greater palatine artery, a branch of the descending palatine artery.
- Branches of the facial artery include the lateral nasal artery and a septal artery, a branch of the superior labial artery.
- Branches of the ophthalmic artery include anterior and posterior ethmoidal arteries.
- Veins that drain the nasal cavity form a submucosal venous plexus that drains into the ophthalmic, facial, and sphenopalatine veins.
- The olfactory nerve (CN I) and the ophthalmic (CN V_1) and maxillary (CN V_2) divisions of the trigeminal nerve innervate the nose **(Fig. 19.24)**.
  - Olfactory nerves, which are responsible for smell, arise from the olfactory epithelium in the roof of the nasal

cavity. They pass through the cribriform plate and end in the olfactory bulbs.
- Infratrochlear and anterior ethmoid branches of CN V_1 and the infraorbital branch of CN V_2 innervate the external nose.
- The anterior and posterior ethmoidal branches of CN V_1 innervate the external nose and the mucosa of the anterosuperior nasal cavity through internal, external, medial, and lateral nasal branches.
- The posterior nasal branches of the nasopalatine nerve on the septum and nasal branches of the greater palatine nerve on the lateral walls (both branches of CN V_2) innervate the mucosa of the posteroinferior nasal cavity.

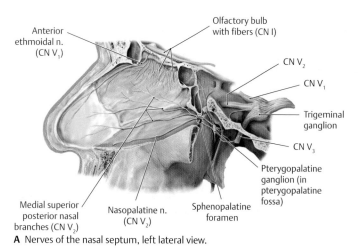

A Nerves of the nasal septum, left lateral view.

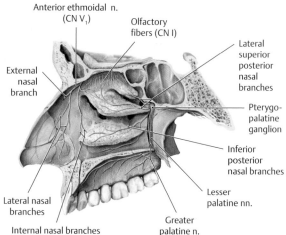

B Nerves of the right lateral nasal wall, medial view.

Fig. 19.24 Nerves of the nasal cavity

19.8 Oral Region

The oral cavity, located below the nasal cavity and anterior to the pharynx, is bounded superiorly by the palate, inferiorly by the tongue and muscular floor, anteriorly by the lips, posteriorly by the uvula, and laterally by the cheeks (**Fig. 19.25**).

Lips, Cheeks, Gingiva, Teeth, and Oral Cavity

— The **lips** frame the mouth and surround the **oral fissure,** the opening into the oral cavity.
- The lips contain the sphincter-like obicularis oris muscle and superior and inferior labial muscles. Externally, they are covered by skin; internally, they are covered by the mucous membrane of the oral cavity.
- The **philtrum,** an external midline depression on the upper lip, extends superiorly to the nasal septum.

- **Labial frenula** are midline folds of mucous membrane that attach the inner surfaces of the upper and lower lips to the gums.

DEVELOPMENT CORRELATION

CLEFT LIP Cleft lip is a congenital defect that occurs early in embryonic life when the maxillary prominence and the median nasal prominence fail to fuse. It is seen in ~ 1:1,000 live births and is more common in males than females. The cleft may be unilateral or bilateral and is described as complete when it extends into the nose and incomplete when it appears as a notch in the lip. Corrective surgery is usually performed when the infant is around 10 weeks old.

— The **cheeks,** continuous with the lips, form the walls of the mouth and the **buccal region** of the face.

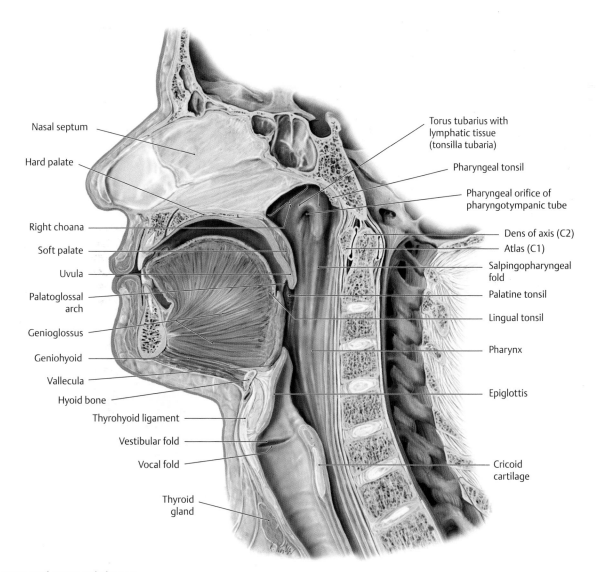

Nasal septum

Hard palate

Right choana

Soft palate

Uvula

Palatoglossal arch

Genioglossus

Geniohyoid

Vallecula

Hyoid bone

Thyrohyoid ligament

Vestibular fold

Vocal fold

Thyroid gland

Torus tubarius with lymphatic tissue (tonsilla tubaria)

Pharyngeal tonsil

Pharyngeal orifice of pharyngotympanic tube

Dens of axis (C2)

Atlas (C1)

Salpingopharyngeal fold

Palatine tonsil

Lingual tonsil

Pharynx

Epiglottis

Cricoid cartilage

Fig. 19.25 Oral cavity and pharynx
Midsagittal section, left lateral view.

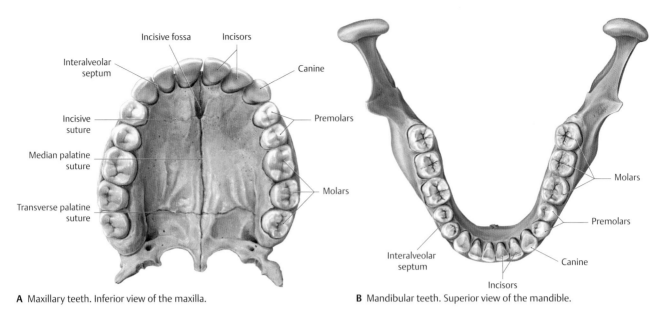

A Maxillary teeth. Inferior view of the maxilla.

B Mandibular teeth. Superior view of the mandible.

Fig. 19.26 Permanent teeth

- The buccinator muscle, innervated by the buccal branch of the facial nerve (CN VII), forms the movable wall of the cheek.
- Buccal fat pads, encapsulated cushions of fat that lie superficial to the buccinator muscles, are proportionately large in infants and reduced in adults.
- The zygomatic bone and zygomatic arch form the "cheek bone."
- Teeth are anchored in **alveoli** (sockets) of the **maxillary** and **mandibular dental arches (Figs. 19.26)**.
  - Children have 20 deciduous teeth, which are replaced at predictable intervals between ages 7 and 25 years.
  - Adult have 32 teeth, consisting of incisors, canines, premolars, and molars.
- The **gingivae**, or gums, made of fibrous tissue covered by the mucous membrane of the oral cavity, are firmly attached to the maxilla and mandible.
- The oral cavity, or mouth, is divided into two regions: the **oral vestibule** and the **oral cavity proper (Fig. 19.27)**.
  - The oral vestibule is the narrow space between the lips and cheeks and the dental arches of the maxilla and mandible.
  - The oral cavity proper is the space bounded anteriorly and laterally by the upper and lower dental arches. Superiorly, the **palate** forms the roof, and inferiorly, the tongue rests on a muscular floor.
- The oral cavity connects posteriorly to the pharynx through a narrow space, the **faucial isthmus.**
- Muscles that form the floor of the mouth, the **suprahyoid muscles**, are attached to the hyoid bone in the neck (**Fig. 19.28; Table 19.9**). They have a complex innervation with contributions from the trigeminal and facial nerves and the C1 spinal nerve via the hypoglossal nerve.
- The lingual, facial, and maxillary branches of the external carotid artery supply the lips, cheeks, floor of the mouth, and upper and lower teeth.
- The trigeminal nerve (CN V) transmits sensation from the mouth (see **Fig. 18.26C**).

- The superior alveolar branch of the maxillary division (CN V$_2$) innervates the upper teeth.
- Inferior alveolar, lingual, and buccal branches of the mandibular division (CN V$_3$) innervate the cheek, lower teeth, and floor of the mouth.
- Visceral motor fibers carried by the chorda tympani (CN VII) synapse in the submandibular ganglion in the floor of the mouth. Postganglionic fibers travel via the lingual nerve to innervate the submandibular and sublingual glands (**Fig. 19.29**).

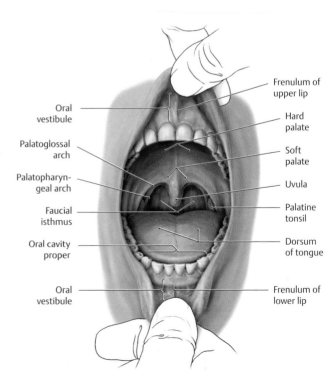

Fig. 19.27 Oral cavity
Anterior view.

A Left lateral view.

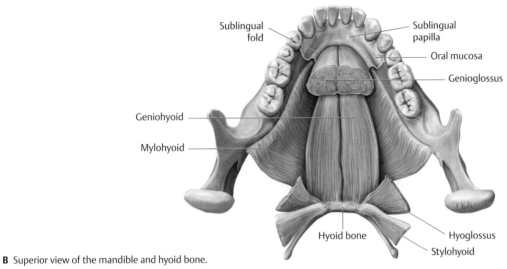

B Superior view of the mandible and hyoid bone.

Fig. 19.28 Muscles of the oral floor: suprahyoid muscles

Table 19.9 **Suprahyoid Muscles**

Muscle		Origin	Insertion/Placement		Innervation	Action
Digastric	Anterior belly	Mandible (digastric fossa)	Hyoid bone (body)	Via an intermediate tendon with a fibrous loop	Mylohyoid n. (from CNV₃)	Elevates hyoid bone (during swallowing), assists in opening
	Posterior belly	Temporal bone (mastoid notch, medial to mastoid process)			Facial n. (CN VII)	
Stylohyoid		Temporal bone (styloid process)		Via a split tendon		
Mylohyoid		Mandible (mylohyoid line)		Via median tendon of insertion (mylohyoid raphe)	Mylohyoid n. (from CN V₃)	Tightens and elevates oral floor, draws hyoid bone forward (during swallowing), assists in opening mandible and moving it side to side (mastication)
Geniohyoid		Mandible (inferior mental spine)		Body of hyoid bone	Anterior ramus of C1 via hypoglossal n. (CN XII)	Draws hyoid bone forward (during swallowing), assists in opening mandible
Hyoglossus		Hyoid bone (superior border of greater cornu)	Sides of tongue		Hypoglossal n. (CN XII)	Depresses the tongue

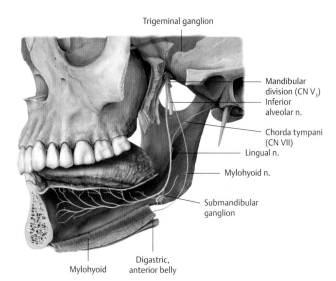

Fig. 19.29 **Nerves in the floor of the mouth**
Left lateral view with left half of the mandible removed.

The Palate

The palate forms the roof of the oral cavity and the floor of the nasal cavity and separates the oral cavity from the pharynx posteriorly.

— Nasal mucosa covers the superior surface, and oral mucosa, densely packed with mucus-secreting palatine glands, covers the inferior surface.
— The palate has anterior and posterior regions.
  • The **hard palate,** formed by the palatine processes of the maxillary bones and the horizontal processes of the palatine bones, makes up the anterior two thirds of the palate (**Fig. 19.30**).
  • The **soft palate,** the posterior third of the palate, has an anterior aponeurotic part that is attached to the hard palate and a posterior muscular part with an unattached posterior margin that ends in a conical projection, the **uvula** (see **Fig. 19.25**).
— During swallowing, muscles of the soft palate can tense and elevate it against the posterior pharyngeal wall to prevent food from passing into the nasal cavity. They can also draw the palate downward against the tongue to prevent food from entering the pharynx. Muscles of the soft palate include the **tensor veli palatini, levator veli palatini, musculus**

DEVELOPMENT CORRELATION

CLEFT PALATE Cleft palate is a congenital defect that occurs early in embryonic life when the lateral palatine processes fail to fuse with each other, with the nasal septum, and/or with the median palatine processes. It is seen in ~ 1:2,500 live births and is more common in females than males. The cleft (a fissure or opening) is described as complete when it involves the soft and hard palate and incomplete when it appears as a "hole" in the roof of the mouth (usually in the soft palate). In each case the uvula is usually also split. The cleft connects the oral cavity directly to the nasal cavity. Initial treatment involves the use of a prosthetic device called a palatal obturator to seal the cleft until corrective surgery is performed when the infant is between 6 and 12 months old.

uvulae, palatoglossus, and **palatopharyngeus (Fig. 19.31**; **Table 19.10**).
— The paired **palatoglossal** and **palatopharyngeal arches,** formed by the **palatoglossus** and **palatopharyngeus muscles,** anchor the soft palate to the tongue and pharynx.
— Greater palatine, lesser palatine, and sphenopalatine branches of the maxillary artery supply the palate (**Fig. 19.32;** see also **Fig. 19.23B**).
— The greater palatine, lesser palatine, and nasopalatine branches of the maxillary division (CN V$_2$) carry sensory innervation from the palate (see **Fig. 19.24B**).

Fig. 19.30 **Hard palate**
Inferior view.

Fig. 19.31 Muscles of the soft palate
Inferior view. The soft palate forms the posterior boundary of the oral cavity, separating it from the oropharynx.

Table 19.10 **Muscles of the Soft Palate**

Muscle	Origin	Insertion	Innervation	Action
Tensor veli palatini	Medial pterygoid plate (scaphoid fossa); sphenoid bone (spine); cartilage of pharyngotympanic tube	Palatine aponeurosis	Medial pterygoid n. (CN V$_3$ via otic ganglion)	Tightens soft palate; opens inlet to pharyngotympanic tube (during swallowing, yawning)
Levator veli palatini	Cartilage of pharyngotympanic tube; temporal bone (petrous part)		Accessory n. (CN XI, cranial part) via pharyngeal plexus (vagus n., CN X)	Raises soft palate to horizontal position
Musculus uvulae	Uvula (mucosa)	Palatine aponeurosis; posterior nasal spine		Shortens and raises uvula
Palatoglossus	Tongue (side)	Palatine aponeurosis		Elevates tongue (posterior portion); pulls soft palate onto tongue
Palatopharyngeus				Tightens soft palate; during swallowing pulls pharyngeal walls superiorly, anteriorly, and medially

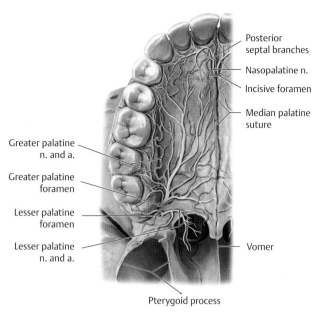

Fig. 19.32 Neurovasculature of the hard palate
Inferior view. The hard palate receives sensory innervation primarily from terminal branches of the maxillary division of the trigeminal nerve (CN V₂). The arteries of the hard palate arise from the maxillary artery.

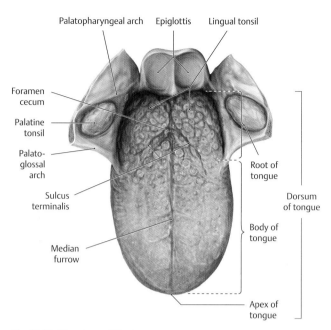

Fig. 19.33 Structure of the tongue
Superior view. The V-shaped sulcus terminalis divides the tongue into an anterior (oral, presulcal) and a posterior (pharyngeal, postsulcal) part.

The Tongue

The tongue is a muscular organ that is involved in speech, taste, and manipulation of food during the initial phase of swallowing. Two thirds of the tongue lies in the oral cavity; the remainder forms the anterior wall of the oropharynx, the part of the pharynx posterior to the oral cavity.

— The tongue has three parts **(Fig. 19.33)**:
 • the **root,** the attached posterior portion;
 • the **body,** the largest portion, between the root and apex; and
 • the **apex,** the anterior tip.
— The **sulcus terminalis,** a groove on the dorsum of the tongue, divides the anterior two thirds of the tongue from the posterior third. A small pit at the center of the groove, the **foramen cecum,** marks the embryonic origin of the thyroid gland.
— Numerous lingual papillae, many containing taste buds, give the mucosa of the anterior two thirds of the tongue its rough texture.
 • **Vallate papillae,** the largest of the lingual papillae, are arranged in a row directly anterior to the sulcus terminalis.
 • **Foliate papillae** are found on the small lateral folds of the lingual mucosa and are not well developed.
 • **Filiform papillae** contain afferent nerve endings that are sensitive to touch but not to taste. These are highly keratinized and facilitate rasplike licking activity.
 • **Fungiform papillae** are most numerous at the apex and margins of the tongue.

— The **lingual tonsil** is a collection of lymphoid nodules distributed over the mucosa of the posterior part of the tongue. Lingual tonsils have crypts that are flushed by glands below them.
— The **frenulum of the tongue,** a midline mucosal fold, attaches the inferior surface of the tongue to the floor of the oral cavity and restricts its movement.
— Extrinsic muscles of the tongue, which originate outside the tongue and are responsible primarily for tongue movements, include the genioglossus, hyoglossus, palatoglossus, and styloglossus muscles **(Fig. 19.34)**.
— Intrinsic muscles of the tongue have no bony attachments and are responsible for changing the shape of the tongue. They include the superior and inferior longitudinal muscles and the transverse and vertical muscles.
— All extrinsic and intrinsic muscles of the tongue, except the palatoglossus, are innervated by the hypoglossal nerve (CN XII). The palatoglossus is innervated by the vagus nerve (CN X).
— The lingual arteries, branches of the external carotid arteries, supply the tongue. The lingual veins accompany the arteries and drain into the internal jugular vein.
— Lymph from the tongue ultimately drains to deep cervical and jugular nodes in the neck, although the drainage from the various parts of the tongue follows four different pathways **(Fig. 19.35; Table 19.11)**. These drainage routes can be clinically important in the metastasis of lingual tumors.
— The five cranial nerves (trigeminal, facial, glossopharyngeal, vagus, and hypoglossal) that innervate the tongue carry motor, general sensory, and special sensory fibers **(Figs. 19.36 and 19.37; Table 19.12)**.

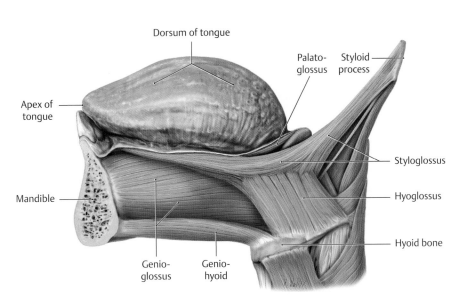

Fig. 19.34 Extrinsic muscles of the tongue
Left lateral view.

Table 19.11 **Lymphatic Drainage of the Tongue**

Area of the Tongue	Drainage Pattern	Primary Nodes
Root	Bilaterally	Superior deep cervical
Medial part of the body	Bilaterally	Inferior deep cervical
Lateral parts of the body	Ipsilaterally	Submandibular
Apex and frenulum	Midline—bilaterally Sides—ipsilaterally	Submental

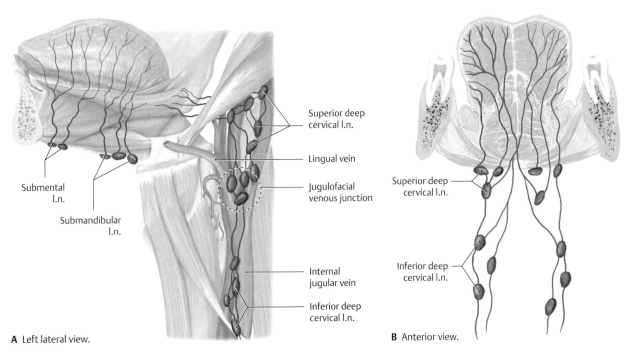

A Left lateral view.

B Anterior view.

Fig. 19.35 Lymphatic drainage of the tongue and oral floor
Lymph flows to the submental and submandibular lymph nodes of the tongue and oral floor, which ultimately drain into the jugular lymph nodes along the internal jugular vein. Because the lymph nodes receive drainage from both the ipsilateral and contralateral sides **(B)**, tumor cells may become widely disseminated in this region (e.g., metastatic squamous cell carcinoma, especially on the lateral border of the tongue, frequently metastasizes to the opposite side).

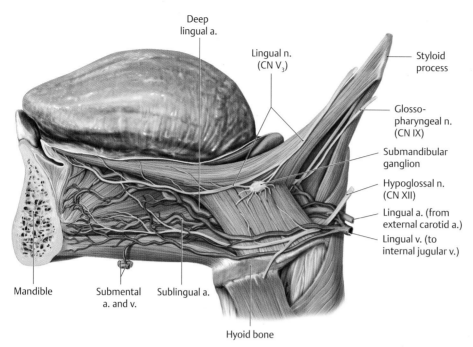

Fig. 19.36 Neurovasculature of the tongue
Left lateral view.

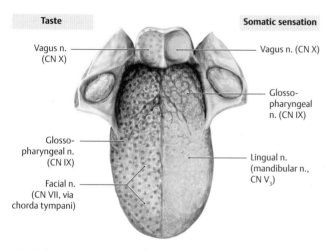

Fig. 19.37 Somatosensory and taste innervation of the tongue
Anterior view.

Table 19.12 **Innervation of the Tongue**

Nerve	Nerve Fibers	Distribution
Lingual nerve (CN V$_3$)	General sensory	Anterior two thirds of the tongue
Chorda tympani (CN VII)	Special sensory	Anterior two thirds of the tongue
Glossopharyngeal nerve (CN IX)	General sensory and special sensory	Posterior third of the tongue
Vagus nerve (CN X)	General sensory and special sensory	Root of the tongue
Hypoglossal nerve (CN XII)	Somatic motor	Muscles of the tongue, except the palatoglossus, which is innervated by the vagus nerve (CN X)

Salivary Glands

Three pairs of salivary glands, the parotid, sublingual, and submandibular, produce and secrete saliva into the mouth (**Fig. 19.38**).

— The **sublingual gland,** the smallest of the three glands, lies deep to the mucosa of the floor of the mouth, forming the **sublingual folds,** onto which it secretes saliva through numerous small ducts.

— The **submandibular gland** has a superficial part located in the neck and a deep part located in the floor of the mouth, which connect around the posterior border of the mylohyoid muscle. The **submandibular (Wharton's) duct** opens via the **sublingual papilla** at the base of the lingual frenulum.

— The parotid gland, the largest of the three glands, is located in the parotid region on the lateral side of the head, anterior to the ear. The parotid duct opens into the vestibule of the mouth at the parotid papilla located adjacent to the second maxillary molar (see Section 19.3).

— The facial, lingual, maxillary, and superficial temporal arteries supply the salivary glands. Veins of similar names accompany the arteries and drain into the retromandibular vein.

— The sublingual and submandibular glands receive parasympathetic secretomotor fibers via the chorda tympani (a branch of CN VII) and submandibular ganglion.

— The parotid gland receives secretomotor (parasympathetic) fibers of the glossopharyngeal nerve (CN IX) that synapse in the otic ganglion.

— Sympathetic innervation to the glands arises from the superior cervical ganglion and follows the branches of the external carotid artery.

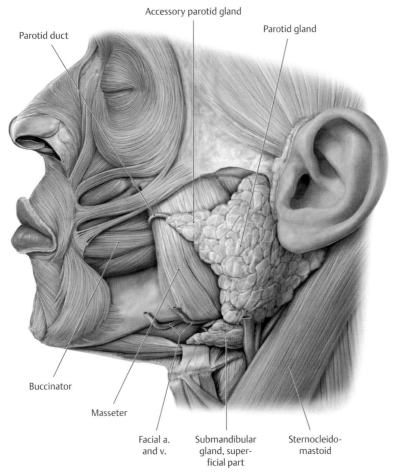

Accessory parotid gland

Parotid duct

Parotid gland

Buccinator

Masseter

Facial a. and v.

Submandibular gland, superficial part

Sternocleidomastoid

A Parotid gland, left lateral view.

Sublingual papilla

Sublingual fold

Oral mucosa

Genioglossus

Sublingual gland

Geniohyoid

Submandibular duct

Mylohyoid

Lingual n.

Inferior alveolar n.

Submandibular gland

Mylohyoid n.

Lingual a.

Hyoid bone

Hyoglossus

Stylohyoid

B Submandibular and sublingual glands, superior view with tongue removed.

Fig. 19.38 Salivary glands

19.9   Pharynx and Tonsils

The **pharynx,** a fibromuscular tube that forms part of the upper airway and the upper digestive tract, transmits air from the nasal cavity to the trachea and food from the oral cavity to the esophagus.

Regions of the Pharynx

The pharynx, which extends from the base of the skull to the inferior aspect of the larynx (cricoid cartilage), is divided into three regions (**Figs. 19.39** and **19.40**; see also **Fig. 19.26**): the nasopharynx, the oropharynx, and the laryngopharynx.

— The **nasopharynx,** the uppermost part of the pharynx, lies posterior to the nasal cavity and above the soft palate. Anteriorly, the nasopharynx communicates with the nasal cavity through the paired choanae.

  • The orifices (openings) of the pharyngotympanic tubes are located on the lateral pharyngeal wall. Above the orifice, the cartilaginous part of the tube protrudes into the pharynx to form a bulge, the **torus tubarius.**

  • A **salpingopharyngeal fold,** formed by the **salpingopharyngeus muscle** deep to the mucosa, extends inferiorly from the torus tubarius.

— The **oropharynx,** which lies posterior to the oral cavity, extends superiorly to the soft palate and inferiorly to the top of the larynx. The posterior tongue forms the anterior boundary.

  • Two arches, the anterior palatoglossal arch (fold) and the posterior palatopharyngeal arch (fold), formed by the palatoglossus and palatopharyngeal muscles, respectively, separate the oropharynx from the oral cavity (see **Fig. 19.26**). Both muscles are innervated by the vagus nerve (CN X).

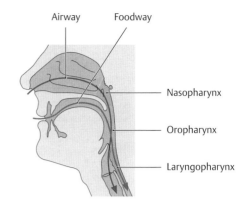

Fig. 19.39 Regions of the pharynx
Midsagittal section, left lateral view. The *blue arrow* indicates flow of air and the *red arrow*, passage of food.

  • The palatine tonsil lies between these arches in the tonsillar fossa.

  • A median fold of mucosa divides the space between the base of the tongue and the epiglottis. The spaces on either side of the fold are called **valleculae.**

— The **laryngopharynx,** which lies posterior to the larynx, extends from the epiglottis to the inferior border of the cricoid cartilage, where it narrows and is continuous with the esophagus.

  • The laryngopharynx communicates with the larynx through the **laryngeal inlet.**

  • **Aryepiglottic folds** separate the laryngeal inlet from mucus-lined fossae on the lateral walls of the pharynx called **piriform recesses.**

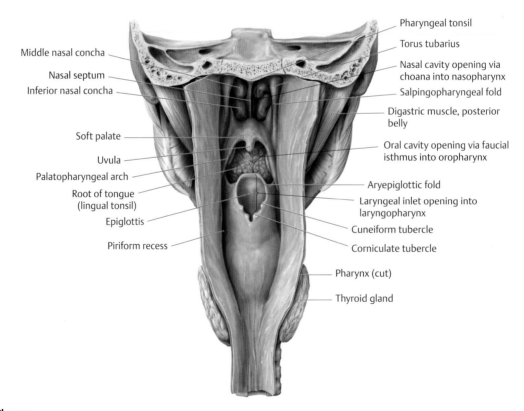

Fig. 19.40 Pharynx
Posterior view of opened pharynx.

Muscles of the Pharynx

An outer circular layer and inner longitudinal layer of skeletal muscles form the walls of the pharynx (**Fig. 19.41; Tables 19.13** and **19.14**). Pharyngeal muscles coordinate with muscles of the floor of the mouth and soft palate during swallowing (**Fig. 19.42**).

— Circular **superior, middle, and inferior pharyngeal constrictor muscles** propel a bolus of food downward through the oropharynx and laryngopharynx.

— Longitudinal muscles, the **salpingopharyngeus** and **palatopharyngeus** innervated by the vagus nerve (CN X) and pharyngeal plexus, and the **stylopharyngeus** innervated by the glossopharyngeal nerve (CN IX), elevate the pharynx to prevent food from entering the nasopharynx.

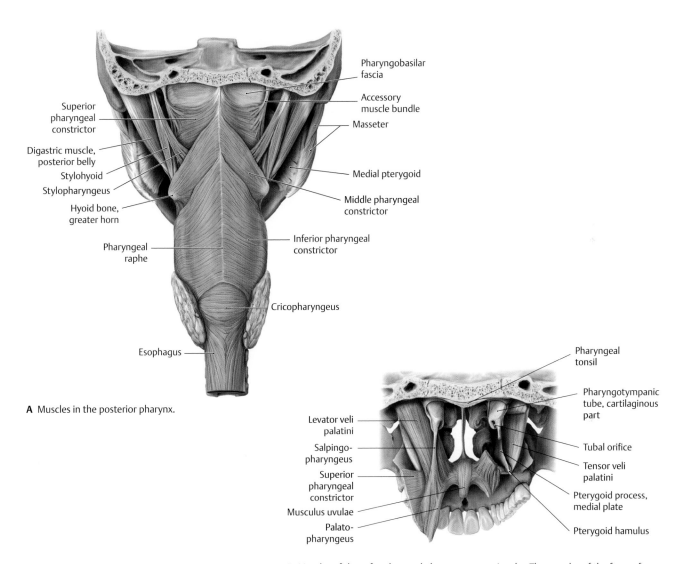

A Muscles in the posterior pharynx.

B Muscles of the soft palate and pharyngotympanic tube. The muscles of the fauces form the posterior boundary of the oral cavity. *Cut on right side:* Levator veli palatini and salpingopharyngeus.

Fig. 19.41 Pharyngeal muscles
Posterior view. (*continued on page 480*)

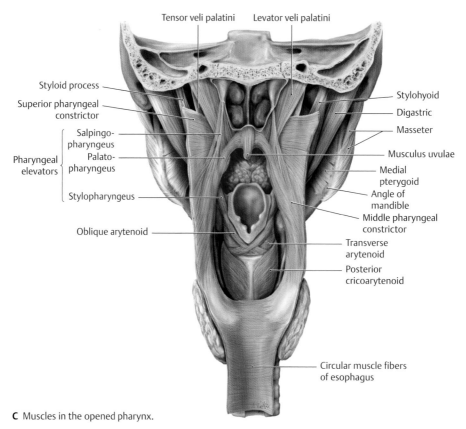

C Muscles in the opened pharynx.

Fig. 19.41 (*continued*) **Pharyngeal muscles**
Posterior view.

Table 19.13 **Muscles of the Pharynx: Pharyngeal Constrictors**

Muscle	Origin	Insertion	Innervation	Action
Superior pharyngeal constrictor	Pterygoid hamulus, pterygomandibular raphe, mylohyoid line of mandible, lateral tongue	Pharyngeal tubercle of occipital bone via median pharyngeal raphe	Vagus n. (CN X) via pharyngeal plexus	Constricts the upper pharynx
Middle pharyngeal constrictor	Greater and lesser horns of the hyoid, stylohyoid lig.	Pharyngeal raphe		Constricts the middle pharynx
Inferior pharyngeal constrictor	Thyroid lamina, inferior horn of hyoid, cricoid cartilage	Pharyngeal raphe; Cricopharyngeus encircles pharyngeal-esophageal junction	Vagus n. via the pharyngeal plexus, recurrent and external laryngeal n (CN X)	Constricts lower pharynx; Cricopharyngeus: sphincter between laryngopharynx and esophagus

Table 19.14 **Pharyngeal Muscles: Pharyngeal Elevators**

Muscle	Origin	Insertion	Innervation	Action
Palatopharyngeus (palatopharyngeal arch)	Palatine aponeurosis (superior surface) and posterior border of palatine bone	Thyroid cartilage (posterior border) or lateral pharynx	Vagus n. (CN X) via pharyngeal plexus	*Bilaterally:* Elevates the pharynx anteromedially.
Salpingopharyngeus	Cartilaginous pharyngotympanic tube (inferior surface)	Along salpingopharyngeal fold to palatopharyngeus		*Bilaterally:* Elevates the pharynx; may also open pharyngotympanic tube.
Stylopharyngeus	Styloid process (medial surface of base)	Lateral pharynx, mixing with pharyngeal constrictors, palatopharyngeus, and thyroid cartilage (posterior border)	Glossopharyngeal n. (CN IX)	*Bilaterally:* Elevates the pharynx and larynx.

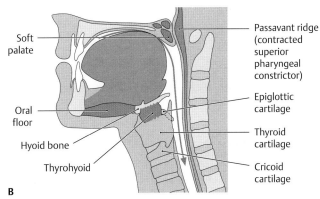

A

B

Fig. 19.42 Anatomy of swallowing
As part of the airway, the larynx in the adult is located at the inlet to the digestive tract **(A)**. During swallowing, therefore, the airway must be briefly occluded to keep food from entering the trachea. During the reflexive phase of swallowing, muscles on the floor of the mouth and the thyrohyoid elevate the larynx while the epiglottis covers the laryngeal inlet, sealing off the lower airway. In addition, the soft palate tightens, elevates, and opposes the posterior pharyngeal wall, sealing off the upper airway **(B)**.

Tonsils

— **Tonsils,** masses of lymphoid tissue found in the mucosal lining of the pharynx, form an incomplete circular ring called the **pharyngeal lymphatic ring** (Waldeyer's ring) around the superior part of the pharynx (**Fig. 19.43**). They include
  • **pharyngeal tonsils** (also known as adenoids) in the mucous membrane of the roof and posterior wall of the pharynx,
  • **tubal tonsils** near the orifices of the pharyngotympanic tube,
  • **palatine tonsils** in the fossae between the palatoglossal and palatopharyngeal arches, and
  • **lingual tonsils** on the posterior one third of the dorsum of the tongue.
— Tonsillar lymphatic vessels drain to the jugulodigastric node near the angle of the mandible before draining to the deep cervical lymph nodes.

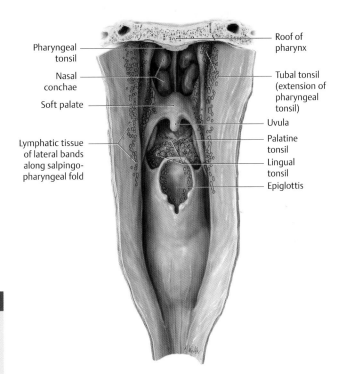

Fig. 19.43 Tonsils: Waldeyer's ring
Posterior view of the opened pharynx.

CLINICAL CORRELATION

TONSILLECTOMY During a tonsillectomy, the palatine tonsils are removed from the tonsillar bed along with their accompanying fascia. The glossopharyngeal nerve, which lies on the lateral wall of the pharynx, is vulnerable to injury during the procedure and may result in loss of sensation and taste from the posterior one third of the tongue. Bleeding may occur from the large external palatine vein or from the tonsillar branches of the facial, ascending pharyngeal, maxillary, and lingual arteries. The internal carotid artery may also be vulnerable because it runs just lateral to the tonsil.

Neurovasculature of the Pharynx

— Direct and indirect branches of the external carotid artery supply the pharynx. These include the facial, lingual, ascending palatine, descending palatine, and ascending pharyngeal arteries (see **Fig. 17.23**).

— Venous drainage of the pharynx passes through the pharyngeal venous plexus to the internal jugular vein (see **Fig. 17.29**).

— Sensory innervation of the pharyngeal mucosa varies by region **(Fig. 19.44)**.
  • The maxillary nerve (CN V_2) innervates the nasopharynx.
  • The glossopharyngeal nerve (CN IX) primarily innervates the oropharynx, although its territory extends into both the nasopharynx and laryngopharynx.
  • The vagus nerve (CN X) via its internal laryngeal branch innervates the laryngopharynx.

CLINICAL CORRELATION

GAG REFLEX The gag reflex is a reflexive contraction of the pharyngeal muscles that protects the airway by preventing accidental ingestion and aspiration. It is elicited by touching the soft palate or back of the tongue. The glossopharyngeal nerve (CN IX) is the afferent limb, and the vagus nerve (CN X) serves as the efferent limb of the reflex.

B Glossopharyngeal n. in the oropharynx.

A Maxillary n. in the nasopharynx.

Fig. 19.44 Sensory innervation of the pharynx

C Vagus n. in the laryngopharynx.

20 The Eye and Ear

The eye, the organ of vision, and the ear, which contains the organs for hearing and balance, are anatomically the most complex of the sense organs. The eyes, enclosed within the bony orbits, are prominent features of the face. The ears have superficial and deep components that are related to the temporal bones on the sides of the head.

20.1 The Eye

The anatomy of the eye includes the bony orbit, the eyelids and lacrimal apparatus, the eyeball, and six extraocular muscles.

The Bony Orbit

The paired **orbits** lie on either side of the superior part of the nasal cavity, above the maxillary sinuses and below the anterior cranial fossae (see **Fig. 17.15**). These cavities are shaped like quadrangular pyramids with the apex directed posteriorly and the base opening onto the face (**Fig. 20.1**).

— Seven bones of the skull form the bony orbit:
  1. the frontal bone, which forms the roof;
  2. the maxilla, which forms the floor;
  3. the ethmoid,

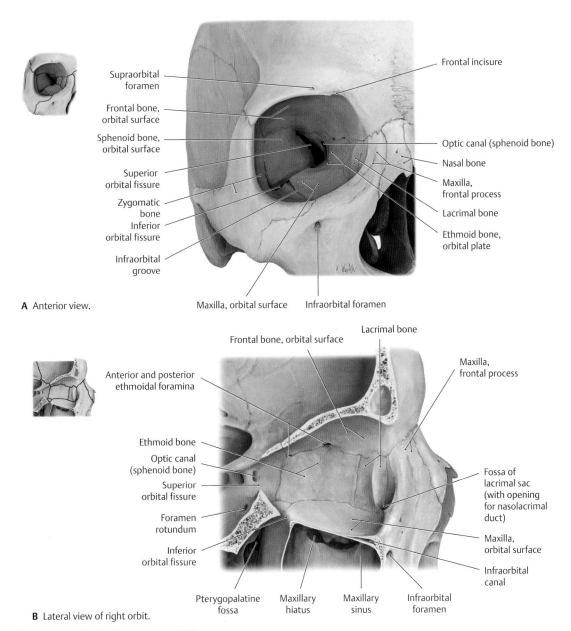

A Anterior view.

B Lateral view of right orbit.

Fig. 20.1 **Bones of the orbit** (*continued on page 484*)

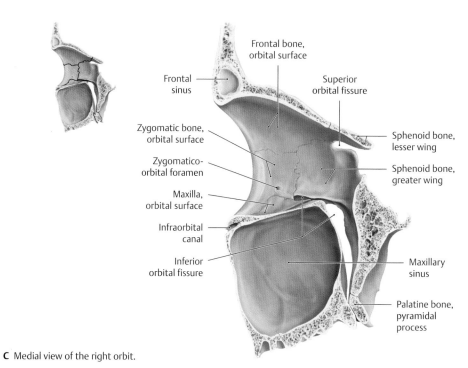

C Medial view of the right orbit.

Fig. 20.1 (*continued*) **Bones of the orbit**

4. lacrimal,
5. palatine, and
6. sphenoid bones, which form the medial wall; and
7. the zygomatic bone, which, along with the sphenoid bone, forms the lateral wall.

— Numerous openings allow nerves and vessels to pass between the orbit and the middle cranial fossa, the nasal cavity, the pterygopalatine fossa, and the face (**Table 20.1**).

— The eyeball occupies the anterior part of the orbit, accompanied by six extraocular muscles, ophthalmic vessels, and five cranial nerves (optic, oculomotor, trochlear, trigeminal, and abducent). Periorbital fat supports and surrounds these structures.

Table 20.1 **Openings in the Orbit for Neurovascular Structures**

Opening*	Nerves	Vessels
Optic canal	Optic n. (CN II)	Ophthalmic a.
Superior orbital fissure	Oculomotor n. (CN III) Trochlear n. (CN IV) Abducent n. (CN VI) Trigeminal n., ophthalmic division (CN V_1) • Lacrimal n. • Frontal n. • Nasociliary n.	Superior ophthalmic v.
Inferior orbital fissure	Infraorbital n. (CN V_2) Zygomatic n. (CN V_2)	Infraorbital a. and v., inferior ophthalmic v.
Infraorbital canal	Infraorbital n. (CN V_2), a., and v.	
Supraorbital foramen	Supraorbital n. (lateral branch)	Supraorbital a.
Frontal incisure	Supraorbital n. (medial branch)	Supratrochlear a.
Anterior ethmoidal foramen	Anterior ethmoidal n., a., and v.	
Posterior ethmoidal foramen	Posterior ethmoidal n., a., and v.	

* The nasolacrimal canal transmits the nasolacrimal duct.

Eyelids and Lacrimal Apparatus

The upper and lower **eyelids** are movable folds of skin that protect the eyeball from injury, irritation, and light. They are separated from each other by the **palpebral fissure (Fig. 20.2).**

— The eyelids are covered externally by skin and internally by the **palpebral conjunctiva**. This thin inner membrane reflects at the **superior** and **inferior fornices** onto the anterior eyeball as the **bulbar (ocular) conjunctiva**. When the eyes are closed, the palpebral and bulbar conjunctivae form the **conjunctival sac.**

— **Tarsal plates** or **tarsus**, bands of dense connective tissue that provide support for both the upper and lower eyelids, are attached to **medial** and **lateral palpebral ligaments**, which connect to the medial and lateral margins of the orbit, respectively. Tarsal glands within the tarsal plates lubricate the edges of the eyelids to prevent them from sticking together.

— The **orbicularis oculi muscle** (see **Fig. 19.2**), innervated by the facial nerve (cranial nerve [CN] VII), closes the eye in a sphincter-like fashion. The **levator palpebrae superioris muscle**, innervated by the oculomotor nerve (CN III) and attached to the superior tarsal plate, opens the eye by lifting the upper eyelid.

— An **orbital septum**, which connects the tarsal plates to the margins of the orbit, holds the orbital fat within the orbit and helps to limit the spread of infection to and from the orbit.

The **lacrimal apparatus** produces and drains tears that cleanse and lubricate the outer surface of the eye (**Fig. 20.3**).

— The **lacrimal gland**, which produces and secretes tears, resides in the lacrimal fossa in the supralateral aspect of the orbit. Secretomotor parasympathetic fibers from the facial nerve (CN VII) stimulate the gland (see **Fig. 18.27**).

— Blinking of the eye sweeps the tears across the eye toward the medial angle, where they drain via **superior** and **inferior puncta** (openings) into **lacrimal canaliculi** and the **lacrimal sac**, the dilated superior part of the nasolacrimal duct.

— The **nasolacrimal duct** is a membranous structure that begins in the medial angle of the eye and terminates in the inferior meatus of the nasal cavity. Tears drain into the nasal cavity via this duct.

Paries superior orbitae
Periorbita
M. levator palpebrae superioris
M. rectus superior
Septum orbitale
Fornix conjunctivae superior
Pars orbitalis musculi orbicularis oculi
M. tarsalis superior
Tarsus superior with gll. tarsales
Palpebra superior
Lens
Cornea
Iris
Corpus ciliare
Tarsus inferior
Gll. ciliares and sebaceae
Retina
Sclera
M. tarsalis inferior
Palpebra inferior
Pars palpebralis musculi orbicularis oculi
N. infraorbitalis

Fornix conjunctivae superior
Tunica conjunctiva bulbi
Tunica conjunctiva palpebrarum (tarsal conjunctiva)
Fornical conjunctiva
Fornix conjunctivae inferior

A Sagittal section through the anterior orbital cavity.

B Anatomy of the conjunctiva.

Fig. 20.2 Eyelids and conjunctiva

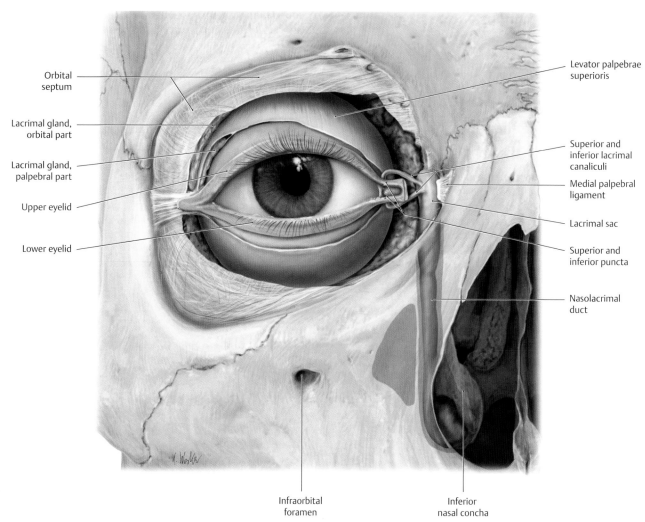

Orbital
septum

Lacrimal gland,
orbital part

Lacrimal gland,
palpebral part

Upper eyelid

Lower eyelid

Levator palpebrae
superioris

Superior and
inferior lacrimal
canaliculi

Medial palpebral
ligament

Lacrimal sac

Superior and
inferior puncta

Nasolacrimal
duct

Infraorbital
foramen

Inferior
nasal concha

Fig. 20.3 Lacrimal apparatus
Right eye, anterior view.
Removed: Orbital septum (partial). *Divided:* Levator palpebrae superioris (tendon of insertion).

The Eyeball

The eyeball, the organ of vision, has three concentric layers that form its outer walls: the sclera, the choroid, and the retina (**Fig. 20.4**).

— The **sclera**, the white part of the eye, forms the posterior five sixths of the outer fibrous layer of the eye; the **cornea**, the transparent part of the sclera, forms the anterior sixth. This outer layer is largely avascular but provides structure to the eyeball.

— The **choroid**, the middle vascular layer, provides oxygen and nutrients to the underlying retina (**Fig. 20.5**).

• The **ciliary body** connects the choroid with the circumference of the iris. Short, smooth muscle fibers, **zonular fibers**, which attach the ciliary body to the lens, control the thickness and refractive power of the lens and therefore the focus of the eye.

• The **iris**, an adjustable muscular diaphragm, surrounds a central aperture, the **pupil**.

    ○ The **pupillary sphincter muscle** of the iris responds to parasympathetic stimulation to constrict the pupil.

    ○ The **pupillary dilator muscle** of the iris responds to sympathetic stimulation to dilate the pupil.

— The **retina**, the inner sensory layer, has a posterior **optic part** that is sensitive to light and a **nonvisual part** that continues anteriorly over the ciliary body and iris.

• The **optic disk**, a point on the retina where the optic nerve exits the eyeball, lacks photoreceptors and therefore is insensitive to light and is known as the **blind spot**.

• The **macula** of the retina, a spot lateral to the optic disk, is an area of intense visual acuity.

• The **fovea centralis**, a depression in the macula, is the area of greatest visual acuity.

— Light passes through four refractive media before focusing on the retina of the eye:

1. The cornea, the primary refractive medium for light entering the eye

2. The **aqueous humor**, a watery solution that fills the **anterior** and **posterior chambers** of the eye that lie anterior to the lens and ciliary body. The balance between its production and drainage determines the intraocular pressure.

3. The **lens**, a transparent biconcave disk that focuses objects on the retina by changing its thickness. In the process of **accommodation**, which is mediated by parasympathetic

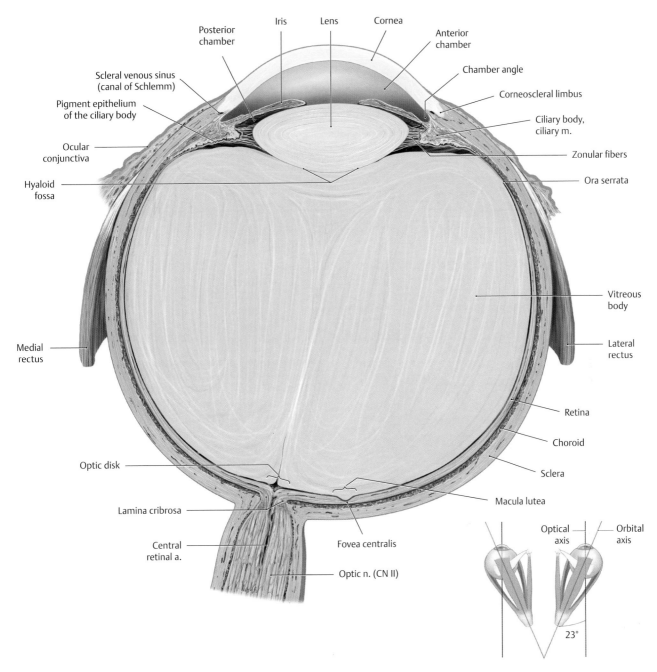

Fig. 20.4 Structure of the eyeball
Transverse section through the right eyeball, superior view.

stimulation, the ciliary muscle contracts, causing the lens to thicken and bring near objects into focus.

4. The **vitreous body**, a jelly-like substance that fills the chamber of the eye posterior to the lens.

CLINICAL CORRELATION

CORNEAL REFLEX A positive corneal reflex is the bilateral contraction of the orbicularis oculi muscles (a blink) when the cornea is touched or exposed to bright light. The afferent limb is the nasociliary nerve of the ophthalmic division of the trigeminal nerve (CN V$_1$); the efferent limb is the facial nerve (CN VII). The reflex protects the eye from foreign bodies and bright light.

CLINICAL CORRELATION

PUPILLARY LIGHT REFLEX The pupillary light reflex is rapid constriction (miosis) of both pupils (via the constrictor pupillae muscle) in response to shining a light into the eye. The afferent limb of the reflex is the optic nerve (CN II). The efferent limb is the parasympathetic fibers of the oculomotor nerve (CN III). Both pupils constrict because each retina sends fibers into the optic tracts of both sides. If the parasympathetic fibers are interrupted, both pupils dilate (mydriasis) as a result of the unopposed sympathetic outflow to the dilator pupillae muscle. This reflex mediates papillary aperture variation and is therefore one of the means by which the eye adapts to changes in light intensity **(Fig. 20.6)**.

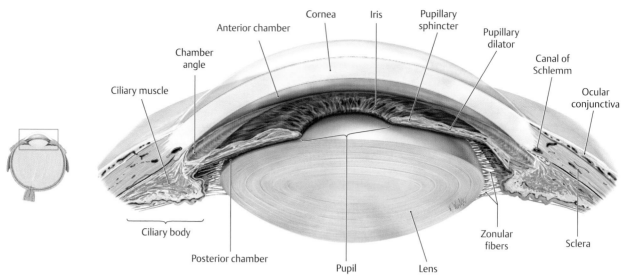

Fig. 20.5 Cornea, iris, and lens
Transverse section through the anterior segment of the eye, anterosuperior view.

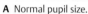

A Normal pupil size.   **B** Maximum constriction (miosis).

C Maximum dilation (mydriasis).

Fig. 20.6 Pupil
Pupil size is regulated by two intraocular muscles of the iris: the pupillary sphincter, which narrows the pupil (parasympathetic innervation), and the pupillary dilator, which enlarges it (sympathetic innervation).

CLINICAL CORRELATION

PRESBYOPIA AND CATARACTS The lens of the eye undergoes age-related changes that affect vision in the older patient. The loss of elasticity of the lens, and the subsequent loss of accommodation, diminishes a patient's ability to focus on near objects, a condition known as presbyopia. Opacities of the lens or its capsule, known as cataracts, reduce the amount of light that reaches the retina, resulting in blurred, cloudy vision. Treatment involves surgical removal of the affected lens and replacement with a plastic lens implant.

CLINICAL CORRELATION

GLAUCOMA Glaucoma refers to a group of eye diseases that involve increased intraocular pressure and atrophy of the optic nerve. In primary open-angle glaucoma, the most common form, venous channels in the angle between the cornea and the iris that allow drainage of the aqueous humor from the anterior and posterior chambers are blocked. The subsequent buildup of aqueous humor results in raised intraocular pressure and eventual damage to the optic nerve. This leads to a gradual loss of peripheral vision that progresses to tunnel vision. Pressure on the retina can lead to blindness.

Extraocular Muscles

— The six extraocular muscles that control the movement of the eyeball (**Fig. 20.7**; **Table 20.2**) include
  • four rectus muscles, the **superior rectus**, **medial rectus**, **inferior rectus**, and **lateral rectus**, that originate from a **common tendinous ring** at the apex of the orbit; and

  • two oblique muscles, the **superior oblique** that arises near the apex and reflects back via the trochlea to attach to the eyeball, and the **inferior oblique** that arises from the medial aspect of the orbital floor.
— The muscles allow six cardinal directions of gaze, which are the normal movements of the eyeball tested during clinical evaluation of ocular mobility (**Fig. 20.8**).

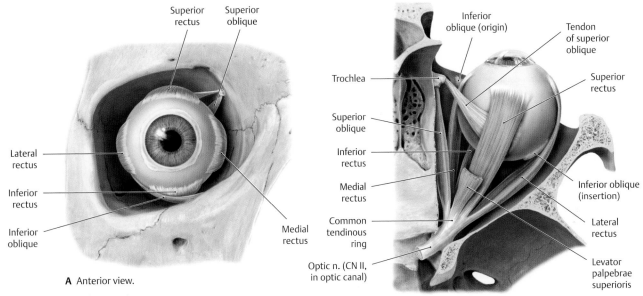

A Anterior view.

B Opened orbit, superior view.

Fig. 20.7 Extraocular muscles
Right eye.

A Superior rectus. **B** Medial rectus. **C** Inferior rectus. **D** Lateral rectus. **E** Superior oblique. **F** Inferior oblique.

Table 20.2 **Actions of the Extraocular Muscles**

Muscle	Origin	Insertion	Action* Vertical Axis (red)	Action* Horizontal Axis (black)	Action* Anteroposterior Axis (blue)	Innervation
Superior rectus	Common tendinous ring (common annular tendon)	Sclera of the eye	Elevates	Adducts	Rotates medially	Oculomotor n. (CN III), superior branch
Medial rectus			–	Adducts	–	Oculomotor n. (CN III), inferior branch
Inferior rectus			Depresses	Adducts	Rotates laterally	
Lateral rectus			–	Abducts	–	Abducent n. (CN VI)
Superior oblique	Sphenoid bone⁺		Depresses	Abducts	Rotates medially	Trochlear n. (CN IV)
Inferior oblique	Medial orbital margin		Elevates	Abducts	Rotates laterally	Oculomotor n. (CN III), inferior branch

*Starting from gaze directed anteriorly.
⁺The tendon of insertion of the superior oblique passes through a tendinous loop (trochlea) attached to the superomedial orbital margin.

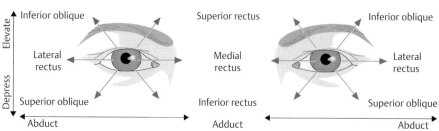

A Starting with the eyes directed anteriorly, movement to any of the cardinal directions of gaze (*arrows*) requires activation of two extraocular muscles, each of which is innervated by a different cranial nerve, thus testing the function of those pairs of muscles.

B Starting with the eyes adducted or abducted, elevating or lowering the eyes activates only the oblique or rectus muscles, respectively, allowing for the testing of the function of individual muscles.

Fig. 20.8 Testing the extraocular muscles

Neurovasculature of the Orbit

— The ophthalmic artery supplies most structures of the orbit (**Fig. 20.9**). One of its branches, the **central retinal artery**, runs within the optic nerve and is the sole arterial supply to the retina through its terminal branches.
  • The ophthalmic artery anastomoses with the facial artery through its supratrochlear branch and with the maxillary artery through its anterior and posterior ethmoidal and middle meningeal branches.
— The **superior** and **inferior ophthalmic veins**, which drain structures in the orbit, primarily drain into the cavernous sinus but also communicate with the facial vein and pterygoid venous plexus (**Fig. 20.10**).

— Six cranial nerves (optic, oculomotor, trochlear, trigeminal, abducent, and facial) innervate structures in the orbit (**Table 20.3**; **Figs. 20.11** and **20.12**).
  • The optic nerve (CN I) transmits images from the retina.
  • The oculomotor nerve (CN III), trochlear nerve (CN IV), and abducent nerve (CN VI) innervate the extraocular muscles.
  • The ophthalmic division of the trigeminal nerve (CN V$_1$) carries general sensory fibers from structures in the orbit and distributes postganglionic autonomic fibers to target organs of the orbit and face.
  • The facial nerve (CN VII) provides secretomotor (parasympathetic) innervation to the lacrimal gland.

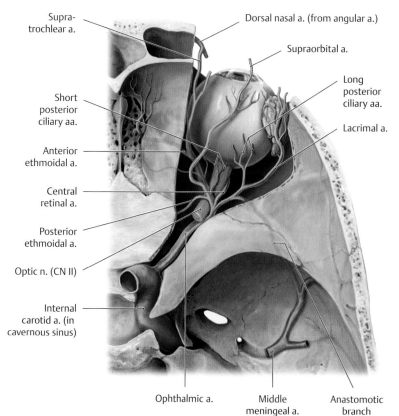

Fig. 20.9 Arteries of the orbit
Right orbit, superior view. *Opened:* optic canal and orbital roof.

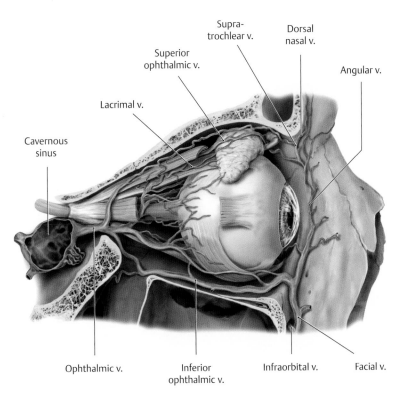

Fig. 20.10 Veins of the orbit
Right orbit, lateral view. *Removed:* lateral orbital wall.
Opened: maxillary sinus.

Table 20.3 **Nerves of the Orbit**

Nerve	Nerve Fibers	Distribution
Optic (CN II)	Special sensory for vision	Retina
Oculomotor (CN III)	Somatic motor	Muscles of the orbit, except the lateral rectus and superior oblique muscles
	Parasympathetic: synapse in ciliary ganglion; postsynaptic fibers travel with nasociliary n. (CN V₁)	Pupilary sphincter muscle and ciliary body
Trochlear (CN IV)	Somatic motor	Superior oblique muscle
Ophthalmic (CN V)		
Lacrimal	General sensory	Lacrimal gland, upper lateral eyeball
Frontal		
- Supratrochlear	General sensory	Anterior scalp
- Supraorbital	General sensory	Anterior scalp
Short ciliary	General sensory	Ciliary body and iris
	Parasympathetic (CN III) and sympathetic	
Nasociliary		
- Anterior and posterior ethmoidal	General sensory	Nasal cavity, ethmoid and sphenoid sinuses
- Infratrochlear	General sensory	External nose, conjunctiva, lacrimal sac
- Long ciliary	General sensory	Iris and cornea
	Sympathetic (carotid plexus)	Pupil dilator
Abducent (CN VI)	Somatic motor	Lateral rectus muscle
Facial (CN VII)	Parasympathetic: synapse in pterygopalatine ganglion; postsynaptic fibers travel with zygomatic n. (CN V₂)	Lacrimal gland

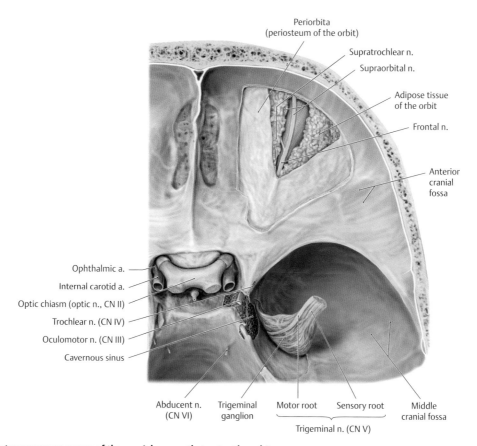

Fig. 20.11 Intracavernous course of the cranial nerves that enter the orbit

Superior view of the anterior and middle cranial fossae, right side. The lateral and superior walls of the cavernous sinus have been opened and the trigeminal ganglion has been retracted laterally. The orbital roof has been removed and the periorbita has been fenestrated. The three cranial nerves that supply the ocular muscles (CN III, CN IV, and CN VI) pass through the cavernous sinus with CN V$_1$ and CN V$_2$ and the internal carotid artery. All of the nerves course along the lateral wall of the sinus except CN VI, which runs directly through the sinus in close proximity to the artery. Because of this relationship, the CN VI may be damaged as a result of a sinus thrombosis or an intracavernous aneurysm of the internal carotid artery.

Fig. 20.12 Innervation of the orbit

Right orbit, lateral view. *Removed:* Temporal bony wall.

OCULOMOTOR NERVE INJURY The oculomotor nerve innervates most of the extraocular muscles. With paralysis of these muscles, the eye is directed downward and outward because of the unopposed action of the lateral rectus (innervated by the abducent nerve) and superior oblique (innervated by the trochlear nerve). The dilator pupillae is also unopposed, so the pupil remains fully dilated. Paralysis of the levator palpebrae superior causes the superior eyelid to droop.

— Autonomic innervation of structures in the orbit includes the following:
  • Sympathetic fibers from the carotid plexus innervate the ciliary body and pupillary dilator muscle (responsible for pupil dilation).
  • Parasympathetic fibers from the oculomotor nerve (CN III) synapse in the ciliary ganglion and travel via the short ciliary nerves to innervate the ciliary body and pupillary sphincter muscles (responsible for pupil constriction).

HORNER'S SYNDROME Horner's syndrome is a kaleidoscope of symptoms resulting from disruption of the cervical sympathetic trunk in the neck. The absence of sympathetic innervation is manifested on the affected side of the face as pupillary constriction (miosis), a sunken eye (enophthalmos), drooping of the upper eyelid (ptosis), loss of sweating (anhydrosis), and vasodilation.

  • Parasympathetic fibers from the facial nerve (CN VII) synapse in the pterygopalatine ganglion and travel via the zygomatic nerve (CN V_2) to innervate the lacrimal gland (responsible for tear secretion).

20.2 The Ear

The ear, which contains the organs for hearing and equilibrium, is divided into external, middle, and internal parts (**Fig. 20.13**).

The External Ear

The external ear collects and conducts sound.
— The **auricle**, the visible external part of the ear, has a skeleton composed of elastic cartilage that is covered by skin.
— The **external acoustic meatus** (external auditory canal), a canal that extends 2 to 3 cm from the auricle to the tympanic membrane, conducts sound waves toward the middle ear. The outer third of the canal is cartilaginous, and the inner two thirds are formed by the temporal bone. Ceruminous and sebaceous glands in the subcutaneous tissue lining the cartilaginous part secrete earwax.
— The **tympanic membrane**, a thin, transparent membrane, separates the external and middle ear.
  • Skin covers the tympanic membrane externally, and a mucous membrane lines it internally.
  • The concave outer surface of the membrane has a central conelike depression, the **umbo**.

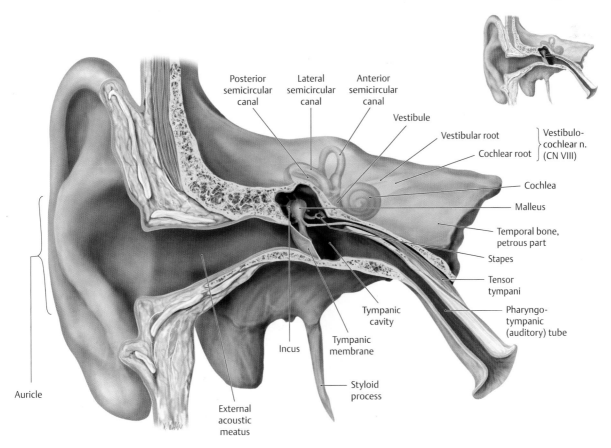

Fig. 20.13 Ear
Coronal section through the right ear, anterior view.

Auriculotemporal n.
(trigeminal n., CN V)

Vagus n. (CN X) and
glossopharyngeal n.
(CN IX)

Facial n. (CN VII)

Facial n.

Lesser occipital nn. and great
auricular n. (cervical plexus)

A Right auricle, lateral view.

B Right auricle, posterior view.

Fig. 20.14 **Innervation of the auricle**

- A thin, superior portion of the membrane, the **flaccid part** (pars flaccida), is distinct from the rest of the membrane, the **tense part** (pars tensa).
— Posterior auricular and anterior auricular arteries, branches of the superficial temporal artery, supply the external ear.
— Sensation from the external ear is transmitted by the cervical plexus and three cranial nerves **(Fig. 20.14)**:
  - the great auricular nerve (cervical plexus) from the auricle;
  - the auriculotemporal nerve, a branch of CN V_3, from the auricle and external surface of the tympanic membrane;
  - the auricular branch of the vagus nerve (CN X) from the external surface of the tympanic membrane; and
  - the glossopharyngeal nerve (CN IX) from the internal surface of the tympanic membrane.

The Middle Ear

— The middle ear, also known as the **tympanic cavity**, is an air-filled chamber housed in the petrous portion of the temporal bone **(Figs. 20.15, 20.16, 20.17)**.
  - Anteriorly, a **pharyngotympanic tube**, which connects the tympanic cavity to the nasopharynx, helps equalize pressure in the middle ear.
  - Posteriorly, the **aditus** (inlet) to the **mastoid antrum** (a cavity in the mastoid process of the temporal bone) connects the tympanic cavity to the bony meshwork of **mastoid air cells**.
  - A thin bony plate, the **tegmen tympani**, forms the roof of the tympanic cavity and separates it from the middle cranial fossa.

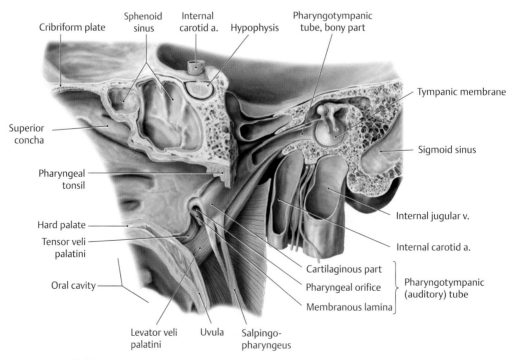

Cribriform plate

Sphenoid sinus

Internal carotid a.

Hypophysis

Pharyngotympanic tube, bony part

Tympanic membrane

Superior concha

Sigmoid sinus

Pharyngeal tonsil

Hard palate

Internal jugular v.

Tensor veli palatini

Internal carotid a.

Oral cavity

Cartilaginous part

Pharyngeal orifice

Pharyngotympanic (auditory) tube

Membranous lamina

Levator veli palatini

Uvula

Salpingo-pharyngeus

Fig. 20.15 **Tympanic cavity and pharyngotympanic tube**
Medial view of opened tympanic cavity.

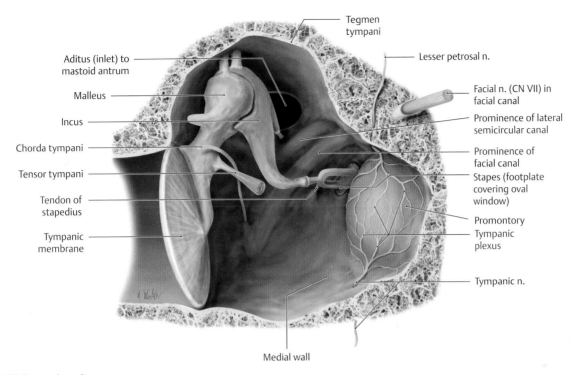

Fig. 20.16 Tympanic cavity
Right tympanic cavity, anterior view. *Removed:* Anterior wall.

- The medial wall, which separates the tympanic cavity from the internal ear, has a **promontory**, covered by the tympanic nerve plexus, and two openings, the **oval** and **round windows** (see **Fig. 20.19**).
— The **auditory ossicles**, the **malleus**, **incus**, and **stapes** bones of the middle ear, articulate with each other through synovial joints and form a bony chain between the tympanic membrane and the oval window of the internal ear.
- The handle of the malleus is embedded in the tympanic membrane, and its head articulates with the incus.
- The **incus** articulates with the malleus and stapes.

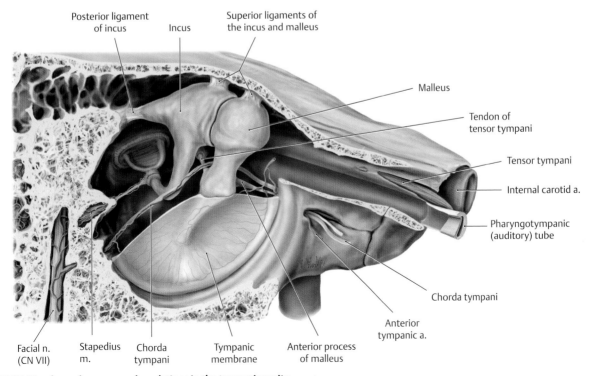

Fig. 20.17 Muscles and neurovascular relations in the tympanic cavity
Right middle ear, lateral view.

- The head of the **stapes** articulates with the incus, and its base fits into the oval window of the bony labyrinth of the internal ear.
— Muscles of the middle ear dampen the movements of the auditory ossicles, thereby lessening the sound transmitted from the external ear.
  - The **tensor tympani**, which is innervated by a branch of the mandibular nerve (CN V$_3$), lessens the damage from loud sounds by tensing the tympanic membrane.
  - The **stapedius**, which is innervated by a branch of the facial nerve (CN VII), dampens the vibrations of the stapes on the oval window.
— The ascending pharyngeal, maxillary, and posterior auricular branches of the external carotid artery and a small branch of the internal carotid artery supply the middle ear.
— The chorda tympani, a branch of the facial nerve (CN VII), has no branches in the middle ear but passes between the malleus and incus to exit the cavity through a small opening in the temporal bone.
— The glossopharyngeal nerve (CN IX) transmits sensation from the tympanic cavity and pharyngotympanic tube. Preganglionic parasympathetic fibers carried in the tympanic nerve (a branch of the glossopharyngeal nerve) synapse in the otic ganglion. The postganglionic fibers join with sympathetic fibers of the internal carotid plexus to form the tympanic plexus (see **Fig. 18.31**).

CLINICAL CORRELATION

OTITIS MEDIA Otitis media is an infection of the middle ear that occurs commonly in children often following an upper respiratory tract infection. Fluid that accumulates in the middle ear can temporarily diminish hearing, and inflammation of the lining of the tympanic cavity can block the pharyngotympanic tube.

CLINICAL CORRELATION

HYPERACUSIS The stapedius muscle protects the delicate inner ear by modifying the vibrations of very loud sounds as they are transmitted through the middle ear to the stapes. Paralysis of the muscle resulting from a lesion of the facial nerve causes an extreme sensitivity to sound, a condition known as hyperacusis.

The Internal Ear

— The internal ear, which contains the organ for hearing, the auditory apparatus, and the organ for balance, the vestibular apparatus, is encased within the petrous part of the temporal bone (**Figs. 20.18** and **20.19**) and consists of the following:
  - A bony **otic capsule**, which forms the walls of the bony labyrinth
  - A **bony labyrinth**, a series of chambers and canals within the otic capsule containing the fluid **perilymph**. It includes the **cochlea**, the **vestibule**, and the **semicircular canals**.
  - A **membranous labyrinth**, a series of sacs and ducts suspended within the bony labyrinth, and filled with a fluid, **endolymph**. The membranous labyrinth is made up of
    ◦ the **cochlear duct** contained within the cochlea,
    ◦ the **utricle** and **saccule** contained within the vestibule, and

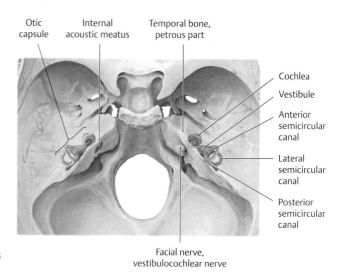

Fig. 20.18 **Projection of the otic capsule of the inner ear onto the skull** Petrous part of the temporal bone, superior view.

◦ the **semicircular ducts** contained within the semicircular canals.
— The auditory apparatus consists of the following:
  - The **cochlea**, a space within the bony labyrinth that includes the bony **cochlear** (spiral) **canal**, which makes 2.5 turns around its axis, the **modiolus** (**Fig. 20.20A**). The basal turn of the cochlea forms the promontory on the medial wall of the middle ear and contains the round window, which is closed by a membrane.

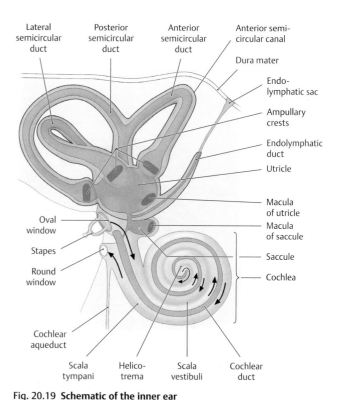

Fig. 20.19 **Schematic of the inner ear**
Right lateral view. The inner ear is embedded within the petrous part of the temporal bone. It is composed of a membranous labyrinth filled with endolymph floating within a similarly shaped bony labyrinth filled with perilymph.

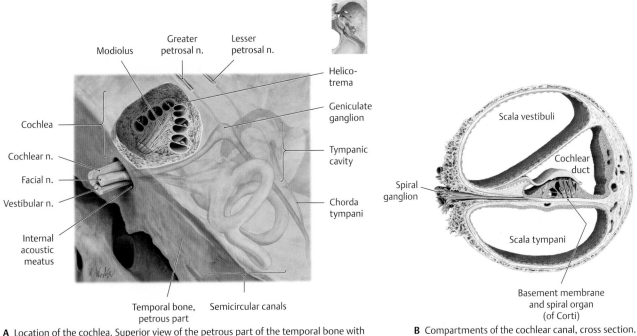

A Location of the cochlea. Superior view of the petrous part of the temporal bone with the cochlea sectioned transversely.

B Compartments of the cochlear canal, cross section.

Fig. 20.20 Auditory apparatus

- The **cochlear duct**, part of the membranous labyrinth, which is a blind-ended duct filled with endolymph and suspended within the cochlear canal **(Fig. 20.20B)**:
  - The cochlear duct divides the cochlear canal into two channels, the **scala vestibuli** and **scala tympani**, which are continuous with each other at the helicotrema, a space at the apex of the canal.
  - At the base of the cochlea, the scala vestibuli lies against the oval window, and the scala tympani lies against the round window.
- The **spiral organ** (of Corti), which contains the sensory receptors for hearing, and is embedded in the **basement membrane** on the floor of the cochlear duct

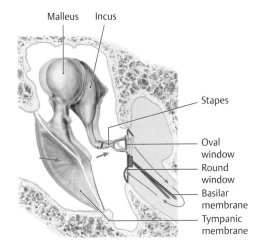

Fig. 20.21 Propagation of sound waves by the ossicular chain

— The sequence of sound transmission through the ear involves **(Fig. 20.21)** the following:
  1. Transmission of sound waves from the external ear and external acoustic meatus to the tympanic membrane of the middle ear. The waves vibrate the auditory ossicles and, in turn, the oval window that is attached to the base of the stapes.
  2. Transmission of vibrations of the oval window to the perilymph of the scala vestibuli, which creates pressure waves that displace the basement membrane and spiral organ of the cochlear duct. Nerve endings in the spiral organ transmit impulses to the brain along the cochlear nerve.
  3. Transmission of the pressure waves of the perilymph from the scala vestibuli along the scala tympani to the round window, with dissipation into the tympanic cavity.
— The vestibular apparatus consists of the following (see **Fig. 20.19**):
  - The vestibule of the bony labyrinth that communicates with the cochlea and semicircular canals
    - A small extension, the **vestibular aqueduct**, communicates with the posterior cranial fossa and contains the **endolymphatic sac**, a membranous storage space for excess endolymph.
  - The utricle and saccule, part of the membranous labyrinth, which lie within the vestibule
    - The utricle communicates with the semicircular ducts; the saccule communicates with the cochlear duct.
    - Both the utricle and saccule contain specialized sensory fields called **maculae**, which occupy different positions in space and are sensitive to movement of the endolymph in the horizontal and vertical planes.

- Three semicircular canals of the bony labyrinth, which are arranged perpendicular to one another and communicate with the vestibule. Each canal has a swelling at one end, the **bony ampulla**.
- Three semicircular ducts, parts of the membranous labyrinth contained within the semicircular canals, that communicate with the utricle
  - An **ampulla** at one end of each semicircular duct contains the **ampullary crest**, an area of sensory epithelium. The ampullary crests respond to motion of the endolymph within the ducts caused by rotation of the head.
— The membranous labyrinth receives its blood supply from the internal auditory artery, a branch of the basilar artery via its anterior inferior cerebellar artery.
— The **vestibular** and **cochlear nerves** within the internal acoustic meatus form the vestibulocochlear nerve (CN VIII) (see **Fig. 18.30**)
- The vestibular nerve innervates organs of the vestibular apparatus: the maculae of the utricle and saccule and the ampullary crests of the semicircular canals. Neuron cell bodies lie within the vestibular ganglion in the internal acoustic meatus.

- The cochlear nerve innervates the spiral organ (of Corti) in the cochlea. Neuron cell bodies lie in the spiral ganglion of the cochlea at the modiolus.

CLINICAL CORRELATION

MENIERE'S DISEASE Meniere's disease is an inner ear disorder resulting from blockage of the cochlear duct. Recurring episodes are characterized by tinnitus (ringing or buzzing in the ear), vertigo (the illusion of movement), and hearing loss. The hearing loss may fluctuate in intensity and from ear to ear but eventually becomes permanent.

CLINICAL CORRELATION

VERTIGO, TINNITUS, AND HEARING LOSS Trauma to the ear can cause three types of symptoms: vertigo, tinnitus, and hearing loss. Vertigo refers to the illusion of movement, or dizziness, and results from injury to the semicircular canals. Tinnitus refers to a ringing in the ears and is a disorder involving the cochlear duct. Causes of hearing loss can be either peripheral or centrally located. Conductive hearing loss occurs when there is impaired transmission of sound waves through the auditory canal to the auditory ossicles. Sensorineural hearing loss occurs when there is damage to the pathway between the cochlea and the brain.

21 The Neck

The neck extends from the base of the skull to the clavicles and manubrium. It contains vital neurovascular structures that supply the head, the thorax, and the upper limb. The neck also contains viscera of the gastrointestinal, respiratory, and endocrine systems.

21.1 Regions of the Neck

The regions of the neck, defined by muscular and skeletal boundaries, are largely descriptive rather than functional, but they are useful for understanding the topographic relationships in the neck, which often play a significant role in medical practice (**Table 21.1; Figs. 21.1**). Refer to Section 21.8 for detailed anatomic relations of these regions.

— The **anterior cervical region** (anterior triangle) extends from the midline of the neck to the anterior border of the sternocleidomastoid muscle.
  • The region is further divided into **submandibular, submental, muscular,** and **carotid triangles.**
  • The anterior region contains most of the cervical viscera, which includes the lower pharynx, esophagus, larynx, trachea, thyroid, and parathyroid glands.
— The **sternocleidomastoid region** is a narrow area defined by the anterior and posterior borders of the sternocleidomastoid muscle.
  • Inferiorly, the sternal and clavicular heads of the muscle define the small **lesser supraclavicular fossa.**
  • This region contains parts of the major vascular structures of the neck.
— The **lateral cervical region** (posterior triangle) extends from the posterior border of the sternocleidomastoid muscle to the anterior border of the trapezius muscle.
  • The posterior belly of the omohyoid muscle divides this region into **omoclavicular** and **occipital triangles.**
  • The scalene muscles and cervical and brachial plexuses are located in this region.
— The **posterior cervical region** extends from the anterior border of the trapezius muscle to the posterior midline of the neck.
  • It contains the trapezius and suboccipital muscles, the vertebral artery, and posterior branches of the cervical plexus.
— The **root of neck,** a transition area for structures passing between the thorax and neck, is enclosed by the superior thoracic aperture, which is formed by the manubrium, the first ribs and their costal cartilages, and the first thoracic vertebra.
  • It contains the trachea, esophagus, common carotid and subclavian arteries, brachiocephalic veins, vagus and phrenic nerves, the sympathetic trunk, the thoracic duct, and the apex of each lung.

A Right anterior oblique view.

B Left posterior oblique view.

Table 21.1 **Regions of the Neck**

Region	Divisions	Contents
① Anterior cervical region (triangle)	Submandibular (digastric) triangle	Submandibular gland and lymph nodes, hypoglossal n. (CN XII), facial a. and v.
	Submental triangle	Submental lymph nodes
	Muscular triangle	Sternothyroid and sternohyoid muscles, thyroid and parathyroid glands
	Carotid triangle	Carotid bifurcation, carotid body, hypoglossal (CN XII) and vagus (CN X) nn.
② Sternocleidomastoid region*		Sternocleidomastoid, common carotid a., internal jugular v., vagus n. (CN X), jugular lymph nodes
③ Lateral cervical region (posterior triangle)	Omoclavicular (subclavian) triangle	Subclavian a., subscapular a., supraclavicular l.n.
	Occipital triangle	Accessory n. (CN XI), trunks of brachial plexus, transverse cervical a., cervical plexus (posterior branches)
④ Posterior cervical region		Nuchal muscles, vertebral a., cervical plexus

* The sternocleidomastoid region also contains the lesser supraclavicular fossa.

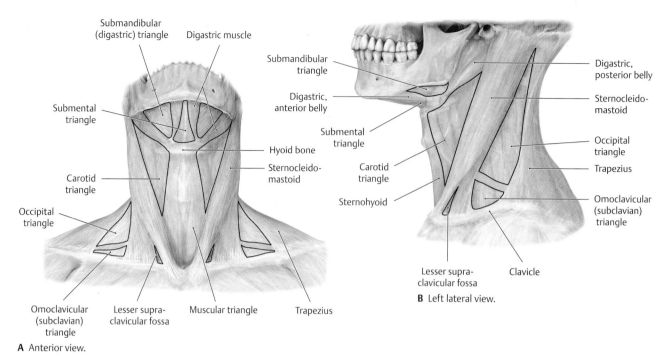

A Anterior view.

Fig. 21.1 Cervical regions

21.2   Deep Fascia of the Neck

Layers of **deep cervical fascia** surround and compartmentalize the structures of the neck **(Fig. 21.2; Table 21.2)**.

— The **investing** (superficial) **layer of the deep fascia** of the neck, a thin layer that lies deep to the skin, surrounds the entire neck but splits to enclose the sternocleidomastoid and trapezius muscles and contains cutaneous nerves, superficial vessels, and superficial lymphatics of the neck.
— The **pretracheal fascia** in the anterior neck has a muscular lamina (layer) that encloses the infrahyoid muscles and a visceral lamina that encloses the viscera of the anterior neck.

— The **prevertebral fascia** surrounds the vertebral column and the deep neck muscles and is continuous with the **nuchal fascia** posteriorly.
— The **carotid sheath,** a condensation of the pretracheal, prevertebral, and investing fasciae, forms a narrow cylindrical tube that encloses the neurovascular bundle of the neck: the internal jugular vein, common carotid artery, and vagus nerve.
— The **retropharyngeal space,** a potential space between the visceral layer of the pretracheal fascia and the prevertebral fascia, extends from the base of the skull superiorly to the superior mediastinum inferiorly.

Fig. 21.2 Fascial layers in the anterior neck

A Transverse section at level of C5 vertebra.

Retro-pharyngeal phase ④

Nuchal ligament

Spinal cord

B Midsagittal section, left lateral view.

Table 21.2 **Deep Cervical Fascia**

Layer	Type of Fascia	Description
① Investing (superficial) layer	Muscular	Envelopes entire neck; splits to enclose sternocleidomastoid and trapezius muscles
Pretracheal layer	② Muscular	Encloses infrahyoid muscles
	③ Visceral	Surrounds thyroid gland, larynx, trachea, pharynx, and esophagus
④ Prevertebral layer	Muscular	Surrounds cervical vertebral column and associated muscles
⑤ Carotid sheath	Neurovascular	Encloses common carotid artery, internal jugular vein, and vagus nerve

Note: The deep cervical fascia is divided into four layers that enclose the structures of the neck.

21.3 Muscles of the Neck

— Three muscles form the most superficial muscular layer of the neck (**Fig. 21.3; Table 21.3**):
  - The **platysma,** a muscle of facial expression, and therefore a subcutaneous muscle, that extends onto the anterolateral surfaces of the neck
  - The **sternocleidomastoid muscle,** a visible landmark that divides the neck into anterior and lateral cervical regions
  - The trapezius, a muscle of the shoulder girdle that extends onto the neck and forms the posterior border of the lateral cervical region

---

CLINICAL CORRELATION

CONGENITAL TORTICOLLIS Congenital torticollis (wryneck) is a condition in which one of the sternocleidomastoid (SCM) muscles is abnormally short, causing the head to tilt to one side with the chin pointing upward to the opposite side. This shortening is thought to be the result of trauma at birth (tears or stretching of the SCM muscle) causing bleeding and swelling within the muscle and subsequent scar tissue formation.

— Muscles attached to the hyoid bone lie between the superficial and deep neck muscles.
  - Suprahyoid muscles, the **digastric, stylohyoid, mylohyoid, geniohyoid,** and **hyoglossus,** form the floor of the mouth and elevate the hyoid and larynx during swallowing and phonation (see **Table 19.9**).
  - **Infrahyoid muscles** in the neck, **omohyoid, sternohyoid, sternothyroid,** and **thyrohyoid,** depress the hyoid and larynx during swallowing and phonation (**Fig. 21.4; Table 21.4**).
— The deep muscles of the neck lie deep to the prevertebral fascia and include the prevertebral and scalene muscles (**Fig. 21.5; Table 21.5**).

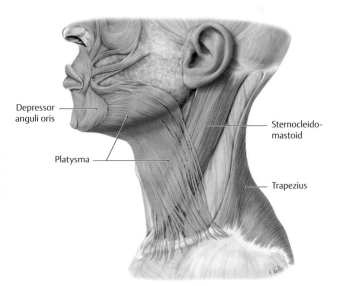

Depressor anguli oris

Platysma

Sternocleidomastoid

Trapezius

Fig. 21.3 Superficial musculature of the neck
Left lateral view.

Table 21.3 **Superficial Neck Muscles**

Muscle		Origin	Insertion	Innervation	Action
Platysma		Skin over lower neck and upper lateral thorax	Mandible (inferior border), skin over lower face and angle of mouth	Cervical branch of facial n. (CN VII)	Depresses and wrinkles skin of lower face and mouth, tenses skin of neck, aids forced depression of mandible
Sternocleidomastoid	Sternal head	Sternum (manubrium)	Temporal bone (mastoid process), occipital bone (superior nuchal line)	*Motor:* accessory n. (CN XI) *Pain and proprioception:* cervical plexus (C2, C3)	*Unilateral:* Tilts head to same side, rotates head to opposite side *Bilateral:* Extends head, aids in respiration when head is fixed
	Clavicular head	Clavicle (medial one third)			
Trapezius	Descending part	Occipital bone, spinous processes of C1–C7	Clavicle (lateral one third)		Draws scapula obliquely upward, rotates glenoid cavity superiorly

Fig. 21.4 Suprahyoid and infrahyoid muscles
Anterior view. The sternohyoid has been cut on the right side. See **Table 19.9** for the suprahyoid muscles.

Table 21.4 **Infrahyoid Muscles**

Muscle	Origin	Insertion	Innervation	Action
Omohyoid	Scapula (superior border)	Hyoid bone (body)	Ansa cervicalis of cervical plexus (C1–C3)	Depresses (fixes) hyoid, draws larynx and hyoid down for phonation and terminal phases of swallowing*
Sternohyoid	Manubrium and sternoclavicular joint (posterior surface)			
Sternothyroid	Manubrium (posterior surface)	Thyroid cartilage (oblique line)	Ansa cervicalis (C2–C3)	
Thyrohyoid	Thyroid cartilage (oblique line)	Hyoid bone (body)	C1 via hypoglossal n. (CN XII)	Depresses and fixes hyoid, raises the larynx during swallowing

*The omohyoid also tenses the cervical fascia (with an intermediate tendon).

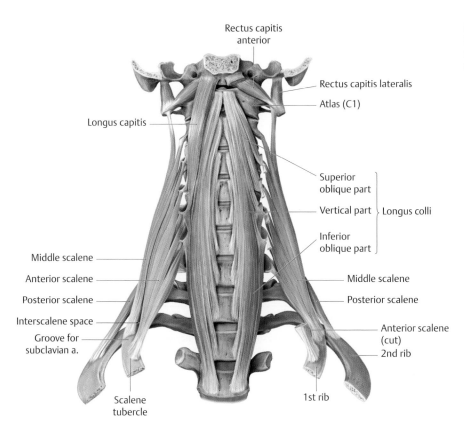

Fig. 21.5 Deep muscles of the neck
Prevertebral and scalene muscles, anterior view. *Removed:* Longus capitis and anterior scalene.

Table 21.5 **Deep Muscles of the Neck**

Muscles	Origin	Insertion	Innervation	Action
Prevertebral				
Longus capitis	Cervical and upper thoracic vertebrae	Cervical vertebrae and basilar part of occipital bone	Anterior rami of C1–C6 (cervical plexus)	Flex the head and cervical spine
Longus colli				
Rectus capitis anterior				
Rectus capitis lateralis				
Scalene				
Anterior scalene	Cervical vertebrae	1st and 2nd ribs	Anterior rami of C3–C8	Flex the cervical spine and elevate the ribs during inspiration
Middle scalene				
Posterior scalene				

21.4   Nerves of the Neck

Nerves of the neck include cervical and thoracic spinal nerves, nerves from the cervical sympathetic trunk, and cranial nerves.

Cervical Nerves

The C1–C4 spinal nerves supply the regions of the neck (**Table 21.6**).

— Anterior rami of C1–C4 cervical spinal nerves form the **cervical plexus,** which has sensory and motor components.

• The sensory nerves of the plexus, the **lesser occipital** (C2), **great auricular** (C2–C3), **transverse cervical** (C2–C3), and **supraclavicular nerves** (C3–C4), innervate the skin of the anterior and lateral neck and lateral scalp. They emerge from behind the midpoint of the posterior border of the SCM muscle, a location known as the **nerve point of the neck** (or Erb's point) (**Fig. 21.6**).

• The **ansa cervicalis** (C1–C3), the motor part of the plexus, which has a superior and inferior root, innervates all of the infrahyoid muscles except the thyrohyoid and usually lies anterior to the internal jugular vein (**Fig. 21.7**).

— The phrenic nerve, which arises from anterior rami of C3–C5 spinal nerves, descends on the surface of the anterior scalene muscle and enters the thorax, where it supplies the diaphragm with sensory and motor innervation.

— Posterior rami of cervical spinal nerves C1 through C3 form three nerves that provide motor and cutaneous innervation to the posterior neck and scalp: the **suboccipital** (C1), **greater occipital** (C2), and **3rd occipital nerves** (C3) (**Fig. 21.8**).

Table 21.6 **Branches of the Spinal Nerves in the Neck**

Posterior (Dorsal) Ramus

	Nerve	Sensory Function	Motor Function
C1	Suboccipital n.	No C1 dermatome	Innervate intrinsic nuchal muscles
C2	Greater occipital n.	Innervate C2 dermatome	
C3	3rd occipital n.	Innervate C3 dermatome	

Anterior (Ventral) Ramus

	Sensory Branches	Sensory Function	Motor Branches	Motor Function
C1	–	–	Form ansa cervicalis (motor part of cervical plexus)	Innervate infrahyoid muscles (except thyrohyoid)
C2	Lesser occipital n.	Form sensory part of cervical plexus, innervate anterior and lateral neck		
C2–C3	Great auricular n.			
	Transverse cervical n.			
C3–C4	Supraclavicular nn.		Contribute to phrenic n.*	Innervate diaphragm and pericardium*

* The anterior roots of C3–C5 combine to form the phrenic nerve.

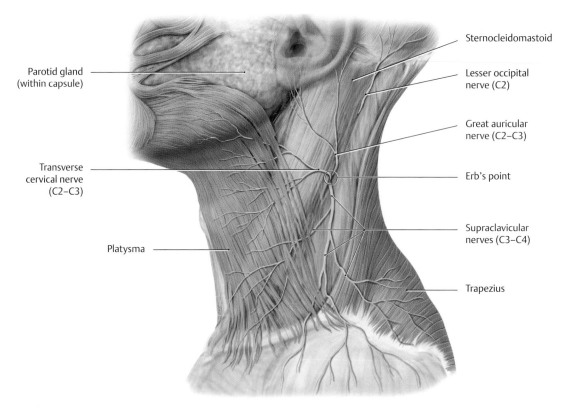

Fig. 21.6 **Sensory nerves of the cervical plexus**
Left lateral view.

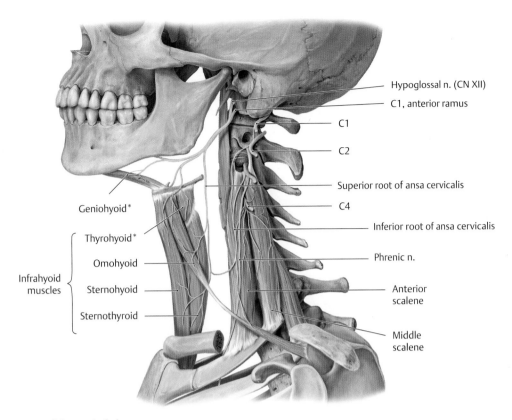

Fig. 21.7 Motor nerves of the cervical plexus
Left lateral view.
*Innervated by the anterior ramus of C1 (distributed by the hypoglossal n.).

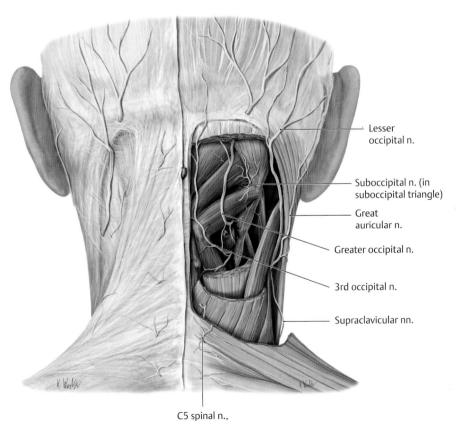

Fig. 21.8 Innervation of the nuchal region
Posterior view.

Brachial Plexus

The brachial plexus, which innervates the upper limb, forms from the anterior rami of C5–T1. It emerges through the **interscalene groove** (the space between the anterior and middle scalene muscles) in the lateral region of the neck before continuing into the axilla (see Section 13.4). Normally four branches arise from the supraclavicular part of plexus to supply muscles of the shoulder and pectoral girdle as it traverses the neck: the dorsal scapular n., suprascapular n., n. to the subclavius, and long thoracic n.

The Cervical Sympathetic Trunk

The cervical sympathetic trunk, a continuation of the thoracic sympathetic trunk, extends into the neck to the level of the C1 vertebra, where it lies anterolateral to the vertebral column and posterior to the carotid sheath.

- The cervical sympathetic trunk receives no white rami communicans from cervical spinal nerves. The preganglionic fibers that synapse in the cervical ganglia originate in thoracic spinal nerves and ascend in the sympathetic trunk to the cervical region.
- Postganglionic fibers from the cervical sympathetic ganglia are distributed along three routes:
  - Via gray rami communicans to join cervical spinal nerves
  - Via cervical cardiac (cardiopulmonary) nerves to the cardiac plexus in the thorax
  - Via sympathetic nerve plexuses surrounding vessels (periarterial plexuses), especially along the external carotid, internal carotid, and vertebral arteries, to supply structures of the head and neck
- The cervical sympathetic trunk has superior, middle, and inferior ganglia.
  - The **superior cervical ganglion** lies anterior to C1 vertebra and posterior to the internal carotid artery. Its branches include
    - the **superior cervical sympathetic cardiac nerve,**
    - branches to the **pharyngeal nerve plexus,**
    - an **internal carotid nerve** that forms the **internal carotid plexus,** and
    - an **external carotid nerve** that forms the **external carotid plexus.**
    - gray rami communicans that join anterior rami of C1–C4 spinal nerves.
  - The **middle cervical ganglion** lies at the level of the C6 vertebra and gives off the **middle cervical sympathetic cardiac nerve,** which joins the cardiac plexus in the thorax, and gray rami communicans to anterior rami of C5 and C6 spinal nerves.
  - The **inferior cervical ganglion** usually combines with the most superior thoracic ganglion (T1) to form the **stellate ganglion,** which lies anterior to the transverse process of the C7 vertebra. It gives off the **inferior cervical sympathetic cardiac nerve,** which descends into the thorax, and gray rami communicans to anterior rami of C7 and C8 spinal nerves.

Cranial Nerves in the Neck

Four of the cranial nerves are found in the neck.

- The glossopharyngeal nerve (cranial nerve [CN] IX) sends branches to the tongue and pharynx in the head and descends into the neck to innervate the carotid body and carotid sinus (see **Fig. 18.31**). It innervates one muscle, the stylopharyngeus.
- The vagus nerve (CN X) descends within the carotid sheath in the neck before entering the thorax. Its branches to cervical structures arise from both thoracic and cervical parts of the nerve (see **Fig. 18.33**).
  - **A superior laryngeal nerve** arises from the cervical part of each vagus nerve and innervates the upper larynx through its internal and external branches.
  - The **right recurrent laryngeal nerve** arises from the inferior cervical part of the right vagus nerve and recurs around the subclavian artery in the neck.
  - The **left recurrent laryngeal nerve** arises from the thoracic part of the left vagus nerve. It recurs around the arch of the aorta and ascends in the neck between the trachea and esophagus.
  - Cervical **cardiac nerves** carry visceral motor (presynaptic parasympathetic) fibers and visceral sensory fibers to the cardiac plexus.
- The spinal accessory nerve (CN XI), which is derived from roots of the upper cervical spinal cord segments, enters the skull through the foramen magnum. After exiting the skull through the jugular foramen, it innervates the SCM muscle, then crosses the lateral region of the neck to innervate the trapezius muscle (see **Fig. 18.34**).
  - The cranial root joins the vagus nerve.
  - The spinal root innervates the SCM muscle, then crosses the lateral region of the neck to innervate the trapezius muscle.
- The hypoglossal nerve (CN XII), which exits the skull through the hypoglossal canal and courses anteriorly to the submandibular region, enters the oral cavity to innervate muscles of the tongue.
  - Along its course, fibers from C1 join the hypoglossal nerve briefly, eventually diverging from it to innervate the geniohyoid and thyrohyoid muscles and to form the superior root of the ansa cervicalis (see **Fig. 21.7**).

21.5   Esophagus

The esophagus is a muscular tube that connects the pharynx in the neck to the stomach in the abdomen (see Section 5.7 and **Fig. 19.42**).

- The cervical esophagus begins at the C6 vertebral level, which corresponds to the inferior border of the cricoid cartilage. The cervical esophagus is posterior to the trachea, anterior to the cervical vertebrae, and continuous with the laryngopharynx superiorly.
- At the pharyngoesophageal junction, the **cricopharyngeus,** the lowest part of the inferior pharyngeal constrictor, forms the superior esophageal sphincter.
- The inferior thyroid arteries, branches of the subclavian arteries via the thyrocervical trunks, supply the cervical part of the esophagus. Veins of similar name accompany the arteries.
- Lymphatic vessels from the cervical esophagus drain to paratracheal and deep cervical nodes.
- The recurrent laryngeal nerves, branches of the vagus nerve (CN X), and vasomotor fibers from the cervical sympathetic trunk innervate the esophagus in the neck.

21.6   Larynx and Trachea

The larynx, part of the upper airway, is responsible for sound production. It communicates superiorly with the pharynx and inferiorly with the trachea and lies anterior to the C3–C6 vertebrae. The trachea, the upper part of the tracheobronchial tree, descends into the thorax, where it is continuous with the bronchi of the lungs.

Laryngeal Skeleton

Three single cartilages and two sets of paired cartilages form the laryngeal skeleton **(Fig. 21.9)**. All except the epiglottis (elastic cartilage) are formed of hyaline cartilage.

— The **thyroid cartilage,** the largest of the nine cartilages, has two **laminae** that join at the midline to form a **laryngeal prominence** (Adam's apple). The **superior horn** of the thyroid cartilage attaches to the hyoid bone, and the **inferior horn** articulates with the cricoid cartilage at the **cricothyroid joint.**

— The **cricoid cartilage,** the only part of the laryngeal skeleton to form a complete ring around the airway, articulates superiorly with the thyroid cartilage and is attached inferiorly

to the first tracheal ring. The anterior part of the cricoid cartilage, the **arch,** is short, and the **lamina,** its posterior part, is tall.

— The **epiglottis,** a leaf-shaped cartilage that forms the anterior wall of the laryngeal inlet at the root of the tongue, is attached inferiorly to the thyroid cartilage and anteriorly to the hyoid bone.

— The paired pyramidal **arytenoid cartilages,** which articulate with the superior border of the cricoid lamina, have an apex that articulates with the tiny **corniculate cartilages** and a **vocal process** that attaches to the thyroid cartilage through the **vocal ligaments.**

— The small, paired corniculate and **cuneiform cartilages** appear as tubercles within the **aryepiglottic fold.** Although the corniculate cartilages articulate with the arytenoids, the cuneiform cartilages do not articulate with the other cartilages.

A Left anterior oblique view.

B Sagittal section viewed from the left medial aspect. *Removed:* Hyoid bone and thyrohyoid ligament. The arytenoid cartilage alters the position of the vocal folds during phonation.

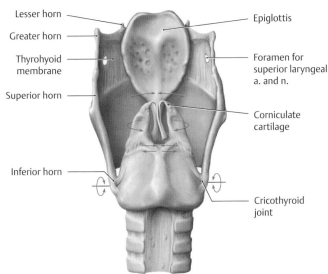

C Posterior view. *Arrows* indicate the direction of movement in the various joints.

D Superior view of thyrohyoid, cricoid, and corniculate cartilages.

Fig. 21.9 Structure of the larynx

Membranes and Ligaments of the Larynx

Membranes of the larynx connect the laryngeal cartilages to each other and to the hyoid bone and trachea (**Figs. 21.10** and **Fig. 21.11;** see also **Fig. 21.9**).

— The **thyrohyoid membrane** attaches the thyroid cartilage to the hyoid bone superiorly.
— The **cricotracheal ligament** attaches the cricoid cartilage to the first tracheal ring inferiorly.
— The **quadrangular membrane** extends posteriorly from the lateral border of the epiglottis to the arytenoid cartilage on each side.
  • The superior free margin of this membrane forms the **aryepiglottic ligament,** which, when covered by mucosa, is known as the **aryepiglottic fold.**
  • The inferior free margin is the **vestibular ligament,** which, when covered by mucosa, is known as the **vestibular fold** or false vocal cord.
— The **cricothyroid membrane** connects the cricoid and thyroid cartilages and extends superiorly deep to the

thyroid cartilage as the **conus elasticus** (see **Figs. 21.9D** and **21.12C**).
— The free superior border of the conus elasticus forms the **vocal ligament,** which extends from the midpoint of the thyroid cartilage to the vocal processes of the arytenoid cartilage. The vocal ligament and the **vocalis muscle** form the **vocal fold** or **vocal cord.**

Laryngeal Cavity

The laryngeal cavity begins at the laryngeal inlet and extends to the inferior border of the cricoid cartilage (see **Figs. 21.10** and **21.11**).
— The vestibular and vocal folds define spaces within the laryngeal cavity.
  • The **supraglottic space** (laryngeal vestibule) or supraglottic space lies above the vestibular folds.
  • The **rima vestibuli** is the aperture between the two vestibular folds.
  • The **laryngeal ventricles** are recesses of the laryngeal cavity between the vestibular and vocal folds.
  • **Laryngeal saccules** are the blind ends of the laryngeal ventricles.
  • The **rima glottidis** is the aperture between the two vocal folds.
  • The **subglottic space** (infraglottic cavity) is the inferior part of the laryngeal cavity, which lies below the vocal folds and extends to the inferior border of the cricoid cartilage.
— Sound is produced as air passes through the laryngeal cavity between the vocal folds. Variations in sound arise from changes in the position, tension, and length of these folds.
— The vestibular folds protect the airway but have no role in sound production.

CLINICAL CORRELATION

TRACHEOSTOMY AND CRICOTHYROIDOTOMY When the upper airway is obstructed, airway access can be reestablished using two different approaches. Tracheostomy is a surgical procedure in which a tracheostomy tube is inserted through an incision in the proximal trachea. This procedure is generally used for long-term management of the airway.

Cricothyroidotomy is a related procedure in which an incision is made in the cricothyroid membrane. This procedure, usually performed in emergency situations, is less technically difficult than tracheostomy and has fewer complications.

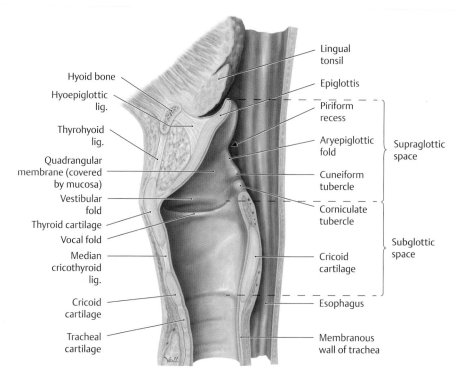

Fig. 21.10 Cavity of the larynx
Midsagittal section viewed from the left side.

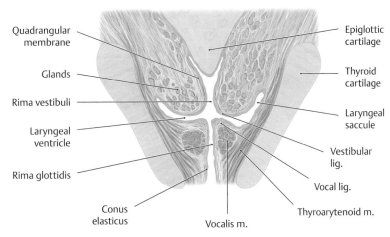

Quadrangular membrane

Glands

Rima vestibuli

Laryngeal ventricle

Rima glottidis

Conus elasticus

Vocalis m.

Epiglottic cartilage

Thyroid cartilage

Laryngeal saccule

Vestibular lig.

Vocal lig.

Thyroarytenoid m.

Fig. 21.11 Vestibular and vocal folds
Coronal section, superior view.

Muscles of the Larynx

The larynx has extrinsic and intrinsic muscle groups.
— Extrinsic muscles are attached to the hyoid bone and move the larynx and hyoid bone together. These include the suprahyoid muscles (see **Table 19.9**), which elevate the larynx, and the infrahyoid muscles (see **Table 21.4**), which depress the larynx.
— Intrinsic muscles move the laryngeal cartilages, which changes the length and tension of the vocal ligaments and size of the rima glottidis (**Table 21.7; Fig. 21.12**).

— Two muscles are particularly clinically and anatomically significant:
  • The **posterior cricoarytenoid muscle** is the only muscle that abducts the vocal folds and opens the rima glottidis.
  • The **cricothyroid muscle,** innervated by the external branch of the superior laryngeal nerve, is the only intrinsic muscle that is not innervated by the inferior laryngeal nerve (a continuation of the recurrent laryngeal nerve).

Table 21.7 **Actions of the Laryngeal Muscles**

Muscle	Action	Effect on Rima Glottidis
① Cricothyroid m.*	Tightens the vocal folds	None
② Vocalis m.		
③ Thyroarytenoid m.	Adducts the vocal folds	Closes
④ Transverse arytenoid m.		
⑤ Posterior cricoarytenoid m.	Abducts the vocal folds	Opens
⑥ Lateral cricoarytenoid m.	Adducts the vocal folds	Closes

*The cricothyroid m. is the only extrinsic laryngeal muscle.

A Laryngeal muscles, superior view.

B Open rima glottidis.

C Closed rima glottidis.

A Extrinsic laryngeal muscles, left lateral oblique view. *Removed:* Epiglottis.

B Intrinsic laryngeal muscles, left lateral view. Removed: Thyroid cartilage (left lamina). *Revealed:* Epiglottis and external thyroarytenoid muscle.

C Left lateral view. *Removed:* Thyroid cartilage (left lamina) and epiglottis.

D Posterior view.

Fig. 21.12 Laryngeal muscles
The laryngeal muscles move the laryngeal cartilages relative to one another, affecting the tension and/or position of the vocal folds.

Neurovasculature of the Larynx (Figs. 21.13 and 21.14)

— The superior and inferior laryngeal arteries are branches of the superior and inferior thyroid arteries, respectively. Veins of the larynx follow the laryngeal arteries and join the thyroid veins.

— The superior and inferior laryngeal branches of the vagus nerve (CN X) provide all of the motor and sensory innervation of the larynx.

• The superior laryngeal nerve splits into an internal sensory branch, which supplies the mucosa of the vestibule and superior surface of the vocal folds, and an external motor branch, which innervates the cricothyroid muscle.

• The **inferior laryngeal nerve,** a continuation of the recurrent laryngeal nerve, supplies the mucosa of the infraglottic larynx and innervates all intrinsic muscles of the larynx except the cricothyroid.

CLINICAL CORRELATION

RECURRENT LARYNGEAL NERVE PARALYSIS WITH THYROIDEC-TOMY The recurrent laryngeal nerves in the neck are vulnerable to damage during thyroidectomy because they run immediately posterior to the thyroid gland. Unilateral damage results in hoarseness; bilateral damage causes respiratory distress and aphonia (inability to speak). Aspiration pneumonia may occur as a complication.

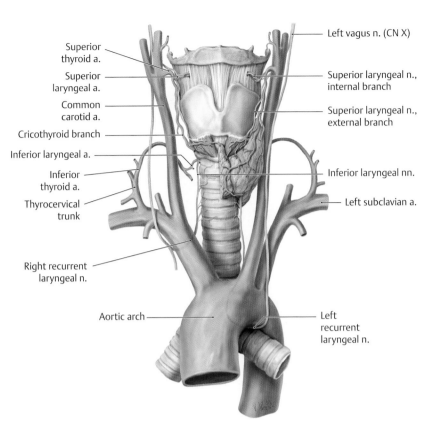

Superior thyroid a.

Superior laryngeal a.

Common carotid a.

Cricothyroid branch

Inferior laryngeal a.

Inferior thyroid a.

Thyrocervical trunk

Right recurrent laryngeal n.

Aortic arch

Left vagus n. (CN X)

Superior laryngeal n., internal branch

Superior laryngeal n., external branch

Inferior laryngeal nn.

Left subclavian a.

Left recurrent laryngeal n.

Fig. 21.13 Arteries and nerves of the larynx, thyroid, and parathyroids
Anterior view.

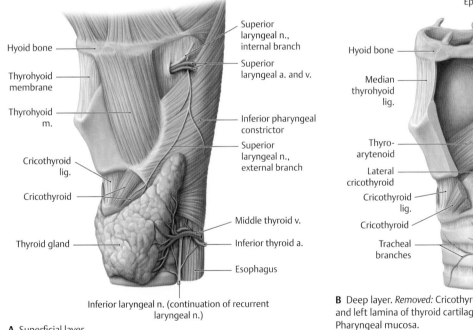

Hyoid bone

Thyrohyoid membrane

Thyrohyoid m.

Cricothyroid lig.

Cricothyroid

Thyroid gland

Superior laryngeal n., internal branch

Superior laryngeal a. and v.

Inferior pharyngeal constrictor

Superior laryngeal n., external branch

Middle thyroid v.

Inferior thyroid a.

Esophagus

Inferior laryngeal n. (continuation of recurrent laryngeal n.)

A Superficial layer.

Hyoid bone

Median thyrohyoid lig.

Thyro-arytenoid

Lateral cricothyroid

Cricothyroid lig.

Cricothyroid

Tracheal branches

Epiglottis

Superior laryngeal n., internal branch

Superior laryngeal a. and v.

Posterior cricoarytenoid

Esophagus

Middle thyroid v.

Inferior thyroid a.

Inferior laryngeal n. (continuation of recurrent laryngeal n.)

B Deep layer. *Removed:* Cricothyroid muscle and left lamina of thyroid cartilage. *Retracted:* Pharyngeal mucosa.

Fig. 21.14 Neurovasculature of the larynx
Left lateral view.

Trachea

The trachea, the extension of the airway inferior to the larynx, extends from the inferior border of the cricoid cartilage to the level of the T4–T5 intervertebral disks in the thorax, where it bifurcates into the two primary bronchi of the lungs (see Section 5.7). In the cervical region (see Section 21.8)

— it lies deep to the superficial and deep cervical fascia, and sternohyoid and sternothyroid muscles.
— the isthmus of the thyroid gland crosses its 2nd to 4th tracheal cartilages. The lobes of the thyroid are lateral to it and descend to the fifth or sixth tracheal cartilage.
— the esophagus lies posterior and separates it from the vertebral column.
— the common carotid arteries ascend lateral to it.
— the recurrent laryngeal nerves ascend lateral or posterolateral to it (in the groove between the trachea and esophagus).
— it is supplied by the inferior thyroid artery and drained by the inferior thyroid veins.
— lymph drains to pretracheal and paratracheal nodes.
— it receives innervation from branches of the vagus n. and the sympathetic trunk.

21.7 Thyroid and Parathyroid Glands

The thyroid and parathyroid glands are endocrine glands that reside in the anterior cervical region.

The Thyroid Gland

The **thyroid gland,** the largest endocrine gland in the body, secretes **thyroid hormone,** which regulates the rate of metabolism, and **calcitonin,** which regulates the metabolism of calcium **(Fig. 21.15A)**.

— The thyroid lies deep to the sternohyoid and sternothyroid muscles (infrahyoid muscles) and anterolateral to the larynx and trachea between C5 and T1 vertebral levels.
— The thyroid has right and left (lateral) lobes connected by a narrow **isthmus** that lies anterior to the second and third tracheal rings.
— A **pyramidal lobe,** present in ~ 50% of the population, is a remnant of the embryonic thyroglossal duct that extends from the isthmus toward the hyoid bone.
— A fibrous capsule encloses the thyroid gland. The pretracheal fascia of the neck lies outside the thyroid capsule.

DEVELOPMENT CORRELATION

THYROGLOSSAL DUCT CYST A thyroglossal duct cyst is a fluid-filled cavity in the midline of the neck, just inferior to the hyoid bone. It results from the proliferation of epithelium left behind from the thyroglossal duct during the descent of the thyroid gland from its embryonic origin on the tongue to its postnatal position in the neck. The cyst can enlarge and press on the trachea and esophagus, in which case it can be surgically removed.

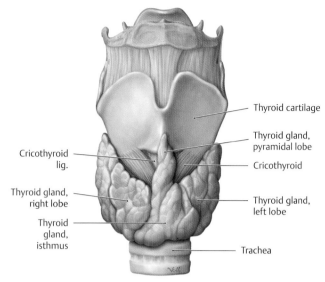

A Thyroid gland. Anterior view.

(labels: Thyroid cartilage; Thyroid gland, pyramidal lobe; Cricothyroid; Thyroid gland, left lobe; Trachea; Cricothyroid lig.; Thyroid gland, right lobe; Thyroid gland, isthmus)

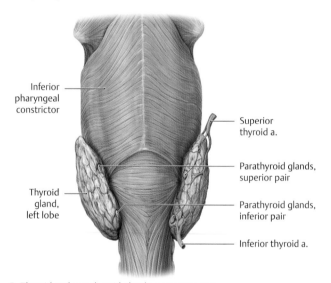

B Thyroid and parathyroid glands, posterior view.

Fig. 21.15 Thyroid and parathyroid glands

(labels: Inferior pharyngeal constrictor; Thyroid gland, left lobe; Superior thyroid a.; Parathyroid glands, superior pair; Parathyroid glands, inferior pair; Inferior thyroid a.)

The Parathyroid Glands

Parathyroid glands, small, ovoid endocrine glands that lie on the posterior surface of the thyroid gland, secrete **parathormone,** which regulates the metabolism of phosphorus and calcium **(Fig. 21.15B)**.

— There are normally four glands, two superior and two inferior, although the number can range from two to six glands.
— The superior parathyroid glands are constant in position near the lower border of the cricoid cartilage. The position of the inferior parathyroid glands may vary, ranging from the lower pole of the thyroid gland to the superior mediastinum.

Neurovasculature of the Thyroid and Parathyroid Glands

— The superior thyroid artery, a branch of the external carotid artery, and the inferior thyroid artery from the thyrocervical trunk supply the thyroid gland (see **Fig. 21.13**). The inferior thyroid artery is usually the main supply to the parathyroid glands.
— **Superior** and **middle thyroid veins** drain into the internal jugular veins; **inferior thyroid veins** drain into the brachiocephalic veins in the mediastinum **(Fig. 21.16)**. Venous drainage from the parathyroid glands joins the thyroid veins.
— Lymphatic vessels of the thyroid may drain directly into the superior and inferior deep cervical nodes or indirectly, passing first through prelaryngeal, pretracheal, and paratracheal nodes.
— The parathyroid glands drain with the thyroid into the inferior deep cervical and paratracheal lymph nodes.
— Cardiac and superior and inferior thyroid sympathetic plexuses arise from the superior, middle, and inferior cervical sympathetic ganglia to supply vasomotor innervation to the thyroid and parathyroid glands.
— The thyroid and parathyroid glands are under hormonal control and therefore lack secretomotor innervation.

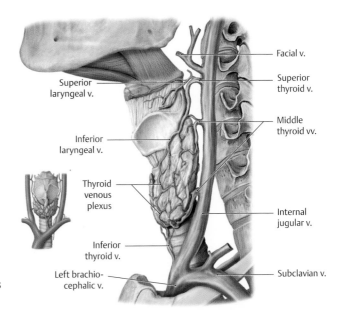

Fig. 21.16 Veins of the larynx, thyroid, and parathyroid glands
Left lateral view. *Note:* The inferior thyroid vein generally drains into the left brachiocephalic vein.

21.8   Topography of the Neck

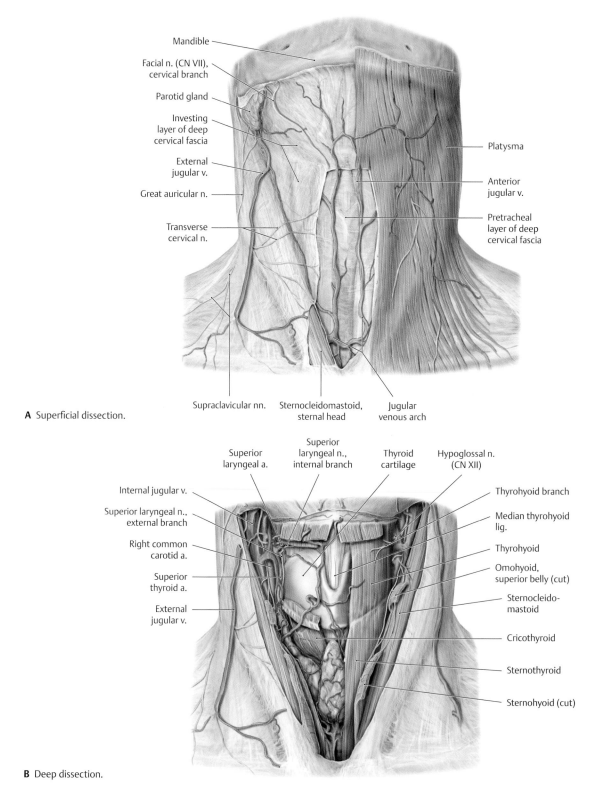

A Superficial dissection.

B Deep dissection.

Fig. 21.17 Topography of the anterior cervical region
Anterior view.

C Deep anterior cervical region.

Fig. 21.17 (*continued*) **Topography of the anterior cervical region**

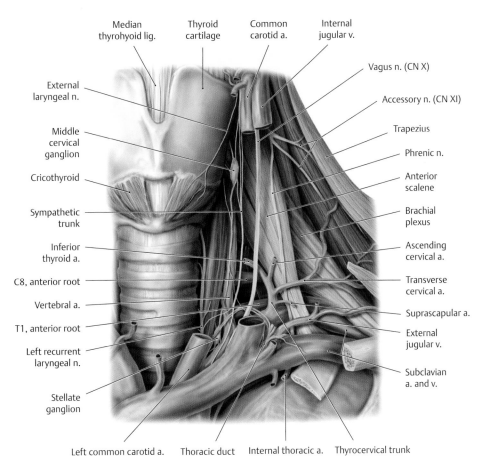

Fig. 21.18 Root of the neck
Anterior view, left side. The thyroid gland has been removed and the common carotid artery and internal jugular vein have been cut to reveal the deep structures in the root of the neck.

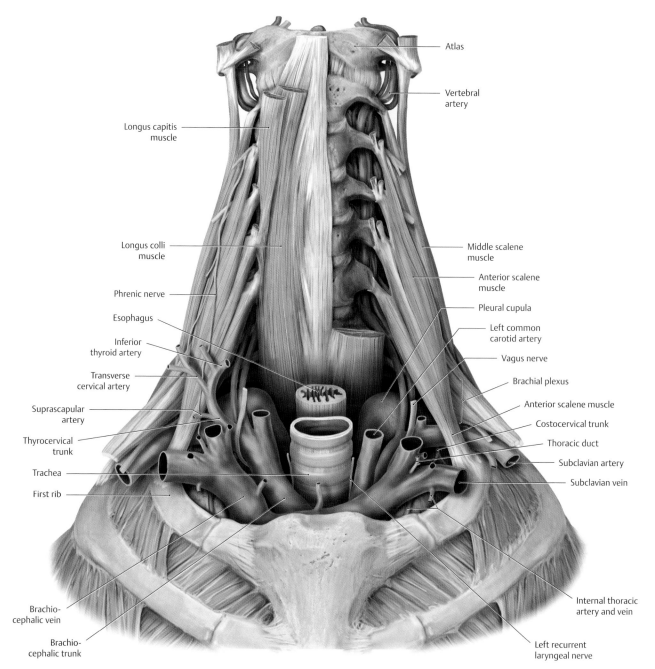

Fig. 21.19 The thoracic inlet

Anterior view. The viscera of the neck have been removed and the esophagus, trachea, common carotid artery and jugular veins have been dissected to show the relations of structures passing through the thoracic inlet. The prevertebral muscles on the left side have been cut to show the course of the vertebral artery.

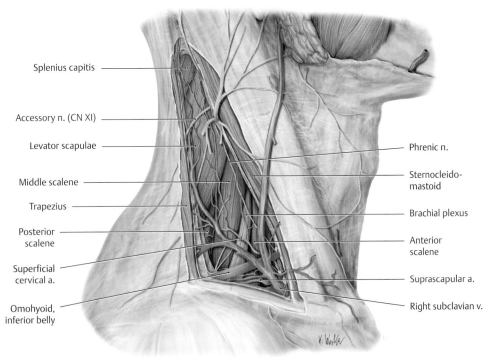

A The superficial, pretracheal, and prevertebral layers of deep cervical fascia have been removed to show the muscles in the floor of the posterior triangle. Note the emergence of the cervical plexus at Erb's point and the brachial plexus in the interscalene groove.

B The sternocleidomastoid has been cut to reveal structures in the carotid triangle and root of the neck.

Fig. 21.20 Lateral cervical region
Right lateral view.

Unit VIII   Clinical Imaging Basics of the Head and Neck

Ultrasound provides excellent high-resolution detail of superficial structures of the neck (such as the thyroid (**Fig. 21.21**) and neck blood vessels) quickly, inexpensively, and safely—that is, without radiation exposure. Evaluation of deeper and intracranial structures requires computed tomography (CT) or magnetic resonance imaging (MRI). CT is fast and best for trauma evaluation, and for bones such as the skull base. MRI's superior soft tissue contrast makes it highly suitable for the brain, and for evaluating tumors of the head and neck (**Table 21.8**).

Vascular structures are an important focus in the radiology of the head and neck anatomy. Vessels can be imaged by ultrasound (**Fig. 21.22**), CT angiogram, MRI angiogram, or fluoroscopic catheter-based angiogram (**Fig. 21.23**). For evaluating the bone and air-filled spaces of the skull, CT provides the clearest detail (**Fig. 21.24**) but the soft tissues of the brain are seen best with MRI (**Figs. 21.25** and **21.26**).

Table 21.8 **Suitability of Imaging Modalities for the Head and Neck**

Modality	Clinical Uses
Radiographs (X-rays)	Used primarily for evaluation of the skull, and the soft tissues of the neck in children. Also used with angiographic studies (fluoroscopy) of the neck and intracranial vessels
CT (computed tomography)	Excellent for high detail evaluation of the skull and skull base, sinuses, cervical spine, and for evaluation of the deeper spaces of the neck
MRI (magnetic resonance imaging)	Excellent for evaluation of the soft tissues of the neck, orbits, cranial nerves and brain
Ultrasound	Used primarily for the thyroid and neck vessels. Also used for evaluation of other abnormalities in the more peripheral soft tissue structures of the neck especially in children (e.g., lymph nodes, branchial cleft cysts, thyroglossal duct cysts).

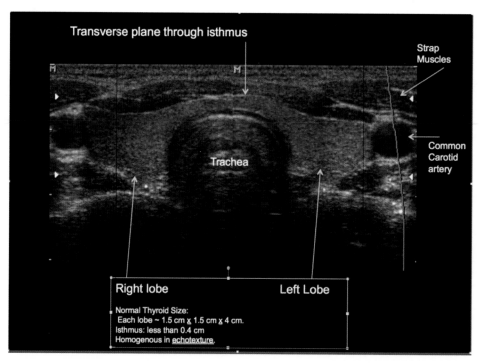

Fig. 21.21 Ultrasound of the thyroid gland
Transverse (axial) plane.
The thyroid gland is perfectly suited for ultrasound because of its position deep to the skin and subcutaneous tissues of the neck. This allows the use of a high-frequency linear transducer probe, which gives the highest resolution possible with ultrasound. The thyroid gland is homogeneously echoic, slightly more echogenic (whiter) than muscle. Note how the echogenic fascial planes delineate the strap muscles. The common carotid artery appears black because of the fluid (blood) it contains. Ultrasound waves do not travel well through air, so the trachea is seen as a curved line anteriorly where the sound waves bounce off the air-filled structure.

A Color Doppler is used to assess motion, more specifically, flow within a blood vessel. The trapezoid-shaped box within the image is the color Doppler "window." Outside of this window is simply gray scale ultrasound. Notice that in gray scale, blood vessels are *black*. The *red* and *blue* color scales indicate direction of flow and give an estimate of velocity.

Fig. 21.22 Ultrasound of the common carotid artery and jugular vein
The skin surface is at the top of the image.

B Spectral ultrasound is used to give a graphical representation of the flow velocity vs. time. In this image, the spectral window is the small parallel lines placed within the deeper vessel. The waveform shown is arterial. Note the systolic peak and diastolic plateau. This deeper vessel is the common carotid artery. (From Schmidt G. Clinical Companions Ultrasound. Stuttgart: Thieme; 2007.)

Left anterior cerebral artery

Left middle cerebral artery

Left internal carotid artery

Fig. 21.23 Angiogram of the left internal carotid artery
Anteroposterior view.
In this fluoroscopic study, bones are digitally subtracted in order to isolate the vessels. The image is a photo negative of the X-ray in which contrast in the vessels appears black. The catheter, inserted into the patient's groin and threaded through the aorta, enters the left internal carotid artery. Note that in the normal condition, blood vessels are smooth and without focal or diffuse dilation and the caliber of the vessels is uniform, tapering slightly as they progress distally, without narrowing or ending abruptly. (From Moeller T, et al. Pocket Atlas of Radiographic Anatomy, 3rd ed. New York: Thieme; 2010.)

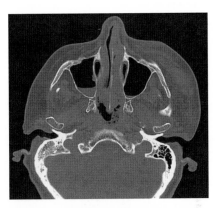

Fig. 21.24 Transverse (axial) section, inferior view
CT is superior for imaging the paranasal sinuses because the high contrast readily differentiates air and bone from other structures. The air-filled sinuses are sharply contrasted against the soft tissues and even more so against the white bones. This feature also makes CT optimal for skull base imaging. Note in this patient there is some fluid in the right maxillary sinus producing an air-fluid level (patient is supine, so the fluid settles in the posterior aspect of the sinus) and the mastoid air cells on the right are filled with fluid instead of air. Compare the normal left side with the abnormal right side. This patient has right maxillary sinusitis and mastoiditis. (From Eastman G, et al. Getting Started in Radiology. Stuttgart: Thieme; 2005.)

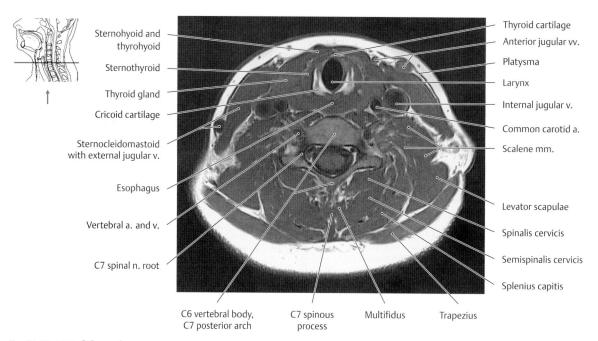

Fig. 21.25 MRI of the neck
Transverse (axial) plane.
In this MRI sequence, fat is bright and muscles are *gray*. The fat planes between muscles allow differentiation of the adjacent muscles and identification of the spaces of the neck.

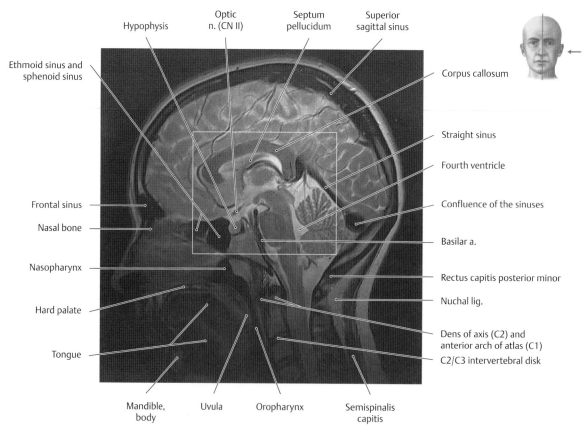

Fig. 21.26 MRI of the head
Midsagittal section.
In this MRI sequence, fluid is bright (note the bright CSF in the 4th ventricle) and soft tissues are shades of *gray*. However, note the subtle differences in gray scale that allow differentiation of the various soft tissues. This feature makes MRI superior to CT for use in imaging the brain. The brainstem structures and corpus callosum are sharply defined. The small amount of fluid interdigitating between the sulci of the cerebrum highlights the gross architecture of the brain. The layers of the scalp and skull are also well differentiated.

Unit VIII   Review Questions: Head and Neck

1. Which bone of the skull contains the optic foramen, foramen ovale, and foramen spinosum?
   A. Frontal
   B. Temporal
   C. Sphenoid
   D. Ethmoid
   E. Occipital

2. The internal jugular vein
   A. is located within the carotid sheath
   B. receives venous drainage from the brain
   C. is a tributary of the brachiocephalic vein
   D. receives blood from the facial vein
   E. All of the above

3. The following structure runs within the falx cerebri.
   A. Inferior sagittal sinus
   B. Transverse sinus
   C. Sigmoid sinus
   D. Cavernous sinus
   E. 3rd ventricle

4. The vertebral artery
   A. ascends through the transverse foramina of all seven cervical vertebra
   B. arises from the first part of the axillary artery
   C. terminates by joining with the posterior cerebellar artery
   D. supplies branches to the thyroid gland
   E. supplies the posterior cerebral circulation

5. A man is taken to the emergency department after his wife noticed something wrong with the left side of his face during breakfast. He is found to have a problem with the nerve exiting the stylomastoid foramen, a disorder called Bell's palsy. Which of the following problems is this patient likely to have?
   A. He is unable to open his left eye.
   B. He is unable to raise his eyebrow on the left side.
   C. He is unable to protrude his tongue to the right.
   D. He is unable to chew.
   E. He is unable to feel pressure on his left cheek.

6. A patient came to the emergency department with a broken mandible resulting from an over-swung baseball bat. Which nerve is most likely affected by this injury?
   A. Lingual nerve
   B. Hypoglossal nerve
   C. Zygomatic branches of facial nerve
   D. Inferior alveolar nerve
   E. Chorda tympani nerve

7. The muscle of mastication that inserts into the condylar process of the mandible and its articular disk and the capsule of the temporomandibular joint (TMJ) is the
   A. medial pterygoid muscle
   B. lateral pterygoid muscle
   C. temporalis muscle
   D. masseter muscle
   E. buccinator muscle

8. A man develops acromegaly secondary to a tumor in his pituitary gland secreting growth hormone. A transsphenoidal resection of the tumor is scheduled. During this process, part of the inferior and posterior nasal septum is removed. Which bone forms this part of the nasal septum?
   A. Vomer
   B. Ethmoid
   C. Palatine
   D. Temporal
   E. Sphenoid

9. The lacrimal gland is innervated by
   A. the facial nerve (VII)
   B. the postganglionic neurons with the cell bodies in the pterygopalatine ganglion
   C. the parasympathetic neurons
   D. the lacrimal nerve
   E. All of the above

10. A 2-year-old boy seen by his pediatrician was noticeably irritable and tugging at his ear. When his mother asked him in a normal tone to sit quietly, he covered his ears screaming in pain and asked her not to shout at him. On exam he was found to have a fever, and his tympanic membrane was red and bulging. He was diagnosed with otitis media and started on antibiotics. The child's extreme sensitivity to sound (hyperacusis) suggests that the infection affected the stapedius muscle. The nerve that innervates this muscle is a branch of what nerve?
    A. Maxillary division of trigeminal nerve
    B. Mandibular division of trigeminal nerve
    C. Facial nerve
    D. Glossopharyngeal nerve
    E. Vagus nerve

11. The innervation for the sternothyroid muscle is the
    A. ansa cervicalis
    B. facial nerve
    C. hypoglossal nerve
    D. accessory nerve
    E. recurrent laryngeal nerve

12. A man was having an animated discussion with his friends when he started coughing after swallowing a piece of chicken at a fast-food restaurant. He soon became unable to speak or cough. Two paramedics who were taking a break at a nearby table quickly came to his help, and one stood behind the man and performed forceful abdominal thrusts (Heimlich maneuver). After several unsuccessful attempts to dislodge the aspirated food, the paramedics decide to perform an emergency airway procedure. What is the most superior site to perform this procedure so that the airway is secured below the vocal folds?
    A. Superior to the hyoid bone
    B. Between the hyoid bone and the thyroid cartilage
    C. Between the thyroid cartilage and the cricoid cartilage
    D. Between the thyroid cartilage and the arytenoid cartilage
    E. Superior to the manubrium in the jugular fossa

13. A man is found to have a nodule in his neck. His calcitonin level is elevated, and a biopsy reveals medullary carcinoma of the thyroid. A thyroidectomy is performed. After surgery the patient's voice is found to be hoarse. What nerve was most likely injured during surgery?
    A. The glossopharyngeal
    B. The hypoglossal
    C. The ansa cervicalis
    D. The recurrent laryngeal
    E. The phrenic

14. A boy who has been vomiting is diagnosed with an obstruction in his gastrointestinal tract. He becomes severely dehydrated, and a sunken anterior fontanelle is felt. What is the youngest age at which this sign no longer would appear in a dehydrated child?
    A. 1 month
    B. 3 months
    C. 6 months
    D. 12 months
    E. 24 months

15. The jugulodigastric lymph nodes that lie near the facial and internal jugular veins are also known as
    A. parotid nodes
    B. superior deep cervical nodes
    C. inferior deep cervical nodes
    D. retroauricular nodes
    E. lateral cervical nodes

16. A patient develops severely elevated intracranial pressure due to a brain tumor obstructing the flow of cerebrospinal fluid (CSF). A shunt is placed to relieve this pressure because the CSF is blocked from being returned to the venous system. Where would this resorption normally take place?
    A. At the choroid plexus
    B. At the interventricular foramen
    C. At the cerebral aqueduct
    D. At the lateral apertures
    E. At the arachnoid granulations

17. The vagus nerve (cranial nerve X)
    A. leaves the skull through the carotid foramen
    B. innervates the carotid sinus
    C. is transmitted through the superior orbital fissure
    D. innervates all of the muscles of the soft palate
    E. None of the above

18. A 40-year-old obese woman has frequent headaches. At an eye exam, she is found to have papilledema (swelling of the optic disk). It is suspected that she has elevated intracranial pressure. CT scan is negative for any strokes or tumors. She is diagnosed with idiopathic intracranial hypertension (pseudotumor cerebri). One complication of this disorder is downward displacement of the brainstem, which leads to stretching of the abducent nerve. How would you diagnose if this complication occurred in this patient?
    A. She would be unable to move her eyes laterally.
    B. She would be unable to move her eyes medially.
    C. She would be unable to move her eyes superiorly.
    D. She would be unable to move her eyes inferiorly
    E. She would be unable to rotate her eyes internally.

19. A 61-year-old firefighter was trapped for 12 hours in a collapsed building following an earthquake. Although he

suffered a fractured tibia, the emergency department physician was also concerned about a deep scalp laceration that extended across the top of the patient's head. Infection from this laceration could spread
    A. to dural venous sinuses through emissary veins
    B. into the neck in the loose areolar tissue
    C. laterally beyond the zygomatic arches
    D. to the epidural space
    E. All of the above

20. A dentist who specializes in relief of facial pain is experimenting with a procedure to inject anesthetic into the pterygopalatine fossa through a lateral approach. The needle passes through the mandibular notch of the mandible, traverses the infratemporal fossa, and enters the pterygomaxillary fissure. Which of the following structures would be at risk during the procedure?
    A. Maxillary artery
    B. Mandibular division of the trigeminal nerve (CN III)
    C. Pterygoid venous plexus
    D. Otic ganglion
    E. All of the above

21. Which of the following drains into the inferior meatus of the nasal cavity?
    A. Nasolacrimal duct
    B. Frontal sinus
    C. Ethmoid sinus
    D. Sphenoid sinus
    E. Maxillary sinus

22. Which of the following vessels accompanies the optic nerve through the optic canal?
    A. Supratrochlear artery
    B. Supraorbital artery
    C. Ophthalmic artery
    D. Ophthalmic vein
    E. Ophthalmic nerve

23. The nerve that innervates the middle ear muscle that changes the shape of the tympanic membrane is the
    A. optic nerve
    B. oculomotor nerve
    C. trochlear nerve
    D. trigeminal nerve
    E. facial nerve

24. The branches of the cervical plexus
    A. originate from the anterior rami of C1 through C4
    B. innervate the sternocleidomastoid
    C. carry preganglionic fibers that synapse in parasympathetic ganglia of the head
    D. include only cutaneous nerves
    E. include the greater occipital nerve

25. Intubation is necessary during surgery because, due to muscle relaxants and other drugs administered during the procedure, patients are unable to fully relax the vocal folds. Paralysis of which muscle prevents the relaxation of the vocal folds?
    A. Thyroarytenoid muscles
    B. Posterior cricoarytenoid muscles
    C. Cricothyroid muscles
    D. Transverse arytenoid muscles
    E. Lateral arytenoids muscles

26. All of the innervation of the larynx, both sensory and motor, is supplied by
    A. the vagus nerve
    B. the glossopharyngeal nerve
    C. the recurrent laryngeal nerve
    D. the superior laryngeal nerve
    E. None of the above

27. Which is the only laryngeal cartilage to completely encircle the airway?
    A. Thyroid
    B. Cricoid
    C. Epiglottic
    D. Arytenoid
    E. Corniculate

28. A man is in a knife fight and receives a stab wound between the sternocleidomastoid muscle and the superior belly of the omohyoid muscle. Profuse bleeding ensues due to penetration of the common carotid artery. Which structure within the same fascial sheath may also have been injured?
    A. External jugular vein
    B. Phrenic nerve
    C. Internal jugular vein
    D. Superior thyroid artery
    E. Sympathetic trunk

29. A man with a long history of tobacco use goes to the dentist for a cleaning. The dentist notices a lesion on the lateral part of the body of the tongue and refers the patient to an otolaryngologist (ENT), who biopsies the lesion and determines that the patient has squamous cell carcinoma of the tongue. A CT of the patient's head and neck demonstrates metastasis to the lymph nodes. The primary group of lymph nodes for the drainage of this patient's cancer is
    A. superior deep cervical
    B. inferior deep cervical
    C. anterior superficial cervical
    D. submandibular
    E. submental

30. All of the following bones form a part of the nasal walls or floor except
    A. Frontal
    B. Ethmoid
    C. Maxilla
    D. Vomer
    E. Palatine

31. The action of the medial pterygoid muscle is to
    A. elevate the mandible
    B. tense the soft palate
    C. elevate the soft palate
    D. elevate the hyoid bone
    E. retract the mandible

32. A 63-year-old man complains of difficulty speaking, chewing, and swallowing. On physical exam, you note that the patient's tongue is atrophied, and when asked to stick out his tongue and say "ahh," the patient's tongue deviates to the left. In obtaining a medical history, you learn that the patient underwent recent surgery on his common carotid artery. Damage to which nerve has most likely caused the observed deficits?
    A. Right glossopharyngeal nerve
    B. Right hypoglossal nerve
    C. Left hypoglossal nerve
    D. Right lingual nerve
    E. Left lingual nerve

33. The mandibular division of the trigeminal nerve (V_3) passes through the foramen ovale into the
    A. infratemporal fossa
    B. pterygopalatine fossa
    C. orbit
    D. nasal cavity
    E. oral cavity

34. A man with hypertension and a long history of smoking suffers a series of transient ischemic attacks (TIAs). In the evaluation, a carotid bruit is heard. Further testing reveals severe stenosis of his internal carotid artery due to atherosclerosis. The TIAs were due to embolism of the atherosclerotic plaque. Which of the following is the first branch of the internal carotid artery likely to be affected by an embolism?
    A. Superior thyroid
    B. Lingual
    C. Facial
    D. Maxillary
    E. Ophthalmic

35. A patient has thrombophlebitis of the right cavernous sinus due to a facial skin infection. The infection traveled via the angular vein to the superior ophthalmic vein and into the cavernous sinus. Which of the following is an additional symptom that this patient might exhibit?
    A. Jugular venous distension on the right
    B. Inability to smile
    C. Inability to chew on the right
    D. Loss of vision in the right eye
    E. Loss of sensation to the right cheek

36. Which of the following arteries is a branch of the internal carotid artery?
    A. Posterior cerebral artery
    B. Occipital artery
    C. Labyrinthine artery
    D. Ophthalmic artery
    E. Middle meningeal artery

Answers and Explanations

1. **C.** The sphenoid forms the posterior orbit and the floor of the middle cranial fossa between the frontal and temporal bones. Foramina of the sphenoid include the optic foramen, foramen ovale, foramen rotundum, foramen spinosum, and superior orbital fissure (Section 17.1).
    A. The frontal bone forms the forehead, the roof and superior rim of the orbit, and the floor of the anterior cranial fossa.
    B. The temporal bone forms part of the middle and posterior cranial fossa. Its foramina include the internal and external acoustic meatuses, carotid canal, and stylomastoid foramen.
    D. The ethmoid bone forms part of the anterior cranial fossa, medial walls of the orbit, and parts of the nasal septum and lateral nasal walls,

E. The occipital bone forms most of the posterior cranial fossa. Its foramina include the foramen magnum, condylar canals, and jugular foramina.

2. **E.** The internal jugular vein is located within the carotid sheath (A), contains venous drainage from the brain (B), is a tributary of the brachiocephalic vein (C), and receives blood from the facial vein (D) (Section 17.4).

   A. The internal jugular vein runs within the carotid sheath with the common carotid artery and vagus nerve. B, C, and D are also correct (E).

   B. Cerebral venous drainage flow primarily to the internal jugular veins. A, C, and D are also correct (E).

   C. The internal jugular veins join the subclavian veins to form the brachiocephalic veins. A, B, and D are also correct (E).

   D. The facial vein is a tributary of the internal jugular vein. A through C are also correct (E).

3. **A.** The inferior sagittal sinus runs in the inferior edge of the falx cerebri and ends as the straight sinus (Section 18.1).

   B. The transverse sinus runs along the posterolateral margins of the tentorium cerebelli.

   C. The sigmoid sinuses run in grooves of the occipital and temporal bones.

   D. The cavernous sinuses lie lateral to the sella turcica between the meningeal and periosteal dura.

   E. The 3rd ventricle lies between the right and left thalami of the diencephalon.

4. **E.** The right and left vertebral arteries join to form the basilar artery. Together these arteries supply the posterior circulation of the brain (Section 18.2).

   A. The vertebral artery ascends through the transverse foramina of C1–C6 vertebrae.

   B. The vertebral artery is a branch of the subclavian artery.

   C. The vertebral artery terminates by joining with the contralateral vertebral artery to form the basilar artery.

   D. The vertebral artery has no branches in the neck.

5. **B.** CN VII, the facial nerve, exits the stylomastoid foramen and is responsible for the muscles of facial expression, including the occipitofrontalis muscle, which elevates the eyebrows (Section 18.3).

   A. The levator palpebrae superioris muscle elevates the eyelid and is innervated by CN III, the oculomotor nerve. In addition to the levator palpebrae superioris, the occipitofrontalis muscle assists in raising the eyebrow, but because CN III is not affected the patient is able to open his eye. He is not, however, able to close his eye completely due to the paralysis of the orbicularis oculi muscle.

   C. CN XII, the hypoglossal nerve, innervates most of the tongue musculature. A left-sided hypoglossal injury would lead to the inability to protrude his tongue to the right.

   D. The muscles of mastication are innervated by the mandibular division of CN V, the trigeminal nerve. Although his ability to chew is unaffected, the patient does have some trouble eating because of paralysis to the buccinator muscle, which assists in positioning food in the oral cavity.

   E. Sensation to the cheek is conveyed through the maxillary division of the trigeminal nerve.

6. **D.** The inferior alveolar nerve courses within the mandibular canal of the mandible and would be injured in this patient (Section 18.3).

   A. The lingual nerve courses through the infratemporal fossa and into the floor of the mouth.

   B. The hypoglossal nerve courses anteriorly below the angle of the mandible before entering the mouth at the posterior border of the mylohyoid muscle.

   C. Zygomatic branches of the facial nerve pass lateral to the masseter muscle as they cross the cheek.

   E. The chorda tympani travels with the lingual nerve in the infratemporal fossa and floor of the mouth.

7. **B.** The lateral pterygoid muscle inserts into the condylar process of the mandible and its articular disk and the capsule of the temporomandibular joint (TMJ) (Section 19.2).

   A. The medial pterygoid inserts into the pterygoid tuberosity on the medial surface of the angle of the mandible.

   C. The temporalis inserts into the apex and medial surface of the coronoid process of the mandible.

   D. The masseter inserts into the masseteric tuberosity at the angle of the mandible.

   E. The buccinator inserts into the angle of the mouth and orbicularis oris.

8. **A.** The vomer makes up the inferior and posterior parts of the nasal septum (Section 19.7).

   B. The ethmoid bone, through its perpendicular plate, makes up the superior and posterior parts of the nasal septum.

   C. The palatine forms the posterior palate and does not contribute to the nasal septum.

   D. The temporal forms the base and lateral side of the skull and does not contribute to the nasal septum.

   E. Although some of the sphenoid bone will be removed as a part of the procedure, it does not contribute to the nasal septum.

9. **E.** The lacrimal gland is innervated by visceral motor fibers (preganglionic parasympathetic [C]) of the greater petrosal branch of the facial nerve (A). The postganglionic neuron is the zygomatic branch of the maxillary nerve (V_2), which has its cell body in the pterygopalatine ganglion (B) and is then distributed to the lacrimal gland. The lacrimal nerve (D) provides sensory innervation to the lacrimal gland, conjunctiva, and upper eyelids (Section 18.3).

   A. The lacrimal gland is innervated by visceral motor fibers (preganglionic parasympathetic of the greater petrosal branch of the facial nerve). B through D are also correct (E).

   B. The zygomatic branch of the facial nerve carries postganglionic parasympathetic fibers from the pterygopalatine ganglion to the lacrimal gland. A, C, and D are also correct (E).

   C. Parasympathetic fibers of the zygomatic nerve innervate the lacrimal gland. A, B, and D are also correct (E).

   D. The lacrimal nerve provides sensory innervation to the lacrimal gland, conjunctiva, and upper eyelids. A through C are also correct (E).

10. **C.** The stapedius nerve arises from the facial nerve in the facial canal to innervate the stapedius muscle, which dampens sound waves transmitted through the middle ear (Section 20.2).

　　A. The maxillary nerve is distributed to the orbit, nasal cavity, and oral cavity, but it has no branches in the middle ear.

　　B. The mandibular nerve innervates the tensor tympani, which tenses the tympanic membrane.

　　D. The glossopharyngeal nerve transmits sensation from the tympanic cavity and pharyngotympanic tube and joins with sympathetic fibers of the internal carotid plexus to form the tympanic plexus.

　　E. The vagus nerve transmits sensation from the external surface of the tympanic membrane.

11. **A.** The ansa cervicalis innervates all of the infrahyoid muscles except the thyrohyoid (Section 21.3 and **Table 21.3**).

　　B. The cervical branch of the facial nerve innervates the platysma.

　　C. The hypoglossal nerve innervates all of the tongue muscles, including the genioglossus, hyoglossus, and intrinsic tongue muscles.

　　D. The accessory nerve innervates the trapezius and the sternocleidomastoid muscles and contributes to the pharyngeal plexus that helps to control the pharyngeal muscles.

　　E. The recurrent laryngeal nerve, a branch of the vagus nerve, innervates the intrinsic muscles of the larynx.

12. **C.** An emergency tracheotomy (or cricothyrotomy) is performed to secure an airway in a patient with respiratory failure who does not have time to have a procedure performed in the operating room. The quickest access to secure an airway is by incising the cricothyroid membrane (Section 21.6).

　　A. Superior to the hyoid bone is superior to the vocal folds and is also a difficult access site given the presence of the mylohyoid muscles.

　　B. The thyrohyoid membrane is between the hyoid bone and the thyroid cartilage and is superior to the vocal folds.

　　D. Between the thyroid and arytenoid cartilages is too posterior to access the airway and is also at the level of the vocal folds.

　　E. Superior to the manubrium in the jugular fossa is a potential site for an airway (tracheostomy) but is more inferior to the cricothyroid membrane. Also, incising the tracheal cartilage or trying to access the airway between the tracheal cartilages is too difficult without the benefit of being in the operating room. Another benefit of a cricothyrotomy versus a tracheostomy is that there are fewer structures at risk for injury such as blood vessels, the recurrent laryngeal nerve, the thyroid gland, and the esophagus.

13. **D.** The recurrent laryngeal nerve is a branch of the vagus nerve, which travels in the tracheoesophageal groove, lateral and posterior to the thyroid gland. Injury to this nerve causes hoarseness, among other complications (Sections 21.6 and 18.3).

　　A., B., C., and **E.** The glossopharyngeal nerve, hypoglossal nerve, nerves of the ansa cervicalis, and the phrenic nerve do not travel close enough to the thyroid gland to be at risk during careful thyroid surgery.

14. **E.** The anterior fontanelle is the fibrous area at the junction of the frontal and parietal bones. It closes at 18 to 24 months of age (Section 17.1).

　　A., B., C., D. The anterior fontanelle remains open until 18 to 24 months of age.

15. **B.** The superior deep cervical nodes lie between the jugular and facial veins and the anterior belly of the digastric (Section 17.5).

　　A. The parotid nodes are superficial nodes that overlie the parotid gland on the side of the face.

　　C. The inferior deep cervical nodes lie in the neck near the inferior part of the internal jugular vein.

　　D. The retroauricular nodes are superficial nodes that lie along the posterior margin of the auricle.

　　E. The lateral cervical nodes are superficial nodes that lie along the external jugular vein in the neck.

16. **E.** The CSF is reabsorbed into the venous system by the arachnoid granulations, which protrude into the superior sagittal sinus (Section 18.2).

　　A. The choroid plexus is the site of CSF production in each of the four ventricles (the first and second [or lateral], the third, and the fourth).

　　B. The interventricular foramen is the communication between the lateral ventricles.

　　C. The cerebral aqueduct is the communication between the third and fourth ventricles.

　　D. The lateral apertures are the communication between the fourth ventricle and the subarachnoid space.

17. **E.** None of the answers above describes the vagus nerve correctly (Section 18.3).

　　A. The vagus nerve leaves the skull through the jugular foramen with the glossopharyngeal and spinal accessory nerves.

　　B. The carotid sinus is innervated by the glossopharyngeal nerve.

　　C. The oculomotor nerve (III), trochlear nerve (IV), abducent nerve (VI), ophthalmic nerve (V_1), and ophthalmic vein are transmitted through the superior orbital fissure.

　　D. The vagus nerve innervates all of the muscles of the soft palate except the tensor veli palatini, which is supplied by the mandibular division of the trigeminal nerve.

18. **A.** The abducent nerves innervate the lateral rectus muscles, which move the eyes laterally (Section 18.3).

　　B. Medial movement of the eyes is controlled by the oculomotor nerves via the medial rectus muscles.

　　C. Superior movement of the eyes is controlled by the oculomotor and trochlear nerves via the superior rectus and inferior oblique muscles.

　　D. Inferior movement of the eyes is controlled by the oculomotor nerves via the inferior rectus and the superior oblique muscles.

　　E. Internal rotation of the eyes, also called intorsion or rotation along the long axis of the eye, is controlled by the trochlear nerves via the superior oblique muscles. This movement is normally prevented by the action of the inferior oblique muscles.

19. A. Emissary veins communicate with veins of the scalp and can carry infections intracranially to the dural venous sinuses (Section 19.1).

B. The attachment of the occipitofrontalis muscle to the skull prevents infections of the scalp from spreading into the neck.

C. The attachment of the epicranial aponeurosis to the zygomatic arches prevents further lateral spread of infection.

D. Spread of infection intracranially occurs through the emissary veins, which communicate with the dural sinuses, not with the epidural space.

E. Not applicable.

20. E. The infratemporal fossa contains the maxillary artery and many of its branches, the mandibular nerve, the pterygoid plexus, and the otic ganglion, as well as the medial and lateral pterygoid muscles (Section 19.5).

A. The infratemporal fossa contains the maxillary artery, but choices B, C, and D are also correct (E).

B. The infratemporal fossa contains the mandibular nerve, but choices A, C, and D are also correct (E).

C. The infratemporal fossa contains the pterygoid plexus, but choices A, B, and D are also correct (E).

D. The infratemporal fossa contains the otic ganglion, but choices A, B, and C are also correct (E).

21. A. The nasolacrimal duct drains tears from the medial corner of each eye into the inferior meatus (Sections 19.7 and 20.1).

B. The frontal sinus drains into the middle meatus through a frontonasal duct.

C. The ethmoid sinus drains into the superior and middle meatuses.

D. The sphenoid sinus drains into the sphenoethmoidal recess in the posterosuperior part of the nasal cavity.

E. The maxillary sinus drains into the middle meatus.

22. C. Only the ophthalmic artery and optic nerve enter the orbit through the optic canal (Sections 17.1 and 20.1).

A. The supratrochlear artery is a branch of the ophthalmic artery in the orbit that supplies the scalp.

B. The supraorbital artery is a branch of the ophthalmic artery in the orbit that supplies the scalp.

D. The ophthalmic vein enters the orbit through the superior orbital fissure.

E. The ophthalmic nerve (CN V_1) enters the orbit through the superior orbital fissure.

23. D. The mandibular division of the trigeminal nerve innervates the tensor tympani muscle, which lessens damage from loud sounds by tensing the tympanic membrane (Section 20.2).

A. The optic nerve carries sensory innervation from the neural retina to the lateral geniculate nucleus.

B. The oculomotor nerve innervates most of the extraocular muscles of the eye and the intrinsic muscles of the eye.

C. The trochlear nerve innervates the superior oblique extraocular muscle of the eye.

E. The facial nerve innervates the stapedius muscle, which dampens the vibrations of the stapes on the oval window.

24. A. The cervical plexus originates from the anterior rami of C1–C4 (Section 21.4).

B. The accessory nerve (CN XI) innervates the sternocleidomastoid.

C. Only the oculomotor, facial, and glossopharyngeal nerves carry preganglionic parasympathetic nerves that synapse in the head.

D. The cervical plexus has both sensory and motor components. The sensory nerves of the plexus, the lesser occipital, great auricular, transverse cervical, and supraclavicular nerves innervate the skin of the anterior and lateral neck and lateral scalp. The ansa cervicalis, the motor part of the plexus, innervates most of the infrahyoid muscles.

E. The greater occipital nerve is supplied by the posterior rami of spinal nerves C1–C3 and is therefore not a branch of the cervical plexus.

25. B. The only muscles that relax the vocal folds are the posterior cricoarytenoid muscles. Note that there are other results of anesthesia that also necessitate intubation (Section 21.6).

A. The thyroarytenoid closes the vocal folds.

C. The cricothyroid muscles do not have direct actions on the vocal folds.

D. The transverse arytenoid muscles close the vocal folds.

E. The lateral arytenoid muscles close the vocal folds.

26. A. All of the innervation of the larynx, both sensory and motor, is supplied by the superior and inferior (recurrent) laryngeal branches of the vagus nerve (CN X) (Section 21.6).

B. The glossopharyngeal nerve (IX) innervates the tympanic cavity and pharyngotympanic (auditory) tube; the pharynx (sensory and motor), the tonsils, palate, posterior one third of the tongue (sensory and taste), and the stylopharyngeus muscle. It also innervates the carotid body and carotid sinus.

C. The recurrent laryngeal nerve is a branch of the vagus nerve that innervates all of the muscles of the larynx except the cricothyroid and carries sensation from the lower half of the larynx (from the vocal cords downward).

D. The superior laryngeal nerve innervates the cricothyroid muscle, which helps to tense the vocal folds and provides sensation to the upper half of the larynx (above the vocal cords).

E. Not applicable.

27. B. The only laryngeal cartilage to completely encircle the airway is the cricoid cartilage (Section 21.6).

A. The U-shaped thyroid cartilage has two laminae that join in the anterior midline to form a laryngeal prominence.

C. The epiglottic cartilage, a single leaf-shaped cartilage, forms the anterior wall of the laryngeal inlet at the root of the tongue.

D. Paired arytenoid cartilages articulate with the superior borders of the cricoid laminae. Their vocal processes attach to the thyroid cartilage through the vocal ligaments.

E. Corniculate cartilages appear as small tubercles within the aryepiglottic fold.

28. **C.** The common carotid artery, internal jugular vein, and vagus nerve are contained within the carotid sheath (Section 21.2).

    A. The external jugular vein is not within the carotid sheath.

    B. The phrenic nerve lies on the anterior scalene muscle behind the carotid sheath.

    D. The superior thyroid artery is a branch of the external carotid artery and does not travel in the carotid sheath.

    E. The sympathetic trunk lies behind the carotid sheath.

29. **D.** The submandibular lymph nodes are the primary nodes of the lateral part of the body of the tongue (Section 19.8).

    A. The superior deep cervical nodes are the primary nodes of the root of the tongue.

    B. The inferior deep cervical are the primary nodes of the medial parts of the body of the tongue.

    C. The anterior superficial cervical nodes are the primary nodes of the skin anterior muscles of the neck and are not the primary lymph nodes of any part of the tongue.

    E. The submental nodes are the primary nodes of the apex and frenulum of the tongue.

30. **A.** The ethmoid, maxilla, vomer, palatine, lacrimal, nasal, and inferior nasal concha form the bony skeleton of the nasal cavity (Section 19.7).

    B. The ethmoid forms the cribriform plate at the roof of the nasal cavity, the superior and middle nasal concha of the lateral walls, and part of the nasal septum.

    C. The maxilla forms the anterior part of the palate on the floor of the nasal cavity.

    D. The vomer forms part of the nasal septum.

    E. The palatine bone forms the posterior part of the palate on the floor of the nasal cavity.

31. **A.** The medial pterygoid muscle forms a sling with the masseter muscle to elevate the mandible (Section 19.2 and **Table 19.3**).

    B. The tensor veli palatini tenses the soft palate.

    C. The levator veli palatini elevates the soft palate.

    D. The suprahyoid muscles, including digastric, geniohyoid, stylohyoid, and mylohyoid, elevate the hyoid. The medial pterygoid can only elevate the hyoid secondarily by first elevating the mandible.

    E. The posterior part of the temporalis muscle retracts the mandible.

32. **C.** The hypoglossal nerve (CN XII) innervates all muscles of the tongue except for the palatoglossus. When damaged, muscles on the affected side atrophy and fail to contribute to protrusion of the tongue. This causes the tongue to deviate to the side of the lesion (left side in this patient). The nerve is at risk during surgery on the common carotid artery because of its proximity to the carotid bifurcation (Section 18.3).

    A. The stylopharyngeus is the only muscle innervated by the glossopharyngeal nerve.

    B. Damage to the left hypoglossal nerve would cause atrophy of the left side of the tongue and deviation to the right side with protrusion.

    D. The lingual nerve, a branch of the mandibular division of the trigeminal nerve, transmits sensation from the anterior tongue. It also carries parasympathetic fibers via the chorda tympani to the submandibular and sublingual glands and taste from the anterior tongue.

    E. The lingual nerve, a branch of the mandibular division of the trigeminal nerve, transmits sensation from the anterior tongue. It also carries parasympathetic fibers via the chorda tympani to the submandibular and sublingual glands and taste from the anterior tongue.

33. **A.** The mandibular division enters the infratemporal fossa where it sends motor branches to muscles of mastication and sensory branches to the tongue, mandibular teeth, oral cavity, and skin of the lower and lateral face (Section 18.3).

    B. The maxillary division of the trigeminal nerve passes through the foramen rotundum to the pterygopalatine fossa.

    C. The ophthalmic branch of the trigeminal nerve passes through the superior orbital fissure to the orbit.

    D. The maxillary branch of the trigeminal nerve innervates the nasal cavity.

    E. The lingual nerve passes from the infratemporal fossa into the oral cavity.

34. **E.** The internal carotid arteries do not have branches in the neck. The ophthalmic arteries are the first major branches of the internal carotid arteries (Section 18.2).

    A. The superior thyroid is a branch of the external carotid artery.

    B. The lingual artery is a branch of the external carotid artery.

    C. The facial artery is a branch of the external carotid artery.

    D. The maxillary artery is a branch of the external carotid artery.

35. **E.** The cavernous sinus contains the oculomotor, trochlear, abducent, and ophthalmic and maxillary divisions of the trigeminal nerve. The maxillary division of the trigeminal nerve supplies sensation to the cheek (Section 18.1).

    A. Jugular venous distension is caused by a decrease of venous return to the heart.

    B. The inability to smile is caused by a lesion to the facial nerve.

    C. The inability to chew is caused by a lesion to the mandibular division of the trigeminal nerve.

    D. Loss of vision is caused by a lesion to the optic nerve, which does not travel through the cavernous sinus. Note that there are additional causes of loss of vision, none of which are related to the cavernous sinus.

36. **D.** The ophthalmic artery is the first major branch of the internal carotid artery in the anterior cranial fossa (Section 17.3).

    A. The posterior cerebral is the terminal branch of the basilar artery.

    B. The occipital artery is a branch of the external carotid artery.

    C. The labyrinthine artery is a branch of the basilar artery.

    E. The middle meningeal artery is a branch of the maxillary artery, which is a branch of the external carotid artery.

Index

Note: Italicized page numbers represent clinical applications. Illustrative and tabular material is indicated by "f" and "t" respectively immediately following the page number.